2010

WM 203.3SAC

369 0285752

KU-763-437

Secondary Schizophrenia

Secondary Schizophrenia

Edited by

Perminder S. Sachdev

Scientia Professor of Neuropsychiatry, School of Psychiatry, University of New South Wales
Director, Neuropsychiatric Institute, Prince of Wales Hospital, Randwick
New South Wales, Australia

Consulting Editor

Matcheri S. Keshavan

Stanley Cobb Professor and Vice Chair for Public Psychiatry
Department of Psychiatry, Beth Israel Deaconess Medical Center,
and Massachusetts Mental Health Center, Harvard Medical School
Boston, Massachusetts, USA

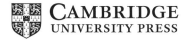

CAMBRIDGE
UNIVERSITY PRESS

CAMBRIDGE UNIVERSITY PRESS
Cambridge, New York, Melbourne, Madrid, Cape Town, Singapore,
São Paulo, Delhi, Dubai, Tokyo

Cambridge University Press
The Edinburgh Building, Cambridge CB2 8RU, UK

Published in the United States of America by
Cambridge University Press, New York

www.cambridge.org
Information on this title:
www.cambridge.org/9780521856973

First published 2010

Printed in the United Kingdom at the University Press, Cambridge

*A catalog record for this publication is available from the British
Library.*

Library of Congress Cataloging in Publication data
Secondary schizophrenia / edited by Perminder S. Sachdev ;
consulting editor, Matcheri S. Keshavan.
    p.   ;   cm.
Includes bibliographical references and index.
ISBN 978-0-521-85697-3 (hardback)
1. Schizophrenia.   2. Psychological manifestations of
general diseases.
I. Sachdev, Perminder S.   II. Keshavan, Matcheri S., 1953–
[DNLM: 1. Psychotic Disorders.   2. Schizophrenia.
WM 200 S445 2010]
RC514.S416   2010
616.89′8 – dc22   2009022571

ISBN 978-0-521-85697-3 Hardback

Contents

Contents

Contributors

Osvaldo P. Almeida MD PhD FRANZCP FFPOA
Director of Research
Western Australian Centre for Health and Ageing
(WACHA),
Western Australian Institute for Medical Research;
Consultant, Department of Psychiatry
Royal Perth Hospital;
and Professor and Chair of Geriatric Psychiatry
School of Psychiatry and Clinical Neurosciences,
Faculty of Medicine, Dentistry and Health Sciences,
University of Western Australia,
Perth, Australia

Rebecca Anglin MD
Resident
Joint Program of Neurology and Psychiatry,
McMaster University,
Hamilton, Ontario, Canada

Vivek Benegal MD DPM
Associate Professor of Psychiatry
Deaddiction Centre,
National Institute of Mental Health and
Neurosciences (NIMHANS),
Bangalore, India

Margaret N. Berry MS CGC
Department of Pediatrics
Section on Medical Genetics,
Wake Forest University School of Medicine,
Winston-Salem, North Carolina, USA

Nash N. Boutros MD
Professor
Department of Psychiatry and Behavioral
Neurosciences,
Wayne State University School of Medicine
Detroit, Michigan, USA

Henry Brodaty MB BS MD DSc FRACP FRANZCP
Professor
Primary Dementia Collaborative Research
Centre,
School of Psychiatry,
University of New South Wales;
and Aged Care Psychiatry,
Euroa Centre, Prince of Wales Hospital,
Randwick, New South Wales, Australia

Alan S. Brown MD MPH
Associate Professor of Clinical Psychiatry and
Clinical Epidemiology
College of Physicians and Surgeons of Columbia
University,
New York State Psychiatric Institute,
New York, New York, USA

Monte S. Buchsbaum MD
Professor of Psychiatry
Neuroscience PET Laboratory,
Mount Sinai School of Medicine,
New York, New York, USA

William Burke PhD
Emeritus Professor of Physiology
Brain Research Laboratory,
Discipline of Anatomy and Physiology,
School of Medical Sciences and Bosch
Institute,
The University of Sydney,
New South Wales, Australia

Kim Burns RN BPsych (Hons)
Research Psychologist
Academic Department for Old Age Psychiatry,
Prince of Wales Hospital, Euroa Centre,
Randwick, New South Wales, Australia

Stanley V. Catts
Professor
School of Medicine,
The University of Queensland;
and Mental Health Centre,
The Royal Brisbane and Women's Hospital,
Herston, Queensland, Australia

Vibeke S. Catts BS MD FRANZCP
School of Medicine,
The University of Queensland,
St. Lucia, Queensland, Australia

Jennifer M. Connolly BSc (Hons)
Research Manager
Kavanagh Research Group,
Institute of Health and Biomedical Innovation,
Queensland University of Technology,
Brisbane, Queensland, Australia

David L. Copolov MB BS PhD DPM MPM FRACP FRANZCP
Professor of Psychiatry
Monash University;
and Professor of Psychiatry
University of Melbourne,
Melbourne, Australia

Louisa Degenhardt BA (Hon) (Psych) MPsychol (Clinical) PhD
Professor of Epidemiology
National Drug and Alcohol Research Centre,
University of New South Wales,
Randwick, New South Wales, Australia

Stewart L. Einfeld MD DCH FRANZCP
Chair of Mental Health
Faculty of Health Sciences;
Senior Scientist
Brain and Mind Research Institute,
University of Sydney,
Sydney, New South Wales, Australia

Anthony Feinstein MPhil PhD FRCPC
Professor
Department of Psychiatry,
Sunnybrook Health Sciences Centre,
University of Toronto,
Toronto, Ontario, Canada

Matt P. Galloway PhD
Department of Psychiatry and Behavioral Neurosciences,
Neuropsychiatry Division,
Wayne State University School of Medicine,
Detroit, Michigan, USA

Bangalore N. Gangadhar MD
Professor and Head
Department of Psychiatry,
National Institute of Mental Health and Neurosciences (NIMHANS),
Bangalore, India

Wayne Hall BSc (Hons) PhD AM
Professor of Public Health Policy
School of Population Health,
University of Queensland,
Herston, Queensland, Australia

Malcolm Hopwood MD FRANZCP
Director
Veterans' Psychiatry Unit;
and Director,
Brain Disorders Program,
Heidelberg Repatriation Hospital,
Heidelberg West, Victoria, Australia

Michael D. Jibson MD PhD
Professor
Director of Residency Education,
Department of Psychiatry,
University of Michigan,
Ann Arbor, Michigan, USA

Ripu D. Jindal MD
University of Pittsburgh School of Medicine,
Pittsburgh, Pennsylvania, USA

David J. Kavanagh
Professor
School of Psychology and Counselling;
and Institute of Health and Biomedical Innovation,
Queensland University of Technology,
Brisbane, Queensland, Australia

Sophie Kavanagh BMed FRANZCP
Croydon Health Group,
Sydney South West Area Health Service,
Croydon, New South Wales, Australia

Matcheri S. Keshavan
Stanley Cobb Professor
and Vice Chair for Public Psychiatry
Department of Psychiatry,
Beth Israel Deaconess Medical Center,
and the Massachusetts Mental Health Center,
Harvard Medical School,
Boston, Massachusetts, USA

Ennapadam S. Krishnamoorthy MD PhD FRCP
Director and TS Srinivasan Chair
The Institute of Neurological Sciences,
Voluntary Health Services Hospital,
Chennai, India

Rajeev Kumar MD FRANZCP PhD
Assistant Professor and Consultant Psychiatrist
Consultation-Liaison Psychiatry Unit, and
Academic Unit of Psychological Medicine,
Yong Loo Lin School of Medicine,
National University of Singapore,
Singapore, Singapore

Alexander F. Kurz MD
Head
Department of Psychiatry and Psychotherapy,
Klinikum rechts der Isar,
Technische Universität Munchen,
Munich, Germany

Nicola T. Lautenschlager MD FRANZCP
Professor and Chair of Psychiatry of Old Age
Department of Psychiatry,
University of Melbourne,
St. George's Campus,
St. Vincent's Hospital,
Kew, Victoria, Australia
Western Australian Centre for Health and Ageing
(WACHA);
School of Psychiatry and Clinical Neurosciences,
University of Western Australia,
Perth, Australia

Edward C. Lauterbach MD FANPA DFAPA
Professor of Psychiatry, Neurology and Radiology;
Director
Neurodegenerative Disease Program;
Chief
Division of Adult and Geriatric Psychiatry,
Department of Psychiatry and Behavioral Sciences,
Mercer University School of Medicine,
Macon, Georgia, USA

Leslie Lester-Burns, BS
Mercer University College of Liberal Arts
Macon, Georgia, USA

Lyn-May Lim MB BS MPsych FRANZCP Cert POA
St. George's Hospital,
Kew, Victoria, Australia

Jeffrey C. L. Looi MBBS FRANZCP MRACMA
Director
Research Centre for the Neurosciences of Ageing
(RESCENA);
and Associate Professor and Deputy Head
Academic Unit of Psychological Medicine,
Australian National University Medical School,
The Canberra Hospital,
Canberra, Australia

Michael Mazurek MD
Associate Professor
Department of Neurology,
McMaster University,
Hamilton, Ontario, Canada

Serge A. Mitelman MD
Assistant Professor of Psychiatry
Mount Sinai School of Medicine,
Neuroscience Positron Emission Tomography
Laboratory,
New York, New York, USA

Ramon Mocellin MB BS MSc MMed FRANZCP
Consultant Neuropsychiatrist
Neuropsychiatry Unit,
Royal Melbourne Hospital;
Research Fellow
Melbourne Neuropsychiatry Centre,
University of Melbourne,
Melbourne, Australia

Bryan Mowry MB BS BA (Hons) MD FRANZCP
Professor
Queensland Brain Institute,
University of Queensland,
Brisbane, Queensland, Australia;
and Executive Director
Queensland Centre for Mental Health Research,
The Park – Centre for Mental Health,
Wacol, Queensland, Australia

Kim T. Mueser PhD
Professor of Psychiatry and Community and Family
Medicine
Dartmouth Medical School,
Hanover, New Hampshire, USA

Anand K. Pandurangi MBBS MD
Professor of Psychiatry, Medical Director, and
Chairman
Division of Inpatient Psychiatry,
Virginia Commonwealth University,
Richmond, Virginia, USA

Eric M. Pihlgren PhD
Department of Psychiatry and Behavioral
Neurosciences,
Neuropsychiatry Division
Wayne State University School of Medicine
Detroit, Michigan, USA

Seethalakshmi Ramanathan MBBS DPM
Clinical Research Fellow
Department of Psychiatry,
KEM Hospital,
Mumbai, India

Patricia I. Rosebush MScN MD FRCP(C)
Professor
Department of Psychiatry and Behavioural
Neurosciences,
McMaster University,
Hamilton, Ontario, Canada

Perminder S. Sachdev MD PhD FRANZCP
Scientia Professor of Neuropsychiatry
School of Psychiatry
University of New South Wales;
Director
Neuropsychiatric Institute,
Prince of Wales Hospital,
Randwick, New South Wales, Australia

Richard D. Sanders MD
Associate Professor
Departments of Psychiatry and Neurology,
Boonschoft School of Medicine and Wright State
University
and the VA Medical Center
Dayton, Ohio, USA

Vandana Shashi MD
Assistant Professor of Pediatrics
Department of Pediatrics,
Section on Medical Genetics,
Wake Forest University School of Medicine,
Winston-Salem, North Carolina, USA

Arabella Smith MBBS DipRCPath FHGSA FRCPA
Department of Cytogenetics,
Children's Hospital Westmead,
Westmead, New South Wales, Australia

Sergio E. Starkstein MD FRANZCP
Professor of Psychiatry
School of Psychiatry,
University of Western Australia
Perth, Australia

Ezra S. Susser MD
Department Chair, Epidemiology,
and Anna Cheskis Gelman and Murray Charles
Gelman Professor of Epidemiology
Mailman School of Public Health;
Professor of Psychiatry
College of Physicians and Surgeons;
and Co-Director
Statistics and Epidemiology,
HIV Center for Clinical and Behavior Studies
(NYSPI),
New York, New York, USA

Rajiv Tandon MD
Professor of Psychiatry
University of Florida College of Medicine,
McKnight Brain Institute,
Gainesville, Florida, USA

Jagadisha Thirthalli MD
Associate Professor of Psychiatry
National Institute of Mental Health and
Neurosciences (NIMHANS),
Bangalore, India

Bruce J. Tonge MBBS MD DPM FRANZCP
Professor
Centre for Developmental Psychiatry and
Psychology,
Monash University,
Clayton, Victoria, Australia

Julian Trollor MB BS MD FRANZCP MFPOA
Chair, Intellectual Disability Mental Health
School of Psychiatry, University of New South Wales;
and Staff Specialist
Neuropsychiatric Institute,
Prince of Wales Hospital, Euroa Centre,
Randwick, New South Wales, Australia

Dennis Velakoulis MB BS FRANZCP
Clinical Director
Melbourne Neuropsychiatry Centre,
North Western Mental Health and
University of Melbourne;
Director
Neuropsychiatry Unit,
Royal Melbourne Hospital,
Parkville, Victoria, Australia

Mark Walterfang MB BS (Hons) FRANZCP
Consultant Neuropsychiatrist
Neuropsychiatry Unit,
Royal Melbourne Hospital;
and Research Fellow
Neuroimaging Laboratory,
Melbourne Neuropsychiatry Centre, University of
Melbourne,
Carlton South, Victoria, Australia

Jane Zhang PhD
Mount Sinai School of Medicine,
New York, New York, USA

Preface

For any mental health researcher, finding the *cause* of schizophrenia would be the ultimate prize. The impact of schizophrenia on our society is immense. Even though it is a low-prevalence disorder relative to depression and anxiety disorders, it has captured the focus of most psychiatric services worldwide. It devastates individuals in the prime of their lives and overwhelms families by its persistent challenge to most things we hold dear about our social existence. For researchers, it is the ultimate challenge and the most frustrating snare. It has a bewitching presence that many find too tempting to resist. Yet, it gives away few secrets. Neuropathologists, who recognize that it is a brain disease, have long regarded it as their graveyard. Neuroscientists often come away with the feeling that they are clutching at straws.

Some of us would like to believe that the answer, once we do stumble upon it, will be simple indeed. Perhaps we are only one step away from a gene that will unravel the mystery. Maybe a misfolded protein will open its cloak to reveal its nakedness. Many others believe, however, that the answer will never be simple – schizophrenia, after all, is about our very nature as human beings and what can go wrong with our existence. My own position is somewhere in between. I believe that eventually we will find genetic determinants of the brain abnormalities that underlie schizophrenia. This will help us understand that what we now regard as schizophrenia is a *potpourri* of disorders. There may well be many phenocopies of the *true* schizophrenia. On the other hand, there may not be a real schizophrenia in any case, but a medley of disorders we naively lump together.

This book is about chipping away at the large lump we presently call schizophrenia. The defining characteristics are broad indeed – the presence of delusions and hallucinations in clear consciousness. A quick browse through the leaves of this book will convince you that the brain responds to many injuries and threats with this response. It could be electrical discharges, traumatic injury, subtle beginnings of neurodegeneration, or the effects of psychoactive drugs. The list is mind-boggling, and each presents a slightly different mechanism of its causation. Could it be that the brain has a limited repertoire of responses to multiple challenges, and schizophrenia is that final pathway? The hope of this book is that many little secrets about schizophrenia will be revealed so that there is nowhere for it to hide. Psychiatry has a proud tradition of arguing about terminology, but I decided to stick with the DSM-IV refuge of *secondary schizophrenia* in this book. It has much to commend it, as discussed in one of the chapters. More than anything else, it makes no false pretense and recognizes our ignorance.

This book has been a collective effort. I am grateful to all the contributors not only for the hours of labor, but also for the infinite patience for the long delays in bringing it to fruition. There are very few experts on secondary schizophrenia. The writing of the chapters has therefore taken many authors outside their comfort zones, and the results are consequently more exciting. In particular, I would like to thank Matcheri Keshavan for his wisdom and generosity in guiding various aspects of the book. His consultations have left me in a considerable debt of gratitude. As always, my assistant Angie Russell has been tenacious in her determination to complete *her* project, and has worked untiringly to give me editorial support. She accepted that not all contributors would follow the guidelines for submission, and had the unenviable task of changing reference styles and crossing the '*t*'s. It is as much her book as that of the authors. The Cambridge University Press has been a solid backer throughout the process. The life of this manuscript has seen a number of changes in the editorial staff, but their support has been unwavering.

In the age of electronic publishing and rapid communication, this book is but a tortoise. I hope that it will hold steadfast, and intermittently poke its little head out to urge all players to move on. The road is long and there is no time to rest.

Perminder Sachdev
Sydney, Australia

Section 1

Introduction

Introduction

Neurobiology and etiology of primary schizophrenia: current status

Matcheri S. Keshavan and Ripu D. Jindal

Facts box

1. Whereas this book focuses on secondary (or "organic") schizophrenia, the neurobiological basis of primary (or "idiopathic") schizophrenia is important to understand.

2. Converging data suggest that cognitive impairments are not epiphenomena but reflect the core pathology of schizophrenia.

3. Functional imaging studies point to abnormalities in prefrontal, cingulate, and medial temporal lobe function in the early stages of schizophrenia.

4. Structural brain abnormalities are present at the onset of illness and appear to be persistent.

5. Siblings and offspring of schizophrenic patients also show structural brain changes.

6. Structural brain changes in individuals with prodromal symptoms may predict development of psychosis.

7. Diffusion tensor imaging studies in schizophrenia have documented reduced structural integrity of white matter tracts.

8. Radioligand studies support the view that psychosis may be related to dopaminergic hyperfunction in mesolimbic brain regions.

9. Genetic factors interact with both early and late environmental factors in affecting neurodevelopment that may be the basis of schizophrenia.

10. The study of "secondary" schizophrenia is likely to provide novel insights into the pathogenesis of the primary disorder.

Organic/functional versus the primary/secondary categorization: a historical perspective

The fourth edition of the Diagnostic and Statistical Manual of Mental Disorders (DSM-IV) dropped the terms "organic" and "functional" used in the earlier editions. The change in terminology in DSM-IV reflected a change in emphasis from the presence or absence of discernible brain pathology (which is often difficult to identify, even in many neurological disorders) to etiology (presumed or actual). This resulted from a growing realization that it is better to categorize psychiatric disorders based on whether the neurobiological alterations are due to a known medical illness ("secondary") or whether they cannot be explained by another illness ("primary" or idiopathic). In this book, this approach has been taken to understand schizophrenia because the term "primary" has the advantage of not ruling out a neurobiological (or "organic") basis. Although a variety of secondary schizophrenias are described throughout this text, it is important to have an understanding of the neurobiological substrates that may underlie primary (or idiopathic) schizophrenic illness. In this chapter, we seek to provide an overview of what is known in this regard, and offer an approach to the differential diagnosis between primary and secondary schizophrenias.

Schizophrenia as a quintessential "primary" psychotic disorder

Schizophrenia is a severe and chronic mental disorder with a lifetime prevalence of approximately 1%. Onset is typically in adolescence to early adulthood, but very rarely before age 11. Symptoms of schizophrenia are classified into *positive symptoms*, that is, false fixed beliefs that cannot be reasoned away (delusions), abnormal perceptions (hallucinations), disorganized speech and behavior, and *negative symptoms* (i.e. deficits in motivation, affect, and socialization). A given patient may exhibit some or all of these symptoms. The course and severity of the illness are also variable. In many patients, some cognitive and social difficulties can be traced back to early childhood, long before the development of symptoms that meet the criteria for schizophrenia. Sometimes, mood, thought, and personality changes are followed by gradual development of subthreshold psychotic symptoms. Even after the development of acute symptoms, the course is variable. In most cases, acute psychotic states are interspersed by periods of remission. Even the periods of remission are not entirely free from negative symptoms and cognitive deficits. The persistence and pervasiveness of the cognitive impairments in schizophrenia led early thinkers like Kraepelin to view schizophrenia as primarily a cognitive brain disorder that begins early in life, hence the term "Dementia Praecox." In this chapter, we review the evidence for and the nature of the brain abnormalities in schizophrenia. Specifically, we address the questions of *whether* there is a neurobiological substrate to the illness, *how* the dysfunctions originate at a physiological level, *where* in the brain the alterations are seen, *what* the nature of the abnormalities may be at neurochemical and neuropathological levels, *why* they may occur (etiology), and *when* in the life course of the individual the pathophysiology may evolve.

Is there brain dysfunction in schizophrenia? Evidence from the prominent cognitive and neurologic impairments

Over the past few decades, converging data suggest that cognitive impairments are not epiphenomena but reflect the core pathology of schizophrenia [1]. This evidence has greatly enhanced our understanding of the neurobiology of the disease. Increased frequency of "soft" neurological signs, detectable on routine bedside neurological examinations, is also seen early in schizophrenia and tends to persist during the illness (Chapter 4).

Schizophrenia patients have a broad range of cognitive impairments, as summarized by the mnemonic SMART (Table 1.1). Cognitive deficits have attracted attention from investigators and clinicians after their major role in predicting functional outcome in schizophrenia became known [2]. Among mediators of functional outcome, social cognition (which

Table 1.1 Cognitive domains (note the mnemonic SMART) commonly affected in schizophrenia, and recommended tests to assess these domains

Speed of processing: Category Fluency; Brief Assessment of Cognition in Schizophrenia (BACS) – Symbol-Coding; Trail Making A

Memory: *Working Memory*: Letter-Number Span; Wechsler Memory Scale (WMS) – III Spatial Span; *Verbal learning/memory*: Hopkins Verbal Learning Test (HVLT) – Revised; *Visual learning/memory*: Brief Visuospatial Memory Test (BVMT) – Revised

Attention: Continuous Performance Test – Identical Pairs (CPT-IP)

Reasoning: Neuropsychological Assessment Battery (NAB) – Mazes

Tact (socal cognition): Mayer-Salovey-Caruso Emotional Intelligence Test (MSCEIT) – Managing Emotions

Source: http://www.matrics.ucla.edu/matrics-psychometrics-frame.htm.

encompasses the different cognitive processes involved in what people think of themselves, others, and social situations [3, 4]) is perhaps the most important. This domain of cognition facilitates interpersonal interactions, and deficits in this domain have been implicated as the core pathology in autism and schizophrenia [5]. Emotional processing, a key component of social cognition, is commonly assessed by responses to emotive facial stimuli [6]. Although regions in the brain associated with social cognition are distinct from those involved with nonsocial cognition, social cognition also depends on the integrity of nonsocial domains of cognition. For example, attention is needed to focus on salient features in a stimulus; working memory is needed for generating appropriate social responses to context information, and executive function is needed to generate and revise hypotheses regarding the meaning of social situations [7].

Cross-sectional comparisons between first-episode and chronic patients suggest some decline in function; however, longitudinal studies show no decrement [8, 9, 10] or modest decreases in cognitive function [11]. Furthermore, a meta-analytic study of memory impairment showed comparable effect sizes in the studies of first-episode and chronic patients [12]. In a longitudinal study, deficits in social cognition were stable over 1 year of follow up [13]. Relationships between clinical symptoms and neuropsychological performance have also been investigated. Some studies [8, 14, 15] found an association between changes in neuropsychological scores and positive symptoms, whereas another [10] found a similar association with change in positive symptoms. Taken together, the longitudinal and some cross-sectional studies and the lone meta-analysis previously described support the view that extensive cognitive deficits are present by the first episode of psychosis and are likely to be a stable, ongoing, traitlike feature of the person's illness.

Studies of cognition in prepsychotic individuals at genetically high risk for psychosis provide a way to determine the static versus progressive nature of the cognitive deficits in schizophrenia. Neuropsychological investigations have been done as part of longitudinal studies of children at genetically high risk of developing psychosis in different parts of the world (i.e. Edinburgh [16], New York [17], Copenhagen [18], and Israel [19]). The New York High-Risk Study demonstrated that deficits in attention, motor skills, and short-term memory detected between the ages of 7 and 12 years predicted development of schizophrenia-related psychosis in 58%, 75%, and 83% of cases, respectively [20]. Similarly, verbal memory and executive function predicted later development of psychosis in the Edinburgh High Risk Study [21]. Together, these observations suggest that cognitive impairments precede the emergence of typical symptoms by several years.

How do neurocognitive alterations originate? Studies of brain function

Alterations in brain function in schizophrenia have been documented on functional neuroimaging studies, such as Positron Emission Tomography (PET) and Blood Oxygenation Level Dependent (BOLD)-based functional MRI (fMRI) performed while the subject is engaged in cognitive tasks. In approximately half of patients with schizophrenia, decreased frontal metabolism and blood flow are evident during cognitive activation tasks. N-back task, which involves the subject observing a sequence of letters and responding to a reappearance of a letter after n trials (i.e., $n = 0, 1, 2$, and so on) is one of the most commonly used tasks. In general, functional neuroimaging studies have demonstrated reduced activation of lateral prefrontal regions during the task performance [22]. Recently, a meta-analysis indicated that even subjects at genetic risk for schizophrenia show abnormalities on functional neuroimaging studies [23]. An fMRI study has also noted that auditory hallucinations are associated with activation in many brain areas, such as

the inferior frontal/insular, anterior cingulate and temporal cortex bilaterally, the right thalamus and inferior colliculus, and the left hippocampus and parahippocampal cortex [24].

An early PET study in schizophrenia detected abnormalities in regional brain function during rest [25]. As stated earlier, impaired working memory is a well-replicated finding in schizophrenia [26], and working memory tasks have been widely used in fMRI studies in schizophrenia to examine responses to cognitive tasks. fMRI studies in healthy humans suggest that the dorsolateral prefrontal cortex (DLPFC) plays a major role in working memory. Approximately 60% of the studies in schizophrenia have shown hypo-activation in the prefrontal cortex during various working memory tasks [27]. However, abnormalities of prefrontal cortical function in schizophrenia are not reducible to simply too much or too little activity and may reflect a compromised effort in processing information mediated by the DLPFC [28].

Some of the electrophysiological abnormalities in patients with schizophrenia and their relatives include abnormal smooth-pursuit eye movements, persistent deficit in performance on the antisaccade tasks [29], abnormalities in the auditory evoked potential (i.e. diminished amplitude and increased latency in the P300 response to an "oddball" auditory stimulus), prepulse inhibition of the startle reflex (which measures the ability of a preceding weak prestimulus to transiently inhibit the response to a closely following strong sensory stimulus), and reduced high frequency (in the gamma range, i.e., 30–70 Hz) oscillatory power in response to auditory stimulation [30].

In recent years, the role of the anterior cingulate cortex in cognitive control and self-monitoring has been well recognized [31]. Using a test of selective attention (i.e. the Stroop task), patients with schizophrenia showed reduced error monitoring and reduced anterior cingulate activity compared to controls [32, 33]. Earlier, Fletcher and colleagues had shown disruption of the normal anterior cingulate modulation of prefrontotemporal integration in patients with schizophrenia [34].

The amygdala and hippocampus seem to have complementary roles in cognitive processing with the former regulating emotion and affect and the latter, episodic and associative memory [35, 36]. Subjects with amygdala damage have been shown to have an impaired ability to interpret facial expressions in a pattern similar to what was shown earlier in autism

[37]. Most fMRI studies of amygdala function indicate that dysfunction of the emotional aspect of the brain is the hallmark of schizophrenia [38]. For instance, patients performed poorly on affect labeling tasks [39] and displayed reduced responsivity of the amygdala [6, 40]. The relationship between these deficits and social functioning and the trajectory of these deficits in at-risk populations are prime areas for further investigation. Taken together, functional imaging studies point to abnormalities in prefrontal, cingulate, and medial temporal lobe function early in the illness. Much work remains to be done to understand the full implications of each of these observations.

In which part of the brain can abnomalities be found? Structural brain imaging studies

The early manifestations of cognitive neurofunctional deficits, as previously outlined, strongly point to neuroanatomical alterations in patients with schizophrenia. *In vivo* neuroimaging studies demonstrate a number of brain structural abnormalities in schizophrenia. Systematic reviews and meta-analyses of MRI studies in schizophrenia indicate reductions in volume of whole brain, as well as grey matter volumes and increases in ventricular volume [41, 42, 43, 44]. More prominent reductions are seen in temporal lobe structures, especially in the hippocampus, amygdala, and the superior temporal gyri [45, 46], the prefrontal cortex, and the thalamus [47]. Automated regional parcellation and voxel-based morphometry (VBM) techniques have largely validated this region of interest (ROI)-based findings. Reductions in medial temporal lobes and the superior temporal gyrus (STG) are well-replicated findings in VBM studies [48]. Moreover, STG volumes and reductions in medial temporal volumes correlate with positive symptoms and memory impairment, respectively [49, 50].

Studies of first-episode schizophrenia show that brain structural alterations are present at illness onset [51] (Figure 1.1). Two recent meta-analyses of such studies [41] show whole brain and hippocampal volume reductions. Brain structural changes evident at illness onset appear to persist during the course of the schizophrenic illness. Some [52, 53], but not all [54], found evidence for further progression of the structural deviations. Collectively, imaging studies suggest that brain structural alterations are a persistent trait of schizophrenia.

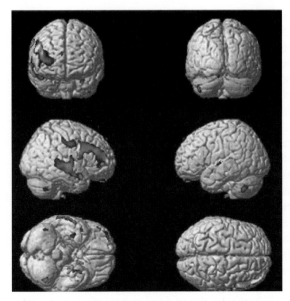

Figure 1.1 Brain MRI images showing grey-matter volume reductions in first-episode schizophrenia subjects compared to healthy controls using Voxel Based Morphometry (VBM). [From the University of Pittsburgh.] (See color plate section.)

Studies of relatives of patients with schizophrenia provide further insight into the illness. ROI studies of offspring and siblings of patients show volumetric reductions in amygdala and hippocampus [55, 56, 57]. Similarly, computational VBM studies have shown reduced grey matter in the PFC in that population [58, 59]. A longitudinal VBM study demonstrated that a spatial pattern of reductions in grey matter density in the left temporal lobe and right cerebellum could predict onset of psychotic symptoms in those at genetic risk [60].

Structural changes have also been shown to predict development of psychosis in those with prodromal symptoms. For instance, Pantelis and colleagues [61] showed that lesser grey matter in the right medial temporal, lateral temporal, inferior frontal cortex, and the cingulate cortex bilaterally predicted the one-third of individuals with prodromal symptoms who developed psychosis on follow-up. This MRI follow-up study suggests an ongoing disease process during the transition from prodrome to psychosis. Prospective MRIs in childhood-onset schizophrenia [62, 63] reveal a relatively more rapid loss in superior frontal and temporal cortices (~3–4% loss per year as opposed to a more subtle 1–2% decrease per year in matched controls). A recent review of the literature suggests that all of the reduction may not be accounted for by the neurons but could be related to white matter changes, that is, demyelination and changes in the lipid metabolism [64]. Many studies of childhood-onset schizophrenia support the post-illness onset progression model.

A follow-up study of the nonpsychotic siblings of patients with childhood-onset schizophrenia has yielded thought-provoking results [65]. It was not entirely surprising to find grey matter deficits in right prefrontal and inferior parietal cortices or even greater reductions in the left prefrontal and bilateral temporal cortices. But it was striking to note that these cortical deficits in siblings disappeared by age 20 and that attenuation of deficits over time correlated with overall functioning at the last scan. Thus, early prefrontal and temporal grey matter loss appears to be a trait marker with differential subsequent trajectory of development among siblings and between those who do and do not develop the disease.

As outlined above, structural abnormalities in schizophrenia are evident in multiple interconnected brain regions, perhaps suggesting disrupted connectivity. Diffusion tensor imaging (DTI) [66], a reliable method of studying brain connectivity and white matter integrity, measures the orientation of water diffusion along the axis of tissue elements, such as axons, and has provided further evidence of parallels between regional development of prefrontal connectivity and cognitive development. DTI studies suggest that working memory capacity and performance on cognitive control tasks correlate with prefrontal–parietal connectivity [67] and frontostriatal connectivity, respectively [68].

Although limited by small sample sizes and other methodological constraints, most DTI studies in schizophrenia document reduced structural integrity of white matter tracts, as measured by fractional anisotropy (FA) in a number of areas, such as the corpus callosum, the arcuate, and the unicinate fasciculi [69]. Similarly, one study of childhood-onset schizophrenia found lesser FA in frontal WM bilaterally, as well as in right occipital WM [70].

What is the neurochemical nature of the brain abnormalities in schizophrenia?

Neurochemical brain imaging using PET and single photon emission computed tomography (SPECT) can inform us about receptors and neurotransmitters such as dopamine (DA) that are critical for understanding psychoses. A small number of studies of PET scans in first-episode schizophrenia have produced suggestive evidence of increased dopamine turnover [71]. An early review of 17 PET and postmortem studies revealed a substantive effect size (1.47) for increases in D2 receptor density and affinity in schizophrenia [72]. Presynaptic DA turnover, as measured by striatal Fluoro-DOPA uptake, also appears to be increased in schizophrenia, especially during psychotic exacerbations [73]. These findings provide support to the long-held view that psychosis may be related to dopaminergic hyperfunction in mesolimbic brain regions [74].

The hyperdopaminergic model of schizophrenia, however, does not explain the cognitive impairments and the negative symptoms that characterize this illness. Weinberger [75] suggested that schizophrenia may be characterized by a deficit in the mesocortical dopaminergic system, which leads to a disinhibition of the mesolimbic dopaminergic system, accounting for positive psychotic symptoms.

Magnetic resonance spectroscopy (MRS) has emerged as an important noninvasive tool to longitudinally evaluate neurochemical changes in schizophrenia. The majority of MRS studies in schizophrenia have employed ^{1}H (Proton) MRS. A recent meta-analysis and systematic review of in vivo ^{1}H spectroscopy studies in schizophrenia shows reduced N acetyl aspartate (NAA), a marker of neuronal integrity, primarily in the PFC and hippocampus both in first-episode and chronic schizophrenia patients [76]. However, there are negative studies as well [77, 78].

NAA reductions may also be present prior to the illness onset. An early study [56] detected a trend toward NAA/choline ratio reductions in the anterior cingulate region in adolescent offspring at genetic risk for schizophrenia. Furthermore, reduced NAA/choline in anterior cingulate predicted conversion to psychosis in those with prodromal symptoms of schizophrenia [79].

A relatively smaller number of studies have employed in vivo ^{31}P spectroscopy in schizophrenia. In an early study [80], decreased phosphomonoesters (PME) in the prefrontal region of first-episode, antipsychotic-naive schizophrenia subjects was observed, suggesting a reduction in synthesis of membrane phospholipids (MPLs). The results seemed to support Feinberg's hypothesis of abnormal neurodevelopment in schizophrenia because of an exaggerated preadolescent synaptic pruning in the

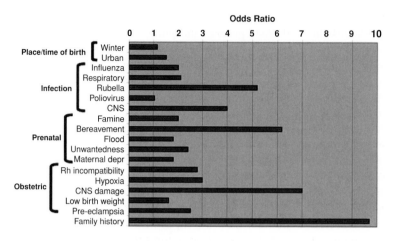

Figure 1.2 Environmental factors in the pathogenesis (abbreviations: CNS, central nervous system; depr, depression; Rh, Rhesus) [91].

prefrontal region [80, 81]. Subsequent studies of first-episode schizophrenia patients largely confirmed these alterations [82, 83, 84, 85, 86, 87]. Nevertheless, collectively, there is compelling evidence of diminished mass or content of MPL at the early stage of schizophrenia (i.e., neurophil), which is consistent with the findings of postmortem studies [88]. Work by our group shows reduced prefrontal PME in adolescent offspring at genetic risk for schizophrenia, suggesting that these alterations may precede symptomatic manifestations [89].

What factors cause brain dysfunction? Genetic and environmental influences

Although the pathophysiology of schizophrenia is progressively being better understood, thanks to the advent of neuroimaging and neuropathological studies, our knowledge of the etiology of this illness is still limited. What is well known, however, is the strong genetic contribution to schizophrenia supported by family, adoption, and twin studies. Several genes have recently been identified that may hold the key to finally understanding the causes of schizophrenia [90]. However, the fact that the concordance for schizophrenia in monozygotic twins is about 50% suggests an important role for environmental factors. Many environmental factors, all of relatively small effects, have been reported to influence risk for schizophrenia (Figure 1.2).

Even the presence of genetic and early environmental risk factors does not always predict who is at a later risk for schizophrenia. Among those at genetic risk, such as offspring of parents with this illness, many

vulnerable individuals develop features of schizophrenia spectrum psychopathology (e.g., schizotypy) but only a small proportion (~10%) go on to develop the full-blown manifestations of schizophrenia. Later environmental risk factors such as psychosocial stress, hormonal factors, and drug abuse may interact to result in the pathophysiologic substrate underlying the vulnerability to schizophrenia and increase risk.

When does the illness develop? Schizophrenia as a progressive neurodevelopmental disorder

Schizophrenia is being increasingly viewed as a disorder of brain development. Circa 2007, it was well established that brain development starts in intrauterine life and continues into early adulthood. Multiple lines of research have detected evidence of neurogenesis and neuronal migration during pre- and perinatal periods. Synaptic proliferation that follows these changes seems to continue into childhood. Subsequent development during late childhood and adolescence is characterized by programmed elimination or pruning of redundant synapses and myelination that continues into adulthood.

Derailments in these developmental and degenerative processes have been proposed as possible mechanisms underlying schizophrenia. Evidence from multiple lines of research has resulted in more than one model for the pathogenesis of schizophrenia. For example, findings of increased rates of birth complications, minor physical abnormalities, neurological soft signs, and subtle behavioral abnormalities in those who later develop schizophrenia has led to the *early developmental* (or "doomed from the womb") model, which proposes that abnormalities in brain development around or before birth cause the failure of brain functions in early adulthood. Defective neuronal migration during the second trimester of pregnancy has been proposed as one of such mechanisms [92]. One argument against this model is the low positive predictive value, that only a small proportion of people who exhibit these risk factors eventually develop schizophrenia.

The typical delay in the onset of salient symptoms of schizophrenia until adolescence or early adulthood is often cited as evidence of derailed *late development in schizophrenia*. According to this model, excessive programmed neuronal pruning and pronounced loss of synapses have a role in the emergence of the illness. This model is supported by the evidence of reductions in dendrite density in cortical brain regions in postmortem studies of schizophrenia [93].

Deterioration in the first few years of the illness in many patients has been attributed to a *post-illness onset* degenerative process [94]. The three pathophysiological models mentioned above are not necessarily considered mutually exclusive; a sequential combination of these processes has also been proposed. The effect of environmental factors, such as illicit drug use and psychosocial stressors as potential triggers, has also been recognized.

Investigating primary versus secondary schizophrenia

Virtually any substance, prescribed drugs, or medical condition affecting nervous system function can present with psychiatric symptoms. This can be said with some confidence to be true for psychosis as well (Table 1.2). Establishing a cause–effect relationship between substance use/medical illness and psychosis, however, is not easy. Suspecting an underlying medical illness is a logical initial step when encountering psychosis in general medical settings. Comorbid medical illnesses are also quite common in patients presenting with psychotic symptoms, especially among the elderly. However, suspecting and identifying an underlying medical illness in younger, newly presenting patients with psychosis in mental health settings (in which the base rate of medical illnesses is low) is more challenging.

In making the distinction between primary and secondary psychosis, it is important to first establish the presence of the general medical condition. The next step, establishing the cause–effect relationship between medical condition and psychosis, is often difficult, but can be helped by considering the following factors:

1. The temporal relationship between the psychosis and the medical condition:

The psychosis begins following the onset of the medical condition, varies in severity with the severity of the medical condition, and resolves when the medical condition gets better. This rule has many exceptions, however. For example, psychosis may sometimes be an early indicator of a medical illness that becomes evident later. Conversely, a medical illness may simply trigger a protracted schizophrenia illness without necessarily causing it.

2. Atypicality of presentation:

A medical cause for psychosis should be especially considered if the presentation is atypical. A later age of onset, severe disorientation and/or confusion, and the presence of multimodality hallucinations (e.g. visual and tactile) increase the possibility of an organic cause.

Specific aspects of psychotic symptoms may sometimes provide clues to regional alterations in brain function and trigger suspicion of neurological disease. For example, denial of blindness that may appear delusional should trigger suspicion of Anton's Syndrome (cortical blindness, due to visual cortex lesions) and denial of paralysis should lead to a consideration of anosognosia (due to lesions in nondominant parietal cortex). Likewise, an isolated delusion of misidentification (Capgras Syndrome), as well as olfactory hallucinations, should point to a temporal lobe disease.

3. The psychosis is not better explained by a primary psychotic disorder or another mental disorder:

For example, even if a concomitant medical illness may raise suspicion of a secondary psychosis, the presence of a strong family history of schizophrenia and a premorbid schizoid personality should raise the suspicion of a primary schizophrenic illness.

In every case, a detailed history and complete physical, including a neurological examination and laboratory evaluation is an essential first step (Table 1.3). In light of emerging knowledge about secondary causes of schizophrenia, one needs to conduct additional investigations such as neurocognitive examinations, brain imaging, and electrophysiological

Table 1.2 Possible causes of secondary schizophrenia: well known disorders that may present with psychosis and approaches* to investigate them

Category	Example of well known causes	Investigations that may help diagnosis
Trauma	Penetrating or closed head injury	CT/MRI
Autoimmune	Systemic lupus erythematosus	Autoantibody titres (e.g. antinuclear antibodies for lupus)
Congenital/cytogenetic	Agenesis of corpus callosum Velocardiofacial syndrome	MRI/CT Karyotyping
Toxic	Drug intoxication: cocaine, 3–4 methylenedioxymethamphetamine (MDMA), amphetamines, phencyclidine (PCP), alcohol, lead poisoning	Urine drug screen Urine heavy metal screen
Iatrogenic	Steroids, antimalarials, isoniazid	Careful medication history; trial off the offending agent
Cerebrovascular	Small strokes in association cortices or subcortical regions	MRI/CT/EEG
Space occupying lesions	Cerebral tumors	MRI/CT/EEG
Metabolic	Metachromatic leucodystrophy Wilson's disease	Arylsulphatase – A levels, copper, and ceruloplasmin levels
Dietary	Pellagra, B12 deficiency	B12, Folate levels
Sepsis	Neurosyphilis, Toxoplasmosis, HIV disease	RPR to rule out syphilis (rapid plasma reagin) HIV antibody titres; lumbar puncture (glucose, protein in CSF)
Unknown/Degenerative/Demyelinating	Lewy body dementia, Parkinson's disease	MRI, CT, EEG, Evoked potentials
Seizures	Partial complex seizures	EEG, including sleep deprivation; telemetric EEG as indicated
Endocrine	Hyper, or hypothyroidism; hyperparathyroidism	Serum calcium

* The mnemonic "TACTICS MDs USE" can be useful in clinical practice.

Table 1.3 Workup to rule out secondary schizophrenia

A. First line assessments in every new patient with psychosis:

1. Neuropsychiatric and medical history

2. Neurological /physical exam

3. Neuropsychological testing

4. Laboratory investigations: complete and differential blood count, erythrocyte sedimentation rate, glucose, electrolytes, thyroid function tests, liver function tests, electroencephalography, urinary drug screen

B. Second-line assessments in patients with high index of suspicion

1. *Blood*: Rapid Plasma Reagin (RPR) to rule out syphilis; HIV testing; serum heavy metals; copper and ceruloplasmin levels, serum calcium levels, autoantibody titres (e.g. antinuclear antibodies for lupus); B12, folate levels; arylsulphatase – A levels

Karyotyping

2. *Urine*: culture and toxicology; urine drug screen; heavy metal screen

3. *Imaging*: MRI/CT/ PET/ SPECT of the brain

4. *Electrophysiological studies*: EEG, polysomnography; evoked potentials

5. *Cerebrospinal fluid analyses*: glucose, protein cultures; cryptococcal antigen

studies, especially in those in their earlier years of the disease, those with atypical presentations, and those in whom there is reason to suspect a primary disorder. Even in those with an established diagnosis of schizophrenia, a neurocognitive examination can be of value in characterizing the deficits and setting treatment goals and priorities that address the concerns of the patients and their caregivers. In future neurocognitive examinations and neuroimaging, assessments are likely to emerge as valuable parameters to predict and monitor treatment response for all patients with schizophrenia.

No clinical feature, singly or as part of a cluster of features, reliably distinguishes between primary and secondary schizophrenia. Early studies, many flawed in design by contemporary standards of research methodology, suggested that catatonic symptoms, altered states of consciousness (i.e. confusional or "dream-like" states), and visual hallucinations are more frequent in secondary schizophrenia, which also tended to have later age of onset. Certain delusions such as those involving beliefs of mistaken identity of others (i.e. Capgrass delusions) are thought to be more common in secondary than in primary schizophrenia.

Whether to conduct a brain scan in a patient with schizophrenia on a routine basis is debatable. When brain scans (commonly structural, e.g., MRI or CT) have been used clinically as part of the workup of a psychotic patient, the purpose is to rule out a space-occupying lesion or developmental malformation as the potential cause of the psychosis. Although incidental findings have been reported in MRI studies of even healthy people [95] and patients who present with psychosis [96], such findings are rare. Thus, in the absence of quantitative analysis, routine brain imaging cannot aid in the differential diagnosis of psychosis without considering the clinical presentation [97].

Conclusions

The contemporary view of schizophrenia as a neuropsychiatric disorder has been shaped by converging data from multiple lines of research. The paradigm shift was hastened by the availability of newer investigational tools such as neuroimaging, as well as advances in histopathological and gene analysis techniques. The old distinction between organic (or structural) and functional (purely psychological) disease misled the field and stunted systematic investigation in the disorders that were earlier deemed purely psychological. Classification of psychiatric disorders into those with or without identifiable etiology has been more meaningful clinically. Even in those without an identifiable etiology, multiple lines of investigation provide robust evidence of diffuse alterations in brain structure and connectivity. Many of these abnormalities are also evident in asymptomatic individuals at genetic predisposition to the disorder, and often evolve during the prodromal phase of the illness –sometimes progress early in the illness – and are usually more prominent in early onset forms of the disorder. A greater understanding of the trait and state-related features of schizophrenia raises the hope of development of successful early interventions that stop or slow, and possibly reverse, the progression of disease pathology in schizophrenia.

References

1. Nuechterlein K. H., *et al.* Identification of separable cognitive factors in schizophrenia. *Schizophr Res*, 2004. **72**(1):29–39.

2. Green M. G., *et al.* Neurocognitive deficits and functional outcome in schizophrenia: are we measuring the "right stuff"? *Schizophrenia Bull*, 2000. **26**:119–36.

3. Penn D. L., *et al.* Cognition and social functioning in schizophrenia. *Psychiatry*, 1997. **60**(4):281–91.

4. Penn D. L., *et al.* Social cognition in schizophrenia. *Psychol Bull*, 1997. **121**(1):114–32.

5. Insel T. R., Fernald R. D. How the brain processes social information: searching for the social brain. *Annu Rev Neurosci*, 2004. **27**:697–722.

6. Gur R. E., *et al.* An fMRI study of facial emotion processing in patients with schizophrenia. *Am J Psychiatry*, 2002. **159**(12):1992–9.

7. Silverstein S. M. Information processing, social cognition, and psychiatric rehabilitation in schizophrenia. *Psychiatry*, 1997. **60**(4):327–40.

8. Censits D. M., *et al.* Neuropsychological evidence supporting a neurodevelopmental model of schizophrenia: a longitudinal study. *Schizophr Res*, 1997. **24**(3):289–98.

9. Gold S., *et al.* Longitudinal study of cognitive function in first-episode and recent-onset schizophrenia. *Am J Psychiatry*, 1999. **156**(9):1342–8.

10. Hoff A.L., *et al.* Longitudinal neuropsychological follow-up study of patients with first-episode schizophrenia. *Am J Psychiatry*, 1999. **156**(9):1336–41.

11. Waddington J. L., Youssef H. A., Cognitive dysfunction in chronic schizophrenia followed prospectively over 10 years and its longitudinal relationship to the emergence of tardive dyskinesia. *Psychol Med*, 1996. **26**(4):681–8.

12. Aleman A., *et al.* Memory impairment in schizophrenia: a meta-analysis. *Am J Psychiatry*, 1999. **156**(9):1358–66.

13. Addington J., Saeedi H., Addington D. Influence of social perception and social knowledge on cognitive and social functioning in early psychosis. *Br J Psychiatry*, 2006. **189**:373–8.

14. Brewer W. J., *et al.* Stability of olfactory identification deficits in neuroleptic-naive patients with first-episode psychosis. *Am J Psychiatry*, 2001. **158**(1):107–15.

15. Schuepbach D., *et al.* Negative symptom resolution and improvements in specific cognitive deficits after acute treatment in first-episode schizophrenia. *Schizophr Res*, 2002. **53**(3):249–61.

16. Hodges A., *et al.* People at risk of schizophrenia: sample characteristics of the first 100 cases in the Edinburgh high-risk study. *Br J Psychiatry*, 1999. **174**:547–53.

17. Erlenmeyer-Kimling L., *et al.* The New York High-Risk Project. Psychoses and cluster A personality disorders in offspring of schizophrenic parents at 23 years of follow-up. *Arch Gen Psychiatry*, 1995. **52**(10):857–65.

18. Parnas J., *et al.* Lifetime DSM-III-R diagnostic outcomes in the offspring of schizophrenic mothers. Results from the Copenhagen High-Risk Study. *Arch Gen Psychiatry*, 1993. **50**(9):707–14.

19. Marcus J., *et al.* Review of the NIMH Israeli Kibbutz-City Study and the Jerusalem Infant Development Study. *Schizophr Bull*, 1987. **13**(3):425–38.

20. Erlenmeyer-Kimling L., *et al.* Attention, memory, and motor skills as childhood predictors of schizophrenia-related psychoses: the New York High-Risk Project. *Am J Psychiatry*, 2000. **157**(9):1416–22.

21. Cosway R., *et al.* Sustained attention in young people at high risk for schizophrenia. *Psychol Med*, 2002. **32**(2):277–86.

22. Glahn D. C., *et al.* Beyond hypofrontality: a quantitative meta-analysis of functional neuroimaging studies of working memory in schizophrenia. *Hum Brain Mapp*, 2005. **25**(1):60–9.

23. Fusar-Poli P., *et al.* Neurofunctional correlates of vulnerability to psychosis: a systematic review and meta-analysis. *Neurosci Biobehav Rev*, 2007. **31**(4):465–84.

24. Shergill S. S., *et al.* Mapping auditory hallucinations in schizophrenia using functional magnetic resonance imaging. *Arch Gen Psychiatry*, 2000. **57**(11):1033–8.

25. Liddle P. F., *et al.* Patterns of cerebral blood flow in schizophrenia. *Br J Psychiatry*, 1992. **160**:179–86.

26. Lencz T., *et al.* Impairments in perceptual competency and maintenance on a visual delayed match-to-sample test in first-episode schizophrenia. *Arch Gen Psychiatry*, 2003. **60**(3):238–43.

27. Wolf R. C., Vasic N., Walter H. The concept of working memory in schizophrenia: current evidence and future perspectives. *Fortschr Neurol Psychiatry*, 2006. **74**(8):449–68.

28. Callicott, J. H., *et al.* Complexity of prefrontal cortical dysfunction in schizophrenia: more than up or down. *Am J Psychiatry*, 2003. **160**(12):2209–15.

29. Harris M. S., *et al.* Longitudinal studies of antisaccades in antipsychotic-naive first-episode schizophrenia. *Psychol Med*, 2006. **36**(4):485–94.

30. Wilson T. W., *et al.* Cortical gamma generators suggest

abnormal auditory circuitry in early-onset psychosis. *Cereb Cortex*, 2008. **18**(2):371–8. [Epub Jun 8, 2007.]

31. Kerns J. G., *et al.* Anterior cingulate conflict monitoring and adjustments in control. *Science*, 2004. **303**(5660):1023–6.

32. Carter C. S., *et al.* Anterior cingulate cortex activity and impaired self-monitoring of performance in patients with schizophrenia: an event-related fMRI study. *Am J Psychiatry*, 2001. **158**(9):1423–8.

33. Kerns J. G., *et al.* Decreased conflict- and error-related activity in the anterior cingulate cortex in subjects with schizophrenia. *Am J Psychiatry*, 2005. **162**(10):1833–9.

34. Fletcher P., *et al.* Abnormal cingulate modulation of fronto-temporal connectivity in schizophrenia. *Neuroimage*, 1999. **9**(3):337–42.

35. LeDoux J. The emotional brain, fear, and the amygdala. *Cell Mol Neurobiol*, 2003. **23**(4–5):727–38.

36. Eichenbaum H. Hippocampus: cognitive processes and neural representations that underlie declarative memory. *Neuron*, 2004. **44**(1):109–20.

37. Adolphs R., Baron-Cohen S., Tranel D. Impaired recognition of social emotions following amygdala damage. *J Cogn Neurosci*, 2002. **14**(8):1264–74.

38. Aleman A., Kahn R. S. Strange feelings: do amygdala abnormalities dysregulate the emotional brain in schizophrenia? *Prog Neurobiol*, 2005. **77**(5):283–98.

39. Hempel A., *et al.* Impairment in basal limbic function in schizophrenia during affect recognition. *Psychiatry Res*, 2003. **122**(2):115–24.

40. Takahashi H., *et al.* An fMRI study of differential neural response to affective pictures in schizophrenia. *Neuroimage*, 2004. **22**(3):1247–54.

41. Steen R. G., *et al.* Brain volume in first-episode schizophrenia: systematic review and meta-analysis of magnetic resonance imaging studies. *Br J Psychiatry*, 2006. **188**:510–8.

42. Ward K. E., *et al.* Meta-analysis of brain and cranial size in schizophrenia. *Schizophr Res*, 1996. **22**(3):197–213.

43. Wright I. C., *et al.* Meta-analysis of regional brain volumes in schizophrenia. *Am J Psychiatry*, 2000. **157**(1):16–25.

44. Woodruff P. W., McManus I. C., David A. S. Meta-analysis of corpus callosum size in schizophrenia. *J Neurol Neurosurg Psychiatry*, 1995. **58**(4):457–61.

45. Nelson M. D., *et al.* Hippocampal volume reduction in schizophrenia as assessed by magnetic resonance imaging: a meta-analytic study. *Arch Gen Psychiatry*, 1998. **55**(5):433–40.

46. Lawrie S. M., Abukmeil S. S. Brain abnormality in schizophrenia. A systematic and quantitative review of volumetric magnetic resonance imaging studies. *Br J Psychiatry*, 1998. **172**:110–20.

47. Konick L. C., Friedman L. Meta-analysis of thalamic size in schizophrenia. *Biol Psychiatry*, 2001. **49**(1):28–38.

48. Honea R., *et al.* Regional deficits in brain volume in schizophrenia: a meta-analysis of voxel-based morphometry studies. *Am J Psychiatry*, 2005. **162**(12):2233–45.

49. Antonova E., *et al.* The relationship between brain structure and neurocognition in schizophrenia: a selective review. *Schizophr Res*, 2004. **70**(2–3):117–45.

50. Lawrie S., Johnstone E., Weinberger D. (Eds.) (2004). *Schizophrenia: from neuroimaging to neuroscience*, Oxford: Oxford University Press.

51. Keshavan M. S., *et al.* Neurobiology of early psychosis. *Br J Psychiatry*, 2005. **48**(Suppl): s8–18.

52. Ho B. C., *et al.* Progressive structural brain abnormalities and their relationship to clinical outcome: a longitudinal magnetic resonance imaging study early in schizophrenia. *Arch Gen Psychiatry*, 2003. **60**(6):585–94.

53. DeLisi L. E., *et al.* Cerebral ventricular change over the first 10 years after the onset of schizophrenia. *Psychiatry Res*, 2004. **130**(1):57–70.

54. Whitworth A. B., *et al.* Longitudinal volumetric MRI study in first- and multiple-episode male schizophrenia patients. *Psychiatry Res*, 2005. **140**(3):225–37.

55. Lawrie S. M., *et al.* Magnetic resonance imaging of brain in people at high risk of developing schizophrenia. *Lancet*, 1999. **353**(9146):30–3.

56. Keshavan M. S., *et al.* Magnetic resonance imaging and spectroscopy in offspring at risk for schizophrenia: preliminary studies. *Prog Neuropsychopharmacol Biol Psychiatry*, 1997. **21**(8):1285–95.

57. Boos H. B., *et al.* Brain volumes in relatives of patients with schizophrenia: a meta-analysis. *Arch Gen Psychiatry*, 2007. **64**(3):297–304.

58. Job D. E., *et al.* Voxel-based morphometry of grey matter densities in subjects at high risk of schizophrenia. *Schizophr Res*, 2003. **64**(1):1–13.

59. Diwadkar V. A., *et al.* Genetically predisposed offspring with schizotypal features: an ultra high-risk group for schizophrenia? *Prog Neuropsychopharmacol Biol Psychiatry*, 2006. **30**(2):230–8.

60. Job D. E., *et al.* Grey matter changes over time in high risk subjects developing schizophrenia. *Neuroimage*, 2005. **25**(4):1023–30.

61. Pantelis C., *et al.* Neuroanatomical abnormalities before and after onset of psychosis: a cross-sectional and longitudinal MRI comparison. *Lancet*, 2003. **361**(9354): 281–8.

62. Thompson P. M., *et al.* Mapping adolescent brain change reveals dynamic wave of accelerated gray matter loss in very early-onset schizophrenia. *Proc Natl Acad Sci USA*, 2001. **98**(20):11650–5.

63. Thompson P. M., *et al.* Structural MRI and brain development. *Int Rev Neurobiol*, 2005. **67**:285–323.

64. Toga A. W., Thompson P. M., Sowell E. R. Mapping brain maturation. *Trends Neurosci*, 2006. **29**(3):148–59.

65. Gogtay N., *et al.* Cortical brain development in nonpsychotic siblings of patients with childhood-onset schizophrenia. *Arch Gen Psychiatry*, 2007. **64**(7): 772–80.

66. Klingberg T., *et al.* Myelination and organization of the frontal white matter in children: a diffusion tensor MRI study. *Neuroreport*, 1999. **10**(13): 2817–21.

67. Nagy Z., Westerberg H., Klingberg T. Maturation of white matter is associated with the development of cognitive functions during childhood. *J Cogn Neurosci*, 2004. **16**(7): 1227–33.

68. Liston C., *et al.* Frontostriatal microstructure modulates efficient recruitment of cognitive control. *Cereb Cortex*, 2006. **16**(4): 553–60.

69. Kanaan R. A., *et al.* Diffusion tensor imaging in schizophrenia. *Biol Psychiatry*, 2005. **58**(12): 921–9.

70. Kumra S., *et al.* Reduced frontal white matter integrity in early-onset schizophrenia: a preliminary study. *Biol Psychiatry*, 2004. **55**(12):1138–45.

71. Lindstrom L. H., *et al.* Increased dopamine synthesis rate in medial prefrontal cortex and striatum in schizophrenia indicated by L-(beta-11C) DOPA and PET. *Biol Psychiatry*, 1999. **46**(5):681–8.

72. Zakzanis K. K., Hansen K. T. Dopamine D2 densities and the schizophrenic brain. *Schizophr Res*, 1998. **32**(3):201–6.

73. Erritzoe D., *et al.* Positron emission tomography and single photon emission CT molecular imaging in schizophrenia. *Neuroimaging Clin N Am*, 2003. **13**(4):817–32.

74. Laruelle M. The role of endogenous sensitization in the pathophysiology of schizophrenia: implications from recent brain imaging studies. *Brain Res Brain Res Rev*, 2000. **31**(2–3):371–84.

75. Weinberger D. R. The biological basis of schizophrenia: new directions. *J Clin Psychiatry*, 1997. **58**:22–7.

76. Steen R. G., Hamer R. M., Lieberman J. A. Measurement of brain metabolites by 1H magnetic resonance spectroscopy in patients with schizophrenia: a systematic review and meta-analysis. *Neuropsychopharma-cology*, 2005. **30**(11):1949–62.

77. Keshavan M. S., Stanley J. A., Pettegrew J. W. Magnetic resonance spectroscopy in schizophrenia: methodological issues and findings–part II. *Biol Psychiatry*, 2000. **48**(5): 369–80.

78. Stanley J. A., Pettegrew J. W., Keshavan M. S. Magnetic resonance spectroscopy in schizophrenia: methodological issues and findings-part I. *Biol Psychiatry*, 2000. **48**(5):357–68.

79. Jessen F., *et al.* Proton magnetic resonance spectroscopy in subjects at risk for schizophrenia. *Schizophr Res*, 2006. **87**(1–3): 81–8.

80. Pettegrew J. W., *et al.* Alterations in brain high-energy phosphate and membrane phospholipid metabolism in first-episode, drug-naive schizophrenics. A pilot study of the dorsal prefrontal cortex by in vivo phosphorus 31 nuclear magnetic resonance spectroscopy. *Arch Gen Psychiatry*, 1991. **48**(6):563–8.

81. Feinberg I. Schizophrenia and late maturational brain changes in man. *Psychopharmacol Bull*, 1982. **18**:29–31.

82. Stanley J. A., *et al.* An in vivo study of the prefrontal cortex of schizophrenic patients at different stages of illness via phosphorus magnetic resonance spectroscopy. *Arch Gen Psychiatry*, 1995. **52**(5): 399–406.

83. Williamson P., *et al.* Localized phosphorus 31 magnetic resonance spectroscopy in chronic schizophrenia patients and normal controls. *Arch Gen Psychiatry*, 1991. **48**:578.

84. Fukuzako H., *et al.* Changes in levels of phosphorus metabolites in temporal lobes of drug-naive schizophrenic patients. *Am J Psychiatry*, 1999. **156**(8):1205–8.

85. Volz H. R., *et al.* Reduced phosphodiesters and high-energy phosphates in the frontal lobe of schizophrenic patients: a (31)P chemical shift spectroscopic-imaging study. *Biol Psychiatry*, 2000. **47**(11):954–61.

86. Smesny S., *et al.* Metabolic mapping using 2D (31)P-MR spectroscopy reveals frontal and thalamic metabolic abnormalities in schizophrenia. *Neuroimage*, 2007. **35**(2):729–37. [Epub Dec 29, 2006.]

87. Stanley J. A., Pettegrew J. W. A post-processing method to segregate and quantify the broad components underlying the phosphodiester spectral region of

in vivo 31P brain spectra. *Magn Reson Med*, 2001. **45**:390–396.

88. Selemon L. D., Goldman-Rakic P. S. The reduced neuropil hypothesis: a circuit based model of schizophrenia. *Biol Psychiatry*, 1999. **45**(1):17–25.

89. Keshavan M. S., *et al.* Prefrontal membrane phospholipid metabolism of child and adolescent offspring at risk for schizophrenia or schizoaffective disorder: an in vivo 31P MRS study. *Mol Psychiatry*, 2003. **8**(3):316–23, 251.

90. Harrison P. J., Owen M. J. Genes for schizophrenia? Recent findings and their pathophysiological implications.

Lancet, 2003. **361**(9355):417–9.

91. Sullivan P. F. The genetics of schizophrenia. *PLoS Med*, 2005. **2**(7):e212.

92. Akbarian S., *et al.* Altered distribution of nicotinamide-adenine dinucleotide phosphate-diaphorase cells in frontal lobe of schizophrenics implies disturbances of cortical development. *Arch Gen Psychiatry*, 1993. **50**(3):169–77.

93. Glantz L. A., Lewis D. A., Decreased dendritic spine density on prefrontal cortical pyramidal neurons in schizophrenia. *Arch Gen Psychiatry*, 2000. **57**:65–73.

94. Lieberman J. A., *et al.* The early stages of schizophrenia: speculations on pathogenesis, pathophysiology, and therapeutic approaches. *Biol Psychiatry*, 2001. **50**(11):884–97.

95. Illes J., *et al.* Ethics. Incidental findings in brain imaging research. *Science*, 2006. **311**(5762):783–4.

96. Lisanby S. H., *et al.* Psychosis Secondary to Brain Tumor. *Semin Clin Neuropsychiatry*, 1998. **3**(1):12–22.

97. Lawrie S. M., *et al.* Qualitative cerebral morphology in schizophrenia: a magnetic resonance imaging study and systematic literature review. *Schizophr Res*, 1997. **25**(2):155–66.

2

The concept of organicity and its application to schizophrenia

Perminder S. Sachdev

Facts box

1. The term "organic" psychiatric disorder has a number of problems that can be described as problems of duality, method, practice, scholasticism, semantics, and stigma.

2. The term "functional" disorders is inadequate as all disorders are associated with functional impairment.

3. The term "secondary," implying idiopathic or as yet insufficiently understood etiology, overcomes some of the problems of "organic."

4. A definitive classification of the psychoses must await a greater understanding of etiopathogenetic mechanisms.

Introduction

This book is on "secondary" schizophrenia, and it is important to examine what constitutes a secondary rather than a primary psychiatric syndrome. This term has a tortuous history that is worth revisiting, both for its explanatory power and its limitations. In many minds, "secondary" equates with the older concept of "organicity." The term "organic" was a product of the move in late-nineteenth and early-twentieth centuries to distinguish "functional" (or psychological) disorders from real "brain" disorders, which was rooted in Cartesian dualism and propelled by the increasing influence of psychodynamic theory. Since then, we have moved further both in the philosophy of mind and in the major paradigms that guide the discipline of psychiatry.

Why not "organic"?

We have chosen not to use "organic psychosis" as a title for this book, even though it is still commonly used in practice. The use of "organic" is a legacy of

the schism between the brain and the mind, and it has a certain power to maintain the philosophical baggage of Cartesian dualism (*the duality problem*). The dichotomy of mind and body (or brain) has a long tradition in Western thought and it has shaped much of our earlier thinking and the terminology we use. Cartesian dualism presents a polarity in the mind–brain problem that is seemingly impossible to bridge. This polarity is reflected in the other dichotomies we have come to accept: structure and function, psychological and biological, organic and functional. Most recent philosophers have abandoned property dualism and accept some shade of materialist monism, according to which they either attempt to "naturalize" consciousness and intentionality, that is, reduce them to some form of physical phenomena [1], or at the very least accept that the basis of the mind and consciousness is in the neurophysiologic processes occurring in the brain. There are many shades of materialism with which we do not have to concern ourselves, but in all of these, there is no place for an organic–functional dichotomy. There is, on the other hand, an interaction between structure and function, whereby no disorder of the brain (or mind) is based solely on disturbance of structure *or* function. The term "organic" steadfastly persists in maintaining the dichotomy against all reasoned argument.

Then there is the *problem of method*. The distinction between organic and functional disorders carries with it an implication that different methodologies are applicable to the two: those of natural science to the former and those of the humanities or social science to the latter. There are tensions between these methods that are not easily reconcilable [2], but for true psychiatry, both aspects are important. The mental lives of individuals have their origins in the brain but belong equally in a phenomenal world, and the study of the two aspects complement each other. The brain mechanisms underlying psychotic disorders are important, but they present an incomplete picture if the nature and content of the symptoms, their meaning to the individual, and his or her adaptation to them are not examined. Any term, such as "organic," that implies a polarity and incompatibility and thwarts the process of application of both the natural and social science methodologies to psychiatric disorders, has outlived its usefulness.

"Organic" also presents a serious problem in its practical usage (the *practice problem*). What is an "organic mental disorder"? ICD-10 [3] attempts to define it as "a range of mental disorders grouped together on the basis of their having in common a demonstrable etiology in cerebral disease, brain injury, or other insult leading to cerebral dysfunction." It further goes on to say that "the term 'organic' means no more and no less than that the syndrome so classified can be attributed to an independently diagnosable cerebral or systemic disease or disorder." The working hypothesis is that the cerebral or systemic dysfunction is directly responsible for the disorder and not a "fortuitous association with such a disease or dysfunction, or a psychological reaction to its symptoms" [3]. In practice, however, the situation is hardly as clear-cut as this may suggest.

First, consider the case in which a cerebral disease is clearly demonstrable and a psychiatric disorder such as psychosis is present. How does one establish that the former is etiologically related to the latter? For instance, when is a psychosis that develops in a patient with temporal lobe epilepsy organic? Is the schizophrenia-like psychosis that develops in someone after traumatic brain injury, even though full clinical recovery from the injury has occurred, organic in origin? These questions are not easy to answer. One guideline often repeated is the temporal association (weeks or months) between the psychiatric syndrome and the putative organic factor. An examination of the psychiatric disorders associated with epilepsy, cerebrovascular disease, Parkinson's disease, and so on, invalidates such an approach. We recognize that cerebral disease may be present for years before a psychiatric disorder develops, and yet the two may be etiologically related. The so-called "organic psychosis" associated with epilepsy may antedate, occur concurrently or postdate the onset of the clinical features of epilepsy [4].

A second guideline has been "common association," such that a particular psychiatric syndrome is recognized to commonly occur in association with a cerebral disorder and more often than chance would have it. This was the approach used by Slater and colleagues [5] in attempting to establish an etiological relationship between epilepsy and chronic schizophrenia-like psychosis. It has produced uncertain results, and many important relationships are still controversial, including that of epilepsy and psychosis. Moreover, a group association is only diffidently applied by the clinician to an individual case, as evidenced by the difficulty one encounters in addressing the question: Is the psychosis in my patient due to epilepsy, cannabis use, or the head trauma he/she suffered some years ago?

A third guideline hopes to yield insight in retrospect, that is, if the treatment of the cerebral or systemic disorder leads to an improvement in the psychiatric syndrome, the two were probably etiologically related. Not only is such retrospective diagnosis useless clinically, in practice, this guideline frequently fails. It is not uncommon for the schizophrenia-like psychosis associated with, for example, cannabis abuse to persist after the latter has been discontinued. In another case, the patient may improve, only to relapse after a short interval in spite of normal laboratory data. That the attribution of "significance" to a recognized "organic" factor is not a very reliable process is indicated by the results of the field trials of ICD-10 [6] in which the kappa coefficients for the organic syndromes were lower than their nonorganic counterparts, contrary to what one might anticipate.

The practical difficulty in establishing the "real" role of a "physical" disorder is compounded by the varying opinions among clinicians regarding which disorders to look for, in which situations, and how hard to search. Further, does the suggested need to exclude "organicity" imply that every patient with psychosis, depression, or anxiety should undergo an extensive battery of tests before a firm diagnosis can be made? And, how does one deal with the "enlarged ventricles" in a patient with "nonorganic schizophrenia"? Diagnosticians have differing views on this, and not everyone digs to the same depth in the search for "organic" gold. Extensive exploration, using the latest technology, often yields "findings" that may be incidental and can be difficult to interpret. Investigating elderly psychiatric patients with MRI is likely to yield abnormalities that may be no different from those seen in a nonpsychiatric population, and yet may be impossible to ignore, thus producing a major dilemma. The problem is again because of the false dichotomy that "organic" tends to perpetuate. We know that

17

psychiatric illnesses have multiple etiological factors – genetics, coarse cerebral disease, personality, stress – some of which would be recognized as organic in most cases. We are, therefore, not dealing with discrete etiological categories, and it is wrong to treat them as such. It was this tendency that led to the paradoxical situation that an apology had to be included in ICD-10: "use of the term 'organic' does not imply that conditions elsewhere in this classification are 'nonorganic'." It begs the question: What is "organic" and what is not? A categorical answer is impossible because the dichotomy itself is false. Birley [7] calls it the *problem of scholasticism*, that is, treating what is vague as if it were precise.

I have already referred, in part, to the *semantic problem*. Proponents of "organic" have had to seek suitable antonyms. "Functional" is much used but is disliked by some because of its long association with physiological function, and the argument that function is impaired in organic disorders as well. The term "nonorganic" was suggested to cover everything that fell into the other basket, but the proponents were apologetic for it, as mentioned above. Furthermore, what is considered "organic" has been referred to by many other terms including brain damage, cerebral damage, brain dysfunction, and brain injury. It seems there is no term that will satisfy us all.

The *problem of stigma* remains. However loudly patients and professionals have demanded destigmatization of mental disorders, society's attitudes have been slow to change. A dichotomy between "organic" and "nonorganic" certainly does not assist the process. Nor does it help the remedicalization of psychiatry.

The final problem I can identify is the *threat of takeover*. Although psychiatrists continue their affair with Descartes, other professions are waiting in the wings – neurologists to take over our "organic" disorders and psychologists and social workers to take over our "nonorganic" ones. Psychiatry must consider this when defining its territory, as that will determine how solid the fences are.

The alternative

Having listed so many problems with "organic," I must argue, like Spitzer and colleagues [8], that it is now "time to retire the term…" But what must take its place? Two terms that have been considered seriously are "symptomatic" and "secondary," the latter having won out in DSM-IV. Primary psychiatric disorders are, thereby, the disorders that were previously "functional" or "nonorganic." This alternative deals with some of the identified problems. Although a primary–secondary dichotomy remains, it does not have the connotation of a duality of mind and brain. "Primary" implies (or so I hope) "idiopathic," that is, the cause is not known, which in general is an accurate acknowledgment of our ignorance. It does not connote lack of cerebral dysfunction of some kind. It groups psychiatric disorders more logically, yielding classes that are characterized by phenomenology and not putative etiology. It makes all psychiatric disorders secure within the field of psychiatry. It has many parallels in medicine in which "idiopathic or primary" and "secondary" categories of hypertension, respiratory failure, hyperparathyroidism, and other disorders are recognized.

But this strategy only goes some of the way. The dichotomy between "functional" and "organic" that is present in the minds of mental health professionals is not necessarily addressed. As Spitzer and colleagues [7] admit, "the (ICD-10) definition of 'organic' is in complete agreement with our definition of 'secondary'." The only hope DSM-IV has is to leave behind the baggage associated with "organic," but it is perhaps only a question of time before "secondary" assumes this burden. The practical problem of deciding what constitutes "secondary," and the problems of method and scholasticism remain. We exchange old semantic problems with new ones. A more radical change is necessary for these problems to go away; we need to change paradigms rather than replace terms with others that signify the same concepts. One suggestion is to treat neurobiological causes of mental disorders on a continuum, which comments the degree to which known neurobiological etiology is attributable to a particular disorder. The known neurobiological disorders or causes could be separately listed, as on Axis III. This strategy is certainly an adequate response to the problem of dichotomy, and with it the problems of method and scholasticism. The major problem it does not deal with, and perhaps the one that makes it a worse choice is that of practice. First, the difficulty of deciding upon the significance of an identifiable cerebral disorder in the causation of a psychiatric syndrome is not helped by this change. That will have to await an increase in our knowledge of brain function – normal and abnormal. Second, the proposed strategy is likely to prove very unreliable, as one would expect a low agreement between psychiatrists regarding the relative significance of neurobiology in individual cases.

Classifiers are unlikely, therefore, to adopt the suggestion. An alternative is to regard all psychotic disorders as being neurobiological, and indicate on a separate axis what contributions – on a continuum again – interpersonal, social, and cultural factors may have made in a particular case. This position is complementary to the above, and the associated difficulties are similar.

I feel that we are condemned to an unsatisfactory position, and the reasons are not difficult to understand: i) positron emission tomography notwithstanding, our understanding of brain function and that of the etiology of psychiatric disorders is still very rudimentary; ii) even as neuroscience is progressing, the realization is prevalent that we have to continue conceptualizing brain function at multiple levels because molecular mechanisms remain inadequate to explain higher-level phenomena in their entirety; and iii) our dialogue occurs in a language born in a dualist age, and this is difficult to transform. This may seem to be the position of a pessimist, but the hope that I see is in the debate that has already been generated. The initial moves, as in DSM-IV, are in the right direction, but we have further to travel. For this book, the prefix "secondary" to schizophrenia will have to suffice because it acknowledges the contribution of the "organic" factor while at the same time accepting that the syndrome may be no different from the idiopathic schizophrenic disorder. It challenges us to rethink schizophrenia while providing clues to its pathophysiology. My hope is that these clues will lead to insights that will provide a deeper understanding of this enigmatic disorder.

References

1. Searle J. R. (1992). *The Rediscovery of the Mind*. Cambridge, Mass: The MIT Press.

2. Slavney P. R., McHugh P. R. (1987). *Psychiatric Polarities: Methodology and Practice*. Baltimore: The Johns Hopkins University Press.

3. World Health Organization (1992). *The ICD-10 Classification of Mental and Behavioural Disorders: Clinical Descriptions and Diagnostic Guidelines*. Geneva: WHO.

4. Starkstein S. E., Mayberg H. S. (1993). Depression in Parkinson disease. In *Depression in Neurologic Disease*, Starkstein S. E., Robinson R. G. (Eds.). Baltimore: The Johns Hopkins University Press, pp. 97–116.

5. Slater E., Beard A. W., Glither E. The schizophrenia-like psychosis of epilepsy. *Br J Psychiatry*, 1963. **109**:95–150.

6. Sartorius N., Kaelber C. T., Cooper J. E., *et al.* Progress toward achieving a common language in psychiatry: Results from the field trials accompanying the clinical guidelines of mental and behavioural disorders in ICD-10. *Arch Gen Psychiatry*, 1993. **50**:115–24.

7. Birley J. L .T. DSM-III: from left to right or right to left? *Br J Psychiatry*, 1990. **157**:116–8.

8. Spitzer R. L., First M. B., Williams J. B. W., *et al.* Now is the time to retire the term "organic mental disorders." *Am J Psychiatry*, 1992. **149**:240–4.

Introduction

3

Secondary hallucinations

Mark Walterfang, Ramon Mocellin, David L. Copolov, and Dennis Velakoulis

Facts box

1. Infrequent hallucinations – auditory as well as visual – are common in the general population and do not necessarily signify a psychiatric disorder.
2. Hallucinations occur in a number of psychiatric disorders, and are most common in schizophrenia.
3. Hallucinations in the setting of brain disease, that is, of organic etiology, are uncommon in general practice but are frequently encountered on hospital wards, especially among the elderly.
4. Although hallucinations may occur in a number of modalities within the individual, the etiological, biological, and treatment facets differ somewhat for auditory, visual, olfactory, gustatory, and tactile hallucinations.
5. A number of neurological or systemic disorders have been associated with hallucinations of different modalities.
6. The models of pathogenesis of hallucinations are drawn from a range of different disorders such as delirium, dementia, and substance-induced states, and bear significant homology to some of the emergent neurobiology of schizophrenia-spectrum disorders.

Introduction

The term "hallucination," which derives from the Greek *alyein* via the Latin *hallucinari*, to "wander in the mind" [1], was first used in the English language in 1572 to describe visual phenomena – "ghostes and spirites walking by nyghte" [2]. The essential feature of hallucinations is that they are percepts in the absence of external stimuli, although they possess other char-

acteristics that distinguish them from related phenomena such as imagery and pseudohallucinations. Slade and Bentall [2] crystallized these features in their definition, proposing that hallucinations are perceptual experiences that occur in the absence of appropriate stimuli, have the full force or impact of the corresponding real perception, and are not amenable to direct and voluntary control. This definition, although widely used, has been subject to suggested amendments, for example, by David [3] who defines hallucinations as "sensory experiences which occur in the absence of corresponding external stimulation of the relevant sensory organ, have a sufficient sense of reality to resemble a veridical perception, over which the subject does not feel that he or she has direct and voluntary control and which occur in the awake state." By providing a less rigid boundary in relation to the reality-like aspect of the symptom, this definition takes into account the spectrum along which such stimulus-independent perceptions are described. It also accommodates the fact that a significant minority of hallucinators are able to use coping mechanisms to modulate their hallucinations [4] even though they may not feel they can control them.

Epidemiology of hallucinations in the community

In the community, hallucinations most commonly occur in the absence of psychiatric or neurological disorders. Several major studies have revealed a higher community prevalence of hallucinations than would be expected if they were only reflective of psychiatric or neurological disease. Ohayon found that 18% of a large sample of 13,057 subjects in the nonhospitalized population across three countries – the UK, Germany and Italy – experienced daytime hallucinations [5]. Among this group, infrequent daytime hallucinations (less than once a week) occurred in 16% and frequent hallucinations in 2%. In contrast to the hallucinations occurring in schizophrenia – in which auditory hallucinations are more common [6] – among Ohayon's group of interviewees who hallucinated more than once a week during the daytime, the frequency was greatest in the olfactory modality, followed by the tactile, and then auditory and visual modalities. In a large nonclinical population, Johns and colleagues found auditory and visual hallucinations occurred in approximately 4% of the sample [7]. Such data support the proposition that just as there is a range of mood and anxiety symptoms in the general population, there is a continuum of psychotic symptoms [8–9]. This is strongly advocated by van Os and colleagues [10]. Evidence from a number of cognitive neuropsychiatric studies suggests that individuals with hallucination-proneness appear to attribute internal events as external, and to have an external locus of control for internal and interpersonal events [11–13]. This appears to occur for both auditory and visual hallucinations [14].

Prevalence of hallucinations in psychiatric disorders

The disorder in which hallucinations are most common is schizophrenia. It is generally well accepted that 60% to 70% of individuals with this disorder experience hallucinations [15]. Auditory hallucinations are most common, followed by visual hallucinations followed by tactile, olfactory and gustatory hallucinations: in 117 consecutively admitted patients studied by Mueser and colleagues, the lifetime prevalence of hallucinations for auditory, visual, tactile, and olfactory/gustatory hallucinations was 72%, 16%, 17%, and 11%, respectively [6]. Another study by Bracha and colleagues suggested that the rate of visual hallucinations in chronic schizophrenia might be as high as 32% [16]. Rates described for auditory hallucinations range from 47% to 98% of schizophrenia patients [6, 16–19], visual hallucinations from 14% to 69% [6, 16–18], and tactile hallucinations from 4% to 25% of patients [6, 16].

Hallucinations also occur in mood disorders. One study of 4,972 hospitalized patients [20] showed that the prevalence of hallucinations in mood disorder patients was considerably greater for bipolar patients than for those with unipolar disorder (23% bipolar mixed, 11% bipolar manic, 11% bipolar depressed, and 6% unipolar vs. 61% schizophrenia). As in schizophrenia, in bipolar disorder, auditory hallucinations were

most common – but in comparison to schizophrenia the hallucinations in that disorder were less severe and more commonly visual.

Hallucinations occur in a wide range of disorders, as adverse reactions to or following intoxication with medications and nonprescription drugs and alcohol and in response to sensory deprivation. Comprehensive compendia of these causes associated with hallucinations in different modalities can be found in Brasic [21] and Cummings [22].

Prevalence of hallucinations in organic disorders

In contrast to the relatively high prevalence of hallucinations in populations of psychiatric patients, especially those with serious psychiatric disorders, secondary or organic hallucinations are uncommon in general psychiatric practice. Cornelius and colleagues reviewed more than 14,800 patients over a four-year period who had been assessed at the Western Psychiatric Clinic, Pittsburgh, Pennsylvania, USA, where retrospective analyses revealed only 11 patients with organic hallucinosis [23]. These patients were distinguished from those with schizophrenia in that visual hallucinations were the only symptom that was present to a significantly greater degree in the organic group. Other distinguishing symptoms including flat affect, thought disorganization, self-neglect, speech pressure, and bizarre behavior all occurred more frequently in schizophrenia.

Although there is extensive literature on hallucinations in individual modalities – as reflected in the sections that follow – there are relatively few papers that compare the phenomenology of organic hallucinosis and hallucinations due to primary psychiatric disorders such as schizophrenia and bipolar disorder. The best information on the distinction between these two broad classes of hallucinations comes from older studies that contrast the presenting features of organic and nonorganic psychosis. One of the most quoted studies in this regard is the investigation by Cutting of 74 patients who suffered from acute organic psychosis and 74 patients with acute schizophrenia [24]. The causes of the organic psychosis included stroke, epilepsy, carcinoma, respiratory failure, and alcohol abuse. Of the 74 patients with organic psychosis, 25 had visual hallucinations compared with 13 with auditory hallucinations. In subjects with schizophrenia the frequencies were reversed – 25 patients had auditory hallucinations and 12 had visual hallucinations [24]. Additionally, first-rank auditory hallucinations occurred in 22% of patients with schizophrenia and only 4% of patients with organic disorders. In contrast, a study by Johnstone and colleagues on 328 recently admitted psychotic patients – 23 of whom had underlying organic disorder – failed to demonstrate major phenomenological differences between patients with primary psychiatric disorders and those with organic disease in a manner that would allow such differences to stand as mainstays in the differential diagnosis of these two sets of disorders [25]. This study highlights the fact that astute clinic judgement is critical in determining if hallucinations are secondary to neurological and other diseases or are due to psychiatric disorders.

Although hallucinations may occur in a number of modalities within the one individual, it is useful to consider them on a modality-by–modality basis, in view of the differing etiological, biological, and treatment facets associated with each type of hallucination.

Secondary visual hallucinations

Throughout history, visual hallucinations (VHs) have long been associated with concepts of insanity [26]. Like other forms of aberrant sensory experience, VHs can occur in healthy individuals, functional psychiatric disorders, and organic states. An understanding of their experience in the latter can inform an understanding of the neurobiology of mental disorders as well as the anatomy of normal human perception.

Spectrum of visual perceptual disturbances

As in other sensory modalities, VHs have been considered to fall at one extreme of a spectrum of perceptual experience. This spectrum extends from normal visual experience, through intense/vivid internal visual imagery to illusions (a misperception of a true percept), and finally frank hallucinations (a percept-like experience in the absence of an external stimulus, experienced as a true percept). This spectral model has served psychiatry well in categorizing auditory hallucinations. It has generally allowed cleavage of functional psychotic disorders, with their characteristic external auditory phenomena and features of first-rank, from nonpsychotic or post-traumatic syndromes where phenomena are more internal, "as if" experiences with content often relating to past emotionally-

laden experience. However, such a one-dimensional model does not capture the full range of possible abnormal visual experiences that occur across a range of functional and organic disorders, such as polyolpia/pallinopsia – where true percepts are experienced multiple times – or metamorphopsia, where true percepts are dimensionally altered; each of these could be considered both an illusion and a hallucination [27]. Additionally, the distinction between hallucination and pseudohallucination has been driven by an assessment of the sufferer's attribution – external versus internal, "like" a true percept versus "is" a true percept, or insight versus insightlessness; in reality, the sufferer's experience is not so readily dichotomized, and it may be that the content and phenomenology of the experience is more closely tied to the underlying pathology than its associated experiential quality.

One model of visual hallucinations is provided by ffytche and colleagues. They propose that visual pathway disorders produce characteristic simple VHs, unfamiliar/malformed figures and landscape scenes, whereas disorders involving the brainstem and/or cholinergic dysfunction result in familiar figures, animals, and frequent delusional elaboration. The clinical utility of this model is supported by the fact that the two groups tend to respond to different treatments [27, 28]. Furthermore, we would argue that an understanding of the anatomy of visual experience, and how lesion location at least partially predicts phenomenology, leads to more appropriate investigation and management of VHs syndromes [29].

Visual hallucinations in normal individuals

Individuals in the community who experience VHs in the absence of a psychiatric or neurological disorder are more likely to experience VHs of people, whereas those with functional psychiatric illness experience nonpersonal VHs [30]. It is not uncommon that the experience of VHs has been incorporated into many cultural understandings of human spiritual experience, whereby VHs may be experienced in religious or spiritual rituals and are attributed to visions or spirit possession [1, 31].

Visual hallucinations occur in a number of nondisease-associated states, perhaps the most common in the community being at the periphery of sleep, known as hypnagogic (entering sleep) and hypnopompic (awakening) hallucinations; this is the most prevalent form of hallucinations in any modality in the community [5]. Sleep-associated hallucinations are far more common than daytime VHs, which occur in less than 1% of the population [5]. Hypnagogic VHs are three to four times more common than hypnopompic VHs in the general population, occurring in up to 5% of individuals, who most commonly see another individual in the room [5, 32]. The strongest predictors of sleep-associated VHs are disorders associated with disregulation of sleep, such as narcolepsy-cataplexy and the synucleinopathies (discussed later), as well as primary sleep disorders, use of alcohol and substances, and psychiatric disorders *other* than psychotic disorders [5].

VHs also occur as normal phenomena throughout the lifecycle. The "imaginary friend" occurs in 15% to 30% of children aged 2 to 10 [33, 34], and is considered a nonpathological developmental phase where reality testing is generally preserved [34, 35] but which may be predictive of adolescent/adulthood emotional disturbance [36]. Similarly, in bereavement, brief VHs of a deceased individual may form part of a normal grief reaction in both children [37, 38] and adults [39–41]. VHs may also occur in healthy adults under periods of sensory deprivation [42], sleep deprivation [43], and starvation [44].

Neurobiology of visual hallucinations

The initial understanding of the pathophysiology of VHs postulated that VHs originated in irritative foci, such as those causing epileptiform activity after infection or trauma in cortical regions involved in vision [45]. These VHs are usually brief, intermittent, and stereotyped, meeting criteria for "simple" VHs [22], and were informed by the cortical stimulation studies by Penfield and Perot, whereby occipital stimulation induced simple VHs, with temporo-occipital and parieto-occipital stimulation resulting in more complex scenes [46]. Simple VHs however are perhaps the least common form of VHs; this model does not account for more complex nonstereotyped and continuous (or more "complex") VHs. These types of hallucinations were most particularly seen in the blind, leading to the theory, first postulated by West [47], that loss of afferent input "releases" the visual and nearby cortex. The theory of VHs as release phenomena, elaborated by Cogan [48], provides a model for understanding how VHs following lesions to more "proximal" structures occur, particularly in circumstances of visual loss, such as the Charles Bonnet Syndrome [28, 29, 49, 50] (Chapter 30). This has been supported by functional magnetic resonance imaging (fMRI) studies, which show selective tonic activity in visual cortical regions, even when not hallucinating [51, 52].

Lesions anywhere in the visual system, from ocular structures through optic nerve, chiasm, and tract structures, including ascending modulatory midbrain structures, can produce VHs, which are usually complex in form [29, 53, 54]. To correlate lesion location to type of VHs, Santhouse and colleagues used factor analysis in patients with complex visual hallucinations (CVHs) to establish anatomical–phenomenological correlates, and demonstrated that landscapes and groups of figures reflected pathologically increased activity in the ventral temporal lobe, distorted faces activity around the superior temporal sulcus, and visual perseveration and palinopsia in the visual parietal lobe [28]. Thus, at the anatomical level, although simple VHs are most likely related to focal lesions of the ocular apparatus or occipital cortex, complex VHs occur when the quality or flow of information moving through the visual system is disrupted.

Although lesion-based models afford some understanding of the anatomy of normal and abnormal visual processing, they do not shed light on functional or neurochemical changes that occur as a result, and do not account for VHs that relate to substance intoxication or withdrawal, medication-related VHs, or VHs seen in global neurometabolic or neurodegenerative disorders such as delirium and dementia. In particular, pharmacologically induced hallucinations suggest that medications with anticholinergic (particularly antimuscarinic) properties are the most visually hallucinogenic [55], particularly in the elderly who generally have lower cholinergic tone than younger adults [56]. VHs occur, although less commonly, with perturbations to serotonergic transmission with hallucinogen use, although visual distortions and an exaggerated sense of reality are more frequent [57, 58]. Additionally, altered dopaminergic transmission in stimulant misuse and dopaminergic treatment of Parkinson's disease (PD) and other synucleinopathies suggest a role for dopamine transmission in VHs [59, 60]. However, psychotogenic stimulants tend to produce more auditory hallucinations and paranoia than VHs. When VHs occur in PD, they tend to occur in advanced disease when cholinergic deficit is more profound [61]. The cortical serotonin to acetylcholine ratio is significantly increased [62], and respond to cholinergic medication [63], tending to suggest an interaction between the dopaminergic and cholinergic (and possibly serotonergic) systems underpinning VHs [49]. This interaction between dopaminergic and cholinergic systems probably also results in the characteristic VHs of delirium, where metabolic stress results in dopamine release and subsequent spreading neuronal depression [64, 65]. Cholinergic systems may be most vulnerable to these effects, resulting in attentional and memory deficits in addition to VHs. Finally, alterations in the GABAergic system that occur in benzodiazepine and alcohol withdrawal, often associated with CVHs, implicate a loss of GABAergic cortical inhibition in withdrawal-associated VHs [66], although this is likely to be mediated through other monoaminergic systems [49].

These otherwise disparate anatomical and neurochemical models of VHs have been united in the perception and attentional deficit (PAD) model of Collerton and colleagues, which focuses on deficits in object-based attention due to dysfunction in lateral frontal cortical systems combined with object-based perceptual deficits due to dysfunction in the ventral ("what") as opposed to dorsal ("where") visual stream [67]. Unlike other models, this can account for VHs whose origin is either predominantly lesion-based or neurochemically driven, in addition to VHs that occur in states of sensory deprivation or in hypogogic or hypnopompic states.

Visual hallucinations in psychiatric disorders

Schizophrenia

Traditionally, VHs have been thought to be relatively uncommon in schizophrenia in comparison to auditory hallucinations, due to work published by Goldberg in 1965 suggesting that only 18% of patients experience this phenomenon [19], and the belief that higher prevalence rates only occurred in specific cultures [17, 68]. However Bracha and colleagues, examined rates of VHs in patients enrolled for schizophrenia studies at the National Institutes of Mental Health in the United States, and showed that VHs were present in approximately half of all patients but were often not inquired about by clinicians [16]. When VHs occur, they tend to occur with auditory hallucinations and delusions, usually as part of a relatively systematized psychotic experience where hallucinatory phenomena

trigger, and are maintained by, a delusional system [69]. The higher rate of auditory hallucinations in schizophrenia may reflect a greater pathoplastic effect on anterior rather than posterior corticocortical systems, and hence affect attribution of speech to a greater degree than visual phenomena.

Whereas the neurocognitive origins of auditory hallucinations in schizophrenia are slowly being elucidated [70], few models exist for the generation of VHs in schizophrenia; it is likely, however, that the core neurocognitive processes are similar. Patients with schizophrenia show deficits in shifting spatial attention [71], which is strongly correlated with positive symptoms including hallucinations [72]. The perceptual-attentional model (discussed later) suggests that hallucinations require attentional deficits combined with visual processing deficits [67]; the former is established as a core deficit of schizophrenia, and visual processing deficits are seen in schizophrenia in "dorsal stream" functions such as motion detection, backward masking, and recognition of atypical objects [73, 74, 75]. In schizophrenia, widespread cellular structural abnormalities that also affect the visual cortex [76], combined with subtle impairments in dorsal stream processes to degrade early visual processing and render it vulnerable to attentional deficits [77].

Delirium

One of the cardinal features of delirium, in addition to attentional dysfunction and impairments in consciousness, is the presence of psychotic symptoms, particularly VHs. The wide range of insults that can result in delirium is illustrative that VHs in delirium can result from perturbations in most of the neurotransmitter systems described above, including glutamatergic, GABAergic, cholinergic, dopaminergic and cholinergic function – as exemplified by alcohol withdrawal, anticholinergic delirium, and the serotonin syndrome [78, 79]. Other substances that stimulate ventral tegmental area dopaminergic neurons, such as opioids and corticosteroids, result in increasing nucleus accumbens dopamine release and consequent reductions in thalamic and cortical acetylcholine [80, 81]. One integrative model of psychotic symptoms, including VHs, in delirium proposes that the thalamus is the final common pathway for most of these insults, impairing the thalamic filtering/modulation function on information flow to sensory cortex from thalamocortical afferents and thus producing attentional

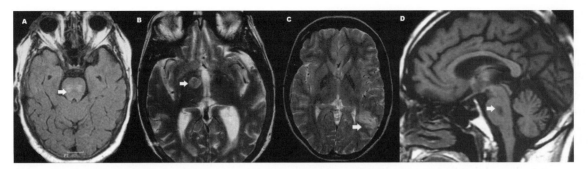

Figure 3.1 Lesions giving rise to VHs, marked with white arrows. (A) An 85-year-old woman with bilateral pontine infarcts who saw Lilliputian figures and the face of a famous actor superimposed on others' heads. (B) A 68-year-old woman with a right thalamic infarct who presented with VHs of small children wearing colorful uniforms. (C) A 33-year-old woman who had a previously embolized left temporoparietal arteriovenous malformation – which recurred, and caused focal epileptiform activity – who described seeing the letters W, R, and K on people's faces, spikes coming from the floor, and disembodied heads and torsos floating 10 feet above the ground. (D) A 52-year-old man with central pontine myelinolysis in the setting of chronic alcohol abuse, who presented with VHs of faces emerging from the walls with grotesque, "alien-like" features and of multiple animals.

disturbance and psychotic symptoms such as VHs [82].

Visual hallucinations in neurological disorders

Localized pathology

As previously described, lesions that affect the visual pathway from retina to occipital cortex, in addition to lesions affecting ascending brainstem/midbrain structures, can cause visual hallucinations [27, 28, 29, 50]. An analysis by Braun and colleagues demonstrated that occipital and occipitoparietal regions were the most commonly implicated cortical regions, and the midbrain, peduncles, pons, and thalamus were the most affected subcortical structures [83]. A wide range of developmental, acquired and iatrogenic lesions have been implicated, including vascular, neoplastic, traumatic, and infectious lesions, migraine, compression, demyelination, and surgical and angiographic intervention [29]. Some examples of the lesion types that may give rise to visual hallucinations are described in Figure 3.1. Two relatively well-described lesion-related syndromes are the *Charles Bonnet Syndrome* and *peduncular hallucinosis*.

The Charles Bonnet Syndrome (CBS) has generally been used to describe a syndrome of complex visual hallucinations in individuals with visual deprivation (usually ocular disease) and preserved cognitive status [84]. In 1769, Charles Bonnet described complex VHs in his cataract-affected grandfather of people, fantastical birds and buildings [85]. In CBS, characteristic

VHs are usually clear, colorful and often Lilliputian images of people, animals, and inanimate objects. They tend to disappear on eye closure (unlike drug-induced states, which worsen with eye closure) and occur in low light [84]. In peduncular hallucinosis (PH) [86], vivid complex VHs occur in the presence of lesions to the midbrain or thalamus, which alter the modulation and flow of information through the visual system [29]. Jean Lhermitte first described PH in a 72-year-old woman with hallucinations of strangely, colorfully attired people and groups of children which occurred at dusk [87]. Common hallucinations include animals, people or children, grotesque and deforming faces or heads, landscapes and tessellated patterns, and groups of people walking in file [29].

Neurodegenerative disorders

Alzheimer's disease (AD), the most common form of dementia in the community, not uncommonly presents with VHs, with a prevalence higher than for auditory hallucinations (19% vs. 12%) and which tend to occur with more advanced disease [88]. VHs in AD may be a result of pathology in the visual (association) cortex [52], particularly periventricular white matter lesions [89] and occipital atrophy [86]. This may relate to the predilection of neurofibrillary tangles for visual association, rather than primary visual, cortex [90]; stimulation of the former, but not the latter, results in complex, lifelike visual phenomena [91]. However, much like CBS, visual acuity appears to play a key role, with Chapman and colleagues showing that impaired visual acuity was highly predictive of VHs and that optical correction and cataract surgery improved outcome the most [92].

The synucleinopathies such as Lewy Body dementia (DLB) and Parkinson's disease with dementia (PDD) also show elevated rates of VHs, with a prevalence of 9% to 45%, and are associated with cognitive impairment and disease severity but generally not medication [93]. In a study matching DLB and PDD patients with AD sufferers on degree of cognitive impairment and visual acuity, Mosimann and colleagues [94] showed that PDD and DLB sufferers had significantly impaired visual processing compared to AD and commensurately higher rates of VHs (PDD 75%, DLB 90%, AD 8%). Both PDD and DLB are associated with cortical Lewy bodies and marked cholinergic deficit in areas involved in visual perception [95, 96], loss of serotonergic and cholinergic neurons in brainstem nuclei that modulate transmission of visual information [97, 98], and impaired contrast vision due to disrupted retinal dopaminergic function [99], each of which have already been described as factors in the development of VHs. Additionally, visual perceptual changes in DLB and PDD are suggestive of a deficit in the ventral ("what") visual pathway [94], which when combined with the cholinergic deficits in attention, satisfy criteria for the PAD model – a combination of visuoperceptual and attentional-executive impairments – of VHs, as previously described [100].

Visual hallucinations in substance-related states

Substance intoxication

The most potent hallucinogenic substances are those that produce significant alterations in serotonergic and cholinergic activity. Lysergic acid (LSD) is perhaps the most well-known of the hallucinogenic serotoninergic compounds, whose hallucinogenic potential is directly proportional to their affinity for $5HT_{2A}$ postsynaptic receptors [57]. Hallucinations caused by LSD and the related serotonergic compound mescaline characteristically begin as intensification of experience, visual distortions and colored shapes, progressing to complex VHs of people and animals [101]. Their partial agonist effect at these receptors in the locus ceruleus – that receives an array of somatosensory information which it projects on to the neocortex – enhances sensory responses and the salience of external stimuli; its effect at cortical receptors increases excitatory thalam-

ocortical glutamatergic afferent stimulation of layer V pyramidal cortical neurons [102, 103]. This results in the characteristic intensification and distortion of sensory experience respectively [103].

Humans have used anticholinergic substances in cultural and religious rituals to attach and enhance meaning to experience and seek "enlightenment," particularly through the VHs induced by *belladonna* or *datura* species, which contain anticholinergic compounds such as scopolamine and atropine. Anticholinergic intoxication may result in hallucinations through modulation of thalamocortical flow as well as through a direct action on the cortex. Acetylcholine in the cortex may act to increase signal to noise ratio, and blockage of this may result in increased cortical "noise" and the intrusion of background cortical activity into perception as well as affecting central cholinergic mechanisms of attention, consistent with the PAD model of VHs [104]. Those antidepressants with prominent anticholinergic properties have also been implicated in causing complex VHs, particularly those which also enhance serotonergic transmission [105], and this may occur through an imbalance in relative serotonin:acetylcholine activity much like that described in Parkinson's disease and other synucleinopathies [105]. Disregulated acetylcholine release may also underlie the hallucinogenic potential of some dopaminergic compounds, such as the amphetamines, through D2 agonism in the nucleus accumbens and resultant disregulation of mesolimbic dopamine transmission [106].

Substance withdrawal

Visual hallucinations are common in both alcohol [107] and benzodiazepine [108] withdrawal states, as well as withdrawal from the increasingly used illicit substance, gamma-hydroxybutyrate [109]. The common mechanism appears to be alterations to the balance between inhibitory gamma amino butyric acid (GABA)-ergic and excitatory glutamatergic receptor systems, as chronic administration of these compounds causes downregulation of inhibitory GABA receptors [110, 111], and chronic alcohol use in particular results in regionally-specific upregulation of the NMDA-subtype of the glutamatergic system [112]. Similar NMDA and GABA receptor changes have been seen in the visual cortical system after deafferentation [113], and it has been suggested that these neurotransmitter changes are central to the deafferentation hypothesis of VHs in CBS [114], with GABAergic medication being one recognized treatment for CBS [115]. Downregulation of the GABAergic system may "release" the excitatory neurotransmitter system, resulting in (particularly) dopamine release [109]. An "illness model" for GABAergic withdrawal hallucinations exists in the form of the extremely rare enzyme disorder, succinic semialdehyde dehydrogenase (SSADH) deficiency, where a defect in the catabolic pathway of GABA results in decreased gabaergic inhibition and increased glutamatergic excitatory activity; in adult SSADH deficiency sufferers, VHs and other psychotic symptoms are a very common presenting symptom [116].

Secondary auditory hallucinations: Spectrum of auditory perceptual disturbances

Just like visual hallucinations occur on a spectrum from simple to complex, and indicate differing underlying pathology, auditory hallucinations also appear to be dimensional in their complexity and the degree to which the individual perceives them as a true percept. Simple auditory hallucinations comprise basic, unstructured sounds that are usually unformed and tonally uncomplicated. They may include whistling, buzzing, and ringing sounds or simple environmental sounds such as running water or vehicular traffic. Tinnitus is perhaps the most commonly reported form of simple auditory disorder of perception. Complex auditory hallucinations involve music, voices (single or multiple), or spoken words. Auditory hallucinations involving spoken words are known as hallmarks of psychiatric illness such as schizophrenia. However, disorders of auditory perception occur in a number of normal and disease states.

Auditory hallucinations in normal individuals

Perception of sound without a source can occur in normal or nondisease physiological states. Perhaps the best-described circumstance is abnormalities of auditory perception associated with sleep. As with VHs, auditory hallucinations (AHs) can be experienced both on waking (hypnopompic) or on falling asleep (hypnogogic) and are reported in general population samples [117]. The prevalence of AHs increases

with sleep disorders such as narcolepsy [118] and REM sleep behavior disorder [119].

Abnormalities of auditory perception in which there is misperception or distortion may also occur in CNS disease. Hyperacusis is reported in a number of organic states such as delirium, migraine, epilepsy, and alcohol withdrawal [120, 121, 122]. Common sounds may be misinterpreted in delirium. For example, the noise of a busy hospital ward can be interpreted as a crowd discussing the patient's poor prognosis. Auditory perceptions can also be split from accompanying visual cues in CNS disorders such as delirium – for instance, the sound from a television may not be associated with the images of its source [123]. Auditory illusions may also occur but are less well defined [124] and often relate to abnormalities of sound location rather than identification.

Simple auditory hallucinosis

Simple sounds lack the multifaceted structure of more complex sounds such as music or the spoken voice. The quality of simple sounds depends on basic characteristics such as pitch (or sound-wave frequency), tone and intensity (loudness). Combinations of frequencies are responsible for harmonics or overtones which give sounds their recognizable character, sometimes referred to as timbre. Sound processing involves a complex interaction of perception, memory, and emotion in order for a sound to be identified. This complex interaction can be different in each individual, generating different perceptions of sounds, often to the extent that the same sounds may be perceived as pleasant or unpleasant in different persons.

Simple auditory hallucinosis can occur in a variety of disorders. This includes alcohol withdrawal [125] and other forms of intoxication, delirium, CNS infections, complex partial seizures, brainstem lesions, and deafness [126, 127]. The best-studied phenomenon is tinnitus.

Tinnutus may be perceived in one or both ears or in the head. Although the term tinnutus is derived from the Latin *tinnire* (to ring) it may also present as buzzing, hissing, humming, beeping, whistling, clicking, or roaring sounds [128]. Tinnitus can have many different causes, but most commonly results from otologic disorders – the same conditions that cause hearing loss. The most common cause is noise-induced hearing loss, resulting from exposure to excessive or loud noises. Ototoxic medications may also be responsible [129]. Neuropathy as well as brainstem and central lesions (such as demyelination in MS) may also produce tinnitus. Unilateral tinnitus is a hallmark of tumors of the cerebellopontine angle such as acoustic neuroma. Pulsatile tinnitus is associated with glomus tumors of cranial nerves and other vascular tumors such as haemangiomas of the middle ear, or arteriovenous malformations [130]. Patients with temporomandibular joint dysfunction [131] and palatal myoclonus [132] may also report tinnitus. This may result from intermittent deformation of the structures of middle and inner ear by muscle contraction. Transient tinnitus can also occur after irritation of the auditory system (loud music) but also in near to absolute silence in the absence of any central or peripheral pathology [133].

Although extensively investigated, the underlying mechanisms involved in producing tinnitus remain unconfirmed [134]. The structures of the inner ear transform acoustic waves into mechanical vibrations and then change fluid pressure in the organ of corti. The mammalian chochlea tranduces these changes in fluid pressure, via stereocilia, into neural activity [135]. The eighth cranial nerves project bilaterally via the inferior colliculus and medical geniculate nucleus to the primary auditory cortex in the superior temporal gyrus as well as other areas such as the limbic system. Although receptor cells can be regenerated from the adjacent supporting Deiters' cells after injury in birds, reptiles, and amphibians, in mammals it is believed they can be produced only during embryogenesis [136]. Hence damage to the hair cell array is not reparable and may result in faulty or false input into central pathways.

A number of well-replicated observations challenge receptor damage as the sole mechanism [133]. First, many sufferers of hearing loss do not describe chronic tinnitus [128]. Second, tinnitus usually persists after the division of the eighth cranial nerve [137]. Last, reports of distress and disability has not been shown to correlate with measures of tinnitus loudness, implying significant emotional factors [138]. Hence it is more likely that tinnitus involves alteration in the central auditory pathway and changes in limbic mechanisms that link emotions to sensory experiences as well peripheral receptor injury [139].

Evidence for such a model is in evolution. Animal models have demonstrated increased activity in the inferior colliculus (after salicylate toxicity) [140] and dorsal cochlear nucleus (high intensity injury) [141].

Functional neuroimaging studies have shown changes in the auditory cortex using positron emission tomography (PET) [142], magnetoencephalography (MEG) [143] and fMRI [144] in tinnitus patients as well as the inferior colliculus [145]. Using high resolution MRI and voxel-based morphometry, Muhlau and others were able to show changes in subcallosal grey matter, in particular the ventral striatum and nucleus accumbens [133].

It is likely that simple auditory hallucinations can arise from both central and peripheral lesions. Most at risk are those whose CNS disease (for example, white matter changes in the elderly) represents a vulnerable substrate onto which a further insult, such as hearing loss, is superimposed. Given that generation of simple auditory hallucinosis may involve lesions in the cochlea, brainstem, cortical and limbic structures, careful history, examination and investigations should evaluate all of these structures.

With respect to tinnitus, exclusion of a structural lesion in unilateral or pulsatile symptoms is important. Evidence for use of psychotropic medication [128] and herbal remedies such as ginko biloba [146] is limited. Education, provision of adequate support, and white-noise masking devices can be effective [147].

Complex auditory hallucinosis

Changes in pitch or frequency, timbre and harmonics, can make a sound more complex. Further complexity is introduced by combinations of frequencies and individual sounds and the characteristics of the sound envelope (attack or beginning, sustain or main component and decay, or the transition to silence). The changes in a sound over time, for example, in a repeating pattern or rhythm can introduce musical qualities. Another layer of complexity is the interpretation of complex sounds. Difference between input to left and right cochlea can introduce spatial characteristics. Complex sounds may construct words and the tone or context of spoken language may convey emotions and affect. Similarly, music can also convey emotion, often linked to memory and previous experience of that piece of music. Perception and comprehension of language involve complex cortical and subcortical mechanisms which are well described elsewhere [135].

Hallucinations of complex sounds are experienced in a variety of organic states. These tend to be transient, associated with disorders of perception in other modalities and phenomenologically distinct from those that characterize psychiatric illness such as schizophrenia. For example, in delirium, auditory hallucinosis is characterized by sounds or voices which accompany VHs [148], such as sounds and speaker announcements of a train station the patient feels is next to his or her hospital bed. This form of hallucinosis can occur in alcohol withdrawal [125], usually within the first 24 hours [149], epilepsy, acute renal or hepatic failure, or other encephalopathies [150].

Auditory hallucinations in psychiatric disorders: schizophrenia

In contrast to the relatively sparse descriptions of the phenomenology of auditory hallucinations in secondary psychoses, there is a reasonably rich description of the form and content of hallucinations in schizophrenia. Two medium-sized, fine-grained phenomenological studies – one published [151] and involving 100 subjects, and one unpublished (Trauer, Mackinnon, and Copolov, personal communication) and involving 199 subjects – have shown that in schizophrenia and related disorders, auditory hallucinations involve a number of voices (the mean being three [151]) that are frequently but not always negative in content (e.g., derogatory, critical, and intrusive), and more often of known identity and of the male gender. Voices are heard inside the head, outside the head, or both inside and outside in roughly equal proportions (34%, 28%, and 38%) [152]. There is mixed evidence as to whether externally heard hallucinated voices are more likely to be judged to be real, [151, 152, 153] but they both appear to evoke similar levels of negative feelings [152]. Most hallucinated voices are heard clearly and are either loud or very loud, and address the hearer in the second or third person [154]. Approximately 50% of adult psychiatric patients with auditory hallucinations experience command hallucinations, with approximately 50% being associated with dangerous behavior [155]. The majority (66%) of patients with auditory hallucinations report using coping strategies to deal with them; such strategies include distraction, auditory competition, or trying to relax or sleep, which are often at least partially successful [4].

A large body of research has explored the neurobiological basis for the high rate of auditory hallucinations in schizophrenia. Consensus is emerging that aberrant speech mechanisms underlie these symptoms in most psychotic patients [156], resulting in inner speech identified as external due to defective self-

monitoring [157]. Functional neuroimaging has suggested involvement of Broca's area and the supplementary motor area, primary and higher-order auditory and association cortex (particularly on the left), and Wernicke's area [157, 158, 159, 160]. Some evidence suggests that the experience of external auditory hallucinations in schizophrenia is due to pathology affecting the planum temporale, a temporal cortical region posterior to the primary auditory cortex in Heschl's gyrus involved in analysis of spatially determined speech properties [161] and this may be at least partially mediated by disrupted dopaminergic transmission in cortical-subcortical circuitry [162].

Auditory hallucinations in neurologic disorders

Epilepsy

All forms of auditory hallucinations have been reported in seizure disorders for many years, but are usually associated with complex partial seizures. As many as 16% of patients with temporal lobe seizures have been reported as experiencing some form of auditory hallucination [163]. In a large retrospective study of more than 3,000 patients with complex partial seizures, Mauguiere and colleagues [164] reported a frequency of auditory ictal phenomena in 2.4% This included hyperacusis (19%), elementary noises (14%) speech (18%), and music (23%).

Auditory hallucinations can comprise some of the symptoms of a schizophrenia-like psychosis in epilepsy. Most (∼ 70%) of these seizure disorders have a temporal focus [165] and have the clinical pattern of complex partial seizures. The psychoses of epilepsy are currently defined as ictal (concurrent with seizure), postictal (within 1–2 days of seizure) and brief (days to weeks post seizure) or chronic interictal [166]. Although ictal psychoses most closely resemble a delirium as described above, often with preserved, if delayed insight, the other presentations may include auditory hallucinations, particularly of the spoken voice, which mimic those of schizophrenia.

Traumatic brain injury

Auditory hallucinations are also reported in traumatic brain injury. Although psychotic symptoms are described in up to 8% with some form of traumatic brain injury, delusions are more common than hallucinations, of which auditory hallucinations are the most common, particularly if the psychotic symptoms are of delayed onset [167]. Frontal and temporal lobe abnormalities on neuroimaging are more common in patients with traumatic brain injury and psychosis, but there was no association with left or right lesions or the severity of hallucinations. Unfortunately, the precise nature of auditory hallucinations is poorly characterized in the literature, although derogatory spoken words are described [168]. Auditory hallucinations and schizophrenia-like psychosis are also described in patients who have undergone temporal lobectomy, with the hallucinations most often taking the form of second person spoken voices [169]. In this group, bilateral temporal lobe lesions are a risk factor for the development of psychotic symptoms.

Musical hallucinosis

One of the most interesting forms of isolated auditory hallucinosis is musical hallucinosis. Musical hallucinosis can be defined as the perception of music without the presence of an external musical stimulus in which the subject maintains insight. Although these phenomena have been described in psychotic illness, epilepsy, and a variety of brain lesions including intracerebral haemorrhage [170], they more often are seen in elderly patients with acquired deafness [171].

Some authors have reported patients with musical hallucinosis later developing auditory hallucinations characteristic of schizophrenia [172]. However, musical hallucinosis is most commonly seen in persons with hearing loss, advanced age, brain disease, cognitive impairment, female gender, and social isolation. Although the relative importance of each of these factors is not well understood [173], deafness is one of the most common associations.

Mechanisms underlying the generation of musical hallucinosis remain poorly understood. The most compelling neurobiological model is one of spontaneous activity arising in a deafferented auditory system, which is then involved in recognition of stimulus by a cortical pattern recognition system [174]. During normal listening to patterned sound such as music, auditory input is processed by two mechanisms, which operate in a hierarchical manner. The pattern is first perceived, and then encoded into memory or recognized. It is possible that reduced auditory input because of deafness allows spontaneous activity within the system. This may take the form of positive feed-

back between the perception and recognition modules resulting in a percept without a stimulus. This, in turn, would allow inputs to be misinterpreted or act as triggers for musical hallucinosis.

Some anatomical substrates for this model have been suggested by functional neuroimaging. Although perception of simple sounds may involve primary auditory cortex (Heschl's gyrus) [175], perception of complex sounds seems to be more widely distributed. The right planum temporale and bilateral frontal areas seem to be involved in determination of melody [176], whereas the cerebellum and basal ganglia seem to have a role in the processing of rhythmic sound [177].

Lesions in the brainstem [178, 179], either hemisphere [180], and the occipital lobe [181] have been reported in musical hallucinosis. However, multiple vascular lesions suggested by white matter hyperintensities on neuroimaging are also common associations [173, 182]. The presence of central vascular lesions may represent the additional risk factor that distinguishes patients with musical hallucinosis from those with deafness without these symptoms. It is possible that vascular lesions may disconnect afferent inputs or cortical networks increasing the threshold for spontaneous activity. The wide variety nature and location of lesions in the auditory system that may result in musical hallucinosis mirrors the heterogeneous lesions associated with complex visual hallucinations [183].

Unfortunately, there is little evidence available to guide treatment apart from the appropriate treatment of the underlying lesion. Pharmacological treatments are usually ineffective; most authors recommend audiological assessment and appropriate amplification [172] when deafness is the trigger. Prognosis is usually guarded with musical hallucinosis persisting and worsening as deafness progresses. Evolution to AHs and paranoid delusions characteristic of late onset schizophrenia-like illnesses have also been reported [184].

Secondary olfactory and gustatory hallucinations

The literature relating to gustatory hallucinations occurring in organic disorders consists mainly of case reports in which the nature of the experiences varies considerably. In contrast, the olfactory experiences of patients with a range of "organic" pathologies are much more uniform in their quality. As described by patients with epilepsy, the perceived smells are unpleasant and usually of burning, rotting, fecal, or other organic material. Patients who describe olfactory or gustatory hallucinations are likely to describe or exhibit other symptoms depending on the underlying condition. Isolated hallucinations in either modality are very rare in either psychiatric or organic states.

Olfactory and gustatory hallucinations in psychiatric illness

Schizophrenia

Olfactory and gustatory hallucinations occur in a significant minority of patients with schizophrenia. For example, Pearlson and colleagues [185] studied 131 patients with schizophrenia and identified olfactory/gustatory hallucinations in 17%/12% of the patients. In schizophrenia, olfactory, gustatory, and tactile hallucinations are usually "fellow travellers" with auditory hallucinations. In one study, 2% of patients with olfactory/gustatory hallucinations, 84% of patients with tactile hallucinations, and 84% of patients with VHs also described auditory hallucinations [6]. The presence of tactile and olfactory/gustatory hallucinations was highly correlated to each other and both types, but not with auditory or visual hallucinations, nor with the severity of delusions.

Other psychiatric disorders

The diagnostic specificity of olfactory hallucinations in patients with psychiatric illness was addressed in a study of 131 patients with schizophrenia, 21 patients with depression, 31 patients with eating disorders, and 77 normal control subjects [186]. Olfactory hallucinations (OHs) were described by patients from the three patient groups but not in the control group (schizophrenia 35%, depression 19%, and eating disorders 29%) and the prevalence was not significantly different by group. Patients with schizophrenia and depression generally described unpleasant smells whereas the eating disorder patients described hallucinations that were food related and generally pleasant.

Cultural variables

Olfactory hallucinations have also been noted in non-Western cultures. Teggin and colleagues [187] reported olfactory hallucinations in 59% of black African patients compared to 20% of white and 27% of patients of color. The black African description of the hallucinations was often related to death or decay. Ndetei and Singh [188] identified olfactory hallucinations in 25% (13/51) of Kenyan patients with schizophrenia but in none of the 29 patients with other psychiatric diagnoses. In a second Kenyan study, only 3% of 141 patients with schizophrenia were found to have olfactory hallucinations [189]. None of these studies examined for the presence of gustatory hallucinations. The World Health Organization ten-country study of 1,288 patients with first-episode schizophrenia, published in 1992, identified OHs in 13% of patients in developed countries and 9% of those patients from developing countries [190].

In summary, OHs have been described in patients with differing diagnoses including schizophrenia, affective disorders, and eating disorders. Gustatory hallucinations have been found in patients with schizophrenia but few studies have investigated for their presence in other psychiatric conditions. The hallucinations tend to be of an unpleasant nature though good descriptive accounts of the quality of the smells is lacking in the psychiatric literature.

Olfactory and gustatory hallucinations in neurological disorders

Epilepsy

An epileptic aura is "that portion of the seizure which occurs before consciousness is lost and for which memory is retained afterwards" [191]. Early studies found that 750 of 1,039 epilepsy patients described 226 different types of epileptic aura [192] whereas a more recent study identified an aura in 64% of 290 patients [193]. The commonest auras described by patients across these studies were of epigastric sensations, motor phenomena, affective states, déjà vu, and vertiginous sensations. In patients unselected for the type of epilepsy, about 1% describe OHs [192, 194], whereas in studies of patients with temporal lobe epilepsy the figures range from 0.03% to 13% [156, 193, 195, 196, 197, 198, 199]. Gustatory hallucinations are also relatively uncommon with prevalence rates of ranging from 0.2% [192], to 2% [193], to 11% [195].

Daly [196] coined the term "uncinate fits" in a description of 55 patients of whom 20 (36%) had olfactory and gustatory phenomena associated with seizures of various etiology. Daly postulated that the uncus, which he considered to the cortical center for smell was the common anatomical structure for these seizures. Patients with olfactory hallucinations usually described neutral, unrecognisable odors, although both pleasant and unpleasant odors were experienced. In the patients with olfactory auras, associated auras and sensations were common but not quantified by the author. Sixteen patients described gustatory hallucinations with their descriptions, including unpleasant, sour/bitter, salty, metallic, or neutral.

Lennox and Cobb conducted a survey of U.S. neurologists and physicians and showed that 56.2% of the 1,527 cases described 327 different sensations which met the author's criteria for an aura [192]. There were no differences in the experience of an aura identified by gender or epilepsy etiology. Auras were found to be more frequently associated with intellectual disability ("mental deterioration") and duration of epilepsy. Fifteen patients (1.0%) had OHs that were described as disagreeable (9), peculiar (2), like bananas, camphor, or the smell of ironing (1 each), whereas only 2 patients described gustatory phenomena. It is not possible from the data available or the text of the article to ascertain the relationship of the olfactory auras to any clinical variables.

Fried and colleagues investigated the relationship between auras and focal epilepsy pathology before and after epilepsy surgery [156]. The 90 patients in the study (43 patients with hippocampal sclerosis, 30 patients with other temporal lobe lesions, and 17 patients with extratemporal lesions) described 125 auras. Of the 11 patients (12.2%) who experienced olfactory/gustatory auras (the study grouped these two together), nine had hippocampal sclerosis. The quality of the auras was not described in the study. Following surgical resection, only 1 of these 11 patients experienced ongoing olfactory/gustatory auras. This patient had a pathological diagnosis of hippocampal sclerosis.

Chen and colleagues also assessed 217 patients who had undergone temporal lobectomy for intractable temporal lobe epilepsy before and after surgery [197]. Twelve (5.5%) of the patients described olfactory auras, but only one patient had a gustatory aura. At postsurgical follow-up, no patients had ongoing auras. All patients described the olfactory experience as unpleasant with descriptions of the smell as "fetid, rotten, or stinking" food, burning, charred things, alcohol, or medicine. One patient had isolated olfactory hallucinations, whereas the other 11 patients most commonly described abdominal sensations, fear, auto-

nomic, or visual symptoms. Based on their observations and their review of the literature, the authors speculate that amygdala pathology is critical in the generation of olfactory auras.

Acharya and colleagues identified 14 patients with OHs in a group of 1,423 patients (0.9%) [198]. Seven patients described the smell as unpleasant (burning, sulphur), five were neutral, and two said the smell was pleasant (e.g., flowers). Five of the patients had associated gustatory auras, one had abdominal aura, one visual, four had psychic auras, and one heard the sound of the ocean. Only 2 of 14 (14%) of patients had isolated olfactory hallucinations and 12 of 14 (86%) of patients described associated auras. Eight of nine patients who went on to surgery were free of seizures and aura following surgery. Like Chen and colleagues [197] the authors propose that the amygdala is the site of the olfactory auras and that the presence of an olfactory aura provides potential anatomical localization to the amygdala.

Other neurological disorders

Olfactory hallucinations have been more commonly described than olfactory associations in the context of other neurological disorders. Olfactory hallucinations have been reported to precede the motor manifestations of Parkinson's disease [199] and to have benefited from l-dopa treatment. A longitudinal study of Parkinsonian patients treated with l-dopa found that the early development of hallucinations (predominantly visual but also tactile, auditory, and olfactory) signaled either a comorbid psychotic illness or an evolving parkinsonism-plus syndrome [200]. In contrast, a study of 98 patients with Parkinson's disease did not identify any patients with OHs and only one patient with gustatory hallucinations [201].

Olfactory hallucinations have been reported as the presenting symptom for cluster headaches [202] and migraines [203]. The smells reported by migraine sufferers tended to be unpleasant and include descriptions such as decaying animals, burning cookies, cigars, peanut butter, and cigarette smoke. Olfactory hallucinations have been reported as an unexpected complication of the administration of intravenous [204] and oral [205] caffeine boluses in normal and panic disorder subjects during research studies of panic and anxiety disorders.

Olfactory hallucinations of gasoline, feces, urine, and garbage have been described in patients with chronic cocaine use [206], whereas a smaller proportion of this group described an inability to detect strong tastes in food, which the authors termed "negative gustatory hallucinations." In all subjects, the hallucinations occurred in association with hallucinations in other modalities.

Secondary tactile hallucinations
Tactile hallucinations in normal individuals

The only strong data set revealing the likely rate of tactile (also known as "somatic" or "haptic") hallucinations in the population comes from the Epidemiological Catchment Area (ECA) study conducted in the United States, and the rates of hallucinations in various modalities has been analysed by Tien [207]. The ECA study noted that tactile ("somatic") hallucinations were perhaps the most common, albeit most benign, form of hallucinations, occurring in rates slightly higher than auditory and significantly higher than visual and olfactory hallucinations across the lifespan. For both genders, this declined until the middle of the seventh decade [207].

Tactile hallucinations in psychiatric disorders

Schizophrenia

Tactile hallucinations have only been occasionally described in schizophrenia [208, 209, 210], usually in the setting of complex hallucinatory phenomena whereby the tactile hallucination is associated with hallucinations in other modalities (particularly visual). One study used functional magnetic resonance imaging (fMRI) in a patient with schizophrenia and painful tactile hallucinations, and noted an increased activation in hallucinations compared to the non-hallucinating state in the precuneus and supplementary motor area region [211]. Shergill and colleagues also used fMRI in a schizophrenia patient experiencing both tactile and auditory hallucinations, and noted increased activation in the primary somatosensory and posterior parietal cortex – regions mediating somatic perception – whereas auditory hallucinations were associated with activation in areas associated with processing external speech [212].

Delusional parasitosis

The role of tactile hallucinations in the delusional parasitosis is contested. In this disorder, the patient experiences a monohypochondriacal conviction that he or she is infested with insects [213, 214]. Some authors believe that tactile hallucinations are the primary disorder in this condition [215, 216] whereas others [217, 218] view the delusion to be primary. In one of the largest samples of subjects reported [219], the presenting complaint in the majority of 52 subjects was insects crawling over the head or body, although this report does not allow the determination of whether sensations preceded the delusional explanation, if the delusions triggered the sensation, or if both commenced simultaneously.

Delirium

Tactile hallucinations are often associated with delirium, although studies are lacking that clearly outline their prevalence as most studies focus on visual and auditory phenomena associated with the delirious state. One descriptive series of consecutive patients suggests the prevalence in an unselected delirious population is less than 5% [148], although these symptoms may be more characteristic of and common in alcohol-withdrawal delirium (discussed later).

Tactile hallucinations in neurological disorders

Tactile hallucinations have been described in a number of organic states including dementia, diabetes, and brain injury [21, 220]. Their most frequent association has been with the synucleinopathies, in particular Parkinson's disease (PD). In the early twentieth century, postencephalitic Parkinsonian states were described as frequently featuring tactile hallucinations [221]. Goetz found 7% of PD patients treated for at least one year with dopaminergic medication experienced tactile hallucinations [59], and features associated with abnormal tactile experiences in PD include cognitive impairment and daytime somnolence [222]. Fenelon described tactile hallucinations, generally intimately associated with visual hallucinations, in a series of eight patients with Parkinson's disease [223], which were frequently of animals, insects, or human figures. Tactile hallucinations have also been described in association with midline tumors, although the mechanism remains unclear [224].

Tactile hallucinations in substance abuse/withdrawal

Tactile hallucinations are relatively frequent in alcohol withdrawal states [225], and are markers of a prolonged and severe withdrawal [226]. Visual hallucinations are often associated with alcohol withdrawal states and as alterations in the dopamine transporter have been associated with VHs in alcohol withdrawal [227], this is suggestive of a dopaminergic role in withdrawal-related THs. Supporting the role of dopaminergic systems, up to 15% of cocaine users may report tactile hallucinations [206]. Tactile hallucinations in cocaine users tend to commence after a number of months of heavy use and are often preceded by migratory itching experiences [220]. They have similarly been associated with chronic use of another dopaminergic compound, amphetamine [228, 229].

Discussion

Understanding the biological basis of hallucinatory experience can shed significant light on the underlying pathophysiology of major mental disorders in which hallucinations are common, most particularly the psychotic disorders such as schizophrenia. A number of the underpinning models described in this chapter, drawn from a range of different disorders such as delirium, dementia, and substance-induced states, bear significant homology to some of the emergent neurobiology of schizophrenia-spectrum disorders.

There are a number of common threads that can be drawn from the preceding sections describing hallucinations in organic states. The strongest evidence for neurochemical disturbance in secondary hallucinatory states revolves around abnormalities in dopaminergic transmission, and disregulation of dopaminergic systems may be the "final common pathway" for psychotic symptoms in schizophrenia [162, 230]. However the role of cholinergic pathology in the attentional, memory, and perceptual disturbances in dementia has also been suggestive of cholinergic pathology underlying positive, negative, and cognitive symptoms in schizophrenia, and this has been supported by a range of studies suggestive of muscarinic cholinergic pathology in primary psychotic illness [231, 232]. The involvement of frontal and temporal cortical zones in a number of hallucination-prone organic disorders also suggests that frontotemporal pathology is implicated in schizophrenia, and again this is borne out by a range of imaging and neuropathological studies [233, 234].

References

1. Sarbin T. R., Juhasz J. B. (1975).The social context of hallucinations. In *Hallucinations: behavior, experience and theory*, Siegel R. and West L. (Eds). New York: John Wiley & Sons.

2. Slade P., Bentall R. (1988). *Sensory definition: a scientific analysis of a hallucination*. Baltimore: Johns Hopkins University Press.

3. David A. The cognitive neuropsychiatry of auditory verbal hallucinations: an overview. *Cogn Neuropsychiatry*, 2004. **9**:107–23.

4. Carter M., Mackinnon A., Copolov D. Patients' strategies for coping with auditory hallucinations. *J Nerv Ment Dis*, 1996. **184**:159–64.

5. Ohayon M. Prevalence of hallucinations and their pathological associations in the general population. *Psychiatry Res*, 2000. **97**:153–64.

6. Mueser K. T., Bellack A. S., Brady E. U. Hallucinations in schizophrenia. *Acta Psychiatr Scand*, 1990. **82**:26–9.

7. Johns L., *et al.* Occurrence of hallucinatory experiences in a community sample and ethnic variations. *Br J Psychiatry*, 2002. **180**:174–8.

8. Johns L., van Os J. The continuity of psychotic experiences in the general population. *Clin Psychol Rev*, 2001. **21**:1125–41.

9. Krabbendm L., *et al.* Explaining transitions over the hypothesized psychosis continuum. *Aust NZ J Psychiatry*, 2005. **39**:180–6.

10. van Os J. , *et al.* Prevalence of psychotic disorder and community level of psychotic symptoms: an urban–rural comparison. *Arch Gen Psychiatry*, 2001. **58**:663–8.

11. Levine E., Jonas H., Serper M. Interpersonal attributional biases in hallucinatory-prone individuals. *Schizophr Res*, 2004. **69**:23–8.

12. Laroi F., Collignon O., Van Der Linden M. Source monitoring for actions in hallucination proneness. *Cogn Neuropsychiatry*, 2005. **10**:105–23.

13. Aleman A., *et al.* Mental imagery and perception in hallucination-prone individuals. *J Nerv Ment Dis*, 2000. **188**:830–6.

14. Morrison A., Wells A., Nothard S. Cognitive factors in predis-position to auditory and visual hallucinations. *Br J Clin Psychol*, 2000. **39**:67–78.

15. Sartorius N., Shapiro R., Jablensky A. The international pilot study of schizophrenia. *Schizophr Bull*, 1974. **1**:21–5.

16. Bracha H., *et al.* High prevalence of visual hallucinations in research subjects with chronic schizophrenia. *Am J Psychiatry*, 1989. **146**:526–8.

17. Zarroug E. The frequency of visual hallucinations in schizophrenic patients in Saudi Arabia. *Br J Psychiatry*, 1975. **127**:553–5.

18. Suhail K., Cochrane R. Effect of culture and environment on the phenomenology of delusions and hallucinations. *Int J Soc Psychiatry*, 2002. **48**:126–38.

19. Goldberg S., Klerman G., Cole J. Changes in schizophrenic psychology and ward behaviour as a function of phenothiazine treatment. *Br J Psychiatry*, 1965. **111**:120–33.

20. Baethge C., *et al.* Hallucinations in bipolar disorder: characteristics and comparison to unipolar depression and schizophrenia. *Bipolar Disord*, 2005. 7: 136–45.

21. Brasic J. Hallucinations. *Percept Mot Skills*, 1998. **86**:851–77.

22. Cummings J., Miller B. Visual hallucinations: clinical occurrence and use in differential diagnosis. *West Med J*, 1987. **146**:46–51.

23. Cornelius J., *et al.* Characterizing organic hallucinosis. *Compr Psychiatry*, 1991. **32**:338–44.

24. Cutting J. The phenomenology of acute organic psychosis. Comparison with acute schizophrenia. *Br J Psychiatry*, 1997. **151**:324–32.

25. Johnstone E., *et al.* Phenomenology of organic and functional psychoses and the overlap between them. *Br J Psychiatry*, 1988. **153**:770–6.

26. Asaad G., Shapiro B. Hallucinations: theoretical and clinical overview. *Am J Psychiatry*, 1986. **143**:1088–97.

27. ffytche D. Visual hallucination and illusion disorders: a clinical guide. *Adv Clin Neurosci Rehabil*, 2004. **4**:16–18.

28. Santhouse A., Howard R., ffytche D. Visual hallucinatory syndromes and the anatomy of the visual brain. *Brain*, 2000. **123**:2055–64.

29. Mocellin R., Walterfang M., Velakoulis D. The neuropsychiatry of complex visual hallucinations. *Aust NZ J Psychiatry*, 2006. **40**:742–51.

30. Lindal E., Stefansson J., Stefansson S. The qualitative difference of visions and visual hallucinations: a comparison of a general-population and clinical sample. *Compr Psychiatry*, 1994. **35**:405–8.

31. LaBarre W. (1975). Anthropological perspectives on hallucination and hallucinogens. In *Hallucinations: Behaviour, Experience and Theory*, Siegel R. and West C. (Eds.). New York: John Wiley & Sons.

32. Ohayon M., *et al.* Hypnagogic and hypnopompic hallucinations: pathological phenomena? *Br J Psychiatry*, 1996. **169**:459–67.

33. Hurlock E., Burnstein M. The imaginary playmate: a questionnaire study. *J Genet Psychol*, 1932. **41**:380–92.

34. Svendsen M. Children's imaginary companions. *Arch Neurol Psychiatry*, 1934. **12**:985–9.

35. Schaeffer C. Imaginary companions and creative adolescents. *Dev Psychol*, 1969. **1**:747–9.

36. Bonne O., *et al.* Childhood imaginary companionship and mental health in adolescence. *Child Psychiatry Hum Dev*, 1999. **29**:277–86.

37. Simonds J. Hallucinations in nonpsychotic children and adolescents. *J Youth Adolesc*, 1975. **4**:171–82.

38. Balk D. Adolescents' grief reactions and self-concept perceptions following sibling death: a study of 33 teenagers. *J Youth Adolesc*, 1983. **12**: 137–61.

39. Adair D., Keshavan M. The Charles Bonnet Syndrome and grief reaction. *Am J Psychiatry*, 1988. **145**:895.

40. Olson P., Suddeth J., Peterson P. Hallucinations of widowhood. *J Am Geriatr Soc*, 1985. **33**: 543–7.

41. Grimby A. Bereavement among elderly people: grief reactions, post-bereavement hallucinations and quality of life. *Acta Psychiatr Scand*, 1993. **87**:72–80.

42. Mullaney D., *et al.* Effects of sustained continuous performance on subjects working alone and in pairs. *Percept Mot Skills*, 1983. **57**:819–32.

43. Mullaney D., *et al.* Sleep loss and nap effects on sustained continuous performance. *Psychophysiology*, 1983. **20**:643–51.

44. Forrer G. Benign auditory and visual hallucinations. *Arch Gen Psychiatry*, 1964. **3**:95–8.

45. Walsh F., Hoyt W. (1969). *Clinical neuro-ophthalmology*. 3rd ed. Baltimore: Williams & Wilkins.

46. Penfield W., Perot P. The brain's record of auditory and visual experience: a final summary and discussion. *Brain*, 1963. **86**: 595–96.

47. West C. (1962). *Hallucinations*. New York: Grune & Stratton.

48. Cogan D. Visual hallucinations as release phenomena. *Graefes Arch Clin Exp Opthal*, 1973. **188**: 139–50.

49. Manford M., Andermann F. Complex visual hallucinations: clinical and neurobiological insights. *Brain*, 1998. **121**: 1819–40.

50. ffytche D., Howard R. The perceptual consequences of visual loss: 'positive' pathologies of vision. *Brain*, 1999. **122**: 1247–60.

51. ffytche D., *et al.* The anatomy of conscious vision: an fMRI study of visual hallucinations. *Nature Neurosci*, 1998. **1**:738–42.

52. Howard R., *et al.* Seeing visual hallucinations with functional magnetic resonance imaging. *Dement Geriatr Cogn Disord*, 1997. **8**:73–77.

53. Lepore F. Spontaneous visual phenomena with visual loss: 104 patients with lesions of retinal and neural afferent pathways. *Neurology*, 1990. **40**: 444–7.

54. Galasko D., Kwo-On-Yuen P., Thal L. Intracranial mass lesions associated with late-onset psychosis and depression. *Psychiatr Clin North Am*, 1988. **11**:151–66.

55. Perry E., Perry R. Acetylcholine and hallucinations: disease-related compared to drug-induced alterations in human consciousness. *Brain Cogn*, 1995. **28**:240–58.

56. Perry E., *et al.* Convergent cholinergic activities in aging and Alzheimer's disease. *Neurobiol Aging*, 1992. **13**:393–400.

57. Glennon R., Titeler M., McKenney J. Evidence for 5HT2 involvement in the mechanism of action of hallucinogenic agents. *Life Sci*, 1984. **35**:2505–11.

58. Abraham H., Aldridge A., Gogia P. The psychopharmacology of hallucinogens. *Psychopharmacology*, 1996. **14**:285–98.

59. Goetz C., *et al.* Early dopaminergic drug-induced hallucinations in Parkinsonian patients. *Neurology*, 1998. **51**:811–14.

60. Angrist B., *et al.* Amphetamine psychosis: behavioural and biochemical aspects. *J Psychiatr Res.*, 1974. **11**:13–23.

61. Dubois B., *et al.* Cholinergic dependent cognitive deficits in Parkinson's disease. *Ann Neurol.*, 1987. **22**:26–30.

62. Perry E., *et al.* Evidence of a monoaminergic–cholinergic imbalance related to visual hallucinations in Lewy body dementia. *J Neurochem.*, 1991. **55**:1454–6.

63. McKeith I., *et al.* Efficacy of rivastigmine in dementia with Lewy bodies: a randomised, double-blind, placebo-controlled international study. *Lancet*, 2000. **356**:2031–6.

64. Packard R. Delirium. *Neurologist*, 2001. **7**:327–40.

65. Brown T. (2000). Basic mechanisms in the pathogenesis of delirium. In *Psychiatric care of the medical patient*, Stoudemire A., Fogel B., Greenberg D. (Eds.). New York: Oxford University Press, pp. 571–80.

66. Nevo I., Hamon M. Neurotransmitter and neuromodulatory mechanisms involved in alcohol abuse and alcoholism. *Neurochem Int.*, 1995. **26**:305–36.

67. Collerton D., Perry E., McKeith I. Why people see things that are not there: a novel perception and attention deficit model for recurrent complex visual

hallucinations. *Behav Brain Sci.*, 2005. **28**:737–94.

68. Ndetei D., Singh A. Hallucinations in Kenyan schizophrenic patients. *Acta Psychiatr Scand.*, 1983. **67**:144–7.

69. Roberts J. (1984). *Differential diagnosis in neuropsychiatry*. New York: John Wiley & Sons.

70. David A. Auditory hallucinations: phenomenology, neuropsychology and neuroimaging update. *Acta Psychiatr Scand Suppl*, 1999. **395**:95–104.

71. Posner M., *et al.* Asymmetries in hemispheric control of attention in schizophrenia. *Arch Gen Psychiatry*, 1988. **45**: 814–21.

72. DiGirolamo G., Posner M. Attention and schizophrenia: a view from cognitive neuroscience. *Cogn Neuropsychiatry*, 1996. **1**:95–102.

73. Chen Y., *et al.* Motion perception in schizophrenia. *Arch Gen Psychiatry*, 1999. **56**: 149–54.

74. Gabrovska V., *et al.* Evidence for an associative visual agnosia in schizophrenia. *Schizophr Res*, 2002. **59**:277–86.

75. Slaghuis W., Bakker V. Forward and backward visual masking of contour by light in positive symptom and negative symptom schizophrenia. *J Abnorm Psychol*, 1995. **104**:41–54.

76. Selemon L., Rajkowska G., Goldman-Rakic P. Abnormally high neuronal density in the schizophrenic cortex: a morphometric analysis of prefrontal area 9 and occipital area 17. *Arch Gen Psychiatry*, 1995. **52**:805–18.

77. Tadin D., *et al.* Believing is seeing in schizophrenia: the role of top-down processing. *Behav Brain Sci*, 2005. **28**:775.

78. Trzepacz P. Is there a final common neural pathway in delirium? Focus on acetylcholine and dopamine. *Semin Clin Neuropsychiatry*, 2000. **5**: 132–48.

79. Flacker J., Lipsitz L. Neural mechanisms of delirium: current hypotheses and evolving concepts. *J Gerontol*, 1999. **54**:8239–46.

80. Cowen M., Lawrence A. The role of opioid–dopamine interactions in the induction and maintenance of ethanol consumption. *Prog Neuropharmacol Biol Psychiatry*, 1999. **23**:1171–212.

81. Piazza P., Le Moal M. Glucocorticoids as a substrate of reward: physiological and pathophysiological implications. *Brain Res Brain Res Rev*, 1997. **23**:359–72.

82. Gaudreau J., Gagnon P. Psychogenic drugs and delirium pathogenesis: the central role of the thalamus. *Med Hypotheses*, 2005. **64**:471–5.

83. Braun C., *et al.* Brain modules of hallucination: an analysis of multiple patients with brain lesions. *J Psych Neurosci*, 2003. **28**:432–9.

84. Teunisse R., *et al.* Visual hallucinations in psychologically normal people: Charles Bonnet's Syndrome. *Lancet*, 1996. **347**:794–7.

85. Bonnet C. (1769). Essai Analytique Sur les Facultés de L'âme. 2nd ed., Copenhague: Philbert.

86. Holroyd S., Shepherd M., Downs J. Occipital atrophy is associated with visual hallucinations in Alzheimer's disease. *J Neuropsychiatry Clin Neurosci*, 2000. **12**:25–8.

87. Lhermitte M. Syndrome de la calotte du penduncule cerebral. Les troubels psycho-sensoriels dans les lesions du mesocephale. *Revue de Neurologique* (Paris), 1922. **38**:1359–65.

88. Bassiony M., Lyketsos C. Delusions and hallucinations in Alzheimer's disease: review of the brain decade. *Psychosomatics*, 2003. **44**:388–401.

89. Lin S., Yu C., Pai M. The occipital white matter lesions in Alzheimer's disease patients with visual hallucinations. *Clin Imaging*, 2006. **30**:388–93.

90. Lewis D., *et al.* Laminar and regional distributions of neurofibrillary tangles and neuritic plaques in Alzheimer's disease: a quantitative study of visual and auditory cortices. *J Neurosci*, 1987. 7:1799–1808.

91. Foerster O. The cerebral cortex in man. *Lancet*, 1931. **2**:309–19.

92. Chapman F., *et al.* Association among visual hallucinations, visual acuity, and specific eye pathologies in Alzheimer's disease: treatment implications. *Am J Psychiatry*, 1999. **156**:1983–5.

93. Barnes J., David A. Visual hallucinations in Parkinson's disease: a review and phenomenological survey. *J Neurol Neurosurg Psychiatry*, 2001. **70**:727–33.

94. Mosimann M., *et al.* Visual perception in Parkinson disease dementia and dementia with Lewy bodies. *Neurology*, 2004. **63**:2091–6.

95. Bohnen N., *et al.* Cortical cholinergic function is more severely affected in Parkinsonian dementia than in Alzheimer disease: an in vivo positron emission tomographic study. *Arch Neurol Psychiatry*, 2003. **60**:1745–8.

96. Harding A., Broe G., Halliday G. Visual hallucinations in Lewy body disease relate to Lewy bodies in the temporal lobe. *Brain*, 2002. **125**:391–403.

97. Halliday G., *et al.* Loss of brainstem and serotonin- and substance P-containing neurons in Parkinson's disease. *Brain Res*, 1990. **510**:104–7.

98. Jellinger K. New developments in the pathology of Parkinson's disease. *Adv Neurol*, 1990. **53**:1–16.

99. Bodis-Wollner I., Tagliati M. The visual system in Parkinson's disease. *Adv Neurol*, 1993. **60**:390–4.

100. Collerton D., *et al.* Systematic review and meta-analysis show that dementia with Lewy bodies is a visual–perceptual and attentional–executive dementia. *Dement Geriatr Cogn Disord*, 2003. **16**:229–37.

101. Young B. A phenomenological comparison of LSD and schizophrenic states. *Br J Psychiatry*, 1974. **124**:64–74.

102. Marek G., *et al.* A major role for thalamocortical afferents in serotonergic hallucinogen receptor function in the rat neocortex. *Neuroscience*, 2001. **105**:379–92.

103. Aghajanian G., Marek G. Serotonin and hallucinogens. *Neuropsychopharmacology*, 1999. **21**:S16–S23.

104. Sarter M., Bruno J. Cortical acetylcholine, reality distortion, schizophrenia and Lewy body dementia: too much or too little acetylcholine? *Brain Cogn*, 1998. **38**:297–316.

105. Cancelli I., Marcon G., Balestrieri M. Factors associated with complex visual hallucinations during antidepressant treatment. *Hum Psychopharmacol*, 2004. **19**:577–84.

106. Moore H., *et al.* Role of accumbens and cortical dopamine receptors in the regulation of cortical acetylcholine release. *Neuroscience*, 1998. **88**:811–22.

107. Lipowski Z. (1980). Delirium due to alcohol and drug withdrawal. In *Delirium: Acute Brain Failure in Man*, Lipowski Z. (Ed.). Charles Springfield: C. Thomas, pp. 317–43.

108. MacKinnon G., Parker W. Benzodiazepine withdrawal syndrome: a literature review and evaluation. *Am J Drug Alcohol Abuse*, 1982. **9**:19–33.

109. Dyer J., Roth B., Hyma B. Gamma-hydroxybutyrate withdrawal syndrome. *Ann Emerg Med*, 2001. **37**:147–53.

110. Krystal J., *et al.* Gamma-aminobutyric acid type A receptors and alcoholism: intoxication, dependence, vulnerability, and treatment. *Arch Gen Psychiatry*, 2006. **63**:957–68.

111. Malcolm R. GABA systems, benzodiazepines, and substance dependence. *J Clin Psychiatry*, 2003. 64 Suppl 3:36–40.

112. Faingold C., Gouemo P. N., Riaz A. Ethanol and neurotransmitter interactions – from molecular to integrative effects. *Prog Neurobiol*, 1998. **55**:509–35.

113. Eysel U., *et al.* Reorganization in the visual cortex after retinal and cortical damage. *Restor Neurol Neurosci*, 1999. **15**:153–64.

114. Burke W. The neural basis of Charles Bonnet hallucinations: a hypothesis. *J Neurol Neurosurg Psychiatry*, 2002. **73**:535–41.

115. Paulig M., Mentrup H. Charles Bonnet's Syndrome: complete remission of complex visual hallucinations treated by gabapentin. *J Neurol Neurosurg Psychiatry*, 2001. **70**:813–14.

116. Gibson K., *et al.* Significant behavioral disturbances in succinic semialdehyde dehydrogenase (SSADH) deficiency (gamma-hydroxybutyric aciduria). *Biol Psychiatry*, 2003. **54**:763–8.

117. Ohayon M. M., *et al.* Hypnagogic and hypnopompic hallucinations: pathological phenomena? *Br J Psychiatry*, 1996. **169**(4):459–67.

118. Cheyne J. A., Rueffer S. D., Newby-Clark I. R. Hypnagogic and hypnopompic hallucinations during sleep paralysis: neurological and cultural construction of the nightmare. *Conscious Cogn*, 1999. **8**(3):319–37.

119. Takata K., *et al.* Night-time hypnopompic visual hallucinations related to REM sleep disorder. *Psychiatry Clin Neurosci*, 1998. **52**(2):207–9.

120. Baguley D.M. Hyperacusis. *J R Soc Med*, 2003. **96**(12):582–5.

121. Gothelf D., *et al.* Hyperacusis in Williams Syndrome: characteristics and associated neuroaudiologic abnormalities. *Neurology*, 2006. **66**(3):390–5.

122. Lee H., *et al.* Hearing symptoms in migrainous infarction. *Arch Neurol*, 2003. **60**(1):113–6.

123. Sims A. P. (2002). *Symptoms in the mind. An introduction to descriptive psychopathology*. 3rd ed. London: W. B. Saunders Company.

124. Yagcioglu S., Ungan P. The 'Franssen' illusion for short duration tones is preattentive: a study using mismatch negativity. *Brain Res*, 2006. **1106**(1):164–76.

125. Glass I. B. Alcoholic hallucinosis: a psychiatric enigma–1. The development of an idea. *Br J Addict*, 1989. **84**(1):29–41.

126. Lanska D. J., Lanska M. J., Mendez M. F. Brainstem auditory hallucinosis. *Neurology*, 1987. **37**(10):1685.

127. Cascino G. D., Adams R. D. Brainstem auditory hallucinosis. *Neurology*, 1986. **36**(8):1042–7.

128. Lockwood A. H., Salvi R. J., Burkard R. F. Tinnitus. *N Engl J Med*, 2002. **347**(12):904–10.

129. Waddell A. Tinnitus. *Clin Evid*, 2004(12):798–807.

130. Weissman J. L., Hirsch B. E. Imaging of tinnitus: a review. *Radiology*, 2000. **216**(2):342–9.

131. Chan S. W., Reade P. C. Tinnitus and temporomandibular pain-dysfunction disorder. *Clin Otolaryngol Allied Sci*, 1994. **19**(5):370–80.

132. Fox G. N., Baer M. T. Palatal myoclonus and tinnitus in children. *West J Med*, 1991. **154**(1):98–102.

133. Muhlau M., *et al.* Structural brain changes in tinnitus. *Cereb Cortex*, 2006. **16**(9):1283–8.

134. Eggermont J. J., Roberts L. E. The neuroscience of tinnitus. *Trends Neurosci*, 2004. **27**(11):676–82.

135. Kandel E. R., Schwartz J. H., Jessell T. H. (2000). *Principles of neural science*. 4th ed. New York: McGraw-Hill Medical.

136. White P. M., *et al.* Mammalian cochlear supporting cells can divide and trans-differentiate into hair cells. *Nature*, 2006. **441**(7096):984–7.

137. Wiegand D. A., Ojemann R. G., Fickel V. Surgical treatment of acoustic neuroma (vestibular schwannoma) in the United States: report from the Acoustic Neuroma Registry. *Laryngoscope*, 1996. **106**(1 Pt 1):58–66.

138. Henry J. A., Meikle M. B. Psychoacoustic measures of tinnitus. *J Am Acad Audiol*, 2000. **11**(3):138–55.

139. Jastreboff P. J. Phantom auditory perception (tinnitus): mechanisms of generation and perception. *Neurosci Res*, 1990. **8**(4):221–54.

140. Chen G. D., Jastreboff P. J. Salicylate-induced abnormal activity in the inferior colliculus of rats. *Hear Res*, 1995. **82**(2):158–78.

141. Kaltenbach J. A., Zhang J., Finlayson P. Tinnitus as a plastic phenomenon and its possible neural underpinnings in the dorsal cochlear nucleus. *Hear Res*, 2005. **206**(1–2):200–26.

142. Lockwood A. H., *et al.* The functional neuroanatomy of tinnitus: evidence for limbic system links and neural plasticity. *Neurology*, 1998. **50**(1):114–20.

143. Muhlnickel W., *et al.* Reorganization of auditory cortex in tinnitus. *Proc Natl Acad Sci USA*, 1998. **95**(17):10340–3.

144. Giraud A. L., *et al.* A selective imaging of tinnitus. *Neuroreport*, 1999. **10**(1):1–5.

145. Melcher J. R., *et al.* Lateralized tinnitus studied with functional magnetic resonance imaging: abnormal inferior colliculus activation. *J Neurophysiol*, 2000. **83**(2):1058–72.

146. Hilton M., Stuart E. Ginkgo biloba for tinnitus. *Cochrane Database Syst Rev*, 2004(2): p. CD003852.

147. Hannan S. A., Sami F., Wareing M. J. Tinnitus. *Br Med J*, 2005. **330**(7485): 237.

148. Webster R., Holroyd S. Prevalence of psychotic symptoms in delirium. *Psychosomatics*, 2000. **41**(6):519–22.

149. Foy A., Kay J., Taylor A. The course of alcohol withdrawal in a general hospital. *QJM*, 1997. **90**(4):253–61.

150. Lishman W. A. (1998). *Organic psychiatry. The psychological consequences of cerebral disorder*. 3rd ed. London: Blackwell Science.

151. Nayani T., David A. The auditory hallucination: a phenomenological survey. *Psychol Med*, 1996. **26**:177–89.

152. Copolov D., Trauer T., Mackinnon A. On the non-significance of internal versus external auditory hallucinations. *Schizophr Res*, 2004. **69**:1–6.

153. Junginger J., Frame C. Self-report of the frequency and phenomenology of verbal hallucinations. *J Nerv Ment Dis*, 1985. **173**:149–55.

154. Oulis P., *et al.* Clinical characteristics of auditory hallucinations. *Acta Psychiatr Scand*, 1995. **92**:97–102.

155. Shawyer F., *et al.* Command hallucinations and violence: implications for detention and treatment. *Psychiatry Psychol Law*, 2003. **10**:97–107.

156. Fried I., Spencer D. D., Spencer S. S. The anatomy of epileptic auras: focal pathology and surgical outcome. *J Neurosurg*, 1995. **83**(1):60–6.

157. McGuire P., *et al.* Abnormal monitoring of inner speech: a physiological basis for auditory hallucinations. *Lancet*, 1995. **346**:596–600.

158. Shergill S., *et al.* Functional anatomy of auditory verbal imagery in schizophrenic patients with auditory hallucinations. *Am J Psychiatry*, 2000. **157**:1691–3.

159. Shergill S., *et al.* Mapping auditory hallucinations in schizophrenia using functional magnetic resonance imaging. *Arch Gen Psychiatry*, 2000. **57**: 1033–8.

160. Lennox B., *et al.* The functional anatomy of auditory hallucinations in schizophrenia. *Psychiatry Res*, 2000. **100**:13–20.

161. Hunter M., *et al.* A neural basis for the perception of voices in external auditory space. *Brain*, 2002. **126**:161–9.

162. Laviolette S. Dopamine modulation of emotional processing in cortical and subcortical neural circuits: evidence for a final common pathway in schizophrenia? *Schizophr Bull*, 2007. **33**: 971–81.

163. Currie S., *et al.* Clinical course and prognosis of temporal lobe epilepsy. *A survey of 666 patients*. *Brain*, 1971. **94**(1):173–90.

164. Mauguiere F. Scope and presumed mechanisms of hallucinations in partial epileptic seizures. *Epileptic Disord*, 1999. **1**(2):81–91.

165. Williamson P. D., Spencer S. S. Clinical and EEG features of complex partial seizures of

166. Sachdev P. Schizophrenia-like psychosis and epilepsy: the status of the association. *Am J Psychiatry*, 1998. **155**(3):325–36.

167. Fujii D., Ahmed I. Characteristics of psychotic disorder due to traumatic brain injury: an analysis of case studies in the literature. *J Neuropsychiatry Clin Neurosci*, 2002. **14**(2):130–40.

168. Stewart B., Brennan D. M. Auditory hallucinations after right temporal gyri resection. *J Neuropsychiatry Clin Neurosci*, 2005. **17**(2):243–5.

169. Shaw P., *et al.* Schizophrenia-like psychosis arising de novo following a temporal lobectomy: timing and risk factors. *J Neurol Neurosurg Psychiatry*, 2004. **75**(7):1003–8.

170. Cerrato P., *et al.* Complex musical hallucinosis in a professional musician with a left subcortical haemorrhage. *J Neurol Neurosurg Psychiatry*, 2001. **71**(2):280–1.

171. Berrios G. E. Musical hallucinations. A historical and clinical study. *Br J Psychiatry*, 1990. **156**:188–94.

172. Ffischer C., Marchie A., Norris M. Musical and auditory hallucinations: a spectrum. *Psychiatry Clin Neurosci*, 2004. **58**(1):96–8.

173. Ffischer C., Ellger T. The clinical spectrum of musical hallucinations. *J Neurol Sci*, 2004. **227**(1):55–65.

174. Griffiths T. D. Musical hallucinosis in acquired deafness. *Phenomenology and brain substrate. Brain*, 2000. 123 (Pt 10):2065–76.

175. Griffiths T. D., *et al.* Analysis of temporal structure in sound by the human brain. *Nat Neurosci*, 1998. **1**(5):422–7.

176. Zatorre R. J., Evans A. C., Meyer E. Neural mechanisms underlying melodic perception and memory for pitch. *J Neurosci*, 1994. **14**(4):1908–19.

177. Penhune V. B., Zattore R. J., Evans A. C. Cerebellar contributions to motor timing: a PET study of auditory and visual rhythm reproduction. *J Cogn Neurosci*, 1998. **10**(6):752–65.

178. Murata S., Naritomi H., Sawada T. Musical auditory hallucinations caused by a brainstem lesion. *Neurology*, 1994. **44**(1):156–8.

179. Schielke E., *et al.* Musical hallucinations with dorsal pontine lesions. *Neurology*, 2000. **55**(3):454–5.

180. Douen A. G., Bourque P. R. Musical auditory hallucinosis from Listeria rhombencephalitis. *Can J Neurol Sci*, 1997. **24**(1): 70–2.

181. Nagaratnam N., Virk S., Brdarevic O. Musical hallucinations associated with recurrence of a right occipital meningioma. *Br J Clin Pract*, 1996. **50**(1):56–7.

182. Stephane M., Hsu L. K. Musical hallucinations: interplay of degenerative brain disease, psychosis, and culture in a Chinese woman. *J Nerv Ment Dis*, 1996. **184**(1):59–61.

183. Mocellin R., Walterfang M., Velakoulis D. Neuropsychiatry of complex visual hallucinations. *Aust NZJ Psychiatry*, 2006. **40**(9):742–51.

184. Baba A., Hamada H. Musical hallucinations in schizophrenia. *Psychopathology*, 1999. **32**(5):242–51.

185. Pearlson G. D., *et al.* A chart review study of late-onset and early-onset schizophrenia.[see comment]. *Am J Psychiatry*, 1989. **146**(12):1568–74.

186. Kopala L. C., Good K. P., Honer W. G. Olfactory hallucinations and olfactory identification ability in patients with schizophrenia and other psychiatric disorders. *Schizophrenia Res*, 1994. **12**(3):205–11.

187. Teggin A. F., *et al.* A comparison of CATEGO class 'S' schizophrenia in three ethnic groups: psychiatric manifestations. *Br J Psychiatry*, 1985. **147**:683–7.

188. Ndetei D. M., Singh A. Hallucinations in Kenyan schizophrenic patients. *Acta Psychiatr Scand*, 1983. **67**(3):144–7.

189. Ndetei D. M., Vadher A. A comparative cross-cultural study of the frequencies of hallucination in schizophrenia. *Acta Psychiatr Scand*, 1984. **70**(6):545–9.

190. Jablensky A., *et al.* Schizophrenia: manifestations, incidence and course in different cultures. *Psychol Med Monogr.*, 1992. Suppl **20**:35–7.

191. Commission on Clasification and Terminology of the Intemational League Against Epilepsy. Proposal for revised clinical and electroencephalographic classification of epileptic seizures. *Epilepsia*, 1981(4). **22**: 489–501.

192. Lennox W. G., Cobb S. Epilepsy. XIII. Aura in epilepsy: A statistical review of 1359 cases. *Arch Neurol Psychiatry*, 1933. **30**:374–87.

193. Gupta A.K., *et al.* Aura in temporal lobe epilepsy: clinical and electroencephalographic correlation. *J Neurol, Neurosurg Psychiatry*, 1983. **46**: 1079–83.

194. Jackson J. H., Stewart P. Epileptic attacks with a warning of a crude sensation of smell and the intellectual aura (dreamy state) in a patient who had symptoms pointing to gross organic disease of the right tempero-sphenoidal lobe. *Brain Inj*, 1899. **22**: 534–50.

195. Taylor D. C., Lochery M. Temporal lobe epilepsy: origin and significance of simple and complex auras. *J Neurol, Neurosurg Psychiatry*, 1987. **50**:673–81.

196. Daly D. Uncinate fits. *Neurology*, 1958. **8**:250–60.

197. Chen C., *et al*. Olfactory auras in patients with temporal lobe epilepsy. *Epilepsia*, 2003. **44**(2):257–60.

198. Acharya V., Acharya J., Luders H. Olfactory epileptic auras. *Neurology*, 1998. **51**(1):56–61.

199. Sandyk R. Olfactory hallucinations in Parkinson's disease. South African Medical Journal. *Suid Afrikaanse Tydskrif Vir Geneeskunde*, 1981. **60**(25): 19.

200. Goetz C. G., *et al*. Early dopaminergic drug-induced hallucinations in Parkinsonian patients. *Neurology*, 1998. **51**(3):811–4.

201. Holroyd S., Currie L., Wooten G. F. Prospective study of hallucinations and delusions in Parkinson's disease. *J Neurol Neurosurg Psychiatry*, 2001. **70**(6):734–8.

202. Silberstein S. D., *et al*. Cluster headache with aura. *Neurology*, 2000. **54**(1):219–21.

203. Fuller G. N., Guiloff R. J. Migrainous olfactory hallucinations. *J Neurol, Neurosurg Psychiatry*, 1987. **50**(12):1688–90.

204. Nickell P. V., Uhde T. W. Dose-response effects of intravenous caffeine in normal volunteers. *Anxiety*, 1994. **1**(4):161–8.

205. Koenigsberg H. W., Pollak C. P., Fine J. Olfactory hallucinations after the infusion of caffeine during sleep. *Am J Psychiatry*, 1993. **150**(12):1897–8.

206. Siegel R. K. Cocaine hallucinations. *Am J Psychiatry*, 1978. **135**(3):309–14.

207. Tien A. Distribution of hallucinations in the population. *Soc Psychiatry Psychiatr Epidemiol*, 1991. **26**:287–92.

208. Heveling T., Emrich H., Dietrich D. Treatment of a rare psychopathological phenomenon: tactile hallucinations and the delusional other. *Eur Psychiatry*, 2004. **19**:387–8.

209. Pfeifer L. A subjective report of tactile hallucinations in schizophrenia. *J Clin Psychol*, 1970. **26**:57–60.

210. Salama A., England R. A case study: schizophrenia and tactile hallucinations, treated with electroconvulsive therapy. *Can J Psychiatry*, 1990. **35**:86–7.

211. Bar K.-J., *et al*. Transient activation of a somatosensory area in painful hallucinations shown by fMRI. *Neuroreport*, 2002. **13**:1–4.

212. Shergill S., *et al*. Modality specific neural correlates of auditory and somatic hallucinations. *J Neurol Neurosurg Psychiatry*, 2001. **71**:688–90.

213. Munro A. Monosymptomatic hypochondriacal psychoses: a diagnostic entity which may respond to pimozide. *Can Psychiatr Assoc J*, 1978. **23**:497–500.

214. Munro A. Monosymptomatic hypochondriacal psychosis manifesting as delusions of parasitosis. A description of four cases successfully treated by pimozide. *Arch Dermatol*, 1978. **114**:940–3.

215. MacNamara P. Cutaneous and visual hallucinations. *Lancet*, 1928. **214**:807–8.

216. Mallet R., Male P. Delire cenesthesique. *Ann Med Psychol*, 1930. **88**:198–201.

217. Dupre E. Les cenestipathies. *Mouvement Medical*, 1913. **23**:3–22.

218. Wilson J., Miller H. Delusions of parasitosis. *Arch Dermatol Syph*, 1946. **54**:39–56.

219. Bhatia M., Jagawat T., Choudhary S. Delusional parasitosis: a clinical profile. *Int J Psychiatry Med*, 2000. **30**:83–91.

220. Berrios G. Tactile hallucinations: conceptual and historical aspects. *J Neurol Neurosurg Psychiatry*, 1982. **45**:285–93.

221. Claude H., Ey H. Troubles psychosensoriels et etats oniriques dans l'encephalite epidemique chronique. *Presse Med* (Paris), 1933. **104**:1281–5.

222. Fenelon G., *et al*. Hallucinations in Parkinson's disease: prevalence, phenomenology and risk factors. *Brain*, 2000. **123**:733–45.

223. Fenelon G., *et al*. Tactile hallucinations in Parkinson's disease. *J Neurol*, 2002. **249**: 1699–703.

224. Murthy P., Jayakumar P., Sampat S. Of insects and eggs: a case report. *J Neurol Neurosurg Psychiatry*, 1997. **63**: 522–3.

225. Chang P., Steinberg M. Alcohol withdrawal. *Med Clin North Am*, 2001. **85**:1191–212.

226. Driessen M., *et al*. Proposal of a comprehensive clinical typology of alcohol withdrawal – a cluster analysis approach. *Alcohol*, 2005. **40**:308–13.

227. Limosin F., *et al*. The A9 allele of the dopamine transporter gene increases the risk of visual hallucinations during alcohol withdrawal in alcohol-dependent women. *Neurosci Lett*, 2004. **362**:9–14.

228. Flaum M., Schultz S. When does amphetamine-induced psychosis become schizophrenia? *Am J Psychiatry*, 1996. **153**:812–15.

229. Nordahl T., Salo R., Leamon M. Neuropsychological effects of chronic methamphetamine use on neurotransmitters and cognition: a review. *J Neuropsychiatry Clin Neurosci*, 2003. **15**:317–25.

230. Di Forti M., Lappin J., Murray R. Risk factors for schizophrenia – all roads lead to dopamine. *Eur*

Neuropsychopharmacol, 2007. **17**:S101–S107.

231. Raedler T., *et al.* Towards a muscarinic hypothesis of schizophrenia. *Mol Psychiatry*, 2007. **12**:232–46.

232. Tandon R. Cholinergic aspects of schizophrenia. *Br J Psychiatry*, 1999. **37**:7–11.

233. Pantelis C., *et al.* Structural brain imaging evidence for multiple pathological processes at different stages of brain development in schizophrenia. *Schizophr Bull*, 2005. **31**:672–96.

234. Keshavan M., *et al.* Neurobiology of early psychosis. *Br J Psychiatry*, 2005. **48**:S8–18.

The neurology of schizophrenia

The neurologic examination in schizophrenia

Richard D. Sanders and Matcheri S. Keshavan

Facts box

1. The neurological examination is important in the assessment of schizophrenia-like psychoses.
2. In the clinical setting, it is conducted with the assumption that abnormal findings will suggest a secondary psychosis.
3. Empirically, it has been studied with the assumption that abnormal findings will suggest that idiopathic psychoses have a neurological base.
4. This review compares schizophrenia with secondary psychoses and with healthy comparison groups.
5. Focus is on specific neurologic tests with some localizing or pathologic significance.

Introduction

Schizophrenia and related conditions have long been regarded as more neurologic or "organic" than other psychiatric conditions such as mood, anxiety, and personality disorders. Correspondingly, published studies of neurological examination in schizophrenia outnumber those in other psychiatric disorders. These studies virtually all conclude that there is an excess of abnormal or anomalous findings in schizophrenia [1, 2, 3, 4, 5, 6]. That they are elevated at the onset of the disorder [7, 8, 9, 10, 11] strongly suggests that they are intrinsic features of the disorder, and not artifacts of medication, institutionalization, or other epiphenomena. Further, clinically recovered patients [12, 13] and symptomatic high-risk subjects [14, 15] have elevated rates of neurological examination abnormality, suggesting that neurological impairment is also not simply a marker of active psychosis. Thus, it is apparent that abnormal neurologic performance in schizophrenia is prevalent and intrinsic to the disease.

Neurologic examinations of people with schizophrenia differ from those of healthy people, but the clinical implications of this are uncertain. The usual clinical purpose of the neurologic examination in the psychotic patient is to rule out secondary or "organic" psychoses. This purpose has been obscured, if anything, by the wealth of data now demonstrating that neurologic signs are prevalent in the "functional" psychoses, so that their very presence cannot be taken as evidence of additional neurologic disorder. Further, we have very little data actually comparing neurologic examination findings from patients with primary and secondary psychoses. Thus, we are left with describing common findings in schizophrenia and the prevalence of abnormalities, providing content for the evaluation of individual patients, and allowing one to judge the likelihood that the case is primary or secondary.

This chapter focuses on "hard" much more than "soft" signs. In this context, "hard" means "strongly indicative of neurologic dysfunction at a specific location or of a specific cause." The term has been used somewhat differently in some schizophrenia research [16, 17, 18]. Although "hard" signs individually are more persuasive than "soft" signs as evidence of discrete lesions, it is really the examination as a whole that provides hard or soft evidence of any particular pathology. Hard signs are included in many neurologic batteries [19, 20, 21, 22] but we cite data using these batteries only when the prevalence of specific signs is reported.

Although the topic of soft signs in schizophrenia has been well-reviewed in recent years, the following will not greatly overlap with those papers [3, 4, 5, 6]. Even our more clinically oriented reviews of the neurologic examination in schizophrenia [23, 24] have not dealt extensively with the question of ruling out secondary schizophrenia. Because the hard signs (as defined herein) have received less attention in recent publications, we tend to focus on older sources. We also include some references to neuropsychological data, as some of these have included localizing tests [25].

Review

Reflexes

Muscle stretch (deep tendon) reflexes can be aberrant in three general ways: hypoactive, hyperactive, and asymmetric. Markedly hypoactive reflexes (including absent reflexes) are uncommon except in the elderly, and most often indicate peripheral neuropathy or hypothyroidism. Markedly hyperactive reflexes (including clonus) are upper motor neuron signs, most often reflecting white matter disease or certain toxic–metabolic states. Markedly asymmetric reflexes are the most localizing of these signs, usually reflecting an upper motor neuron lesion contralateral to the more active side.

Early descriptions and studies of dementia praecox/schizophrenia included hyperactive deep tendon (muscle stretch) reflexes [26, 27, 28]; indeed, Bleuler [27, p. 302] described them as "always exaggerated." Out of 100 patients, Runeberg [29] found reflexes to be hyperactive in 35% and hypoactive in 14%; asymmetry was "very frequent." Among a series of 1,000 preneuroleptic cases, 11% had increased or decreased reflexes, and 10% had asymmetric reflexes; less than 1% of 710 healthy college students had either type of finding [30]. Kennard (1960) [31] examined much smaller numbers of adolescent state hospital patients and found that those who were clinically diagnosed as schizophrenic had less frequent reflex asymmetry (15%) than those diagnosed organic (35%). More recently, diffusely brisk (but not frankly abnormal) reflexes have again been noted in clinical examination [10, 32], but do not discriminate schizophrenia from mood disorders [10]. Either hypoactive or hyperactive reflexes were found in 10.7% of patients, but none had asymmetry [33]. Using what appeared to be a more stringent standard for hyper-reflexia, another study found 3% in schizophrenia and 2% in controls [34]. Chen and colleagues [22] found 3% to 8% prevalence of hyper-reflexia in upper and lower limbs in schizophrenic patients and healthy controls, without significant group differences. Hypo-reflexia was non-significantly more prevalent in the upper extremities (14.5% vs. 10%) and reached significance (ignoring multiple tests of significance) in the lower extremities (14.5% vs. 4%). In summary, hyperactivity has

been described in 3% to 35%, hypoactivity in 14% to 15%, and asymmetry in 10 to 15% of patients with schizophrenia. The variety of findings here may be partly attributable to the fact that clinical muscle-stretch reflex testing is not highly reliable [35], and such studies are not easily blinded. Still, asymmetry is the most diagnostically significant of these findings and has been found consistently at a fairly low frequency in primary schizophrenia.

Pathological reflexes of pyramidal tract integrity were of interest to some twentieth century researchers. The Babinski reflex was present in 1.4% of patients, more than in 0.6% of a comparison group; there were similar results for other related reflexes [30]. Steck (1923) [36] saw the toe rise in only 0.5% of patients with schizophrenia. Quitkin and colleagues [37] noted a Babinski in 3.5% of their schizophrenic patients. Chen and colleagues [22] found it in 6.8% of patients and 5% in healthy controls, whereas Griffiths and colleagues [34] found it in 5% on each side in patients but in no controls on either side. Unequivocal Babinski and related reflexes are not common in schizophrenia.

Pathological nonlocalizing reflexes, often called "frontal, release, primitive, or developmental," usually reflect diffuse impairment. Although intriguing, they have limited utility in clarifying etiology or diagnosis [38, 39, 40].

Motor strength

Hemiparesis can be obvious in the observation of gait (e.g. circumduction of the affected leg) or in reduced spontaneous use of the affected side. Strength testing usually consists of bilateral comparisons, rather than comparisons to external standards. Common upper extremity tests include the pronator drift test, the arm-circling test, and the grip strength test. Drift was found in 12.9% of schizophrenic patients and not in healthy controls (p = 0.0009), nearly significant, even after correcting for about 90 tests of significance [13]. Further, drift was found in a surprising 48% of patients (no control group) in one series [33]. Recent studies found comparable grip strength in schizophrenia and healthy comparison groups [32, 41, 42]. Dynamometer testing may find absolute differences (less power in patients) but normal lateralization [43]. Not surprisingly, schizophrenic patients were less likely to show abnormal strength inequalities than were a group of "organic" patients [44]. Pronator drift is apparently not rare in schizophrenia, so it should not be over-interpreted as an isolated sign. In our experience, false positive results can result from a painful shoulder. The forearm rolling sign uses less time and may be more sensitive and specific [45].

Cranial nerves

The trigeminal/facial corneal reflex was found reduced in 30% and absent in 8% of chronically hospitalized schizophrenic patients. If one excludes the catatonic group, still 5% had no corneal reflex in this series [29].

Facial asymmetry was found in 3% of schizophrenic patients and 0.4% of a comparison group [30]. Similarly, cranial nerve palsies were found in 5% of a schizophrenic sample and none of the control sample [34]. Braun and colleagues noted facial asymmetry in 3.2% of their patient sample [33].

Impaired gag reflex has been found consistently in schizophrenia. In one study, it was found reduced in 29% and absent in 24% [29], whereas in another it was found impaired in 31.3% of unmedicated patients with schizophrenia [46].

Pupils

Earlier studies on neurological findings included numerous observations on pupil size, including reactions to psychological stimuli. Such studies are now generally conducted using tightly controlled conditions and instrumented measures that cannot be matched in usual clinical settings. Irregular pupils were found in 25% and unequal pupils in 11% of a group of patients preselected for having abnormal neurological examinations [28]. Anisocoria was found in 5.6% of patients with schizophrenia and 0.4% of healthy university students [30]. Pupillary findings in general were no more prevalent in first admission schizophrenia (15.6%) than in healthy controls [47]. Abnormal pupillary responses were noted in 9.7% of a group of schizophrenic patients [33]. Anisocoria in the alert patient can reflect any of several problems, including intracranial pathology [48].

Oculomotor

Smooth pursuit abnormalities have been studied for the past century [49], more actively in recent decades [50]. One occasionally notes jerky saccades during unaided observation [1, 22, 32, 34], but smooth pursuit eye movements are now usually the domain of special-

ized laboratories. Elevated blink rates have long been reported in schizophrenia but have no definite diagnostic utility, due partly to numerous other factors that can influence blinking [51, 52].

Marked failure of convergence was present in 6% of never-treated schizophrenic patients compared with 1.2% of healthy controls [8]. In chronic patients, convergence difficulties have been found in 18% to 24% of patients with schizophrenia [15, 53, 54].

Nystagmus was found in only 1.9% of schizophrenic patients and 0.14% of healthy students [3] but elsewhere it was found in 3.3% of schizophrenic patients [33]. Early studies found less nystagmus in response to rotation among schizophrenic patients than was found in healthy subjects [55]. Among adolescent state hospital inpatients, nystagmus was more common in one group diagnosed organic (30%) than schizophrenic (5%) [31]. Phencyclidine intoxication, which can strongly resemble idiopathic psychosis, presents with nystagmus in more than 50% of acute cases [56]. Optokinetic nystagmus was abnormal in 2 of 21 subjects with schizophrenia, compared with none of 20 healthy controls [19].

Strabismus was found to be more frequent in one sample with schizophrenia (13% of 475) than in healthy controls (4.4% of 697); this was particularly true of continuous (as opposed to intermittent) exotropia (8.2% vs. 0.5%) [57].

Motor coordination

The testing of motor coordination roughly checks for the integrity of the cerebellum and associated circuits. These include Romberg and other tests of balance; tandem and other variations on gait; finger-nose, heel-shin, and other tests of motor accuracy; and tasks intended to elicit intention tremor. Peculiarities of spontaneous movement and examination findings characteristic of cerebellar disease were noted in schizophrenia by many early authors [58], including Kraepelin (1919), who even wrote of a "cerebellar form of dementia praecox" [26]. Somewhat in this vein, numerous investigators of the early twentieth century [59] found that patients with schizophrenia showed less response to caloric or rotatory vestibular stimulation than do healthy controls. A failed attempt to replicate such findings [50] triggered modern smooth pursuit eye movements research (discussed above).

Subsequent study of cerebellar examination items has yielded variable results, but individual cerebellar

Table 4.1 Rates (%) of cerebellar signs in groups with schizophrenia and in healthy persons

	Tandem			Romberg			Finger-nose		
Reference	Patient	control	(p)	Patient	control	(p)	Patient	control	(p)
Buchanan & Heinrichs (1989)* (53)	18.4	4	p = .003	7.1	0		45–49	18–26	p < .0005
Griffiths et al. (1998)* (34)	5	0		5	0		3.3	0	
Mohr et al. (1996)* (54)	13	3.5		3	0		16–32	8.8–15.8	
Shibre et al. (2002)* (8)	5	0		1.5	0		4	0	
Lawrie et al. (2001)* (15)	6.7	14.3		0	2.9		13.3	14.3	
Krebs et al. (2000) (62)	44.2	12.5	p = 0.006	28.4	8.3	p = 0.001	43.2	18.8	p = .004
Chen et al. (1995) (22)	9.7	1	p = .018	1.6	0				
Ho et al. (2004) (60)	7.7	0.5	p − .002	9.7	0.6	p = .003	3.9	0.5	NS
Braun et al. (1995) (33)	35.5			0			0		

* Studies using the Neurological Evaluation Scale (53).

signs are fairly common in schizophrenia and usually found to be at least somewhat more common than in healthy comparison groups (Table 4.1). Additionally, the heel-shin test was found abnormal in 1.9% of schizophrenic subjects compared with 0.5% of healthy subjects [60]. Abnormal heel-shin performance was found in 3.2% to 6.5% of an uncontrolled series of patients [33]. One finds that abnormal performance on these tests often bears no resemblance to frank ataxia. One group distinctly specified "gross ataxia" in 5.1% of schizophrenic subjects during the Romberg and in 1.7% during tandem gait [61].

One group [10] found that cerebellar signs separated from other neurological signs in a principal component analysis, and that this factor distinguished schizophrenic subjects from other subjects. Another group [11] found that the posture and oculomotor subscores of an ataxia assessment instrument, but no other summary scores of neurological performance, predicted a diagnosis of schizophrenia. Cerebellar signs are present in a substantial minority of patients with schizophrenia; gross ataxia is uncommon in both primary schizophrenia and in most cases of secondary schizophrenia.

Often linked to cerebellar dysfunction is hypotonia, a finding that is observed periodically in schizophrenia [63]. Observed hypotonia was found in a stunning 63% of subjects in one series, more than 50% of each subtype [29].

Motor Sequencing tests were developed by Luria (1966) [64] to test prefrontal integrity. They were then included in neuropsychological [65] and neurological [19, 53, 66] batteries. Motor sequencing can be quite severely impaired in primary psychosis, enough that testing cannot be completed. Even cooperative subjects can become quite frustrated by these tasks, which include the fist-ring, the fist-edge-palm, and the alternating fist-palm. These are perhaps the most consistent and striking deficits in the psychotic disorders [67]. Motor-sequencing deficits should not point to a secondary schizophrenia.

Motor inhibition deficits, indicated by inappropriate responses to nontarget stimuli, are also common in the primary psychotic disorders. A common example is the Go–No Go test, which has often been studied in schizophrenia [68, 69]. Similarly, impersistence, indicated by failure to maintain an unnatural position past a few seconds, is represented in some soft sign batteries [22, 53]. Neither of these can be expected to reliably distinguish primary from secondary psychosis.

Hypokinetic (Parkinsonian) motor findings

Roughly 10% to 20% of recent-onset, never medicated patients with schizophrenia have Parkinsonian signs [70, 71, 72]. These most often include diminished spontaneous movement of the face and arms, short steps, and diminished arm swing while walking, and "lead pipe" rigidity (that is, a similar degree of resistance throughout the range of motion) of the joints during passive manipulation. When mild and isolated (e.g., when not accompanied by impaired upgaze or overt rest tremor), they have no diagnostic implications, although there may be prognostic significance [71]. Marked or numerous Parkinsonian signs in a person never exposed to dopamine antagonists (or at least 3 months free of oral and 6 months free of depot agents), calcium blockers, or valproate, is quite uncommon in youth [73]. The most common hypokinetic condition of young adulthood associated with psychosis is Wilson disease, and it is around 300 times less common than schizophrenia. Other conditions are even less common, including the Westphal variant of Huntington disease, spinocerebellar ataxia (Friedreich's ataxia, with conspicuous ataxia, usually childhood onset, frequently accompanied by psychosis) and neuroacanthocytosis (more often chorea than Parkinsonism, psychosis not common.).

In later life, Parkinson disease and similar movement disorders will naturally be considered in the differential of Parkinsonian signs, but psychosis is rarely prominent in patients with these entities. In catatonia, rigidity to passive movement is sometimes observed, but the overall setting will generally point to the correct diagnosis. Gegenhalten (i.e. seeming opposition to all passive movement) is sometimes observed in severely disorganized subjects, and spasticity (velocity-dependent resistance to passive movement) may be seen in patients with impaired gross motor control, but these phenomena are distinct from lead-pipe Parkinsonian rigidity.

Hyperkinetic (including choreoathetotic or Huntingtonian) motor findings

Although even less common than Parkinsonism in a never-medicated adult subject with schizophrenia, "tardive-like dyskinesia" [74] may be observed in mild form in acute subjects [71, 72, 75] and more prominently in older and more chronic (but still never-medicated) subjects [76, 77], as well as some normal persons, especially the immature [78] and the elderly [79]. Diagnostically, such movements (particularly chorea) raise the possibilities of Huntington disease (often distinguishable by its precarious gait, the "milk-maid's grip," and definitively by genetic testing). Involuntary movements are very often traceable to drugs, such as the chronic use of dopamine-blocking agents, to cocaine and other stimulants, and occasionally to prescription drugs that are not dopamine antagonists. A lengthy differential includes post-infectious syn-

dromes, Tourette disorder, and a number of uncommon disorders [79].

Gait

Gait has not been well studied as such in schizophrenia but can include signs of hemiparesis and hypokinetic and hyperkinetic movement disorders, as already mentioned. Among other potential information, a wide base is indicative of brain damage, particularly of the hindbrain. A tendency to minimize or not lift feet off the floor ("magnetic gait," now more inclusively termed apraxic gait), is traditionally linked to normal pressure hydrocephalus but is also found in several other conditions, many of which can produce psychosis and call for neuroimaging [48, 80].

Sensory exam

Sensory acuity deficits have been consistently linked to psychosis, first in clinical samples of the elderly [81] and more recently in epidemiologic samples of the young [82, 83, 84]. It is uncertain whether the link between sensory deficits and psychosis may be due to reduced or distorted sensory input, or whether sensory disability is a less specific marker of neurologic handicap. Sensory deficits should be considered together with any other findings as part of a possible neurologic syndrome, and should be corrected if possible.

Visual

Visual acuity problems are of course quite common in the general population, so are unlikely to shed light on differential diagnosis. Visual fields have not been found impaired in schizophrenia [19]. No visual field deficits were found in routine confrontation testing of younger schizophrenia patients [33]. In the elderly, psychosis is associated with visual impairment, or at least uncorrected visual impairment [81]. Studies comparing elderly patients with schizophrenia-like disorder to those with dementia and other organic mental disorders have not found differences in visual acuity [85, 86], although certain other differences in ocular health were noted.

Auditory

Assorted acoustic and related abnormalities have occasionally been associated with schizophrenia [87], but studies of patients with schizophrenia [88, 89] have found no abnormalities on basic acuity measures. In two studies [85, 86], elderly patients with schizophrenia-like disorders had less auditory deficits than those with dementia and other organic mental disorders.

Olfactory

Olfactory identification is impaired in schizophrenia but also in a wide array of other conditions such as ageing, movement disorders, and at least some dementias [90]. This parameter has been studied more than simple olfactory sensitivity, which is intact in schizophrenia [91, 92].

Tactile

In many studies, subjects with schizophrenia have been asked to perform tasks involving the sense of touch, but few of these studies have been of the basic tactile functions. One study using electric stimuli with schizophrenia subjects and healthy controls found elevated tactile thresholds in subjects but no differences in pain thresholds [93]. Bilateral symmetric double simultaneous stimulation is accepted as a subtle test for unilateral sensory loss. One small study found frequent extinctions in several psychiatric groups, including 29% in the schizophrenia group; this was not statistically greater than the 5% in the healthy control group [19]. Some studies [94] list "extinction" among their neurologic tests but are unclear as to whether they refer to this test or the face-hand text (discussed later).

Dorsal column sensory tests

The dorsal column carries vibratory sensations and position sense. Deficits in these may increase suspicion of B_{12} deficiency or CNS syphilis, which are today uncommon mimics of schizophrenia but also can reflect common comorbid problems such as diabetes mellitus. In a sample of schizophrenic subjects it was found that at least 50% had impaired vibratory sensation in their hands, but statistically significant group differences from healthy controls were found only in frequencies of at least 200 Hz (higher than those usually tested at the bedside) [95]. We find no data on the prevalence of abnormal vibratory or position sense, as clinically assessed, in primary schizophrenia.

Higher order sensory tests

Sensory information processed in the posterior association areas of the cortex (temporal, parietal, and occipital association areas) include visuospatial, complex tactile information, and sensory input from multiple modalities. These tests (including right-left orientation, audiovisual integration, graphesthesia) are almost always labeled soft signs. They are found frequently in schizophrenia and have little known significance in diagnosing secondary psychoses. The face-hand test, a form of asymmetric double simultaneous stimulation [96, 97] has a long history of study in schizophrenia, dementia, and other types of brain injury. After minimal instruction, the subject is touched simultaneously on each of four asymmetric combinations of face and hand. In schizophrenia, there may be an increased tendency to neglect the hand stimulus in the first or second of these initial trials [9]. The four asymmetric stimuli are followed by two symmetric stimuli, to both sides of the face and to both hands. If, after reporting only the face stimulus on the first four trials, the subject reports the symmetric stimuli correctly, the asymmetric trials can be repeated. Continuing to report only the face stimulus at this point is indicative of an "organic" mental disorder, rather than schizophrenia [96, 97].

Neurologic exam as an aid in detecting neuromedical etiologies

Specific neurologic exam items most likely to be of value in a "rule-out" exam are those that are least common in (primary) schizophrenia, those that are sensitive and at least moderately specific for particular fairly common causes of secondary schizophrenia, and those that predict a high yield for more expensive or time-consuming diagnostic procedures. Existing studies suggest that the following neurological findings are infrequent in primary schizophrenia and are more common in secondary schizophrenia:

1. Asymmetry of muscle strength reflexes (unless isolated to a single joint)
2. Absent muscle stretch reflexes, except in the elderly [48]
3. Babinski reflex (upgoing toe)
4. Hemiparesis (possibly excepting the flattened nasolabial fold or mild isolated paresis)
5. Absent corneal reflex
6. Nystagmus without other explanation, such as toxicity
7. Marked hearing deficit
8. Anosmia or marked insensitivity to smell

9. Persistent extinction of hand on face-hand test
10. Marked chorea or athetosis without other explanation (e.g., prior drug treatment)
11. Marked ataxia without toxic explanation (current drugs or toxins)

Neurologic examination abnormalities are routinely considered in the aggregate, on an informal basis in clinical practice but can also be aggregated formally. For example, we derived a summary "hard" (i.e. localizing) sign index from a neurologic battery constructed for a family study [98], including the following: Romberg sway, Babinksi reflex, extinctions during symmetric double simultaneous light touch, hemiparesis evident during the arm circling test, facial asymmetry noted at rest, and lateralizing dysgraphesthesia.

The significance of global impairment

Like general cognitive impairment, the presence of a variety of neurologic signs, even if individually nonspecific, increases the likely yield of an organic workup [99]. The overall severity of impairment in a neurologic examination [54, 61], specifically impairment on perceptual tests [100, 101], may predict impairment in a neuropsychological battery. Supporting the importance of "nonspecific" neurologic findings are some studies of imaging in routine general psychiatric practice. In one series of 150 head CT scans [102] neurological examinations were globally abnormal in 15 of 16 subjects for whom abnormal CT results had an impact on treatment. Neurologic findings were localizing in only 8 of the 15 cases. A set of neurologic "soft" signs and cognitive tests, previously found to predict performance on a neuropsychological battery [99] administered to a group of patients referred for MRI, predicted periventricular white matter lesions. Using stepwise multiple regression, a motor sequencing task and visual tracking were highly efficient in predicting this result [103]. Thus, nonspecific and nonfocal signs may prove predictive of imaging results in schizophrenia. One may wonder that there are not more studies relevant to the question of whether the neurologic exam is helpful in selecting psychotic patients for imaging. Although there are many series of research subjects involving both neurologic and imaging studies, cases of secondary schizophrenia are routinely screened out, so that most studies are of little use for our purpose.

Detecting specific etiologies of secondary schizophrenia

There are essentially no neurologic data comparing groups with schizophrenia to those with any particular types of secondary schizophrenia. Certain forms of epilepsy can mimic schizophrenia, but there are no known characteristic neurologic findings. Ischaemic or neoplastic lesions can produce psychosis and in so doing tend to produce findings in accordance with lesion location or by increasing intracranial pressure.

Velocardiofacial syndrome affects approximately 2% of those diagnosed with schizophrenia, can be specifically tested if suspected, and carries with it significant family-planning implications. It has no specific neurologic examination profile [104].

Metachromatic leukodystrophy is a rare white matter disease famous for close simulations of schizophrenia. Adult-onset cases have been divided into cases with quite distinct motor and psychiatric presentations. The psychiatric subgroup presents with a schizophrenia-like illness in adolescence or young adulthood, with no frankly abnormal neurologic findings [105].

Psychotic disorders resembling schizophrenia can complicate chronic alcoholism. These usually feature nonbizarre delusions or hallucinations. There are no known characteristic neurologic features, but chronic alcoholism tends to carry with it findings of polyneuropathy and cerebellar injury [106]. As with any delirium, the alcoholism-related Wernicke's syndrome can superficially resemble psychosis and has characteristic extraocular paresis and ataxia. Complicating this issue (and complicating the recent interest in "cerebellar" deficits in schizophrenia), schizophrenic brains may have an increased incidence of subtle Wernicke pathology, perhaps due to the toxic-metabolic extremes to which they may be prone [107].

Comorbid substance use disorders can also cause diagnostic confusion, by raising the question of substance-induced psychotic disorder, and by potentially contributing additional neurologic impairment. Alcohol is the only popularly abused substance for which there is a significant body of neurologic examination research in schizophrenia. There is some evidence for increased impairment in higher-order perceptual functioning in schizophrenia with comorbid alcoholism [108, 109], but this effect is probably not dramatic enough to be of advantage in clinical diagnosis. Surprisingly, most studies found that alcoholism

Table 4.2 Guide to interpreting results of the examination to rule out a secondary schizophrenia

Neurologic sign	Findings in primary schizophrenia	If abnormal, consider
Muscle stretch reflexes	Occassionally exaggerated or diminished	Asymmetry in focal lesions; diminished or delayed relaxation in hypothyroidism; exaggerated in white matter disease
Babinski (upgoing toe)/hemiparesis	Rare	Focal lesions; white matter disease
Pupils /cornea	Unequal pupils rarely seen; may have diminished corneal reflex	Dilated in PCP/stimulant psychosis; absent light response and other findings in neurosyphilis; unequal pupils may reflect ocular/brainstem pathology
Anosmia	Hyposmia seen in small proportion	Consider Parkinson disease/dementia, head injury
Eye movements	Saccadic/smooth pursuit abnormalities, not obvious at bedside; nystagmus uncommon	Nystagmus in drug toxicity (barbiturate, benzodiazepine, PCP); paresis in Wernicke encephalopathy
Visual field/visual acuity	Normal	Consider contribution of visual deficit to psychosis
Auditory acuity	Normal	Consider contribution of auditory deficit to psychosis
Parkinsonian (hypokinetic) signs	Rigidity in catatonia; mild rigidity in schizophrenia	Consider Parkinson disease, Wilson's Disease
Dyskinetic (hyperkinetic) signs	Mild findings occasional in never-treated schizophrenia	Lond differential; tardive dyskinesia, Sydenham or Huntington chorea, Tourette Syndrome
Vibration/position sense	Normal	Consider B12 deficiency; diabetes mellitus; neurosyphilis
Cerebellar signs (Romberg, finger-nose, heel-shin, tandem gait)	Common in schizophrenia when mild	Consider cerebellar disease; Wernicke encephalopathy or other toxic-metabolic problem
Apraxic gait	Not seen	Structural neuroimaging indicated, often frontal lobe disease

in schizophrenia adds little or no additional cerebellar or other motor impairment to that seen in schizophrenia without alcoholism [54, 60, 108, 110, 111]. Existing studies suggest that the neurological examination will probably not be helpful in distinguishing schizophrenia from the psychotic disorders secondary to alcohol.

Among acute intoxications, phencyclidine (PCP) may most closely resemble schizophrenia. Nystagmus is the most common neurologic sign; extrapyramidal motor signs such as rigidity and dystonia are seen occasionally [56]. PCP should be considered in the differential for acute or even subacute psychosis with nystagmus.

Intoxication with stimulants, such as amphetamines and cocaine, can simulate schizophrenia. Particularly in the acute (intoxicated) phase, one may observe pupillary dilation and hyperkinetic motor signs that may resemble tardive dyskinesia or akathisia [112]. In withdrawal, there is some tendency for patients to develop hypokinetic (Parkinsonian) signs

[113]. These are by no means specific findings, though, and are more helpful if kept in mind as one explanation for such movement disturbances if observed.

Conclusion

Nearly a century of study yields fairly consistent results with respect to the prevalence of the diagnostically important "hard" signs in schizophrenia. Based on this work, a neurologic assessment of patients with psychosis should include:

- Gait*
- Arm circling or drift
- Face hand test
- Symmetric double simultaneous stimulation, including feet
- Muscle stretch reflexes
- Babinski
- Visual fields
- Visual acuity screening

- Auditory acuity screening
- Vibratory sensation
- Involuntary movements (chorea, athetosis, tic)*
- Parkinsonian signs
- Motor asymmetries (gait, face, limbs)*

(*May be observed without specific formal elicitation).

Table 4.2 provides a quick guide to interpreting results of the examination to rule out a secondary schizophrenia.

Although the research cited herein is diverse and interesting, it has severe limitations in helping us distinguish primary from secondary schizophrenia. What we clearly need are studies directly addressing the use of the neurologic exam in detecting secondary schizophrenia. These studies should take two forms: one, better conducted among representative clinical samples, would investigate the yield of a structured examination in detecting neuropathology of potential etiologic significance among psychotic patients.

The second, which would only be feasible in referral centers, would compare the examinations of primary schizophrenia with a group with a schizophrenia-like psychosis of a particular etiology. For example, a group of patients with epilepsy and psychosis could be compared with a group with primary schizophrenia, matched demographically and perhaps for severity of psychosis, with examiner blinding. Another feasible study would compare primary schizophrenia with stimulant-induced psychosis.

It is doubtful, though, that research will remove the need for clinician judgment in interpreting the results of an individual's neurologic exam. Routinely performing the examination (rather than delegating to an extender or to a consultant) is invaluable, as one can then readily distinguish typical from atypical performance for a schizophrenia patient. Finally, the exam should be considered as a whole and in light of all other available information (history, mental state, diagnostic studies, etc.).

References

1. Stevens J. R. The Neuropathology of schizophrenia. *Psychol Med*, 1982. **12**:695–700.

2. Cadet J. L., Rickler K. C., Weinberger D. L. (1986). The clinical neurologic examination in schizophrenia. In *The Neurology of Schizophrenia*, Nasrallah H. A. and Weinberger D. L. (Eds.). New York: Elsevier.

3. Heinrichs D. W., Buchanan R. W. Significance and meaning of neurological signs in schizophrenia. *Am J Psychiatry*, 1988. **145**:11–18.

4. Boks M. P., Russo S., Knegtering R., Van Den Bosch R. J. The specificity of neurological signs in schizophrenia: a review. *Schizophr Res*, 2000. **43**:109–16.

5. Candela S., Manschreck T. Neurological soft signs in schizophrenia. Research findings and clinical relevance. *Psychiatr Ann*, 2003. **33**:157–66.

6. Bombin I., Arango C., Buchanan R. W. Significance and meaning of neurological signs in schizophrenia: two decades later. *Schizophr Bull*, 2005. **31**:962–77.

7. Dazzan P., Murray R. M. Neurological soft signs in first-episode psychosis: a systematic review. *Br J Psychiatry Suppl*, 2002. **43**:S50–7.

8. Shibre T., Kebede D., Alem A., *et al.* Neurological soft signs (NSS) in 200 treatment-naive cases with schizophrenia: a community-based study in a rural setting. *Nord J Psychiatry*, 2002. **56**:425–31.

9. Keshavan M. S., Sanders R. D., Sweeney J. A., *et al.* Diagnostic specificity and neuroanatomical validity of neurological abnormalities in first-episode psychoses. *Am J Psychiatry*, 2003. **160**:1298–1304.

10. Boks M. P., Liddle P. F., Burgerhof J. G., *et al.* Neurological soft signs discriminating mood disorders from first episode schizophrenia. *Acta Psychiatr Scand*, 2004. **110**:29–35.

11. Varambally S., Venkatasubramanian G., Thirthalli J., *et al.* Cerebellar and other neurological soft signs in antipsychotic-naive schizophrenia. *Acta Psychiatr Scand*, 2006. **114**:352–6.

12. Bachmann S., Bottmer C., Schroder J. Neurological soft signs in first-episode schizophrenia: a follow-up study. *Am J Psychiatry*, 2005. **162**:2337–43.

13. Chen E. Y., Hut C. L., Chan R. C., *et al.* A 3-year prospective study of neurological soft signs in first-episode schizophrenia. *Schizophr Res*, 2005. **75**:45–54.

14. Hans S. L., Marcus J., Nuechtereein K. H., *et al.* Neurobehavioral deficits at adolescence in children at risk for schizophrenia: the Jerusalem infant development study. *Arch Gen Psychiatry*, 1999. **56**:741–48.

15. Lawrie S. M., Bye M., Miller P., *et al.* Neurodevelopmental indices and the development of psychotic symptoms in subjects at high risk of schizophrenia. *Br J Psychiatry*, 2001. **178**:524–30.

16. Woods B. T., Kinney D. K., Yurgelun-Todd D. A. Neurological "hard" signs and family history of psychosis in schizophrenia. *Biol Psychiatry*, 1991. **30**:806–16.

17. Kinney D. K., Yurgelun-Todd D. A., Woods B.T. Neurological hard signs in schizophrenia and major mood disorders. *J Nerv Ment Dis*, 1993. **181**:202–4.

18. Whitty P., Clarke M., Browne S., *et al.* Prospective evaluation of neurological soft signs in first-episode schizophrenia in relation to psychopathology: state versus trait phenomena. *Psychol Med*, 2003. **33**:1479–84.

19. Cox S. M., Ludwig A. M. Neurological soft signs and psychopathology: incidence in diagnostic groups. *Can J Psychiatry*, 1979. **24**:668–73.

20. Schroder J., Niethammer R., Geider F. J., *et al.* Neurological soft signs in schizophrenia. *Schizophr Res*, 1991. **6**:25–30.

21. Ismail B., Cantor-Graae E., Mcneil T. F. Neurological abnormalities in schizophrenic patients and their siblings. *Am J Psychiatry*, 1998. **155**:84–9.

22. Chen E. Y., Shapleske J., Luque R., *et al.* The Cambridge neurological inventory: a clinical instrument for assessment of soft neurological signs in psychiatric patients. *Psychiatry Res*, 1995. **56**:183–204.

23. Sanders R. D., Keshavan M. S. Physical and neurologic examinations in neuropsychiatry. *Semin Clin Neuropsychiatry*, 2002. **7**:18–29.

24. Sanders R., Keshavan M., Goldstein G. Clinical utility of the neurologic examination in the psychoses. *Psychiatr Ann*, 2003. **33**:195–200.

25. Goldstein G., Sanders R. (2004). Sensory-perceptual and motor function. In *Comprehensive Handbook of Psychological Assessment*, Goldstein G. and Beers S. (Eds.). New York: Wiley.

26. Kraepelin E. (1919–1971). *Dementia Praecox*. New York: Churchill Livingston Inc.

27. Bleuler E. (1950). *Dementia praecox or the group of schizophrenias [1911]*. New York: International University Press.

28. Muehlig W. Schizophrenia: neurological signs. *J Mich State Med Soc*, 1940. **39**:116–42.

29. Runeberg J. Die Neurologie der schizophrenie. *Acta Psychiatr Neurologica*, 1936. **11**:523–47.

30. Lemke R. Neurological findings in schizophrenics. *Psychiatr Neurol Med Psychol*, 1955. **7**:226–9.

31. Kennard M. The value of equivocal signs in neurological diagnosis. *Neurology*, 1960. **10**:753–64.

32. Flyckt L., Sydow O., Bjerkenstedt L., *et al.* Neurological signs and psychomotor performance in patients with schizophrenia, their relatives and healthy controls. *Psychiatry Res*, 1999. **86**: 113–29.

33. Braun C. M., Lapierre D., Hodgins S., *et al.* Neurological soft signs in schizophrenia: are they related to negative or positive symptoms, neuropsychological performance, and violence? *Arch Clin Neuropsychol*, 1995. **10**:489–509.

34. Griffiths T. D., Sigmundsson T., Takei N., *et al.* Neurological abnormalities in familial and sporadic schizophrenia. *Brain*, 1998. **121**:191–203.

35. Sanders R. D., Keshavan M. S. The neurologic examination in adult psychiatry: from soft signs to hard science. *J Neurospsychiatry Clin Neurosci*, 1998. **10**:395–404.

36. Steck H. Neurologische untersichungen an schizophrenen. *Zeitschr f d ges Neurol u Psychitrie BD*, 1923. **82**:292–320.

36. Quitkin F., Rifkin A., Klein D. F. Neurologic soft signs in schizophrenia and character disorders. Organicity in schizophrenia with premorbid asociality and emotionally unstable character disorders. *Arch Gen Psychiatry*, 1976. **33**:845–53.

38. Keshavan M. S., Kumar Y. V., Channabasavanna S. M. A critical evaluation of infantile reflexes in neuropsychiatric diagnosis. *Indian J Psychiatry*, 1979. **21**:267–70.

39. Vreeling F. W., Houx P. J., Jolles J., Verhey F. R. Primitive reflexes in Alzheimer's disease and vascular dementia. *J Geriatr Psychiatry Neurol*, 1995. **8**:111–17.

40. Kowall N., Berman S. (1999). Primitive reflexes in psychiatry and neurology. In *Movement disorders in neurology and neuropsychiatry*, Joseph A. and Young R. (Eds.). New York: Blackwell Science.

41. Rosofsky I., Levin S., Holzman P. S. Psychomotility in the functional psychoses. *J Abnorm Psychol*, 1982. **91**:71–4.

42. Schwartz F., Carr A., Munich R., et al. Voluntary motor performance in psychotic disorders: a replication study. *Psychol Rep*, 1990. **66**:1223–34.

43. Merrin E. L. Motor and sighting dominance in chronic schizophrenics. Relationship to social competence, age at first admission, and clinical course. *Br J Psychiatry*, 1984. **145**: 401–6.

44. Watson C. G., Thomas R. W., Felling J., *et al.* Differentiation of organics from schizophrenics with the trail making, dynamometer, critical flicker fusion, and light-intensity matching tests. *J Clin Psychol*, 1969. **25**:130–3.

45. Sawyer R. N. Jr., Hanna J. P., Ruff R. L., *et al.* Asymmetry of forearm rolling as a sign of unilateral cerebral dysfunction. *Neurology*, 1993. **43**:1596–8.

46. Craig T. J., Richardson M. A., Pass R., *et al.* Impairment of the gag reflex in schizophrenic inpatients. *Compr Psychiatry*, 1983. **24**:514–20.

47. Rubin P., Vorstrup S., Hemmingsen R., et al. Neurological abnormalities in patients with schizophrenia or schizophreniform disorder at first admission to hospital: correlations with computerized tomography and regional cerebral blood flow findings. *Acta Psychiatr Scand*, 1994. **90**:385–90.

48. McGee S. (2001). *Evidence-based physical diagnosis*. Philadelphia: Saunders.

49. Diefendorf A., Dodge R. An experimental study of the ocular reactions of the insane from photographic records. *Brain*, 1908. **31**:451–89.

50. Levy D. L., Holzman P. S., Proctor L. R. Vestibular responses in schizophrenia. *Arch Gen Psychiatry*, 1978. **35**:972–81.

51. Mackert A., Woyth C., Flechtner K. M., *et al.* Increased blink rate in drug naive acute schizophrenic patients. *Biol Psychiatry*, 1990. **27**:1197–202.

52. Chan R. C., Chen E. Y. Blink rate does matter: a study of blink rate, sustained attention, and neurological signs in schizophrenia. *J Nerv Ment Dis*, 2004. **192**:781–3.

53. Buchanan R. W., Heinrichs D. W. The neurological evaluation scale (NES): a structured instrument for the assessment of neurological signs in schizophrenia. *Psychiatry Res*, 1989. **27**:335–50.

54. Mohr F., Hubmann W., Cohen R., *et al.* (1996). Neurologic soft signs in schizophrenia: assessment and correlates. *Eur Arch Psychiatry Clin Neurosci*, 1996. **246**:240–8.

55. Leach W. W. Nystagmus: An integrative neural deficit in schizophrenia. *J Abnorm Soc Psychol.*, 1960. **60**:305–9.

56. McCarron M. M., Schulze B. W., Thompson G. A., *et al.* Acute phencyclidine intoxication: incidence of clinical findings in 1,000 cases. *Ann Emerg Med*, 1981. **10**:237–42.

57. Yoshitsugu K., Yamada K., Toyota T., *et al.* A novel scale including strabismus and 'cuspidal ear' for distinguishing schizophrenia patients from controls using minor physical anomalies. *Psychiatry Res*, 2006. **145**:249–58.

58. Taylor M. A. The role of the cerebellum in the pathogenesis of schizophrenia. *Neuropsychiatry Neuropsychol Behav Neurol*, 1991. **4**:251–80.

59. Angyal A., Sherman M. Postural reactions to vestibular stimulation in schizophrenic and normal subjects. *Am J Psychiatry*, 1942. **98**:857–62.

60. Ho B. C., Mola C., Andreasen N. C. Cerebellar dysfunction in

neuroleptic naive schizophrenia patients: clinical, cognitive, and neuroanatomic correlates of cerebellar neurologic signs. *Biol Psychiatry*, 2004. **55**:1146–53.

61. Flashman L. A., Flaum M., Gupta S., *et al.* Soft signs and neuropsychological performance in schizophrenia. *Am J Psychiatry*, 1996. **153**:526–32.

62. Krebs M., Gut-Fayand A., Bourdel M., *et al.* Validation and factorial structure of a standardized neurological examination assessing neurological soft signs in schizophrenia. *Schizophr Res*, 2000. **45**:245–60.

63. Cantor S., Pearce J., Pezzot-Pearce T., *et al.* The group of hypotonic schizophrenics. *Schiz Bull*, 1981. **7**:1–11.

64. Luria A. (1966). *Higher cortical functions in man.* New York: Basic Books. (Originally published by Moscow University Press, 1962.)

65. Golden C. J., Hammeke T., Purisch A. (1980). *The Luria-Nebraska battery manual.* Los Angeles, California: Western Psychological Services.

66. Manschreck T. (1989). Motor and cognitive disturbances in schizophrenia disorders. In *Schizophrenia: scientific progress*, Schultz S. and Tamminga C. (Eds.). New York: Oxford University Press.

67. Jahn T., Cohen R., Hubmann W., *et al.* The brief motor scale (BMS) for the assessment of motor soft signs in schizophrenic psychoses and other psychiatric disorders. *Psychiatry Res*, 2006. **142**.177–89.

68. Bates A. T., Liddle P. F., Kiehl K. A., *et al.* State dependent changes in error monitoring in schizophrenia. *J Psychiatr Res*, 2004. **38**:347–56.

69. Kathmann N., Von Recum S., Haag C., *et al.* Electrophysiological evidence for reduced latent inhibition in schizophrenic patients. *Schizophr Res*, 2000. **45**:103–14.

70. Caligiuri M. P., Lohr J. B., Jeste D. V. Parkinsonism in neuroleptic-naive schizophrenic patients. *Am J Psychiatry*, 1993. **150**:1343–8.

71. Chatterjee A., Chakos M., Koreen A., *et al.* Prevalence and clinical correlates extrapyramidal signs and spontaneous dyskinesia in never-medicated schizophrenic patients. *Am J Psychiatry*, 1995. **152**:1724–9.

72. Wolff A. L., Odriscoll G.A. Motor deficits and schizophrenia: the evidence from neuroleptic–naive patients and populations at risk. *J Psychiatry Neurosci*, 1999. **24**:304–14.

73. Paviour D. C., Surtees R. A., Lees A. J. Diagnostic considerations in juvenile Parkinsonism. *Mov Disord*, 2004. **19**:123–35.

74. Ismail B., Cantor-Graae E., McNeil T. F. Neurodevelopmental origins of tardivelike dyskinesia in schizophrenia patients and their siblings. *Schizophr Bull*, 2001. **27**:629–41.

75. Purl B. K., Barnes T. R., Chapman M. J., *et al.* Spontaneous dyskinesia in first episode schizophrenia. *J Neurol Neurosurg Psychiatry*, 1999. **66**:76–8.

76. Fenton W. S., Blyler C. R., Wyatt R. J., *et al.* Prevalence of spontaneous dyskinesia in schizophrenic and non-schizophrenic psychiatric patients. *Br J Psychiatry*, 1997. **171**:265–8.

77. Mckenna P. J., Lund C.E., Mortimer A. M., *et al.* Motor, volitional and behavioural disorders in schizophrenia. 2: The 'conflict of paradigms' hypothesis. *Br J Psychiatry*, 1991. **158**:328–36.

78. Karp B. I., Garvey M., Jacobsen L. K., *et al.* Abnormal neurologic maturation in adolescents with early-onset schizophrenia. *Am J Psychiatry*, 2001. **158**:118–22.

79. Hyde T., Hotson J., Kleinman J. Differential diagnosis of choreiform tardive dyskinesia.

J Neuropsychiatry Clin Neurosci, 1991. **3**:255–68.

80. Della Sal S., Francescani A., Spinnler H. Gait apraxia after bilateral supplementary motor area lesion. *J Neurol Neurosurg Psychiatry*, 2002. **72**:77–85.

81. Prager S., Jeste D. V. Sensory impairment in late-life schizophrenia. *Schizophr Bull*, 1993. **19**:755–72.

82. David A., Malmberg A., Lewis G., et al. Are there neurological and sensory risk factors for schizophrenia? *Schizophr Res*, 1995. **14**:247–51.

83. Schubert E. W., Henrjksson K. M., McNeil T. F. A prospective study of offspring of women with psychosis: visual dysfunction in early childhood predicts schizophrenia-spectrum disorders in adulthood. *Acta Psychiatr Scand*, 2005. **112**:385–93.

84. Stefanis N., Thewissen V., Bakoula C., et al. Hearing impairment and psychosis: a replication in a cohort of young adults. *Schizophr Res*, 2006. **85**:266–72.

85. Sjogren H. Paraphrenic, melancholic and psychoneurotic states in the presenile-senile period of life: a study of 649 patients in the functional division. *Acta Psychiatr Scand*, 1964. **40**: 1–63.

86. Gurian B., Wexler D., Baker E. Late-life paranoia: possible association with early trauma and infertility. *Int J Geriatr Psychiatry*, 1992. **7**:277–84.

87. Gordon A. G. Schizophrenia and the ear. *Schizophr Res*, 1995. **17**: 289–91.

88. Bartlett M. The sensory acuity of psychopathic individuals: a comparison of the auditory acuity of psychoneurotic and dementia praecox cases with that of normal individuals. *Psychiatr Q*, 1935. **9**:422–5.

89. Ludwig A. M., Wood B. S., Jr., Downs M. P. Auditory studies in

schizophrenia. *Am J Psychiatry*, 1962. **119**:122–7.

90. Hawkes C. Olfaction in neurodegenerative disorder. *Adv Otorhinolaryngol*, 2006. **63**: 133–5.

91. Kopala L., Clark C., Hurwitz T. Olfactory deficits in neuroleptic naive patients with schizophrenia. *Schizophr Res*, 1992. **8**:245–50.

92. Sirota P., Davidson B., Mosheva T., *et al.* Increased olfactory sensitivity in first episode psychosis and the effect of neuroleptic treatment on olfactory sensitivity in schizophrenia. *Psychiatry Res*, 1999. **86**: 143–53.

93. Collins L., Stone L. Pain sensitivity, age and activity level in chronic schizophrenics and normals. *Br J Psychiatry*, 1966. **112**:33–5.

94. Nasrallah H. A., Tippin J., Mccalley-Whitters M., *et al.* Neurological differences between paranoid and nonparanoid schizophrenia: Part III. Neurological soft signs. *J Clin Psychiatry*, 1982. **43**:310–2.

95. Detre T., Bunney W. E. Jr. Human vibration perception. II. A preliminary report on vibration perception in psychiatric patients. *Arch Gen Psychiatry*, 1961. **4**:615–8.

96. Fink M., Green M., Bender M. B. The face–hand test as a diagnostic sign of organic mental syndrome. *Neurology*, 1952. **2**:46–58.

97. Patten S. B., Lamarre C. J. The face–hand test: a useful addition to the psychiatric physical examination. *Psychiatr J Univ Ott*, 1989. **14**:554–6.

98. Sanders R. D., Joo Y. H., Almasy L., *et al.* Are neurologic examination abnormalities heritable? A preliminary study. *Schizophr Res*, 2006. **86**:172–80.

99. Jenkyn L. R., Walsh D. B., Culver C. M., *et al.* Clinical signs in diffuse cerebral dysfunction. *J Neurol Neurosurg Psychiatry*, 1977. **40**:956–66.

100. Arango C., Bartko J. J., Gold J. M., *et al.* Prediction of neuropsychological performance by neurological signs in schizophrenia. *Am J Psychiatry*, 1999. **156**:1349–57.

101. Sanders R., Shuepbach D., Keshavan M. S., *et al.* Neurologic exam abnormalities and neuropsychological performances in neuroleptic-naive psychosis. *J Neuropsychiatr Clin Neurosci*, 2004. **16**:480–7.

102. Moles J. K., Franchina J. J., Sforza P. P. Neurological deficits and CT findings in psychiatric patients. *Psychosomatics*, 1998. **39**:394–5.

103. Bae C. J., Pincus J. H. Neurologic signs predict periventricular white matter lesions on MRI. *Can J Neurol Sci*, 2004. **31**:242–7.

104. Murphy K. C. (2002) Schizophrenia and velo-cardio-facial syndrome. *Lancet*, 2002. **359**:426–30.

105. Baumann N., Turpin J. C., Lefevre M., *et al.* Motor and psycho-cognitive clinical types in adult metachromatic leukodystrophy: genotype/phenotype relationships? *J Physiol Paris*, 2002. **96**:301–6.

106. Rubino F. A. Neurologic complications of alcoholism. *Psychiatr Clin North Am*, 1992. **15**:359–72.

107. Casanova M. F. Wernicke's disease and schizophrenia: a case report and review of the literature. *Int J Psychiatry Med*, 1996. **26**:319–28.

108. Allen D. N., Goldstein G., Forman S. D., *et al.* Neurologic examination abnormalities in schizophrenia with and without a history of alcoholism. *Neuropsychiatry Neuropsychol Behav Neurol*, 2000. **13**:184–7.

109. Goldstein G., Allen D. N., Sanders R. D. Sensory-perceptual dysfunction in patients with schizophrenia and comorbid alcoholism. *J Clin Exp Neuropsychol*, 2002. **24**:1010–16.

110. Kinney D. K., Yurgelun-Todd D. A., Woods B. T. Neurologic signs of cerebellar and cortical sensory dysfunction in schizophrenics and their relatives. *Schizophr Res*, 1999. **35**:99–104.

111. Desmukh A., Rosenbloom M., Pfefferbaum A., *et al.* Clinical signs of cerebellar dysfunction in schizophrenia, alcoholism and their comorbidity. *Schizophr Res*, 2002. **57**:281–91.

112. Bartzokis G., Beckson M., Wirshing D. A., *et al.* Choreoathetoid movements in cocaine dependence. *Biol Psychiatry*, 1999. **45**:1630–5.

113. Bauer L. O. Resting hand tremor in abstinent cocaine-dependent, alcohol-dependent, and polydrug-dependent patients. *Alcohol Clin Exp Res*, 1996. **20**:1196–201.

5

Functional neuroimaging in schizophrenia

Serge A. Mitelman, Jane Zhang, and Monte S. Buchsbaum

Acknowledgments: This work was supported by NIMH grants P50 MH 66392–01, MH 60023, and MH 56489 to Dr. Buchsbaum and by NARSAD Young Investigator and NIMH MH 077146 awards to Dr. Mitelman.

Facts box

1. Functional imaging has shown decreases in resting activity and the amount of activation by cognitive tasks in the frontal lobe, temporal lobe, cingulate gyrus, and thalamus in schizophrenia.

2. Decreases in activity appear in regions that also show decreases in volume when anatomical imaging techniques are used.

3. The underlying etiology and pathogenesis of these activities and volume changes remain unclear.

4. Psychotic symptoms include auditory and visual hallucinations, paranoid delusions or paranoid trends, ideas of reference, ideas of influence, catatonia, and atypical features such as complex perceptual distortions. Although a link between psychotic symptoms and basal ganglia, temporal lobe, and frontal lobe pathology is supported, symptoms appear to be variable after the onset of neuronal damage, and remission has also been reported.

5. Treatment is largely symptomatic but links between brain region change and symptom change are being established.

Brain function and schizophrenia

Instruments for observing and assessing organ function have been technical eye-opening scientific advances in understanding of disease in the last 100 years. Although the uniform tissue composition and circulation-borne products of the liver and pancreas have made blood chemistry sampling and postmortem assessment fruitful approaches, the regional complexity and behavioral productions of the brain have made these methods less informative for the brain, the target organ of schizophrenia. In this review, we describe brain–function research in psychiatry from its inception with the electroencephalogram (EEG) to the current advances in regional metabolism, blood flow, receptor chemistry, and most recently, the deficiencies in the dynamic connectivity of circuits.

Electroencephalography, cerebral blood flow, and the earliest functional imaging of schizophrenia

Among the earliest observations in Jena, Germany, of Hans Berger, the developer of the electroencephalogram, was the observation of diminished occipital alpha activity in patients with schizophrenia [1]. This reduction in smooth rhythmic resting activity over the visual cortex, which is observed in normal individuals when they open their eyes, is consistent with modern computer analysis of the electrical signals and with concepts of heightened sensory responsiveness, the symptoms of hallucinations, and complex regional changes in brain function seen in schizophrenia. The earliest cerebral blood oxygen and glucose studies by Joseph Wortis and colleagues [2] at Bellevue Hospital in New York assessed arteriovenous difference and did not find patients with schizophrenia to be different from controls. Seymour Kety and colleagues, in 1948 at the University of Pennsylvania, studied cerebral blood flow (CBF) and similarly did not find differences in total CBF, but suggested that regional blood flow abnormalities might exist [3]. The current regional approach to brain imaging in schizophrenia began with the work of David Ingvar and coworkers in Lund, Sweden [4] who

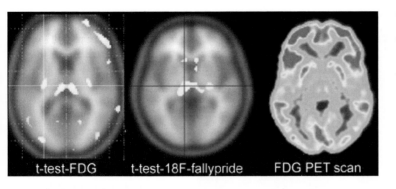

Figure 5.1 Hypofrontality: individual unmedicated patient with schizophrenia showing areas in prefrontal cortex (including Brodmann areas 10, 47, 9, 46) with relative metabolic rate two standard deviations below the normal control comparison group.

introduced regional functional imaging and staged cognitive tasks to identify specific brain regions activated by different mental activities and initiated the current direction of research in functional brain imaging in schizophrenia.

Hypofrontality

Starting with the initial observation using the [133]Xenon inhalation method by Ingvar and Franzen [4], and the first independent confirmation using the newly available positron emission tomography (PET) [5], resting hypofrontality, or reduced frontal-to-occipital metabolic ratios, in patients with schizophrenia has been reported in numerous studies by various methodologies [6, 7, 8, 9, 10]. Initially there were negative studies as well (e.g. [11, 12, 13, 14]). Similarly, task-related hypofrontality under various frontal lobe cognitive tasks in patients with schizophrenia has had almost as many proponents [6, 9, 15, 16, 17, 18] as detractors [19, 20]. Reviews of progress in functional neuroimaging concluded that hypofrontality had been the most consistent finding in schizophrenia [21, 22]; yet another contemporaneous review estimated that hypofrontality was found in only about one-third of published reports [23].

A more stringent meta-analysis of activation patterns in 103 suitable voxel-based [133]Xenon inhalation, single photon emission computed tomography (SPECT), and PET ([15]O$_2$ and FDG) studies of prefrontal activation supported both resting and task-activated hypofrontality in patients with schizophrenia [24]. Moreover, a positive association of resting hypofrontality with duration of illness was also suggested in this analysis and may provide an explanation for some of the earlier discrepancies. Whether this longitudinal pattern reflects the actual chronicity of the illness or disease-independent treatment effects

remains to be elucidated, for although hypofrontality has been demonstrated in neuroleptic-naïve patients [25], treatment with antipsychotic agents may contribute to its severity [26].

The newly emergent imaging technologies have also come to buttress this earliest of the functional neuroimaging findings of schizophrenia research: use of the functional near-infrared spectroscopy (fNIRS), still in its nascency, has already provided support for both the resting [27] and task-induced [28, 29] hypofrontality and for the association of its severity with the duration of illness. As a matter of fact, fNIRS studies in schizophrenia have thus far concentrated mainly on the prefrontal cortex [30, 31, 32, 33], and the findings have been congruent with the extensive body of previously available neuroimaging research.

Cerebral disconnectivity and schizophrenia

Schizophrenia, since its very nosological inception, had generally been considered a grey matter disease. Despite decades of intense neuropathological investigations that failed to establish anatomical basis of the illness, the vast majority of neuroimaging studies for a long time concentrated almost exclusively on the grey matter. Initial limitations of the available neuroimaging methodologies did confine their application mainly to the analysis of the ventricular system and anatomically bounded grey matter. Things began to change only with the advent of the newer tomographic techniques for functional neuroimaging – based on the positron-emission scintigraphy and later on the ultrafast sequences of magnetic resonance signal (MRS) acquisition. These methodological developments were paralleled by a shift of overall emphasis from localization of cerebral function to hodology

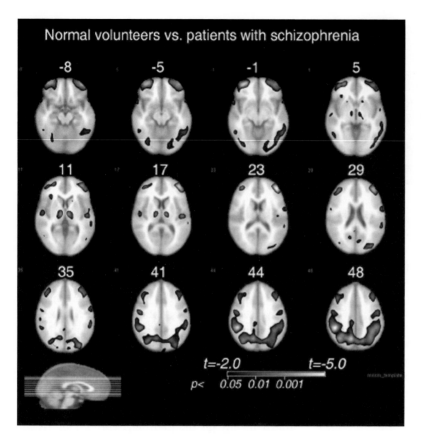

Figure 5.2 Group comparison of patients with schizophrenia and normal controls. Areas where patients (n = 59) are significantly lower than normals (n = 70) are shown with a black edge and light interior corresponding to the t grey-scale bar in the lower right. The Talairach z level is shown in mm above each slice image. The background to the patches identified as statistically significant is the Montreal Neurological Institute anatomical MRI brain.

in neuroanatomy as a scientific discipline [34]. The newly popular hodological, or connectionist, approach to functional neuroanatomy naturally led to refreshed interest in the so-called disconnection syndromes [35] and it did not take long for schizophrenia to be postulated as one [36, 37, 38, 39]. In fact, ideas regarding interhemispheric disconnectivity in schizophrenia had circulated even before the rise of modern neuroimaging techniques [40].

One of the most consistent theoreticians to regard schizophrenia as a disconnection syndrome – Karl Friston – has envisioned it as a disorder of functional integration, the central pathophysiological mechanism being that of disturbed synaptic plasticity [37, 41, 42, 43]. Friston regards schizophrenia as a primary disorder of synaptic transmission resulting in disconnectivity. He emphasizes dysfunctional regional integration as opposed to dysfunctional regional specialization (which he considers to be a secondary feature), and functional as opposed to anatomical disconnectivity. Some other authors suggest that developmental anatomical disconnectivity (i.e. miswiring),

stemming from the disturbed neuronal migration in the second trimester, may be at play [44, 45, 46, 47]. Indeed, supportive of the latter hypothesis, experimental miswiring of prefrontal efferents in Mongolian gerbils was recently induced by methamphetamine intoxication in the early postnatal period [6]. Still others point to the possibility that dysmyelination may be pivotal in the pathophysiology and even etiology of the illness [48], or – in other words – that schizophrenia is a white-matter disease par excellence. This view draws its supportive evidence from a host of recent cerebral gene expression, diffusion-weighted, and magnetization transfer imaging studies [49]. This is further bolstered by a very recent discovery that unlike the many grey-matter findings, relative glucose metabolism in patients with schizophrenia appears to be increased in the white matter [50]. Irrespective of the proposed pathophysiology, the disconnection hypothesis has served to shift the scientific interest away from structural volumetrics to functional interregional interactions. It also helps bridge the gap between the so-called "functional" and "organic" views of schizophrenia as this distinction becomes less clear when disconnection is considered to be the pathophysiological basis.

The neuroimaging methods for studying regional interconnectivity include evaluation of individual regions of interest and use of bivariate correlation coefficients or higher-order factor analysis, path analysis, and other multivariate techniques to infer the interregional relationships among them. Thus, interregional correlation matrices of glucose metabolic rates have been widely used and validated in the assessment of functional neural systems [51, 52, 53, 54, 55, 56]. Pairwise interregional metabolic correlations are thought to reflect *functional connectivity*, but these do not allow any inferences on the directionality of the functional regional interactions. Structural equation modeling based on *a priori* neuroanatomical assumptions has been employed in order to account for the directionality and strength of the interregional influences, that is, the so-called *effective connectivity* [57, 58, 59, 60]. These methods, initially developed for PET, have later been applied to time-series data derived from the functional MRI, and, rather than relying on manually applied regions of interest, now primarily exploit the statistical parametric mapping (SPM) analysis of voxel-to-voxel correlations at rest and under imposed cognitive tasks [61, 62, 63].

Use of continuous cognitive tasks allows for detection of relative activation failures at locations normally activated by a task or aberrant regional recruitment that may be conceptualized as pathological reliance on alternative networks in a compensatory effort. The major difficulty with this approach lies in the comparison of groups of subjects differing in test performance [64], whereby the differences in performance mediate the differential patterns of activation [65]. In addition, association of these pathologically recruited networks with specific clinical symptoms (e.g., hallucinations or specific delusional beliefs) or cognitive deficits (e.g., in short-term memory, implicit learning, or visual recognition) may allow for certain anatomical localization of the clinical semiotics.

Another approach to studying interregional integration in the brain is EEG evaluation of task-induced temporal synchronization of electrical activity across bandwidths and regions of interest. As with other functional neuroimaging methods, this may be accomplished by using bivariate correlative or phase coherence measures of time series data collected from preselected pairs of electrodes or by applying multivariate analytic techniques to the hypothesis-independent voxel-to-voxel measurements with the creation of synchronization maps.

Finally, evaluation of interregional correlations in volumetric data, derived from structural MRI analyses, may also be viewed as providing task-independent information on sustained, tonic activation of functional networks, consistent enough to result in correlated trophic influences and thus point to abnormalities of sustained networking in patients with schizophrenia relative to healthy controls. Theoretically, this approach allows for evaluation of chronically engaged, abnormal cerebral networks independently of a task. In our study comparing volumetric and metabolic thalamocortical intercorrelations in healthy subjects during a ubiquitous verbal learning task, metabolic intercorrelations were much more widespread and numerous in comparison to the correlations of regional volumes [66]. The idea that grey-matter volumetric abnormalities may be mediated by consistent functional activations is preliminarily supported by a recent study reporting that an association of thought disorder in schizophrenics with grey-matter reductions in planum temporale was mediated by posterior temporal hyperactivation in BOLD signal [67]. In group comparisons, significant direct interregional correlations present only in patients with schizophrenia would signify abnormal reliance on alternative strategies for compensatory information processing. The absence of normal interregional correlations in patients would signify reduced interregional connectivity [68, 69]. Following is the review of selected experimental literature on the aforementioned aspects of functional regional integration in schizophrenia.

Aberrant regional recruitment under a task

PET and SPECT

Countless assessments of regional changes in glucose metabolism or oxygen utilization have documented aberrant regional activations in patients with schizophrenia in association with a vast array of cognitive tasks and within a multitude of surveyed cerebral structures [70, 71]. These include the frontal lobe, mainly subregional prefrontal cortex [72, 73], anterior cingulate gyrus [74, 75, 76], temporal lobe [77], parietal lobe, posterior cingulate gyrus [75], occipital lobe

[77], striatum [78], cerebellum [79], thalamus and its subdivisions [80, 79, 81], including the mediodorsal nucleus [82, 83].

In some of the studies, functional disconnections have been inferred for the fronto-temporal [55, 84, 85, 86], prefronto-cingulate [87], prefronto-parietal [88], contralateral prefronto-hippocampal [89], occipito-temporal [77], as well as thalamo-cortical (specifically involving the mediodorsal nucleus in the left hemisphere, [90]), temporo-occipito-cerebellar and fronto-striatal regions [77]. In the more recent of these studies, multiple foci of aberrant activation have been documented.

A possible relationship of functional disconnectivity to acute state of the illness has been suggested by Erkwoh and colleagues [91] who, in a SPECT study, found that fronto-temporal disconnectivity in first-episode neuroleptic-naïve patients improved with symptom remission following antipsychotic treatment.

fMRI

Echoing the earlier metabolic PET studies, fMRI evaluations of task-induced changes in the BOLD signal in patients with schizophrenia have over the last two decades documented abnormal activation patterns involving the prefrontal cortex [92, 93, 94, 95], parietal cortex [96], temporal cortex [97, 94, 98], hippocampal circuitry [99, 100], primary visual areas [101], anterior cingulate [102, 95], thalamus [93], amygdala [103, 104], and cerebellum. Interregional disconnectivities under various tasks have been reported in the prefronto-cingulate and fronto-cerebellar circuitries, anterior cingulate and supplementary motor cortices.

Importantly, the number of negative studies purporting the lack of between-group differences among patients with schizophrenia and healthy controls has thus far been minimal, although these notably pertained to the oft-reported anterior cingulate region [105] and the fusiform gyrus [106]. Whereas poor task performance in many of these studies has been associated with hypoactivations in the relevant circuitries as compared to healthy control subjects, poor patient performance in some other tasks has actually been associated with hyperactivations, deemed reflective of an increased effort on the patients' part [107, 108].

Resting disconnectivity

fMRI

The studies that examined the resting state functional connectivity in patients with schizophrenia in the entire brain reported widespread functional disconnectivity (mainly reductions in connectivity), including within the so-called "default mode" network of brain activity [109, 110, 111]. Other more localized resting state investigations found reduced prefrontal lobe connectivity with the temporal [112] as well as parietal lobes, thalamus and striatum [113]. In this latter study, enhanced fronto-temporal resting connectivity in the left hemisphere was also reported [113]. At least some of the functional disconnectivities may be present even before the overt onset of illness in individuals at high genetic risk [114, 115, 116] and in never-medicated, first-outbreak patients [99, 102, 113], particularly in the prefrontal cortex [117].

Although the vast majority of the functional MRI (fMRI) studies report diminished connectivity in schizophrenia brains either diffusely at rest or as inferred from abnormal regional activations under an assembly of cognitive tasks, one recent study attempted to investigate a general pattern of connectivity between *the core* network engaged by a task (lexical decision making and retrieval in this case) and *the rest* of the brain, viewed as unstructured background noise [118]. The authors report that although the core topography per se did not differ among schizophrenia and healthy subjects, connectivity between *the core* and *the rest*, as well as within *the rest* of the brain, was higher in patients with schizophrenia. Moreover, within *the core*, fronto-parietal correlations in schizophrenia patients were significantly lower than in healthy subjects. The authors conclude that there appears to be diminished separation of the core task-related functional activity from the background noise, as well as diminished antero-posterior interlobar integration within the core. This finding may provide one possible explanation for the complicated patterns of both increased and decreased functional activations found with a variety of tasks as reviewed in the previous chapters. In a similar vein, Winder and colleagues [119] report diminished fronto-temporal connectivity in the left hemisphere and strengthened fronto-temporal connectivity in the right hemisphere during a matching task. Gur and colleagues [120] likewise found that patients not only underactivated target-specific areas to attentional demands, but also displayed an excessive employment of networks apparently committed to processing irrelevant stimuli.

EEG

Gamma-band electrical activity (high-frequency oscillations at ~40 Hz) has in recent years been at the very center of theoretical interest in the pathophysiology of schizophrenia because synchronization of activities in the gamma band is viewed as a likely candidate to account for the mechanism of integrative binding of disparate cerebral activities into unified networks [121]. This unifying mechanism has been considered necessary for the conscious sense of agency dating back to the Kantian theory of apperceptive self-awareness. Disruption in the mechanism of binding would therefore be resonant with the clinical descriptions of schizophrenia in terms of loose associations [122] or cognitive dysmetria [36], the pathophysiological concept of disconnection, and indeed the etymology of the nosological term itself (*schizo* and *phrenia*).

In spite of this theoretical interest in the gamma band, reports of disturbances in the somewhat lower-frequency beta band in the recent literature on schizophrenia have been no less frequent, which may in part be explained by terminological confusion. Thus, a study by Strelets *et al.* [123], which reported disruption of interhemispheric "high-frequency beta-rhythm" integration in the frontal lobes in patients with schizophrenia, in fact focused on the approximately 40 Hz oscillations that by many authors would be considered to lie in the gamma frequency band. Taken together, diminished synchronization of local oscillations in the high-frequency beta and gamma bands has been reported by several groups [124]. Other authors found reduced [125] or increased [126, 127, 128] coherence in the theta and delta frequency bands, generally assessed under resting condition. Widespread, particularly fronto-temporal, disconnectivity was documented using a related technique of low-resolution electromagnetic tomography (LORETA) as well [129, 130, 131, 132]. In addition, microstates of synchronous EEG activity at rest have been noted to be shorter [133, 134], sequentially different [135] and topographically more dispersed [136] in patients with schizophrenia, thus indicating both reduced maintenance of the synchronizations and impairment in their sequential integration.

Studies evaluating changes in correlations of regional EEG activity with cognitive (working memory) tasks have found reduced network recruitments in patients [137, 138]. Similarly, normal gamma-band synchronization preceding a willed motor act, talking or thinking (thought to reflect corollary discharge, important in theorizations on hallucinatory and delusional passivity phenomena, cf. [139]) has recently been reported to be diminished in patients with schizophrenia [140]. These studies generally use techniques akin to evoked response potentials.

The fact that some authors found increased synchronizations (i.e. hyperconnectivity), even in the lower range of the beta rhythm (<30 Hz), in patients with schizophrenia [127, 128, 141] or in their subgroups led Gruzelier [142] to propose that the direction of change may in fact be syndrome dependent, namely, diminished with the predominance of the negative symptoms and increased with the predominance of the positive symptoms. Lee and Cooeagyues [143] observed that although synchronization in gamma-band activity was decreased in the left frontal lobe in schizophrenia patients as a group, dividing the patients into three subgroups by the predominant clinical syndrome revealed decreased synchrony with psychomotor poverty, right hemispheric increase in synchrony with reality distortion, and widespread increase, involving more posterior regions, with disorganization. In a case report, intense tactile hallucinations in a nonschizophrenic patient also were specifically related to increased synchronicity in the gamma band [144]. Yet, in a study by Strelets and colleagues [123], both negative and positive syndrome groups of schizophrenics showed decreased synchronicity in the high-frequency beta/gamma rhythm, so that the issue remains unsettled at this time.

Some of the previous reports apparently evaluated first-episode schizophrenia patients [136, 133, 125, 126, 127, 145, 124, 128, 146] indicating that the abnormalities may already be present close to the clinical onset of the illness [147] or even represent a genetic diathesis for psychosis [148]. Strelets and colleagues [149] found some lateralized differences between the first-episode and chronic schizophrenia patients, although both groups displayed disordered interhemispheric connectivity.

A recent study, utilizing innovative statistical methodology, described differential patterns of fractal, higher-order temporal periodicity in the alpha and theta rhythm fluctuations in the frontal lobes among patients with schizophrenia and healthy comparison subjects, suggesting increased randomness (diminished regularity) in the patients in the alpha rhythm dynamics and, in contrast, diminished complexity (heightened regularity) in the theta rhythm dynamics [150]. Another innovative study [151], which analyzed multivariate S-estimator maps of synchronized electrical activity across a wide range of bandwidths, found a bilateral pattern of increased synchronization in the temporal regions and decreased synchronization in the upper parietal regions, both changes more pronounced with more severe psychopathology.

Structural (volumetric) intercorrelations

Two reports of detailed analyses of regional cortical intercorrelations of grey matter volumes by individual Brodmann areas [68, 69] documented reduced associations among proximate regions within the frontal and temporal lobes, and strengthening of more distant (interlobar) fronto-temporal, as well as fronto-parietal and temporo-occipital intercorrelations, albeit less prominently, in patients with schizophrenia. Fronto-temporal grey matter volume dissociations in schizophrenics have been reported in some other investigations [44, 152, 153].

Thalamo-cortical dissociations in patients with schizophrenia, assessed in another two studies from our laboratory [154, 155], were found to be rather widespread, especially with the prefrontal, medial-temporal, and cingulate-cortical regions in both hemispheres and, for the pulvinar with the occipital and orbito-frontal cortices in the right hemisphere. The latter pulvino-cortical dissociations were proposed to be pathogenetically related to visual attentional deficits amply described in patients with schizophrenia.

Functional imaging correlates of clinical symptomatology

A number of functional neuroimaging studies have in recent years increasingly focused on relationships between regional abnormalities and specific clinical symptoms or syndromes of schizophrenia [156]. Auditory hallucinations have been consistently related to activations in the left superior temporal gyrus and,

in some reports, to the right temporal lobe regions as well [42, 156, 157, 158, 159, 160, 161]. Reduced fronto-temporal connectivity was also associated with auditory hallucinations [162] and there was an observation of an accentuated multiregional response to emotion-laden words in hallucinating patients [163]. Similar to the described activations in auditory cortical areas with auditory hallucinations, a case report of fMRI in a patient with visual hallucinations revealed activation in the visual areas and the hippocampus [164].

Formal thought disorder, specifically disturbance in the train of thought, has been related to underactivation of the posterior (Wernicke's) part of the superior temporal gyrus [165, 166, 167] and Broca's area in the frontal lobe [168]. Receptive prosodic disturbances [169] and misattribution of speech [170, 171] in patients were also associated with primary auditory cortex and its connectivity with the anterior cingulate.

Reality distortion was associated with hyperactivation in the medial prefrontal cortex [172] and a persecutory attributional stance in patients was accompanied by more severe prefronto-amygdalar disconnection [173].

Impaired connectivity between the anterior-cingulate and supplementary motor areas was related to negative symptoms. The poor functional outcome in schizophrenia overall was associated with more severe hypoactivation in the temporal lobe and cingulate gyrus, as well as more significant hypofrontality at rest, as compared to the good-outcome patient group [174]. Finally, one of the often-reported schizophrenia endophenotypes – impaired inhibition of saccadic eye movements – was ascribed to failure to activate the lentiform nuclei, thalami, and the left inferior frontal gyrus in response to an antisaccadic task [175].

Receptor occupancy evaluation with PET

Dopamine D_2 receptor binding in neuroleptic-naive patients with schizophrenia has in recent years been studied using raclopride-^{11}C as the ligand. Reduced ligand binding has been reported in the thalamus [176, 177, 178], especially within the left medio-dorsal and pulvinar nuclei [176], as well as the anterior cingulate [176, 179], amygdala [176], but not the caudate [177]. The biggest effect has thus far been reported in the

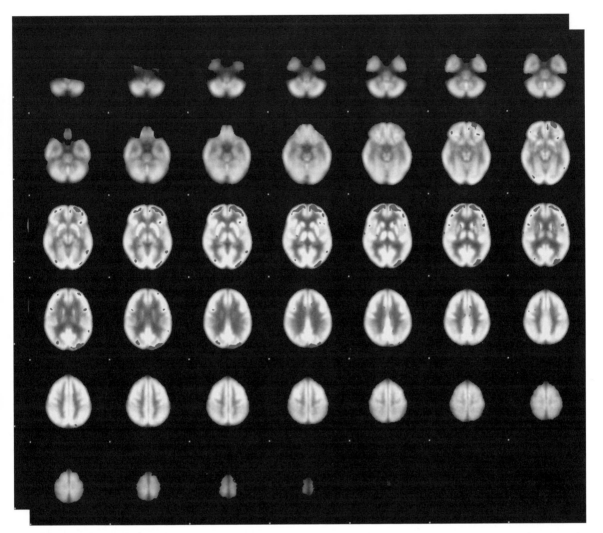

Figure 5.3 Significance probability mapping [184] test areas of decrease in FDG relative metabolic rate and D2 receptor binding. (See color plate section.)

thalamus. One study that found no regional between-group differences in the raclopride C11 binding [180] did report a significant direct correlation between the ligand binding in the frontal lobe and the positive symptom severity in schizophrenics.

Preliminary investigations with some other ligands have been less conclusive, with reports of either no intergroup differences [181] or elevated binding [182] for serotonin 1A receptors, as well as the as-yet unreplicated finding of decreased frontal lobe binding for histamine H1 receptors [183].

Conclusion and new directions

At the present time, all functional neuroimaging modalities are in transition from being strictly research tools to assisting clinical diagnosis and treatment choice. Work is being done on developing fMRI classificatory instruments aimed at image-based identification of patients with schizophrenia [185] and on PET prediction of response to neuroleptic treatment [186]. This may be reasonably expected to eventually make functional neuroimaging clinically useful for diagnosis and treatment.

References

1. Gloor, P. Hans Berger and the discovery of the electro-encephalogram. *Electroencephalography and Clin Neurophysiol*, 1969. (Suppl) **28**:1–36.

2. Wortis J., Bowman K. M., Goldfarb W. Human brain metabolism: normal values and values in certain clinical states. *Am J Psychiatry*, 1940–1. **97**: 552–65.

3. Kety S. S., Woodford R., *et al.* Cerebral blood flow and metabolism in schizophrenia. *Am J Psychiatry*, 1948. **104**: 765–70.

4. Ingvar D. H., Franzen G. Abnormalities of cerebral blood flow distribution in patients with chronic schizophrenia. *Acta Psychiatr Scand*, 1974. **50**: 425–62.

5. Buchsbaum M. S., Ingvar D. H., Kessler R., *et al.* Cerebral glucography with positron emission tomography. Use in normal subjects and in patients with schizophrenia. *Arch Gen Psychiatry*, 1982. **39**:251–59.

6. Andreasen N. C., Rezai K., Alliger R., *et al.* Hypofrontality in neuroleptic-naive patients and in patients with chronic schizophrenia. Assessment with xenon 133 single-photon emission computed tomography and the Tower of London. *Arch Gen Psychiatry*, 1992. **49**:943–58.

7. Bagorda F., Teuchert-Noodt G., Lehmann K.. Isolation rearing or methamphetamine traumatisation induce a "disconnection" of prefrontal efferents in gerbils: implications for schizophrenia. *J Neural Transm*, 2006. **113**:365–79.

8. Farkas T., Wolf A. P., Jaeger J., *et al.* Regional brain glucose metabolism in chronic schizophrenia. A positron emission transaxial tomographic study. *Arch Gen Psychiatry*, 1984. **41**:293–300.

9. Ortuño F., Moreno-Iñiguez M., Millan M., *et al.* Cortical blood flow during rest and Wisconsin Card Sorting Test performance in schizophrenia. *Wien Med Wochenschr*, 2006. **156**:179–84.

10. Wolkin A., Jaeger J., Brodie J. D., *et al.* Persistence of cerebral metabolic abnormalities in chronic schizophrenia as determined by positron emission tomography. *Am J Psychiatry*, 1985. **142**:564–71.

11. Ebmeier K. P., Lawrie S. M., Blackwood D. H. R., *et al.* Hypofrontality revisited: a high resolution single photon emission computed tomography study in schizophrenia. *J Neurosurg Psychiatry*, 1995. **58**:452–6.

12. Gur R. E., Skolnick B. E., Gur R. C., *et al.* Brain function in psychiatric disorders. I. Regional cerebral blood flow in medicated schizophrenics. *Arch Gen Psychiatry*, 1983. **40**:1250–54.

13. Matthew R. J., Duncan G. C., Weinman M. L., *et al.* Regional cerebral blood flow in schizophrenia. *Arch Gen Psychiatry*, 1982. **39**:1121–4.

14. Sheppard G., Gruzelier J., Manchanda R., *et al.* 15O positron emission tomographic scanning of predominantly never-treated acute schizophrenic patients. *Lancet*, 1983. 1448–52.

15. Buchsbaum M. S., Nuechterlein K. H., Haier R. J., *et al.* Glucose metabolic rate in normals and schizophrenics during the continuous performance test assessed by positron emission tomography. *Br J Psychiatry*, 1990. **156**:216–27.

16. Hazlett E. A., Buchsbaum M. S., Jeu L. A., *et al.* Hypofrontality in unmedicated schizophrenia patients studied with PET during performance of a serial verbal learning task. *Schizophr Res*, 2000. 43:33–46.

17. Steinberg J. L., Devous Sr. M. D., Paulman R. G. Wisconsin card sorting activated regional cerebral blood flow in first break and chronic schizophrenic patients and normal controls. *Schizophr Res*, 1996. **19**:177–87.

18. Weinberger D. R., Berman K. F., Zec R. F. Physiological dysfunction in dorsolateral prefrontal cortex in schizophrenia. I. Regional cerebral blood flow evidence. *Arch Gen Psychiatry*, 1986. **43**: 114–24.

19. Callicott J. H., Bretolino A., Mattay V. S., *et al.* Physiological dysfunction of the dorsolateral prefrontal cortex in schizophrenia revisited. *Cereb Cortex*, 2000. **10**;1078–92.

20. Walter H., Wunderlich A. P., Blankenhorn M., *et al.* No hypofrontality, but absence of prefrontal lateralization comparing verbal and spatial working memory in schizophrenia. *Schizophr Res*, 2003. **61**:175–84.

21. Andreasen N. C., O'Leary D. S., Flaum M., *et al.* Hypofrontality in schizophrenia: distributed dysfunctional circuits in neuroleptic-naïve patients. *Lancet*, 1997. **349**:1730–4.

22. Velakoulis D., Pantelis C. What have we learned from functional imaging studies in schizophrenia? The role of frontal, striatal and temporal areas. *Aust N Z J Psychiatry*, 1996. **30**:195–209.

23. Chua S. E., McKenna P. J. Schizophrenia – a brain disease? A critical review of structural and functional cerebral abnormality in the disorder. *Br J Psychiatry*, 1996. **166**:563–82.

24. Hill K., Mann L., Laws K. R., *et al.* Hypofrontality in schizophrenia: a meta-analysis of functional imaging studies. *Acta Psychiatr Scand*, 2004. **110**:243–56.

25. Molina V., Sanz J., Reig S., *et al.* Hypofrontality in males with first-episode psychosis. *Br J Psychiatry*, 2005. **186**:203–8.

26. Molina V., Sanz J., Sarramea F., *et al.* Marked hypofrontality in clozapine-responsive patients. *Pharmacopsychiatry*, 2007. **40**:157–62.

27. Hoshi Y., Shinba T., Sato C., *et al.* Resting hypofrontality in schizophrenia: a study using near-infrared time-resolved spectroscopy. *Schizophr Res*, 2006. **84**:411–20.

28. Shinba T., Nagano M., Kariya N., *et al.* Near-infrared spectroscopy analysis of frontal lobe dysfunction in schizophrenia. *Biol Psychiatry*, 2004. **55**:154–64.

29. Watanabe A., Kato T. Cerebrovascular response to cognitive tasks in patients with schizophrenia measured by near-infrared spectroscopy. *Schizophr Bull*, 2004. **30**:435–44.

30. Fallgatter A. J., Strik W. K. Reduced frontal functional asymmetry in schizophrenia during a cued continuous performance test assessed with near-infrared spectroscopy. *Schizophr Bull*, 2000. **26**:913–19.

31. Kubota Y., Toichi M., Shimuzu M., *et al.* Prefrontal activation during verbal fluency tests in schizophrenia–a near-infrared spectroscopy (NIRS) study. *Schizophr Res*, 2005. **77**:65–73.

32. Okada F., Tokumitsu Y., Hoshi Y., *et al.* Impaired interhemispheric integration in brain oxygenation and hemodynamics in schizophrenia. *Eur Arch Psychiatry Clin Neurosci*, 1994. **244**:17–25.

33. Suto T., Fukuda M., Ito M., *et al.* Multichannel near-infrared spectroscopy in depression and schizophrenia: cognitive brain activation study. *Biol Psychiatry*, 2004. **55**:501–11.

34. ffytche D. H., Catani M. Beyond localization: from hodology to function. *Phil Trans R Soc B*, 2005. **360**:767–79.

35. Catani M., ffytche D. H. The rises and falls of disconnection syndromes. *Brain*, 2005. **128**:2224–39.

36. Andreasen N. C., Paradiso S., O'Leary D. S. "Cognitive dysmetria" as an integrative theory of schizophrenia: a dysfunction in cortical–subcortical–cerebellar circuitry? *Schizophr Bull*, 1998. **24**:203–18.

37. Friston K. J., Frith C. D. Schizophrenia: a disconnection syndrome? *Clin Neurosci*, 1995. **3**:89–97.

38. Goldberg E., Bilder R. M., Hughes J. E., *et al.* A reticulo-frontal disconnection syndrome. *Cortex*, 1989. **25**:687–95.

39. Swerdlow N., Koob G. Dopamine, schizophrenia, mania, and depression: towards a unified hypothesis of cortico-striato-palido-thalamic function. *Behav Brain Sci*, 1987. **10**:197–245.

40. Beaumont J. G., Dimond S. J. Brain disconnection and schizophrenia. *Br J Psychiatry*, 1973. **123**:661–2.

41. Friston K. J. The disconnection hypothesis. *Schizophr Res*, 1998. **30**:115–25.

42. Friston K. J. Schizophrenia and the disconnection hypothesis. *Acta Psychiatr Scand Suppl*, 1999. **395**:68–79.

43. Stephan K. E., Baldeweg T., Friston K. J. Synaptic plasticity and disconnection in schizophrenia. *Biol Psychiatry*, 2006. **59**:929–39.

44. Bullmore E. T., Frangou S., Murray R. M. The dysplastic net hypothesis: an integration of developmental and dysconnectivity theories of schizophrenia. *Schizophr Res*, 1997. **28**:143–56.

45. Bullmore E. T., Woodruff P. W., Wright I. C., *et al.* Does dysplasia cause anatomical dysconnectivity in schizophrenia? *Schizophr Res*, 1998. **30**:127–35.

46. Jones, E. (1995) Cortical development and neuropathology in schizophrenia. In *Development of the Cerebral Cortex*, vol **193**, Block G. (Ed.). New York: J. Wiley, pp. 277–95.

47. Jones, E. Cortical development and thalamic pathology in schizophrenia. *Schizophr Bull*, 1997. **23**:483–501.

48. Davis K. L., Stewart D. G., Friedman J. I., *et al.* White matter changes in schizophrenia: evidence for myelin-related dysfunction. *Arch Gen Psychiatry*, 2003. **60**:443–56.

49. Kubicki M., McCarley R. W., Shenton M. E. Evidence for white matter abnormalities in schizophrenia. *Curr Opin Psychiatry*, 2005. **18**:121–34.

50. Buchsbaum M. S., Buchsbaum B. R., Hazlett E. A., *et al.* Relative glucose metabolic rate higher in white matter in patients with schizophrenia. *Am J Psychiatry*, 2007b. **164**:1072–81.

51. Clark C. M., Kessler R., Buchsbaum M. S., *et al.* Correlational methods for determining regional coupling of cerebral glucose metabolism: a pilot study. *Biol Psychiatry*, 1984. **19**:663–78.

52. Horwitz B., Duara R., Rapoport S. I. Intercorrelations of glucose metabolic rates between brain regions: application to healthy males in a state of reduced sensory input. *J Cereb Blood Flow Metab*, 1984. **4**:484–99.

53. Horwitz B. Simulating functional interactions in the brain: a model for examining correlations between regional cerebral metabolic rates. *Int J Biomed Comput*, 1990. **26**:149–70.

54. Horwitz B. Functional interactions in the brain: use of correlations between regional metabolic rates. *J Cereb Blood Flow Metab*, 1991. **11**:A114–A120.

55. Katz M., Buchsbaum M. S., Siegel B. V. Jr., *et al.* Correlational

patterns of cerebral glucose metabolism in never-medicated schizophrenics. *Neuropsychobiology*, 2006. **33**:1–11.

56. Kessler R. M., Clark C. M., Buchsbaum M. S., *et al.* (1983). Regional correlations in patterns of glucose use in patients with schizophrenia and normal subjects during mild pain stimulation. In *Positron Emission Tomography of the Brain*, W. D. Heiss and M. E. Phelps (Eds.). Berlin: Springer Verlag, pp. 196–200.

57. Friston K. J. Functional and effective connectivity: a synthesis. *Hum Brain Mapp*, 1994. **2**: 56–78.

58. Lagreze H. L. Hartmann A., Anzinger G., *et al.* Functional cortical interaction patterns in visual perception and visuospatial problem solving. *J Neurol Sci*, 1993. **114**:25–35.

59. McIntosh A. R. Gonzalez-Lima F. Network interactions among limbic cortices, basal forebrain, and cerebellum differentiate a tone conditioned as a Pavlovian excitor or inhibitor: fluoro-deoxyglucose mapping and covariance structural modeling. *J Neurophysiol*, 1994. **72**:1717–33.

60. McIntosh A. R., Grady C. L., Ungerleider L. G., *et al.* Network analysis of cortical visual pathways mapped with PET. *J Neurosci*, 1994. **14**:655–66.

61. Rogers B.P., Morgan V.L., Newton A.T., *et al.* Assessing functional connectivity in the human brain by fMRI. *Magn Reson Imaging*, 2007. **25**:1347–57.

62. Schlosser R., Gesierich G. T., Kaufmann B., *et al.* Altered effective connectivity during working memory performance in schizophrenia: a study with fMRI and structural equation modeling *Neuroimage*, 2003a. **19**:751–63.

63. Schlosser R. G., Gesierich T., Kaufmann B., *et al.* Altered

effective connectivity in drug free schizophrenic patients. *Neuroreport*, 2003b. **14**:2233–7.

64. Brown G. G., Eyler L. T. Methodological and conceptual issues in functional magnetic resonance imaging: applications to schizophrenia research. *Annu Rev Clin Psychol*, 2006. **2**: 51–81.

65. Snellenberg J. X. van, Torres I. J., Thornton A.E. Functional neuroimaging of working memory in schizophrenia: task performance as a moderating variable. *Neuropsychology*, 2006. **20**:497–510.

66. Mitelman S. A. Byne W., Kemether E. M., *et al.* Metabolic thalamocortical correlations during a verbal learning task and their comparison with correlations among regional volumes. *Brain Res*, 2006. **1114**:125–37.

67. Weinstein S., Woodward T. S., Ngan E. T. Brain activation mediates the association between structural abnormality and symptom severity in schizophrenia. *Neuroimage*, 2007. **36**:188–93.

68. Mitelman S. A., Shihabuddin L., Brickman A. M., *et al.* Cortical intercorrelations of temporal area volumes in schizophrenia. *Schizophr Res*, 2005. **76**:207–29.

69. Mitelman S. A., Buchsbaum M. S., Brickman A. M., *et al.* Cortical intercorrelations of frontal area volumes in schizophrenia. *Neuroimage*, 2005. **27**:753–70.

70. Buchsbaum M. S. Positron emission tomography studies of abnormal glucose metabolism in schizophrenic illness. *Clin Neurosci*, 1995. **3**:122–30.

71. Buchsbaum M. S., Hazlett E. A. Positron emission tomography studies of abnormal glucose metabolism in schizophrenia. *Schizophr Bull*, 1998. **24**:343–64.

72. Siegel B. V., Jr., Buchsbaum M. S., Bunney W. E., Jr., *et al.*

Cortical-striatal-thalamic circuits and brain glucose metabolic activity in 70 unmedicated male schizophrenic patients. *Am J Psychiatry*, 1993. **150**:1325–36.

73. Volkow N. D., Wolf A. P., Brodie J. D., *et al.* Brain interactions in chronic schizophrenics under resting and activation condition. *Schizophr Res*, 1988. **1**:47–53.

74. Fujimoto T., Takeuch K., Matsumoto T., *et al.* Abnormal glucose metabolism in the anterior cingulate cortex in patients with schizophrenia. *Psychiatry Res*, 2007. **154**:49–58.

75. Haznedar M. M., Buchsbaum M. S., Hazlett E. A., *et al.* Cingulate gyrus volume and metabolism in the schizophrenia spectrum. *Schizophr Res*, 2004. **71**:249–62.

76. Yücel M., Brewer W. J., Harrison B. J., *et al.* Anterior cingulate activation in antipsychotic-naïve first-episode schizophrenia. *Acta Psychiatr Scand*, 2007. **115**: 155–8.

77. Kim J. J., Seok J. H., Park H. J., *et al.* Functional disconnection of the semantic networks in schizophrenia. *Neuroreport*, 2005. **16**:355–9.

78. Shihabuddin L., Buchsbaum M. S., Hazlett E. A., *et al.* Dorsal striatal size, shape, and metabolic rate in never-medicated and previously medicated schizophrenics performing a verbal learning task. *Arch Gen Psychiatry*, 1998. **55**:235–43.

79. Crespo-Facorro B., Paradiso S., Andreasen N. C., *et al.* Recalling word lists reveals "cognitive dysmetria" in schizophrenia: a positron emission tomography study. *Am J Psychiatry*, 1999. **156**:386–92.

80. Buchsbaum M. S., Someya T., Teng C. Y., *et al.* PET and MRI of the thalamus in never-medicated patients with schizophrenia. *Am J Psychiatry*, 1996. **153**:191–9.

81. Hazlett E. A., Buchsbaum M. S., Byne W., *et al.* Three-dimensional

analysis with MRI and PET of the size, shape, and function of the thalamus in the schizophrenia spectrum. *Am J Psychiatry*, 1999. **156**:1190–9.

82. Hazlett E. A., Buchsbaum M. S., Kemether E. M., *et al.* Abnormal glucose metabolism in the mediodorsal nucleus of the thalamus in schizophrenia. *Am J Psychiatry*, 2004. **161**:305–14.

83. Lehrer D. S., Christian B. T., Mantil J., *et al.* Thalamic and prefrontal FDG uptake in never medicated patients with schizophrenia. *Am J Psychiatry*, 2005. **162**:931–8.

84. Meyer-Lindenberg A., Poline J. B., Kohn P. D., *et al.* Evidence for abnormal cortical functional connectivity during working memory in schizophrenia, *Am J Psychiatry*, 2001. **158**:1809–17.

85. Ragland J. D., Gur R. C., Glahn D. C., *et al.* Frontotemporal cerebral blood flow change during executive and declarative memory tasks in schizophrenia: a positron emission tomography study. *Neuropsychology*, 1998. **12**:399–413.

86. Ragland J. D., Gur R. C., Raz J., *et al.* Effect of schizophrenia on frontotemporal activity during word encoding and recognition: a PET cerebral blood flow study. *Am J Psychiatry*, 2001. **158**:1114–25.

87. Spence S. A., Liddle P. F., Stefan M. D., *et al.* Functional anatomy of verbal fluency in people with schizophrenia and those at genetic risk. Focal dysfunction and distributed disconnectivity reappraised. *Br J Psychiatry*, 2000. **176**:52–60.

88. Kim J. J., Kwon J. S., Park H. J., *et al.* Functional disconnection between the prefrontal and parietal cortices during working memory processing in schizophrenia: a [15O]H2O PET study. *Am J Psychiatry*, 2003. **160**:919–23.

89. Meyer-Lindenberg A. S., Olsen R. K., Kohn P. D., *et al.* Regionally specific disturbance of dorsolateral prefrontal-hippocampal functional connectivity in schizophrenia. *Arch Gen Psychiatry*, 2005. **62**:379–86.

90. Mitelman S. A. Byne W., Kemether E. M., *et al.* Metabolic disconnection between the mediodorsal nucleus of the thalamus and cortical Brodmann's areas of the left hemisphere in schizophrenia. *Am J Psychiatry*, 2005d. **162**:1733–5.

91. Erkwoh R., Sabri O., Willmes K., *et al.* Aspects of cerebral connectivity in schizophrenia. A comparative CBF study on treated schizophrenics before and after medication. *Fortschr Neurol Psychiatr*, 1999. **67**:318–26.

92. Kaladjian A., Jeanningros R., Azorin J. M., *et al.* Blunted activation in right ventrolateral prefrontal cortex during motor response inhibition in schizophrenia. *Schizophr Res*, 2007. **97**:184–93.

93. Schlösser R. G., Koch K., Wagner G., *et al.* Inefficient executive cognitive control in schizophrenia is preceded by altered functional activation during information encoding: an fMRI study. *Neuropsychologia*, 2008. **46**:336–47. [Epub Jul 19, 2007.]

94. Schneider F., Habel U., Reske M., *et al.* Neural substrates of olfactory processing in schizophrenia patients and their healthy relatives. *Psychiatr Res*, 2007. **155**:103–12.

95. Weiss E. M., Siedentopf C., Golaszewski S., *et al.* Brain activation patterns during a selective attention test – a functional MRI study in healthy volunteers and unmedicated patients during an acute episode of schizophrenia. *Psychiatry Res*, 2007. **154**:31–40.

96. Barch D. M., Csernansky J. G. Abnormal parietal cortex activation during working memory in schizophrenia: verbal phonological coding disturbances versus domain-general executive dysfunction. *Am J Psychiatry*, 2007. **164**:1090–8.

97. Ragland J. D., Gur R. C., Valdez J., *et al.* Event-related fMRI of frontotemporal activity during word encoding and recognition in schizophrenia. *Am J Psychiatry*, 2004. **161**:1004–15.

98. Walter H., Vasic N., Höse A., *et al.* Working memory dysfunction in schizophrenia compared to healthy controls and patients with depression: evidence from event-related fMRI. *Neuroimage*, 2007. **35**:1551–61.

99. Achim A. M., Bertrand M. C., Sutton H., *et al.* Selective abnormal modulation of hippocampal activity during memory formation in first-episode psychosis. *Arch Gen Psychiatry*, 2007. **64**:999–1014.

100. Weiss A. P., Goff D., Schacter D. L., *et al.* Fronto-hippocampal function during temporal context monitoring in schizophrenia. *Biol Psychiatry*, 2006. **60**:1268–77.

101. Haenschel C., Bittner R. A., Haertling F., *et al.* Contribution of impaired early-stage visual processing to working memory dysfunction in adolescents with schizophrenia. *Arch Gen Psychiatry*, 2007. **64**:1229–40.

102. Boksman K., Theberge J., Williamson P., *et al.* A 4.0-T fMRI study of brain connectivity during word fluency in first-episode schizophrenia. *Schizophr Res*, 2005. **75**:247–63.

103. Das P., Kemp A. H., Flynn G., *et al.* Functional disconnections in the direct and indirect amygdale pathways for fear processing in schizophrenia. *Schizophr Res*, 2007. **90**:284–94.

104. Tregellas J. R., Tanabe J. L., Miller D. E., *et al.* Neurobiology of

smooth pursuit eye movement deficits in schizophrenia: an fMRI study. *Am J Psychiatry*, 2004. **161**:315–21.

105. Harrison B. J., Yücel M., Fornito A., *et al.* Characterizing anterior cingulate activation in chronic schizophrenia: a group and single-subject fMRI study. *Acta Psychiatr Scand*, 2007. **116**: 271–9.

106. Yoon J. H., D'Esposito M., Carter C. S. Preserved function of the fusiform face area in schizophrenia as revealed by fMRI. *Psychiatry Res*, 2006. **148**:201–16.

107. Kuperberg G. R., Deckersbach T., Holt D. J., *et al.* Increased temporal and prefrontal activity in response to semantic associations in schizophrenia. *Arch Gen Psychiatry*, 2007. **64**:138–51.

108. Tregellas J. R., Davalos D. B., Rojas D. C., *et al.* Increased hemodynamic response in the hippocampus, thalamus and prefrontal cortex during abnormal sensory gating in schizophrenia. *Schizophr Res*, 2007. **92**:262–72.

109. Bluhm R. L., Miller J., Lanius R. A., *et al.* Spontaneous low-frequency fluctuations in the BOLD signal in schizophrenic patients: anomalies in the default network. *Schizophr Bull*, 2007. **33**:1004–12.

110. Garrity A. G., Pearslon G. D., McKiernan K., *et al.* Aberrant "default mode" functional connectivity in schizophrenia. *Am J Psychiatry*, 2007. **164**:450–7.

111. Liang M., Zhou Y., Jiang T., *et al.* Widespread functional disconnectivity in schizophrenia with resting-state functional magnetic resonance imaging. *Neuroreport*, 2006. **17**:209–13.

112. Wolf D. H., Gur R. C., Valdez J. N., *et al.* Alterations of fronto-temporal connectivity during word encoding in schizophrenia. *Psychiatry Res*, 2007. **154**:221–32.

113. Zhou Y., Liang M., Jiang T., *et al.* Functional dysconnectivity of the dorsolateral prefrontal cortex in first-episode schizophrenia using resting-state fMRI. *Neurosci Lett*, 2007. **417**:297–302.

114. Li X., Branch C. A., Bertisch H. C., *et al.* An fMRI study of language processing in people at high genetic risk for schizophrenia. *Schizophr Res*, 2007. **91**:62–72.

115. Thermenos H. W., Seidman L. J., Poldrack R. A., *et al.* Elaborative verbal encoding and altered anterior parahippocampal activation in adolescents and young adults at genetic risk for schizophrenia using MRI. *Biol Psychiatry*, 2007. **61**:564–74.

116. Whalley H. C., Simonotto E., Marshall I., *et al.* Functional disconnectivity in subjects at high genetic risk of schizophrenia. *Brain*, 2005. **128**:2097–108.

117. Fusar-Poli P., Perez J., Broome M., *et al.* Neurofunctional correlates of vulnerability to psychosis: a systematic review and meta-analysis. *Neurosci Biobehav Rev*, 2007. **31**:465–84.

118. Foucher J. R., Vidaihet P., Chanraud S., *et al.* Functional integration in schizophrenia: too little or too much? Preliminary results on fMRI data. *Neuroimage*, 2005. **26**:374–88.

119. Winder R., Cortes C. R., Reggia J. A., *et al.* Functional connectivity in fMRI: A modeling approach for estimation and for relating to local circuits. *Neuroimage*, 2007. **34**:1093–107.

120. Gur R. E., Turetsky B. I., Loughead J., *et al.* Visual attention circuitry in schizophrenia investigated with oddball event-related functional magnetic resonance imaging. *Am J Psychiatry*, 2007. **164**:442–9.

121. Lee K. H., Williams L. M., Breakspear M., *et al.* Synchronous gamma activity: a review and contribution to an integrative neuroscience model of schizophrenia. *Brain Res Rev*, 2003. **41**:57–78.

122. Bleuler E. (1911). *Dementia praecox or the group of schizophrenias*. Zinkin J., translator. New York: International Universities Press.

123. Strelets V. B., Novototsky-Vlasov V. Y., Golikova J. V. Cortical connectivity in high frequency beta-rhythm in schizophrenics with positive and negative symptoms. *Int J Psychophysiol*, 2002. **44**:101–15.

124. Symond M. P., Harris A. W., Gordon E., *et al.* "Gamma synchrony" in first-episode schizophrenia: a disorder of temporal connectivity? *Am J Psychiatry*, 2005. **162**:459–65.

125. Koenig T., Lehmann D., Saito N., *et al.* Decreased functional connectivity of EEG theta-frequency activity in first-episode, neuroleptic-naïve patients with schizophrenia: preliminary results. *Schizophr Res*, 2001. **50**:55–60.

126. Merrin E.L., Floyd T.C., Fein G. EEG coherence in unmedicated schizophrenic patients. *Biol Psychiatry*, 1989. **25**:60–6.

127. Nagase Y., Okubo Y., Matsuura M., *et al.* EEG coherence in unmedicated schizophrenic patients: topographical study of predominantly never medicated cases. *Biol Psychiatry*, 1992. **32**:1028–34.

128. Wada Y., Nanbu Y., Kikuchi M., *et al.* Aberrant functional organization in schizophrenia: analysis of EEG coherence during rest and photic stimulation in drug-naïve patients. *Neuropsychobiology*, 1998. **38**:63–9.

129. Kawasaki Y., Sumiyoshi T., Higuchi Y., *et al.* Voxel-based analysis of P300 electrophysiological topography associated with positive and negative symptoms of

schizophrenia. *Schizophr Res*, 2007. **94**:164–71.

130. Mientus S., Gallinat J., Wuebben Y., *et al.* Cortical hypoactivation during resting EEG in schizophrenics but not in depressives and schizotypal subjects as revealed by low resolution electromagnetic tomography (LORETA). *Psychiatry Res*, 2002. **116**: 95–111.

131. Pae J. S., Kwon J. S., Youn T., *et al.* LORETA imaging of P300 in schizophrenia with individual MRI and 128-channel EEG. *Neuroimage*, 2003. **20**:1552–60.

132. Winterer G., Mulert C., Mientus S., *et al. Brain Topogr*, 2001. **13**:299–313.

133. Koenig T., Lehmann D., Merlo M. C., *et al.* A deviant EEG brain microstate in acute, neuroleptic-naïve schizophrenics at rest. *Eur Arch Psychiatry Clin Neurosci*, 1999. **249**:205–11.

134. Strelets V. B., Farber P. L., Golikova J. V., *et al.* Chronic schizophrenics with positive symptomatology have shortened EEG microstate durations. *Clin Neurophysiol*, 2003. **114**:2043–51.

135. Sakkalis V., Oikonomou T., Pachou E., *et al.* Time-significant wavelet coherence for the evaluation of schizophrenic brain activity using a graph theory approach. *Conf Poc IEEE Eng Med Biol Soc*, 2006. **1**:4265–8.

136. Breakspear M., Terry J. R., Friston K. J., *et al.* A disturbance of nonlinear interdependence in scalp EEG of subjects with first episode schizophrenia. *Neuroimage*, 2003. **20**:466–78.

137. Ford J. M., Mathalon D. H. Electrophysiological evidence of corollary discharge dysfunction in schizophrenia during talking and thinking. *J Psychiatr Res*, 2004. **38**:37–46.

138. Peled A., Geva A. B., Kremen W. S., *et al.* Functional connectivity and working memory in

schizophrenia: an EEG study. *Int J Neurosci*, 2001. **106**:47–61.

139. Feinberg I., Guazzelli M. Schizophrenia – a disorder of the corollary discharge systems that integrate the motor systems of thought with the sensory systems of consciousness. *Br J Psychiatry*, 1999. **174**:196–204.

140. Ford J. M., Roach B. J., Faustman W. O., *et al.* Out-of-synch and out-of-sorts: dysfunction of motor-sensory communication in schizophrenia. *Biol Psychiatry*, 2008. **63**:736–43.

141. Whitford T. J., Farrow T. F., Rennie C. J., *et al. Neuroreport*, 2007. **18**:435–9.

142. Gruzelier J. Functional neuropsychological asymmetry in schizophrenia: a review and reorientation. *Schizophr Bull*, 1999. **25**:91–120.

143. Lee K. H., Williams L. M., Haig A. R., *et al.* Gamma (40 Hz) phase synchronicity and symptom dimensions in schizophrenia. *Cogn Neuropsychiatry*, 2001. **6**:7–20.

144. Baldeweg T., Spence S., Hirsch S. R., *et al.* Gamma-band electroencephalographic oscillations in a patient with somatic hallucinations. *Lancet*, 1998. **352**:620–1.

145. Saito N., Kuginuki T., Yagyu T., *et al.* Global, regional, and local measures of complexity of multichannel electroencephalo-graphy in acute, neuroleptic-naïve, first-break schizophrenics. *Biol Psychiatry*, 1998. **43**: 794–802.

146. Yeragani V. K., Cashmere D., Miewald J., *et al.* Decreased coherence in higher frequency ranges (beta and gamma) between central and frontal EEG in patients with schizophrenia: a preliminary report. *Psychiatr Res*, 2006. **141**:53–60.

147. Begré S., Koenig T. Cerebral disconnectivity: an early event in

schizophrenia. *Neuroscientist*, 2008. **14**:19–45.

148. Winterer G., Coppola R., Egan M. F., *et al.* Functional and effective frontotemporal connectivity and genetic risk for schizophrenia. *Biol Psychiatry*, 2003. **54**:1181–92.

149. Strelets V. B., Garakh Z. H. V., Novototskii-Vlasov V. Y., *et al.* Relationship between EEG power and rhythm synchronization in health and cognitive pathology. *Neurosci Behav Physiol*, 2006. **36**:655–62.

150. Slezin V. B., Korsakova E. A., Dytjatkovsky M. A., *et al.* Multifractal analysis as an aid in the diagnostics of mental disorders. *Nord J Psychiatry*, 2007. **61**:339–42.

151. Jalili M., Lavoie S., Deppen P., *et al.* Disconnection topography in schizophrenia revealed with state-space analysis of EEG. *PLoS ONE*, 2007. **2**:e1059.

152. Tien A. Y., Eaton W. W., Schlaepfer T. E., *et al.* Exploratory factor analysis of MRI brain structure measures in schizophrenia. *Schizophr Res*, 1996. **19**:93–101.

153. Woodruff, P. W., Wright I. C., Shuriquie N., *et al.* Structural brain abnormalities in male schizophrenics reflect fronto-temporal dissociation. *Psychol Med*, 1997. **2**:1257–66.

154. Mitelman S. A., Brickman A. M., Shihabuddin L., *et al.* Correlations between MRI-assessed volumes of the thalamus and cortical Brodmann's areas in schizophrenia. *Schizophr Res*, 2005. **75**:265–81.

155. Mitelman S. A. Byne W., Kemether E. M., *et al.* Correlations between volumes of the pulvinar, centromedian, and mediodorsal nuclei and cortical Brodmann's areas in schizophrenia. *Neurosci Lett*, 2006a. **392**:16–21.

73

156. Kircher T. T. J., Thienel R. Functional brain imaging of symptoms and cognition in schizophrenia. *Progress Brain Res*, 2005. **150**:299–308.

157. Dierks T., Linden D. E., Jandl M., *et al.* Activation of Heschl's gyrus during auditory hallucinations. *Neuron*, 1999. **22**:615–21.

158. Jardri R., Pins D., Delmaire C., *et al.* Activation of bilateral auditory cortex during verbal hallucinations in a child with schizophrenia. *Mol Psychiatry*, 2007. **12**:319.

159. Shergill S. S., Brammer M. J., Williams S. C., *et al.* Mapping auditory hallucinations in schizophrenia using functional magnetic resonance imaging. *Arch Gen Psychiatry*, 2000. **57**: 1033–8.

160. Silbersweig D. A., Stern E., Frith C., *et al.* A functional neuroanatomy of hallucinations in schizophrenia. *Nature*, 1995. **378**:176–9.

161. Suzuki M., Yuasa S., Minabe Y., *et al.* Left superior temporal blood flow increases in schizophrenic and schizophreniform patients with auditory hallucinations: a longitudinal case study using 123I-IMP SPECT. *Eur Arch Psychiatr Clin Neurosci*, 1993. **242**:257–61.

162. Lawrie S. M., Buechel C., Whalley H. C., *et al.* Reduced frontotemporal functional connectivity in schizophrenia associated with auditory hallucinations. *Biol Psychiatry*, 2002. **51**:1008–11.

163. Sanjuan J., Lull J. J., Aguilar E. J., *et al.* Emotional words induce enhanced brain activity in schizophrenic patients with auditory hallucinations. *Psychiatry Res*, 2007. **154**:21–9.

164. Oertel V., Rotarska-Jagiela A., van de Ven V. G., *et al.* Visual hallucinations in schizophrenia investigated with functional magnetic resonance imaging.

165. Kircher T. T. J., Liddle P. F., Brammer M. J., *et al.* Neural correlates of format thought disorder in schizophrenia. *Arch Gen Psychiatry*, 2001. **58**: 769–74.

166. McGuire P. K., Quested D. J., Spence S. A., *et al.* Pathophysiology of 'positive' thought disorder in schizophrenia. *Br J Psychiatry*, 1998. **173**:231–5.

167. Weinstein S., Werker J. F., Vouloumanos A., *et al.* Do you hear what I hear? Neural correlates of thought disorder during listening to speech in schizophrenia. *Schizophr Res*, 2006. **86**:130–7.

168. Lahti A. C., Weiler M. A., Holcomb H. H., *et al.* Correlations between rCBF and symptoms in two independent cohorts of drug-free patients with schizophrenia. *Neuropsychopharmacology*, 2006. **31**:221–30.

169. Leitman D. I., Hoptman M. J., Foxe J. J., *et al.* The neural substrates of impaired prosodic detection in schizophrenia and its sensorial antecedents. *Am J Psychiatry*, 2007. **164**:474–82.

170. Allen P., Amaro E., Fu C. H., *et al.* Neural correlates of the misattribution of speech in schizophrenia. *Br J Psychiatry*, 2007. **190**:162–9.

171. Mechelli A., Allen P., Amaro E. Jr., *et al.* Misattribution of speech and impaired connectivity in patients with auditory verbal hallucinations. *Hum Brain Mapp*, 2007. **28**:1213–22.

172. Taylor S. F., Welsh R. C., Chen A. C., *et al.* Medial frontal hyperactivity in reality distortion. *Biol Psychiatry*, 2007. **61**: 1171–8.

173. Williams L. M., Das P., Liddel B. J., *et al.* Fronto-limbic and autonomic disjunctions to

negative emotion distinguish schizophrenia subtypes. *Psychiatry Res*, 2007. **155**: 29–44.

174. Buchsbaum M. S., Nenadic I., Hazlett E. A., *et al.* Differential metabolic rates in prefrontal and temporal Brodmann areas in schizophrenia and schizotypal personality disorder. *Schizophr Res*, 2002. **54**:141–50.

175. Tu P. C., Yang T. H., Kuo W. J., *et al.* Neural correlates of antisaccade deficits in schizophrenia, an fMRI study. *J Psychiatr Res*, 2006. **40**: 606–12.

176. Buchsbaum M. S., Christian B. T., Lehrer D. S., *et al.* D2/D3 dopamine receptor binding with [F-18]fallypride in thalamus and cortex of patients with schizophrenia. *Schizophr Res*, 2006. **85**:232–44.

177. Tavlik M., Nordström A. L., Olsson H., *et al.* Decreased thalamic D2/3 receptor binding in drug-naïve patients with schizophrenia: a PET study with [11C]FLB 457. *Int J Neuropsychopharmacol*, 2003. **6**:261–370.

178. Tavlik M., Nordström A. L., Okubo Y., *et al.* Dopamine D2 receptor binding in drug-naïve patients with schizophrenia examined with raclopride-C11 and positron emission tomography. *Psychiatry Res*, 2006. **148**:165–73.

179. Suhara T., Okubo Y., Yasuno F., *et al.* Decreased dopamine D2 receptor binding in anterior cingulate cortex in schizophrenia. *Arch Gen Psychiatry*, 2002. **59**:25–30.

180. Glenthoj B. Y., Mackeprang T., Svarer C., *et al.* Frontal dopamine D(2/3) receptor binding in drug-naive first-episode schizophrenic patients correlates with positive psychotic symptoms and gender. *Biol Psychiatry*, 2006. **60**:621–9.

181. Frankle W. G., Lombardo I., Kegeles L. S., *et al.* Serotonin 1A receptor availability in patients with schizophrenia and schizo-affective disorder: a positron emission tomography imaging study with [11C]WAY 100635. *Psychopharmacology (Berl)*, 2006. **189**:155–64.

182. Tauscher J., Kapur S., Verhoeff N. P., *et al.* Brain serotonin 5-HT(1A) receptor binding in schizophrenia measured by positron emission tomography and [11C]WAY-100635. *Arch Gen Psychiatry*, 2002. **59**:514–20.

183. Iwabuchi J., Ito C., Tashiro M., *et al.* Histamine H1 receptors in schizophrenic patients measured by positron emission tomography. *Eur Neuropsychopharmacol*, 2005. **15**:185–91.

184. Bartels P., Subach J. (1976). Significance probability mappings and automated interpretation of complex pictorial scenes. In *Digital Processing of Biomedical Imagery*, Preston E. and Onoe M. (Eds.). New York: Academic Press, pp. 101–14.

185. Shi F., Liu Y., Jiang T., *et al.* Regional homogeneity and anatomical parcellation for fMRI image classification: application to schizophrenia and normal controls. *Med Image Comput*, 2007. **10**:136–43.

186. Buchsbaum M. S., Haznedar M. M., Aronowitz J., *et al.* FDG-PET in never-previously medicated psychotic adolescents treated with olanzapine or haloperidol. *Schizophr Res*, 2007. **94**:293–305.

Section 3

Organic syndromes of schizophrenia

Schizophrenia-like psychosis and epilepsy

Perminder S. Sachdev

Facts box

- There is evidence from epidemiological as well as clinical data that schizophrenia-like psychosis is more common in patients with epilepsy and vice versa.
- Psychoses associated with epilepsy have been traditionally categorized into ictal, postictal, and interictal. The interictal psychoses may be brief or chronic in duration.
- Ictal psychosis is generally either a partial complex (psychomotor) status or a petit mal status.
- Postictal psychosis begins a few hours to a few days following a flurry (usually) of seizures and has plaeomorphic symptomatology, a short duration, and often settles spontaneously.
- Brief interictal psychosis has usually been referred to as "alternating psychosis," suggesting that the psychosis and seizures are antithetical; when psychosis is present, seizures are usually in abeyance.
- Alternating psychosis has been associated with the concept of Forced Normalization of EEG (electroencephalograph).
- Brief psychosis has been reported in relation to the use of antiepileptic drugs. Antipsychotics, on the other hand, lower the threshold for epileptic seizures.
- Postictal and brief interictal psychoses share clinical features and may have similar pathogenetic mechanisms. Bimodal psychosis has been described in some patients.
- The overall evidence suggests that chronic schizophrenia-like psychosis is many times higher in epileptic patients than in the general population.
- It is often noted that patients who develop psychosis have a severe form of epilepsy involving multiple seizure types, a history of status epilepticus, and resistance to drug treatment.
- Suggestions that psychosis in epilepsy might be exclusively or preferentially associated with temporal lobe epilepsy (TLE) are supported by a majority of case studies. The evidence also points to a mediobasal rather than neocortical temporal lobe abnormality underpinning psychosis when the focus is in the temporal lobes.
- The laterality issue remains undecided, but the importance of a left-sided focus is not striking.
- Schizophrenia-like psychosis may develop *de novo* many months or years after temporal lobectomy for the treatment of intractable epilepsy.
- Discussion of pathogenesis of chronic psychosis has centered broadly on two mechanisms: 1) the psychosis is due to the repeated electrical discharges, either directly or through the development of neurophysiological or neurochemical abnormalities; or 2) the epilepsy and psychosis share a common neuropathology that may be localized (emphasis on temporal lobe but also frontal lobe and the cerebellum) or widespread in the brain. A synthesis of these two mechanisms may be possible.

The association between epilepsy and schizophrenia has attracted the attention of psychiatrists since the nineteenth century [1]. This clinically observed association was seen as a basis for exploration of the pathogenesis of mental illness, with epilepsy-related psychosis as a possible model of schizophrenia. It was this relationship that prompted the exploration of convulsive therapy in the treatment of psychiatric disorders. The proconvulsant nature of neuroleptic drugs and the occurrence of psychosis with anticonvulsants have further fueled the interest. We have come a considerable distance since the first efforts of understanding this association, but many aspects of this relationship still remain controversial [1, 2, 3, 4, 5, 6]. This chapter reviews the current evidence for the relationship and attempts to synthesize the understanding that emerges from its examination.

Introductory caveats

Any examination of the association must contend with a number of limitations in the literature, conceptual as well as empirical. Some of these limitations are elaborated first.

Problems with definitions

Although the definition of epilepsy has been consistent, the definitions of "psychosis" and "schizophrenia" used in studies have lacked standardization. Clearly, the significance of a confusional postictal psychosis is different from that of a postictal manic psychosis or an interictal schizophreniform psychosis. This problem has been particularly salient in the literature on psychosis following the use of anticonvulsant drugs. In this chapter, I restrict myself to the examination of psychoses that phenomenologically resemble a schizophreniform illness, in which thought and perceptual disturbances, usually in the form of delusions and hallucinations, are the main features. Because the term schizophrenia refers to an idiopathic syndrome, the schizophreniform illness associated with epilepsy is referred to as schizophrenia-like psychosis (SLP) in order to keep the issue of causality open.

The problem of heterogeneity

Both epilepsy and schizophrenia are heterogeneous disorders, and their categorization has varied considerably in the last century. Epilepsy, by definition, is characterized by recurrent seizures that are symptoms of an underlying cortical neuronal abnormality that transiently leads to an electrical discharge in the brain. The cause of this could be a brain malformation, an altered metabolic state, a traumatic lesion, and so on. It is therefore appropriate to refer to the "epilepsies" rather than one disease. The relative proportion of different types of epilepsies is difficult to determine. For example, estimates of the proportion of epilepsy patients who have a temporal lobe focus vary from 30% to as much as 76% [7], and studies have differed in the rigor with which a temporal lobe onset was investigated. This has direct relevance to the question of whether psychosis has a special relationship with TLE. The diagnosis of schizophrenia poses even greater problems. For example, the six-month criterion for schizophrenia used in the Diagnostic and Statistical Manual of Mental Disorders-III (DSM-III) and subsequent classifications had a major impact on the prevalence rates for this disorder, with implications for associations based on previous epidemiological data. In examining the association, therefore, the characteristics of the "schizophrenia" being referred to must be closely examined.

The problem of superficial similarity

A considerable proportion of the discussion on this topic has been influenced by the similarity between temporal lobe phenomena and psychotic symptoms. Auditory hallucinations, depersonalization, altered bodily experiences, labile emotions, and so on are features common to both disorders. This does not necessarily imply a common origin for the two sets of symptoms. Similar brain phenomena may be produced by pathology in different brain regions [8]. This is because the brain is massively interconnected, and there are proximal as well as remote effects of lesions or malfunction.

The focus on seizures

The exclusive focus on seizures in the epileptic patient may be in error as the epileptic brain is not normal between seizures. Even when neuroimaging or interictal EEG abnormalities are lacking, some abnormality at the cellular or molecular level is likely to be present [9], and the psychosis may be related to that underlying abnormality. Furthermore, epilepsy is not a static process, and the brain of the epileptic patient is undergoing structural and neurochemical change before and after the development of seizures, to which ictal events may actually contribute [10, 11].

Is there an affinity between epilepsy and SLP?

Evidence has been presented in the literature on both "affinity" and "antagonism" between the two disorders, which may seem mutually inconsistent on the surface, but must be reconciled in any analysis. The two themes that have dominated psychiatric thought on the association between SLP and epilepsy are: 1) they occur together more often than by chance [10]; and 2) they are antagonistic to each other [12]. Because the evidence suggests that both associations are possible, at least in a modified form, the paradox must be addressed, if not resolved. Is it possible that affinity is explained by one mechanism and antagonism by another, and the two can coexist?

The promise of new insights

Even if we are able to fully understand the association between the disorders, new insights do not necessarily follow. The majority of epilepsies are idiopathic in nature, so that their etiology cannot greatly inform the understanding of schizophrenia. In relation to the genetic mechanisms, more than 200 single gene disorders are known in which epilepsy is an important phenotypic feature [13], and these include neurodegenerative disorders, mental retardation syndromes, neuronal migration disorders, and mitochondrial encephalopathies. To which kind of epilepsy the psychosis relates is therefore important for any meaningful understanding. It is no longer a novel finding simply to demonstrate that psychosis may be related to cerebral dysfunction, and the exercise would be sterile if a deeper understanding of the pathogenetic mechanisms were not forthcoming.

Categorization

How does one best classify SLP associated with epilepsy? A consensus on the classification is lacking, and neither DSM-IV nor International Classification of Diseases (ICD-10) has addressed this issue specifically. Application of DSM-IV criteria results in an ambiguous situation in which one can make the diagnosis of a primary psychotic syndrome or secondary syndrome (due to a general medical condition) depending on whether the nature of the evidence

Table 6.1 Schizophrenia-like psychoses (SLP) and epilepsy: a classification

1. Ictal psychosis:
   a. Partial complex or psychomotor status
   b. Simple partial status
   c. Petit mal status
2. Postictal psychosis:
   a. Single episode
   b. Recurrent
3. Brief interictal psychosis
   a. Alternating psychosis
   b. Nonperiodic
4. Bimodal psychosis
5. Chronic interictal psychosis
6. Antiepileptic drug-induced psychosis
7. Neuroleptic-induced epilepsy in a schizophrenic patient

prompts one to deduce that the psychotic disturbance is etiologically related to the epilepsy "through a physiological mechanism" (p. 316, [14]). Most often, separate diagnoses of epilepsy and the particular psychotic syndrome are appropriate. In such circumstances, note should be made of the relationship of the psychosis with the onset of epilepsy, seizure frequency, recent seizure episodes, current anticonvulsant medication, EEG abnormalities, and the underlying neurological lesion, if known.

Because clinical seizures are the outstanding feature of epilepsy, psychotic syndromes have traditionally been classified according to their temporal relationship to these events, as ictal, postictal (or peri-ictal), and interictal, with the last type being either brief or chronic. For this review, I will retain this classification without implying that these categories are distinct in their pathophysiology or clinical manifestations (see Table 6.1).

Ictal psychosis

A nonconvulsive status epilepticus can result in symptoms resembling psychosis. The psychosis is necessarily brief, usually minutes to hours. When prolonged into days, it is likely to be ictal behavior that extends postictally. The most common association is with *partial complex (or psychomotor) status*, and patients may present a wide range of perceptual, behavioral, cognitive, and affective symptoms, often in association with automatisms involving oral activity, picking at clothes, and paucity of speech or mutism [15, 16]. These episodes of automatisms may be recurrent, with behavior not being normal in the intervening periods, although the patient may respond to simple instructions. Hallucinations may be prominent, and paranoid delusions or overvalued ideas may be present. Consciousness is altered during the episode but may be difficult to test, and patients are amnesic for the episode. The appropriate DSM-IV diagnosis would therefore be delirium. There is generally a history of partial or generalized seizures, with reports of an aura in most cases.

Simple partial status may produce affective, autonomic, and psychic symptoms that may include hallucinations and thought disorder in clear consciousness. Insight is usually maintained, and the manifestation is not that of a true psychosis, but the symptoms may be misinterpreted or embellished by the patient and behavioral disturbance may result [17].

Petit mal status (absence or spike-wave status) results in altered consciousness and such motor symptoms as eyelid fluttering and myoclonic jerks, and it may superficially resemble psychosis with disorganized behavior, but delusions and hallucinations are lacking [16]. Patients almost always have a history of absence seizures or rarely generalized tonic-clonic seizures, and the onset is usually before the age of 20. If it has a later onset, there is frequently an underlying metabolic disturbance [18]. The onset and offset are abrupt, and the episode may last from minutes to several hours or even days. The alteration of consciousness is variable, ranging from slowing of thinking and behavior to marked disorientation to stupor.

Patients with ictal psychosis usually have a history of epilepsy. By definition, ictal psychosis is concurrently associated with epileptic discharges in the brain, and, except in some patients with simple partial status [19], scalp EEG abnormalities are detectable. The majority of discharges in psychomotor status have a focus in the limbic and isocortical components of the temporal lobe, but the focus is extratemporal in about 30% of patients [20], usually in the frontal or cingulate cortex. Because the scalp EEG may be normal in simple partial seizures, the behavioral disturbance may be mistaken to be interictal, and a high index of suspicion is necessary. In such cases, if the patient is on anticonvulsant medication, the dose may have to be reduced, especially if EEG telemetry is planned. Activating techniques such as light sleep or sleep deprivation may be useful, and special recordings (sphenoidal, esophageal, or foramen ovale) may be necessary. Resolution of the disturbance with intravenous diazepam is not diagnostically foolproof as many nonepileptic behaviors may so resolve [17]. Some assistance in diagnosis may come from the examination of serum prolactin levels, which rise after epileptic seizures, peaking at about 20 minutes and returning to baseline around 1 hour [21]. With partial complex seizures, the rise is less than that after generalized convulsions, but rises above 500 mU/L should be considered as suggestive [22]. A rise may be insignificant or absent after a simple partial seizure.

Symptoms may reflect one of two mechanisms [23]: 1) A positive effect of the seizure discharge, that is, the epileptic discharge activates a behavioral mechanism represented in the area subjected to the discharge. This may result in a myriad of symptoms in the behavioral, cognitive, affective, perceptual, or autonomic domains; 2) A negative effect, that is, either: a) the individual is unable to engage in a certain behavior owing to the temporary paralysis of the anatomical substrate of that behavior; or b) some behaviors are released by the inactivation of structures that normally suppress them. Behavioral disturbance due to a negative effect may occur in other situations, for example, when the whole cerebral cortex is subjected to a relatively mild form of seizure activity represented by generalized spike and wave discharges. This negative effect may continue postictally, or it may initiate then. Experiential phenomena in ictal psychosis are likely to be due to positive effects, whereas automatisms may be caused by positive or negative effects.

The question of whether chronic psychoses in clear consciousness can be a direct consequence of continuous seizure activity restricted to deep brain structures has generated much controversy. Most epileptologists consider this to be extremely unlikely, [17] but this long-held idea remains current [3]. Kendrick and Gibbs [24] first used implanted electrodes to study the electrophysiological disturbance in schizophrenia and in the psychoses of psychomotor epilepsy; spike discharges in medial temporal and frontal structures were demonstrated in both patient groups. They reported that surgery on medial temporal structures was nearly always beneficial for schizophrenia. Semp-Jacobsen [25] and Heath [26] noted similar abnormal discharges that did not spread beyond the amygdala, hippocampus, and septal regions, again in both schizophrenic and "epileptic psychosis" patients. Scalp EEGs were normal or only mildly abnormal. These findings have not been further examined, perhaps due to ethical constraints against using depth recordings for research purposes. In patients undergoing depth recording for another purpose such as presurgical evaluation, the chance occurrence of psychotic phenomena may present an opportunity to address this question. Invasive recordings in animals are generally not enough to provide the pathogenetic insights to complex behavioral disorders [27]. A noninvasive neurophysiological technique that may be able to detect deep limbic discharges is magnetoencephalography, arguably an important tool for future attempts to address this issue [28].

Even if continuous ictal activity in depth recordings could be demonstrated, appropriate longitudinal and controlled studies are necessary to establish its significance. First, epileptiform activity in deep structures may be common in nonpsychotic patients with focal epilepsy, especially in the preictal and postictal periods [29]. Neurons in the medial temporal region in temporal lobe epileptic patients have higher firing rates, more frequent burst discharges, and stronger synchrony than neurons in nonepileptic regions, especially during sleep [30]. Second, rapid synchronized neuronal discharges, which form the basis of epileptic discharges, occur normally in the limbic structures, hypothalamus, and brainstem in association with vital functions such as parturition, milk ejection, growth hormone release, and orgasm [5].

Postictal psychosis

The behavioral disturbances that may follow a seizure, or a bout of seizures, have received increased attention in the last two decades [31, 32, 33, 34, 35, 36, 37, 38, 39, 40, 41]. Postictal psychosis (PIP) as a special instance of such disturbance has been recognized for centuries, but its clinical importance has been overshadowed by the interictal psychoses. Indeed, a literary reference to postictal psychosis occurs in Shakespeare's Othello (IV, I, 42, 43, 44, 45, 46, 47, 48):

IAGO: *My Lord is fall'n into a epilepsy. This is his second fit; he had one yesterday.*

CASSIO: *Rub him about the temples.*

IAGO: *No, forbear; the lethargy must have his quiet course; if not, he foams at the mouth; and bye and bye breaks out to savage madness …*

Because PIPs are brief and occur in close proximity with seizures, they are ideal for the investigation of some pathogenetic mechanisms of psychosis. They usually follow seizure clusters or a recent exacerbation in seizure frequency [31] that may be related to withdrawal of anticonvulsants, often as a part of the video-EEG monitoring of patients [33, 35]. Postictal psychoses are common in epilepsy-monitoring facilities; 6.4% of the patients in one study developed this syndrome [35], and nearly 10% did so in another study [37]. If the psychosis develops gradually and in parallel with increasing seizure frequency, it may be referred to as peri-ictal rather than postictal, but there is no reason to believe that this distinction is meaningful clinically or for its pathophysiology. A confounding factor in the evaluation of PIP in video-EEG monitoring facilities is that these patients have often had a withdrawal of their anticonvulsants, and it has been suggested that this itself may result in psychopathology [38], although psychosis is not usual in the absence of seizures.

Between the last seizure and the psychosis there is usually a nonpsychotic period, which ranges from a few hours to a few days. This period lasted 12 to 72 hours in the Kanner study [35] and up to 1 week according to Logsdail and Toone [31]. Some clouding of consciousness is often present in this period, and it may extend to the initial period of psychosis or even the whole episode. The psychotic symptoms are pleomorphic (persecutory, grandiose, referential, somatic, and religious delusions, catatonia, hallucinations, etc.), and affective symptoms (manic or depressive) are often prominent [31, 39]. First-rank symptoms of Schneider can occur but are rare [35]. Postictal psychoses resolve within a few days, with the mean duration in the study by Kanner and colleagues [35] being about 70 hours (range = 24–144), and all resolving within 1 month in the study by Savard and colleagues [33]. A few reports of longer duration of PIP have been published, but at which point the diagnosis should be changed to interictal psychosis is debatable. The proposal of the Subcommission on Classification of the ILAE Commission on Epilepsy and Psychobiology was that PIP lasting more than a month may require reconsideration of diagnosis and a change to interictal psychosis [36].

Although the resolution of PIP is generally spontaneous, it is aided by neuroleptic medication, usually in small doses. A further seizure may exacerbate the psychosis, and anticonvulsant treatment should be carefully monitored. The brief psychosis may recur, at a frequency of 2 to 3 episodes per year in two studies [35, 49], and in some patients (15% in one study

[31]) these episodes may become chronic. More longitudinal studies of patients with PIP are needed to examine its course, its likelihood of recurrence, and factors that predispose a transition into chronic interictal psychosis.

The predisposing factors of PIP are poorly understood. A question that has been frequently posed in the published literature is whether PIP is associated with a specific type of epilepsy, that is, with a temporal focus, and whether independent bilateral disturbance is more commonly represented than unilateral abnormality. The majority of reported patients suffer from partial complex seizures that are secondarily generalized. Epilepsy has often been present for more than 10 years before the onset of psychosis [31, 35, 37]. EEG abnormalities persist in the majority of patients during the psychosis in the majority of cases [31]. In a case report by So and colleagues [32], the patient with postictal psychosis demonstrated frequent bitemporal independent epileptiform discharges on depth recording that were maximal in the mesial limbic regions. On the other hand, another report presented two patients with PIP who had repeated EEGs during the psychosis showing that their habitual focal epileptiform abnormalities were absent [50] – suggestive of "forced normalization" (discussed later). Although Kanner and colleagues [35] found no specific predisposing factors that differentiated their psychotic group from a comparable nonpsychotic epilepsy group, Savard and colleagues [33] were impressed with a high rate of ictal fear, bilateral independent discharges, and gross structural lesions (6 out of 9 patients), including the presence of alien tissue tumors. Kanemoto and colleagues [39] also noted frequent psychic auras, and Umbricht and colleagues [51] noted frequent bitemporal foci in their subjects. In contrast with the other literature, Devinsky and colleagues [52] found similar rates of PIP in partial and primary generalized epilepsies, although they did note bilateral independent interictal discharges in those with partial seizures. PIP has also been associated with frontal lobe epilepsy, accounting for 3 out of 11 cases in one series [53]. Five of the 14 patients studied by Logsdail and Toone [31] had abnormalities on brain computerized tomography (CT). In the MRI study of Kanemoto and colleagues [37], postictal psychosis was most likely to occur in patients with resistant TLE stemming from mesial temporal sclerosis, especially on the left side. These patients with left-side mesial temporal sclerosis were also likely to have atrophy of the temporal

neocortex. Mathern and colleagues [54] reported two patients, one of whom had unilateral postictal discharges, but on autopsy was found to have bilateral hippocampal neuronal loss, although the pathology was asymmetric. Some authors also report low intelligence as a predisposing factor for PIP [39, 50], suggesting the presence of more widespread brain abnormality. In summary, the weight of the evidence supports a stronger association with complex partial epilepsy, especially of temporal lobe origin, in which there is bilateral pathology, although this relationship is not exclusive.

The pathogenetic mechanisms are unclear, although the proximity of these psychoses to seizures and their frequent occurrence in epilepsy centers while patients are being monitored make them ideal candidates for the exploration of underlying mechanisms. The finding of chronic frequent subictal discharges suggests that ictal activity in the temporal lobe may be directly related to this kind of psychosis. Changes in monoamines, particularly postsynaptic dopamine receptor sensitivity, have been suggested as the mediating mechanism [32]. Some support for the dopamine mechanism came from a single photon emission computed tomography (SPECT) study using [(123) I]iodobenzamide that demonstrated low levels of striatal dopamine D2 receptors in patients with periictal psychosis [55]. Low folic acid levels have been suggested to have a role [56], but firm evidence is lacking. The significance of a report of hyponatremia in these patients is also unknown [35].

More importantly, it would be fruitful to examine PIP in the context of the homeostatic mechanisms that are brought about in the brain to control seizures, which have been divided into electrophysiological mechanisms, cerebral blood flow (CBF) changes, and neurotransmitter and receptor changes [40]. Postictal psychosis in this context has been conceptualized as a phenomenon akin to Todd's paralysis, indicating the postictal inactivation of cortical regions involved in the ictal event, which usually include bilateral medial temporal structures [17]. A simple electrophysiological explanation – that the postictal state is caused by "neuronal exhaustion" – is not supported by experimental evidence [57]. A second possible explanation – also lacking evidence – is that of neurotransmitter depletion due to repeated firing [40]. An important aspect of seizure termination is active inhibition, in which a number of mechanisms are involved. A hierarchy of inhibition is produced by fast inhibitory postsynaptic potential (IPSP) mediated by gamma amino butyric acid-A (GABA$_A$) receptors, a later hyperpolarizing potential mediated by GABA$_B$ receptors [40], and after hyperpolarization produced by calcium-activated potassium currents. Although these inhibitory mechanisms are brief, prolonged inhibition of neuronal activity can be produced by hyperpolarizing pumps, whose object is to restore the steady-state ionic balance after neuronal activity. Seizures lead to increased extracellular K+, and levels higher than 20 to 30 mm produce a spreading depression and cessation of neuronal activity, which may account for the postictal state [58]. Seizures also cause lactic acidosis and low pH, and the H+ ions compete with other ions at the ion channel associated with N-methyl-D-aspartic acid (NMDA) receptors.

Seizures cause a release of a number of other neurotransmitters that include acetylcholine, catecholamines, serotonin, opiates, adenosine, and nitric oxide (NO). Endogenous opiates appear to play a special role in the postictal state [43]. Naloxone is noted to reverse post-seizure catalepsy in rats subjected to electroshock [44] and to increase the rate of interictal spiking in humans [45], but the evidence is not entirely consistent [46, 47]. Adenosine and NO are neuromodulators that may act as endogenous anti-seizure agents. It is possible that the repeated release of neurotransmitters during seizure activity leads to post-synaptic receptor changes, as has been demonstrated for benzodiazepine receptors [48], and this may be relevant to PIP.

Seizures lead to substantial changes in CBF that may have a relevance to PIP, although the precise mechanism is unknown. Ipsilateral to the temporal lobe seizure, there is a rise of CBF to twice the baseline at about 5 min, but by 1 hour, the CBF is below baseline. A SPECT study of four patients with TLE and postictal psychosis demonstrated mesial frontal hyperperfusion during the psychosis [34]. Another report from the same group suggested hyperperfusion in both temporal and mesial frontal regions and the left lateral frontal region [59]. Fong and colleagues [60] reported a marked right temporal and left basal ganglia hyperperfusion in PIP in two patients. It is worth considering that the CBF response in patients with PIP is aberrant, and this may in some way be related to the psychosis. A difficulty in the interpretation of these findings is created by the fact that seizures may uncouple cerebral perfusion from metabolic activity by altering cerebrovascular autoregulation, as has been

Table 6.2 Possible pathogenetic mechanisms of the postictal state with relevance to postictal psychosis

1. Electrophysiological:
   a. Continuous ictal discharges leading to psychomotor change
   b. Neuronal "exhaustion" from a seizure cluster
2. Neurotransmitter changes:
   a. Catecholamine depletion
   b. Increased postsynaptic dopamine sensitivity
   c. Increased endogenous opiates
   d. Increased adenosine
   e. Increased nitric oxide
3. Postictal inhibitory mechanisms:
   a. Fast inhibitory postsynaptic potential (GABA$_A$ mediated)
   b. Later hyperpolarizing potential (GABA$_B$ mediated)
   c. After hyperpolarization due to calcium-activated potassium currents
   d. Na-K hyperpolarizing pumps
   e. Increased extracellular K+
   f. H+ induced attenuation of NMDA receptors
   g. Increased opiates, adenosine and NO
4. Cerebral blood flow alterations due to poor autoregulation
5. Other:
   a. Low folic acid
   b. Hyponatraemia

demonstrated for postictal hemiparesis [61]. Hyperperfusion in PIP, therefore, cannot necessarily be construed as hypermetabolism, although regional variations after correction for global change in perfusion cannot be dismissed. Moreover, increased perfusion is equally likely to be related to increased inhibition or excitation, and the primary disturbance may be local or remote. Metabolic studies, combined with neurotransmitter labels, using positron emission tomography (PET) are more likely to help sort out these possibilities.

In summary, understanding the mechanisms of the postictal state can provide useful insights into the pathogenesis of PIP, which may further inform the pathogenesis of psychosis in general. Manipulation of some of these mechanisms with drugs may produce valuable strategies to prevent psychosis and other psychiatric and cognitive disturbances of the postictal state (see Table 6.2).

Brief interictal psychosis

Brief psychotic episodes can also develop when seizures are infrequent or fully controlled. These psychoses last from days to weeks, they are usually self-limiting, and their separation from postictal psychoses may be difficult. The phenomenology is characterized by paranoid delusions and auditory hallucinations, but multiple other features, including affective symptoms, may occur [62, 63, 64, 65]. Tellenbach [62] pointed out the presence of premonitory symptoms such as insomnia, anxiety, feelings of oppression, and withdrawal as heralding the psychosis, and Wolf [66] suggested that treatment with anxiolytics at this stage may prevent development of the psychosis.

The relationship of brief interictal psychoses (BIP) to seizures and EEG abnormality has received much attention. Interictal implies that these psychoses occur in-between seizures rather than in close proximity with them. The favored description is of an *alternating psychosis* [62], that is, a brief psychosis alternating with periods of increased seizure activity such that the seizures and psychosis appear antagonistic. Unlike PIP, this psychosis can be ameliorated by the occurrence of one or more seizures [66]. Alternating psychoses are uncommon, and Schmitz and Wolf [67] reported three cases of alternating psychosis in 697 epilepsy patients.

The concept of forced normalization (forcierte Normalisierung) (FN) was introduced by Landolt [68] for the puzzling observation that the EEGs of epilepsy patients often looked less pathological when their behavior had deteriorated. This phenomenon, also called "paradoxical" or "spurious" normalization [66], has been documented by a number of authors [65, 66, 69] with the additional observations that: 1) the EEG may become more, rather than entirely, normal; 2) the manifestation is not always of psychosis, and other disturbances, such as affective symptoms, an anxiety or dissociative state, and behavioral disturbance, may be present; and 3) not all BIPs manifest this phenomenon [63]. Ramani and Gumnit [63] observed FN in only one of nine epilepsy patients who became psychotic while being treated in the hospital for their epilepsy. Forced normalization is not exclusive to interictal psychosis and has been occasionally described with PIP, suggesting a complexity of the relationship of seizure activity with psychosis. Interestingly, Landolt described this phenomenon in relation to childhood absence seizures, and some authors have suggested that it is more likely to occur with primary generalized epilepsy [70].

The neurophysiological basis of FN is not definitely known. One suggestion is that it reflects ongoing subcortical or mesial temporal epileptic activity with enhanced cortical inhibition [64, 70]. This has been referred to as an "inhibitory surround" in response to ongoing seizures. This explanation argues that ongoing epileptic activity is necessary for the maintenance of inhibition as well as the development of psychosis. Although the role of inhibition in response to seizure activity, as a homeostatic mechanism against ictal activity, is an appealing hypothesis to explain FN, it is possible that it does not represent ongoing epileptiform activity, but is a prolonged response to preceding epileptiform activity. It is known that occasionally patients may develop prolonged unconsciousness after a seizure or a series of seizures, especially in elderly or ill patients [71]. Todd's paralysis has been reported to last for up to 36 hours [72]. It is therefore possible that inhibition after a seizure or a series of seizures may be fairly prolonged. It is also important to understand the sources of the EEG abnormalities. The scalp EEG is a reflection of groups or populations of neurons that fire in a synchronous manner. The pyramidal neurons of layers IV and V of the cortex are considered to be responsible for scalp EEG activity, but both radially and tangentially oriented currents may make a contribution to the EEG signal. Sources of EEG abnormality in epilepsy may lie close to the surface or deep in the brain, and the latter are less likely to be picked up on the scalp. The inhibitory events described previously are most likely to occur in close proximity to the seizure focus, thereby reducing the electrical current generated from the focus, and this may be the basis for the normalization. Even a reduction in the frequency of epileptic events will produce a relative normalization.

Patients with BIP have been reported to suffer from either partial complex epilepsy or primary generalized epilepsy. Although a temporal lobe onset is common, Wolf [66] argued that all of these patients also had generalized seizures. Kanemoto and colleagues [37] reported the frequent presence of mesial temporal sclerosis in patients with interictal psychosis, who also were likely to have experienced the onset of epilepsy before the age of 10 years. Ictal fear and autonomic aura have been more commonly reported in patients who develop BIP [73], but this is not invariably supported.

Special relationships between BIP and two drug classes should be highlighted.

Psychosis and anticonvulsant drugs

Anticonvulsant drugs have been reported to precipitate psychosis, although the published literature is confounded by the inclusion of affective and confusional psychoses in this category. The facts that the control of seizures may induce psychosis in a few patients and that neuroleptic drugs, which are proconvulsant, are useful in treating such a psychosis are consistent with the concept of alternating psychosis and forced normalization. Gibbs [74] first drew attention to this in relation to phenacetylurea, and Landolt [75] implicated the succinimides. Wolf [66] further emphasized the relationship with ethosuximide and reported that valproate did not produce the same result. Others have reported psychosis in association with clobazam, phenytoin, carbamazepine, barbiturates, and benzodiazepines [1]. Psychosis related to vigabatrin, a new antiepileptic drug that is an irreversible inhibitor of GABA aminotransferase, has excited much interest, but the psychoses reported are multiform, and a relationship to seizure control in those who present with psychosis has not been reported [76]. Topiramate has been associated with FN and psychosis, especially in patients who were concurrently on vigabatrin [77]. Forced normalization has also been reported with levetiracetam [78], but is rare with lamotrigine and gabapentin [79]. Another group of drugs that are potent anticonvulsants in animal models is the NMDA antagonists, for example, MK-801, ketamine, and phencyclidine. These drugs are also potent psychotogens [80]. The psychoses related to phenytoin are likely to be toxic in nature.

Antipsychotic drugs and epilepsy

All antipsychotic drugs have the propensity to cause paroxysmal EEG abnormalities and induce seizures, and the effect is related to drug type and dose [81]. The phenothiazines have been the most widely studied for their seizure propensity. They have been reported in 9% of patients who received high-dose phenothiazines (> = 1,000 mg/day chlorpromazine or its equivalent), 0.7% of patients who received moderate doses, and 0.3% of patients who received low doses (> = 200 mg/day chlorpromazine or its equivalent) [82]. From the published literature, the relative risk of seizures with the various typical antipsychotics is difficult to

Table 6.3 The relative risk of seizures with antipsychotic drug used*

High risk	Intermediate risk	Low risk
Clozapine (HD to MD)	Clozapine (LD)	Haloperidol
Chlorpromazine (HD)	Chlropromazine (MD to LD)	Trifluoperazine
	Olanzapine	Fluphenazine
	Quetiapine	Flupenthixol
	Thioridazine	Pimozide
		Molindone
		Risperidone

HD high dose; MD moderate dose; LD low dose
* Adapted from Alldredge, 1999 [82].

establish, but the risk is considered to be lower with haloperidol, trifluoperazine, pimozide, and molindone. Although there is a clear increase of seizure incidence in cases of antipsychotic overdose and with high doses of these drugs, an elevated risk over placebo is generally not established for low to moderate doses. The newer antipsychotics are not free of this effect, and in fact, clozapine is the most epileptogenic of the antipsychotics, with myoclonus or frank seizures reported in 0.3% to 5% of patients treated with therapeutic doses [5]. In the premarketing studies of clozapine, the overall incidence of seizures was 2.9%: 4.4% with high doses (600–900 mg/day), 2.7% with moderate doses (300–599 mg/day), and 1.0% with low doses (299 mg/day or less) [63]. A subsequent postmarketing surveillance study of 5,629 patients reported a rate of 1.3%, which was again dose dependent [83]. The rates are lower with the other atypical drugs, with a seizure rate of 0.9% reported for olanzapine and quetiapine (cf. 0.5% for placebo) and 0.3% for risperidone [84]. The relative risks of commonly used antipsychotic drugs are summarized in Table 6.3. In spite of these increased rates, antipsychotics can be safely used in the management of psychosis in patients with epilepsy, with the preference for low to moderate doses, although this clinical question has rarely been examined in a systematic study. In a study of thioridazine for behavioral disturbance in epilepsy, seizure frequency was improved in 41% of test subjects and unchanged in 20%, with the improvement being attributed to better control of emotional triggers for the seizures [85]. Clozapine can be used in low doses without seizure exacerbation. If a seizure occurs, the dose can be lowered or the patient switched to another drug such as olanzapine.

Are postictal and brief interictal psychoses distinct?

The previous descriptions suggest that there is a classical distinction between PIP and BIP, with the former being closely related to a flurry of seizures, and the latter occurring during a period when seizures are relatively quiescent. However, this distinction may to some extent be arbitrary. Phenomenologically, the two syndromes are very similar, although the PIP is likely to be briefer in duration. The interval between the last seizure and the occurrence of PIP can vary considerably and the interval of up to one week is an arbitrary one [31]. The predisposing factors for the two syndromes appear to be similar as well. The neurophysiological correlates are not necessarily distinctive. Although FN is usually associated with BIP, it is not invariable in this syndrome [63], and can occur in PIP [50]. Patients who experience both PIP and BIP have been said to have *bimodal psychosis* [86], and in these patients either syndrome may appear first.

An examination of possible neurophysiological factors underlying the psychosis suggests that they may share common mechanisms. The inhibitory processes mentioned previously not only bring about the postictal state but are also necessary for maintaining the interictal state. Postictal and brief interictal psychoses may therefore not be as different from each other as is generally thought. As the development of seizures may be due to either disinhibition or hypersynchrony involving enhanced disinhibition [87], the occurrence of a seizure during psychosis may have different pathogenetic mechanisms and may indicate either disinhibition or increased inhibition. The effect on psychosis of a seizure could thereby be either an amelioration of symptoms or their exacerbation. This may explain why seizures during postictal psychosis often exacerbate the psychosis, whereas those during brief interictal psychosis may improve the psychiatric status. Different patterns of excitation and inhibition may also explain why the EEG may show "forced normalization" in some cases of interictal psychosis. These speculations can be tested by the longitudinal examination of patients with brief psychoses, using neurophysiological and neuroimaging methods.

Chronic interictal psychosis

The investigation of the relationship between epilepsy and chronic SLP was brought into the modern era by Slater and colleagues [88]. For some time, there was high expectation that this would become a model psychosis that would reveal the pathogenesis of schizophrenia. Despite a great deal of further work, many aspects of this relationship remain controversial, and the promised insights have been slow to arrive.

Evidence for association

The evidence that there is indeed an affinity between schizophrenia and epilepsy must come from epidemiological data. The epidemiological evidence for this association is summarized in Table 6.4. The rates must be interpreted in light of the general prevalences of psychosis, schizophrenia, and epilepsy in the general population. Schizophrenia is estimated to have a prevalence of 0.5% to 1% in the general population, but if we use a broad concept of psychosis, the prevalence is likely to be much higher [89]. Epilepsy has a point prevalence of 0.4% to 1% in the general population, and the lifetime risk of having at least one unprovoked seizure is 2% to 5% [90, 91]. The prevalence is low in the first decade of life, increases to a plateau in the adult years, and increases further in the elderly [91]. Methodological difficulties in the studies should also be taken into account in the interpretation of the prevalence data. For example, the classic study by Slater and colleagues [88] drew its subjects from tertiary centers in two major London hospitals. The overall evidence suggests that SLP is many times higher in epileptic patients than in the general population. A recent study based on the Danish longitudinal registers is particularly noteworthy for its comprehensive coverage of a population of 2.7 million [92]. The relative risk of schizophrenia in patients with epilepsy was 2.48 (95% CI 2.20–2.8) and of SLP, 2.93 (2.69–3.20). The risk was the same in men and women and increased with age and with a family history of schizophrenia or epilepsy.

Clinical features

Slater and colleagues [88] reported that they had found a mean age at onset of about 30 years and that the symptoms were largely paranoid-hallucinatory, commonly associated with catatonia, affective blunting, and volitional symptoms. Phenomenologically, the

Table 6.4 Epidemiological evidence for the association between epilepsy and schizophrenia-like psychosis (SLP)

Measure and Authors	N	%	Comment
Prevalence of SLP in epilepsy clinic groups:			
Gibbs and Gibbs [93]	11,612	2.8	Reliability of psychiatric diagnosis uncertain; majority of subjects young
Currie et al. [94]	666	1.8	No criteria described; only patients with temporal lobe epilepsy included
Standage and Fenton [95]	37	8.0	Temporal lobe epilepsy not different from other epilepsies
Mendez et al. [4]	1,611	9.25	1.06% of migraine (comparison) subjects had schizophrenia-like psychosis; comprehensive assessment used DSM-III-R criteria
Schmitz and Wolf [67]	697	4.0	Both generalized and focal epilepsies represented
Onuma et al. [96]	1,285	9.1	Point prevalence, 4.0%
Prevalence of SLP in epileptic patients in community-based studies:			
Krohn [97]	—	2.0	Additional 9% had incapacitating behavioral disorder
Gudmundsson [98]	987	8.1	Entire epileptic population of Iceland studied
Qin et al. [92]	2.27 × 106	RR2.93 (2.69–2.20)	Danish longitudinal register. Risk increased with age and family history of schizophrenia and epilepsy.
Prevalence of epilepsy in psychotic patients:			
Kat [99]	50,000	0.33	
Davison and Bagley [100]	1–10	Estimates from published data	
Betts [101]	1,950	2.1	Hospitalized patients
Annual incidence of psychosis in epileptic patients:			
Lindsay et al. [102]	87	10	Temporal lobe epilepsy subjects followed up for 39 years
Onuma et al. [96]	1,285	0.3	up for 39 years

disorder was indistinguishable from schizophrenia, although the authors reported a better preservation of affect, mood swings, mystical experiences, and visual hallucinations. Investigators in two controlled studies from London [103, 104] also noted the largely paranoid-hallucinatory characteristics of the disorder, but they stressed the greater frequency of "organicity." One report commented on the rarity of negative symptoms, formal thought disorder, and catatonic symptoms [105], whereas another reported that visual hallucinations were more prominent than auditory ones [106]. In the study by Mendez and colleagues [4], the epilepsy-with-schizophrenia group did not differ from the nonepileptic schizophrenic comparison subjects on any psychosis item except increased suicidal behavior. In conclusion, except for minor reported differences, which may be accounted for by selection biases in the comparison group, the chronic psychoses of epilepsy are similar to schizophrenia.

Many authors have commented on the relative lack of negative symptoms and a more benign course for epileptic schizophrenia [88, 107], but supportive controlled studies are lacking. Nearly one-half (45%) of the patients of Slater and colleagues [88] had a chronic course. In a 10-year follow-up study in Japan [108], 64% of the patients had a chronic course. In the absence of an appropriate comparison group, it is difficult to know if this outcome is different from that in schizophrenia with a relatively later age at onset.

Risk factors of chronic SLP with epilepsy

Although a number of studies have examined the risk factors, the literature remains contentious, without a clear consensus emerging on many variables. The putative risk factors are summarized in Table 6.5.

Age at onset, duration, and severity of epilepsy

Epilepsy beginning at an early age [109] and enduring through puberty [102, 110, 111] has been associated with SLP. Other studies have found no relationship to age of onset [69, 112] or have associated psychosis with later age of onset of epilepsy [4, 92]. In the large Danish study [92], for every five-year

Table 6.5 Putative risk factors for chronic schizophrenia-like psychosis of epilepsy

1. Age: Early age of onset, but evidence conflicting

2. Sex: A female bias reported by one group but not others

3. Family history: F/H of psychosis or epilepsy

4. Characteristics of epilepsy:

   a. Many years (usually 10–14) between the onset of epilepsy and the onset of psychosis

   b. Severe epilepsy: multiple seizure types, history of status epilepticus, multiple hospital admissions, resistance to drugs

   c. Partial complex epilepsy, especially of mediobasal temporal lobe origin

   d. History of secondary generalization

   e. Left sided focus

5. Neuropathology:

   a. Presence of neuroembryodysplastic lesions, for example, gangliogliomas, hamartomas.

   b. Bilateral pathology

6. Neurological examination: sinistrality

increase in the age at diagnosis of epilepsy, there was an increased relative risk of 1.2 (1.14–1.26, p < 0.0001) of SLP. Many years (usually 10–14) are said to intervene between the onsets of epilepsy and SLP [88, 104, 107], but this period is highly variable and patients who develop epilepsy after the psychosis are usually excluded from such analyses. Moreover, the peak age at onset for epilepsy is in any case earlier than that for schizophrenia [90], thus making the relevance of this observation somewhat ambiguous.

It is often noted that the patients who develop psychosis have a severe form of epilepsy involving multiple seizure types [95], a history of status epilepticus [88], and resistance to drug treatment [6]. The risk was higher in epileptics with multiple admissions in the Danish study [92]. The frequency of seizures at the time of development of the psychosis is variable; some authors report an improvement [102], whereas others report a worsening [4]. Most often, it is not possible in the case of chronic psychosis to relate the onset of the psychosis to any change in seizure frequency [88].

Is greater risk of psychosis particular to temporal lobe epilepsy (TLE)?

Suggestions that psychosis in epilepsy may be exclusively or preferentially associated with TLE are sup-

ported by a majority of case series [74, 88, 103, 104, 113]. Mendez and colleagues [4] reported a higher rate of partial complex seizures, but not temporal lobe foci, in their group with SLP plus epilepsy than in their non-schizophrenic epilepsy comparison subjects. In studies that compared patients with TLE and those with generalized epilepsy [114, 115], the patients with TLE were more likely to be psychotic, but the subject groups in these studies were small. In the large Danish study, the relative risk associated with complex partial epilepsy was slightly but nonsignificantly higher than other types of epilepsy [92] (relative risk, after adjustment for complex partial epilepsy 3.38, for other partial epilepsy 3.18, for generalized epilepsy 2.81). Another argument [89] has been that the proportion of TLE in epilepsy-psychosis patients is no different from that in the adult epileptic population in general, the latter being estimated to be about 60% [90, 91]. This debate, therefore, has not resolved but continues to be in favor of a special but not exclusive relationship between SLP and TLE. Additionally, there are neuroimaging and neuropathological data linking the temporal lobe with psychosis (discussed in later sections).

There is also a suggestion that the phenomenology of the psychosis associated with TLE is somewhat different from that associated with generalized epilepsy. The latter are reportedly relatively mild, shorter in duration, often associated with confusion in the early stages, and lacking in Schneiderian first-rank symptoms [114].

Mediobasal or neocortical temporal lobe epilepsy?

Kristensen and Sindrup [69] reported that psychotic patients had a substantial preponderance of temporal mediobasal spike foci, recorded on sphenoidal electrodes, and an excess of epigastric auras. Hermann and colleagues [116] reported a higher frequency of schizophrenia and other psychopathology in patients with an aura of fear. Mendez and colleagues [4] reported more psychic and autonomic auras in the psychotic patients. The neuropathological literature (see later section) has supported a predominant abnormality in the medial temporal structures, although more widespread damage has also been reported [68, 69]. The majority of the evidence, therefore, points to a mediobasal rather than neocortical temporal lobe abnormality underpinning psychosis when the focus is in the temporal lobes.

Laterality of epileptic focus?

Because the suggestion by Flor-Henry [117] of a preponderance of left-sided pathology in patients with SLP, many studies have examined this issue. In the EEG studies, the majority opinion favors an excess of left temporal foci in the patients with TLE and schizophreniform psychosis [103, 118], although there have been some negative laterality studies [69, 115, 119]. There are many problems with the available data. First, the rigor with which laterality was established differs across studies, and the use of surface EEG recordings to establish laterality is open to question. Second, the presence of an epileptic focus on one side does not mean that pathology is restricted to that side. Third, left-sided preponderance of temporal lobe foci may not be restricted to psychotic individuals, as the evidence supports a left-sided bias for TLE in general [94]. Fourth, there is emerging evidence that epilepsy patients with schizophrenia have generalized seizures even when they have a temporal focus [4, 66]. Fifth, the instruments and diagnostic criteria used for psychosis are language dependent, thus introducing a left-side bias [89].

The neuroimaging studies that examined laterality were inconclusive. The CT [104, 107] and MRI [120] studies failed to demonstrate lateralized lesions, although the patients with hallucinations had higher T1 values in the left temporal lobe. Two small functional imaging studies [121, 122] provided preliminary evidence of greater left medial temporal lobe dysfunction in SLP with epilepsy. A proton magnetic resonance spectroscopy study [123] showed metabolic abnormalities in the left temporal lobe of patients with SLP and epilepsy. The neuropathological studies [109, 110] have not supported lateralization of pathology.

The laterality issue therefore remains undecided, but the importance of a left-sided focus is not striking. It is possible that the structural abnormality in epileptic psychosis is not lateralized, and is possibly bilateral, but that the functional abnormality is predominantly left-sided. However, right-sided abnormality seems to be sufficient, and generalization of the epileptic disturbance is commonly present.

Sex

A female sex bias was reported by one group [111] but is not generally supported [88, 104, 105, 107].

Family history

Patients who have SLP with epilepsy generally have been reported not to have a greater than normal familial aggregation of schizophreniform disorders [88, 104, 107]. In the Danish longitudinal registers study [92], family history of psychosis was associated with a relative risk of 3.12 (2.83–3.43) of schizophrenia-like psychosis associated with epilepsy. Interestingly, a family history of epilepsy also increased the risk of schizophrenia or SLP, even after adjusting for the effects of personal history of epilepsy and other confounding factors. This familiar aggregation of epilepsy and SLP suggests shared genetic and/or environmental factors.

Premorbid personality

Because patients with primary schizophrenic illness often have abnormalities in their premorbid personalities, their assessment has been considered a measure of vulnerability. Slater and colleagues [88] argued that the premorbid personalities of subjects with psychosis related to epilepsy were normal, suggesting that they were different from primary schizophrenics. However, assessments of premorbid personalities are notoriously unreliable, and other studies have not commented on this aspect.

Postlobectomy psychosis

Schizophrenia-like psychosis may develop *de novo* many months or years after temporal lobectomy for the treatment of intractable epilepsy. Rates from 3% to 28% have been reported, as summarized in Table 6.6. The psychosis is usually a paranoid-hallucinatory state with depressive features [102, 111, 119], the neuropathology is diverse, the patients additionally have had generalized seizures, and there is an overrepresentation of right lobectomy [124, 125, 126]. Roberts and colleagues [109] argued that the postoperative onset of psychosis may be an artifact of an earlier age at operation, but the clustering of the onset of psychosis particularly in the 6 months after the lobectomy argues against this [127]. Shaw and colleagues [127] recently summarized the literature on postlobectomy psychosis, noting reports of 50 cases of *de novo* psychosis following temporal lobectomy, and added 11 of their own. They reiterate the excess of congenital lesions such as dysembryoblastic neuroepithelial tumors in the excised lobes rather than the typical mesial temporal sclerosis. They also emphasize

Table 6.6 Schizophrenia-like psychosis in patients with drug-resistant temporal lobe epilepsy before and after temporal lobectomy

						Schizophrenia-like psychosis		
Authors	N	Years	N	%	Duration of follow-up N	Before lobectomy %	After lobectomy N	New occurrence after lobectomy %
Bailey et al. [128]	63	2–6	12	19	19	30	7	11
Taylor [129]	100	>5	16	16	19	19	3	3
Jensen and Larsen [119]	74	2–5	11	15	20	27	9	12
Polkey [124]	40	2–5	0	0	3	8	3	8
Stevens [125]	14	20–30	0	0	4	28	4	28
Roberts et al. [109]	249	–[a]	16	6	25	10	9	4
Shaw et al. [127]	320	8	–	–	–	–	11	3.4

[a] Not Stated

bilateral temporal lobe abnormalities, reporting bilateral EEG abnormalities preoperatively and a small amygdala on the unoperated side, but right-sided lobectomy did not emerge as a significant risk factor in their series. There are some reports of improvement of schizophrenic symptoms with temporal lobectomy; it is interesting that these cases were associated with left-sided surgery [109, 125].

Neuroimaging studies

A few neuroimaging studies must be highlighted in relation to chronic SLP of epilepsy. An MRI study [120] already referred to did not show any difference in T1 relaxation times between epilepsy-psychosis patients and schizophrenic comparison subjects. There is extensive literature on MRI brain morphometry of schizophrenia and TLE, and some of the morphological abnormalities described (large ventricles, small hippocampus) are common to the disorders [130]. A PET study using ^{15}O-H$_2$O demonstrated lower oxygen extraction ratios in the frontal, temporal, and basal ganglia regions of psychotic patients with epilepsy than in nonpsychotic epileptic patients [121], and a small study using SPECT showed lower left medial temporal blood flow in psychotic than nonpsychotic epileptic patients [122]. The left temporal lobe abnormality was supported by another study [131], but a more recent SPECT study of interictal psychosis in patients with TLE failed to find a significant difference from controls, with a trend for increased blood flow in the posterior cingulated region [132]. The PET study of patients with psychosis by Reith and colleagues [133],

which included two patients with chronic and two with postictal SLP, showed higher than normal levels of dopa decarboxylase activity in SLP and schizophrenia, and it was suggested to be due to suppressed tonic release of dopamine in striatum because of low corticostriatal glutamatergic input.

Neuropathological studies

Neuropathological studies of SLP with epilepsy have been limited. A large series from London, drawing on subjects with histories of temporal lobectomies, has been reported [109, 111]. Taylor [111] commented that epilepsy patients with SLP were less likely to have mesial temporal sclerosis and more likely to have alien tissue lesions (small tumors, hamartomas, and focal dysplasias). In the report by Roberts and colleagues [109], 40% of patients with SLP and epilepsy had mesial temporal sclerosis, 20% had alien tissue gangliomas, and 20% had no lesions (49%, 4%, and 15% of the total epileptic group, respectively). Histories of birth injury, head injury, and febrile convulsions were not overrepresented in the group with SLP, but the frequency of alien tissue tumors and early onset of seizures suggested a developmental lesion in the medial temporal structures that had been physiologically active from an early age. Stevens [134], on the other hand, reported widespread pathology in six cases of epilepsy and psychosis; the pathology included the hippocampus, hypothalamus, thalamus, pallidum, and cerebellum. In a study by Bruton and colleagues [110], epileptic patients with SLP had larger ventricles, more periventricular gliosis, more focal damage, and more periventricular white matter softenings than nonpsychotic epileptic comparison subjects, but similar rates of mesial sclerosis, suggesting greater nonspecific neuropathology.

Possible pathophysiological mechanisms for psychosis in epilepsy

Discussion has centered broadly on two mechanisms: i) the psychosis is due to the repeated electrical discharges, either directly or through the development of neurophysiological or neurochemical abnormalities; or ii) the epilepsy and psychosis share a common neuropathology that may be localized (emphasis on temporal lobe but also frontal lobe and the cerebellum) or widespread in the brain. Both mechanisms may be operative, the latter being primary and the former modifying the presentation, determining exacerbations and remissions, or being the proximate cause. The possible roles of psychological factors, neurotoxicity of anticonvulsant drugs, deficiencies (e.g. folic acid), and abnormal experiences seem to be of secondary importance.

Psychosis is a direct consequence of the epileptiform disturbance

I have previously referred to mechanisms by which seizures may directly result in ictal, postictal, and BIP: continuous subictal activity, homeostatic mechanisms that help reduce epileptic excitability, and neurochemical and neuroendocrine changes produced by the seizures. These explanations are inadequate for chronic SLP although they may account for some fluctuation of symptoms.

Kindling has been proposed as one possible mechanism for the occurrence of chronicity. Studies of behavioral and pharmacological kindling in animals, and the development of mirror foci, suggest that the potential exists for repetitive epileptiform discharges to facilitate subsequent propagation along specific pathways that may cause interictal disturbance. Electrical and pharmacological kindling of the ventral tegmentum and amygdaloid kindling by cocaine and apomorphine in the cat [135] have been suggested as model psychoses. The long duration of epilepsy before the onset of psychosis, the frequency of the partial seizures, and the limbic origin of the seizures provide evidence for this hypothesis. Kindling may thus explain some aspects of the relationship between epilepsy and psychosis, especially

Table 6.7 The cellular and molecular consequences of seizures with relevance to the pathogenesis of chronic psychosis

1. Neurogenesis from precursor or stem cells, especially in the granular layer of hippocampus
2. Neuronal cell death by necrosis or apoptosis, especially in various hippocampal sectors
3. Expansion of glutamatergic presynaptic mossy fibers
4. Sprouting and altered dendritic morphology, resulting in "mis-wiring"
5. Increase in perforated postsynaptic densities on granule cell dendrites
6. Glial cell activation and proliferation
7. Change in ion channels, for example, increased expression of the α_{1H}-subunit of the voltage-sensitive Ca^{++} channel
8. Changes in synaptic function.

the antagonism [136], but there are limitations to the hypothesis: the relationship of the psychosis to seizures is variable in terms of age at onset, duration, and frequency; it is uncertain whether kindling can be permanent; patients usually have generalized seizures and widespread pathology; and kindling currently imputes the dopamine hypothesis of psychosis, support for which is inconsistent. Postlobectomy psychosis has been suggested to be a result of downstream kindling due to persistent ictal activity and perhaps decreased seizure frequency [125]. Delayed psychosis after right temporoparietal stroke has been reported in one series of eight patients, seven of whom developed seizures before the psychosis [137].

Another mechanism by which frequent seizures may bring about chronic behavioral disturbance is the production of plastic regenerative changes affecting, in particular, the medial temporal lobes. Some of the cellular and molecular consequences of repeated seizures are summarized in Table 6.7. The consequences may be somewhat different depending upon whether seizures occur in childhood or adulthood. There may also be genetic susceptibility to brain changes. In mice, there are strain-dependent differences in kainite-induced cell death in the hippocampus [138]. It has been shown that stimulation of the hippocampus leads to an anomalous axonal sprouting from dentate granule cells before the development of seizures [139]. Expansion of glutamatergic presynaptic mossy fibers and an increase in perforated postsynaptic densities on granule cell dendrites have been demonstrated in temporal lobectomy specimens [140], changes possibly produced by increased expression of messenger RNA for c-fos and NGF by recurrent limbic seizures.

In addition, there is neurogenesis as well as neuronal loss, in varying combinations. There is also activation and proliferation of glial cells. Synaptic function and ion channel function may be altered. The aberrant regeneration and the resultant "miswiring" alone or in combination with the other morphological and functional changes interact with the baseline neuropathology. This may be the underlying basis for chronic schizophrenia-like psychosis. The superimposition of seizures on this may further modify the expression of the psychopathology, producing both exacerbations and remissions depending upon their nature and frequency.

Both psychosis and epilepsy are symptomatic of an underlying neuropathological or physiological dysfunction

The following major possibilities may be considered: i) neurodevelopmental abnormalities leading to cortical dysgenesis as the common factor; ii) diffuse brain damage causing both epilepsy and psychosis; and iii) an imbalance of excitation and inhibition.

Cortical dysgenesis hypothesis

Neuropathological studies of temporal lobe epilepsy suggest that about two-thirds of the patients show hippocampal cell loss and sclerosis, particularly in the prosubiculum and CA1 regions, and a substantial proportion of TLE patients [141] have other pathologies, in particular gliomas, hamartomas, and heterotopias. The presence of these alien tissue lesions suggests defective neuroembryogenesis. Patients with mesial sclerosis commonly have heterotopias, hippocampal neuronal loss of about 20% to 50% [141], and synaptic reorganization in the hippocampus. Veith [142] reported heterotopias in 37% of TLE patients but only 4% of nonepileptic comparison subjects. Heterotopic abnormalities have also been described in primary generalized epilepsies [143, 144]. Cryptic insults such as childhood viruses, fever, or minor hypoxia may lead to synaptic reorganization in vulnerable brains, exacerbating the problem. There is now considerable evidence that schizophrenia is associated with cortical maldevelopment [145]. More than a decade ago it was demonstrated that schizophrenic patients had a disorganization of the pyramidal cell layer [146], which was thought to represent a problem in the migration of primitive neurons into the presumptive hippocampal plate. Heterotopias have been demonstrated in the

brains of schizophrenic persons [147], and there is also evidence for synaptic reorganization [148]. These disturbances either have a genetic basis or may be due to prenatal, perinatal, or early developmental insults. If similar developmental abnormalities underlie both epilepsy and schizophrenia, it is not surprising that some epilepsy patients develop SLP. The evidence that SLP is more likely to develop in epileptic patients with developmental brain abnormalities [109, 111, 127] is consistent with this suggestion. That epilepsy and psychosis have different ages at onset may be due to different functional consequences of the abnormalities, depending on the stage of neurodevelopment. Epileptic activity may, in addition, exacerbate an underlying dysgenesis, setting the stage for psychosis.

Diffuse brain damage hypothesis

Although there has been extensive neuropathological interest in the temporal lobe, there is evidence that brain abnormalities in the brains of schizophrenic subjects are widespread [115]. Most neuropathological studies of epilepsy and psychosis have been limited to the examination of resected temporal lobes. The studies by Stevens [125] and Bruton and colleagues [110] are exceptions, revealing excess pathology that was widespread and not dissimilar to some of the pathology reported for schizophrenia. These findings argue that SLP may be related to degenerative or regenerative changes in the brain not directly related to the classic epileptic pathology.

Imbalance of cortical excitation and inhibition

Epileptic conditions are presumed to involve a chronic imbalance of excitatory and inhibitory influences [87], whereas increased inhibition plays an important role in the development and maintenance of the interictal state [149]. Human TLE is associated with enhanced inhibition [150], which contrasts it from neocortical epilepsy, in which the epileptogenic regions demonstrate reduced after-discharge thresholds [151]. The role these inhibitory processes play in the genesis of psychosis has not been adequately examined. Active inhibitory processes may produce focal reversible deficits, but is it possible that chronic SLP is a manifestation of similar processes bilaterally in the limbic and frontal cortices?

Abnormalities of cortical inhibition have been implicated in schizophrenia. Patients with schizophrenia have reduced sensorimotor gating, which has been attributed to the disinhibition of cortical inhibitory processes due to excessive dopamine excitation [152]. The motor abnormalities of schizophrenia, which range from excitation to catatonic stupor, have been attributed to reduced cortical inhibition [153]. Schizophrenic patients have impaired inhibition of event-related potentials to paired auditory stimuli [154]. In a direct examination of cortical inhibition using transcranial magnetic stimulation, it was shown that unmedicated schizophrenic patients had deficits of cortical inhibition that was corrected by medication [155].

The important neurotransmitters involved in the inhibitory processes are GABA, opioids, and adenosine, whereas glutamate is the key excitatory amino acid. Both GABA [156] and glutamic acid [157] have been implicated in the development of psychosis. Glutamate is also important for the maintenance of brain plasticity and surges in its levels may be responsible for mossy fiber sprouting in the hippocampus in TLE. These plastic brain changes associated with epilepsy raise the question whether repeated seizures, and indeed the occurrence of PIP, eventually leads to chronic psychosis. There is a suggestion that this may indeed be the case in some subjects [158].

Composite model

An attempt at a synthesis of the various hypotheses is presented in Figure 6.1. According to this view, epilepsy patients who develop chronic SLP have a brain lesion that makes them vulnerable to psychosis. This lesion may be neurodevelopmental, leading to cortical dysgenesis, or be acquired through trauma, hypoxia, infection, and so on. The abnormality may be widespread but is particularly likely to involve the limbic structures, leading to abnormalities of connectivity of these structures to their afferent and efferent projection regions. Because the development of medial temporal structures is asymmetric, it may explain some of the laterality data. The abnormality is likely to cause electrical storms in the limbic cortex, with seizures occurring at an early age. The occurrence of frank seizures or microseizures exacerbates the abnormality owing to kindling mechanisms or the regenerative and neuroplastic changes involving axonal sprouting, synaptic reorganization, dendritic changes, glial changes, and so on. In due course, these result in disruption of anatomically distributed functional systems and lead to SLP, accounting for the "affinity" between epilepsy and SLP. Seizures, either by the presence of continuous subictal activity or by their modulation of

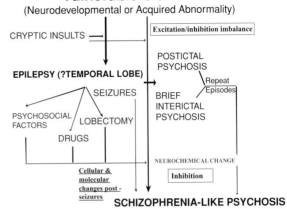

Figure 6.1 Possible pathophysiological mechanisms for the association between epilepsy and schizophrenia-like psychosis.

catecholamine and pre- and post-synaptic glutamatergic and GABAergic activity, modulate the expression of the psychosis or act as brakes, sometimes leading to the impression of antagonism. There may be long-term changes in the balance between excitation and inhibition. The picture is further complicated by drug therapy, with its potential for neurotoxicity, and psychosocial factors related to epilepsy, a chronically disabling and stigmatizing illness.

Future directions

Although the relationship between epilepsy and SLP has in itself been an intriguing clinical issue, it carries within it the potential to provide understanding of the pathogenesis of the schizophrenias in general. The newer epidemiological studies have been more sophisticated, but more work remains to be done. For example, the question of whether SLP is specific to TLE should be further investigated by using extratemporal partial epilepsy and generalized epilepsy patients as comparison subjects and performing longitudinal studies. The determinants of the interval between the onset of epilepsy and that of psychosis should be studied in a longitudinal investigation of TLE patients beginning in the first or early second decade of life. It is important that brief psychoses be distinguished from the chronic psychoses in such investigations. Longitudinal studies are also necessary to determine the factors that lead to chronicity of psychosis in patients with repeated postictal and interictal psychoses. Chronic interictal psychoses studied longitudinally will help determine how seizures modulate the expression of psychotic symptoms. The boundary between postictal and brief interictal psychoses is poorly defined, and a comparison of the clinical features of these subgroups, as currently distinguished, as well as their ictal, EEG, and neuroimaging correlates, will be instructive. Methodologically superior family-genetic studies of SLP will help answer the question of whether the epilepsy patients who become psychotic are so predisposed genetically. Some work of this kind has begun to appear [92].

Newer neurophysiological and neuroimaging techniques have not yet been sufficiently applied to the psychoses of epilepsy. Magnetoencephalography, with its potential to detect deep limbic discharges noninvasively, may help answer the question of whether prolonged psychosis can be produced by continuous subictal activity without abnormalities on scalp EEG. Because both anticonvulsants and antipsychotics may confound such studies, drug-free and preferably drug naive subjects should be studied. Magnetic source imaging is also an excellent technique with which to examine SLP for anomalous cerebral lateralization in view of the intriguing but uncertain literature on laterality of epilepsy and SLP. The application of MRI, with its ability to image mesial sclerosis, heterotopias, and other developmental abnormalities and to perform volumetric assessments, can address a number of questions: Does mesial temporal sclerosis underlie schizophrenia-like psychosis in epilepsy, or is it related to neurodysplastic lesions? Do the patients who develop SLP also have abnormalities of the temporal and/or frontal neocortices? Do they have heterotopias, abnormal gyral patterns, or cortical dysgenesis? Are large ventricles and low volume of the cortex, thalamus, cerebellum, and so on, commonly reported in schizophrenia, also present in the chronic SLP of epilepsy? Functional imaging studies, using PET, SPECT, or functional MRI, should examine the hypothesis of hypofrontality in SLP if a final common pathway for the psychoses is hypothesized. PET and SPECT should be applied to the study of neurotransmitter function in SLP, in particular to examine pre- and post-synaptic dopamine, serotonin, and glutamate functions. Patients who received temporal lobe surgery and had a previous history of psychosis, or developed psychosis subsequently, remain an excellent resource for neuropathological studies. Nonpsychotic patients should be used for comparison, and surgically excised tissue, should be examined for cell disarray, low numbers of certain cells (e.g. neurons containing dinucleotide phosphate diaphorase), small neuronal size, and abnormal cell migration. Newer techniques, such as immunocytochemistry and in situ hybridization for gene expression of messenger RNA, when applied to surgically excised tissue, may help examine the dopamine hyperfunction, glutamate hypofunction, and other neurotransmitter hypotheses of schizophrenia in subjects with SLP. Several techniques are now available to identify candidate genes for cortical development that could be applied to tissue from patients with SLP. Finally, because animal models of epilepsy are well established, they provide a useful entry point to the development of suitable models for schizophrenia or psychotic disturbance.

References

1. Trimble M. (1991). *The Psychoses of Epilepsy*. New York: Raven Press.

2. Taylor D. C. Schizophrenias and epilepsies: Why? When? How? *Epilepsy Behav*, 2003. **4**:474–82.

3. Mace C. J. Epilepsy and schizophrenia. *Br J Psychiatry*, 1993. **163**:439–45.

4. Mendez M. F., Grau R., Doss R. C., *et al.* Schizophrenia in epilepsy: seizure and psychosis variables. *Neurology*, 1993. **43**:1073–7.

5. Stevens J. R. Clozapine: the yin and yang of seizures and psychosis. *Biol Psychiatry*, 1995. **37**:425–6.

6. Trimble M. R., Ring H. A., Schmitz B. (1996). Neuropsychiatric aspects of epilepsy. In *Neuropsychiatry: a Comprehensive Textbook*. Fogel B., Schiffer R., and Rao S. (Eds.). Baltimore: Williams & Wilkins, pp. 771–803.

7. Gastaut H., Gastaut J. L., Goncalves e Silva G. E., *et al.* Relative frequency of different types of epilepsy: a study employing the classification of the International League Against Epilepsy. *Epilepsia*, 1975. **16**:457–61.

8. Cummings J. L. Frontal-subcortical circuits and human behaviour. *Arch Neurol*, 1993. **50**:873–80.

9. Engel J. Jr., Caldecott-Hazard S., Bandler R. Neurobiology of behavior: anatomic and physiologic implications related to epilepsy. *Epilepsia*, 1986; **27**(suppl2):S3–S13.

10. Dichter M. A. Cellular mechanisms of epilepsy and potential new treatment strategies. *Epilepsia*, 1989. **30**(suppl 1):S3–S12.

11. Meldrum B. S. Why and when are seizures bad for the brain? *Trends Pharmacol Sci*, 2001. **22**:445–6.

12. von Meduna L. Uber experimentelle campherepilepsie. *Archiv fur Psychiatrie*, 1934. **102**:333–9.

13. Steinlein O. K. Genetic mechanisms that underlie epilepsy. *Nature Rev Neurosci*, 2004. 400–8.

14. Diagnostic and Statistical Manual of Mental Disorder (4th Edition). (1991). Washington, DC: American Psychiatric Association.

15. Lee S. I. Nonconvulsive status epilepticus. *Arch Neurol*, 1985. **42**:778–81.

16. Scholtes F. B., Renier W. O., Meinardi H. Nonconvulsive status epilepticus: causes, treatment, and outcome in 65 patients. *J Neurol Neurosurg Psychiatry*, 1996. **61**:93–5.

17. Engel J. Jr., Bandler R., Griffith N. C., *et al.* (1991). Neurobiological evidence for epilepsy-induced interictal disturbances. In *Neurobehavioral Problems in Epilepsy: Advances in Neurology*, vol. **55**. Smith D., Treiman D., and Trimble M. (Eds.). New York: Raven Press, pp. 97–111.

18. Fenton G. W. Epilepsy and automatism. *Br J Hosp Med*, 1972. **7**:57–64.

19. Devinsky O., Kelly K., Porter R. J., *et al.* Clinical and electroencephalographic features of simple partial seizures. *Neurology*, 1988. **43**: 1347–52.

20. Williamson P. D., Spencer S. S. Clinical and EEG features of complex partial seizures of extratemporal origin. *Epilepsia*, 1986. **27**(Suppl 2):S46–S63.

21. Trimble M. R. Serum prolactin in epilepsy and hysteria. *Br Med J*, 1978. **2**, 1682.

22. Dana-Haeri J., Trimble M. R., Oxley J. Prolactin and gonadotrophin changes following generalized and partial seizures. *J Neurol Neurosurg Psychiatry*, 1983. **46**:331–5.

23. Gloor P. (1991). Neurobiological substrates of ictal behavioral changes In *Neurobehavioral Problems in Epilepsy: Advances in Neurology*, vol **55**. Smith D., Treiman D. and Trimble M. (Eds.). New York: Raven Press, pp. 1–34.

24. Kendrick J. F., Gibbs F. A. Origin, spread and neurosurgical treatment of the psychomotor type of seizure discharge. *J Neurosurg*, 1957. **14**:270–84.

25. Sem-Jacobsen C. W. Depth electrographic observations on psychotic patients: a system related to emotional behaviour. *Acta Psychiatr Scand*, 1959. **34**:412–16.

26. Heath R. G. Common clinical characteristics of epilepsy and schizophrenia: clinical observation and depth electrode studies. *Am J Psychiatry*, 1962. **118**:1013–26.

27. Engel A. K., Moll C. K. E., Fried I., *et al.* Invasive recordings from the human brain: clinical insights and beyond. *Nat Rev Neurosci*, 2005. **6**:35–47.

28. Fenwick P. (1990). The use of magnetocencephalography in neurology. In *Advances in Neurology*, vol **54**: Magnetoencephalography. Sato S. (Ed.). New York: Raven Press, pp. 271–82.

29. Spencer S. S., Spencer D. D., Williamson P. D., *et al.* The localizing value of depth electroencephalography in 32 patients with refractory epilepsy. *Ann Neurol*, 1982. **12**:248–53.

30. Staba R. J., Wilson C. L., Bragin A., *et al.* Sleep states differentiate single neuron activity recorded from human epileptic hippocampus, entorhinal cortex, and subiculum. *J. Neurosci*, 2002. **22**:5694–704.

31. Logsdail S. J., Toone B. K. Postictal psychosis: a clinical and phenomenological description. *Br J Psychiatry*, 1988. **152**:246–52.

32. So N. K., Savard G., Andermann F., *et al.* Acute postictal psychosis: a stereo EEG study. *Epilepsia*, 1990. **31**:188–93.

33. Savard G., Andermann F., Olivier A., Remillard G. M. Postictal psychosis after partial complex seizures: a multiple case study. *Epilepsia*, 1991. **32**:225–31.

34. Baumgartner C., Podreka I., Benda N., *et al.* Postictal psychosis: a SPECT study (abstract). *Epilepsia*, 1995. **36**(Suppl 3):S218.

35. Kanner A. M., Stagno S., Kotagal P., *et al.* Postictal psychiatric events during prolonged video-electroencephalographic monitoring studies. *Arch Neurol*, 1996. **53**:258–63.

36. Krishnamoorthy E. S. An approach to classifying neuropsychiatric disorders in epilepsy. *Epilepsy Behav*, 2000. **1**:373–7.

37. Kanemoto K., Takenchi J., Kawasaki J., Kawai I. Characteristics of temporal lobe epilepsy with mesial temporal sclerosis, with special reference to psychotic episodes. *Neurology*, 1996. **47**:1199–203.

38. Ketter T. A., Malow B. A., Flamini R., *et al.* Anticonvulsant withdrawal-emergent psychopathology. *Neurology*, 1994. **44**:55–61.

39. Kanemoto K., Kawasaki J., Kawai I. Postictal psychosis: a comparison with acute interictal and chronic psychoses. *Epilepsia*, 1996. **37**:551–6.

40. Fisher R. S., Schachter S. C. The postictal state: a neglected entity in the management of epilepsy. *Epilepsy Behav*, 2000. **1**:52–9.

41. Akanuma N., Kanemoto K., Adachi N., *et al.* Prolonged postictal psychosis with forced normalization (Landolt) in temporal lobe epilepsy. *Epilepsy Behav*, 2005. **6**:456–9.

42. Haglund M. M., Schwartzkroin P. A. Role of Na-K pump, potassium regulation and IPSPs in seizures and spreading depression in immature rabbit hippocampal slices. *J Neurophysiol*, 1990. **63**:225–39.

43. Meldrum B. S. (1991). Neurochemical substrates of ictal behavior. In *Problems in Epilepsy: Advances in Neurology*, vol **55**. Smith D., Treiman D., and Trimble M. (Eds.). New York: Raven Press, pp. 35–45.

44. Holaday J. W., Tortella F. C., Long J. B., *et al.* Endogenous opioids and their receptors: evidence for involvement in the postictal effects of electroconvulsive shock. *Ann NY Acad Sci*, 1986. **462**:124–39.

45. Molaie M., Kadzielawa K. Effect of naloxone infusion on the rate of epileptiform discharges in patients with complex partial seizures. *Epilepsia*, 1989. **30**:194–200.

46. Sperling M. R., Melmed S., McAllister T., *et al.* Lack of effect of naloxone on prolactin and seizures in electroconvulsive therapy. *Epilepsia*, 1989. **30**:41–4.

47. Velisek L., Mares P. Differential effects of naloxone on postictal depression. *Epilepsy Res*, 1992. **12**:37–43.

48. Paul S. M., Skolnik P. Rapid changes in brain benzodiazepine receptors after experimental seizures. *Science*, 1978. **202**:892–4.

49. Lancman M. E., Craven W. J., Asconape J. J., *et al.* Clinical management of recurrent postictal psychosis. *J Epilepsy*, 1994. **7**:47–51.

50. Akanuma N., Kanemoto K., Adachi N., *et al.* Prolonged postictal psychosis with forced normalization (Landolt) in temporal lobe epilepsy. *Epilepsy Behav*, 2005. **6**:456–9.

51. Umbricht D., Degreef G., Barr W. B., *et al.* Postictal and chronic psychoses in patients with temporal lobe epilepsy. *Am J Psychiatry*, 1995. **152**:224–31.

52. Devinsky O., Abramson H., Alper K., *et al.* Postictal psychosis: a case control series of 20 patients and 150 controls. *Epilepsy Res*, 1995. **20**:247–53.

53. Adachi N., Onuma T., Nishiwaki S., *et al.* Inter-ictal and post-ictal psychoses in frontal lobe epilepsy: a retrospective comparison with psychoses in temporal lobe epilepsy. *Seizure*, 2000. **9**:328–35.

54. Mathern G. W., Pretorius J. K., Babb T. L., *et al.* Unilateral hippocampal mossy fiber sprouting and bilateral asymmetric neuron loss with episodic postictal psychosis. *J Neurosurg*, 1995. **82**:228–33.

55. Ring H. A., Trimble M. R., Costa D. C., *et al.* Striatal dopamine receptor binding in epileptic psychosis. *Biol Psychiatry*, 1994. **35**:375–80.

56. Reynolds E. H. (1991). Interictal psychiatric disorders: neurochemical aspects. In *Advances in Neurology*, vol **55**. Smith D., Treiman D., and Trimble M. (Eds.). New York: Raven Press, pp. 47–58.

57. Fisher R. S., Prince D. A. Spike-wave rhythms in cat cortex induced by parenteral penicillin. II. Cellular features. *Electroencephalogr Clin Neurophysiol*, 1977. **42**:625–39.

58. Herreras O., Somjen G. G. Analysis of potential shifts associated with recurrent spreading depression and prolonged unstable spreading depression induced by microdialysis of elevated K+ in hippocampus of anesthetized rats. *Brain Res*, 1993. **610**:284–94.

59. Leutmezer F., Podreka I., Asenbaum S., *et al.* Postictal psychosis in temporal lobe epilepsy. *Epilepsia*, 2003. **44**:582–90.

60. Fong G. C., Fong K. Y., Mak W., *et al.* Postictal psychosis related regional cerebral hyperperfusion.

J Neurol Neurosurg Psychiatry, 2000. **68**:100–1.

61. Kimura M., Sejima H., Ozasa H., *et al.* Technitium-99m-HMPAO SPECT in patients with hemiconvulsions followed by Todd's paralysis. *Pediatr Radiol*, 1998. **28**:92–4.

62. Tellenbach H. Epilepsie als Anfallsleiden und als Psychose: Uber alternative Psychosen paranoider Pragung bei "forcierter Normalisierung" (Landolt) des Elektroencephalogramms Epileptischer. *Nervenarzt*, 1965. **36**:190–202.

63. Ramani V., Gumnit R. J. Intensive monitoring of interictal psychosis in epilepsy. *Ann Neurol*, 1982. **11**:613–22.

64. Wolf P. The clinical syndromes of forced normalization. *Jpn J Psychiatry Neurol*, 1984. **38**:187–92.

65. Pakalnis A., Drake M. E., John K., *et al.* Forced normalization: acute psychosis after seizure control in 7 patients. *Arch Neurol*, 1987. **44**:289–92.

66. Wolf P. (1991). Acute behavioral symptomatology at disappearance of epileptiform EEG abnormality: paradoxical or "forced" normalization. In *Neurobehavioral Problems in Epilepsy: Advances in Neurology*, vol **55**. Smith D., Treiman D., and Trimble M. (Eds.). New York: Raven Press, 1991, pp. 127–42.

67. Schmitz B., Wolf P. Psychosis in epilepsy: frequency and risk factors. *J Epilepsy*, 1995. **8**:295–305.

68. Landolt H. Some clinical electroencephalographical correlations in epileptic psychoses (twilight states). *Electroencephalogr Clin Neurophysiol*, 1953. **5**:121.

69. Kristensen O., Sindrup H. H. Psychomotor epilepsy and psychosis. *Acta Neurol Scand*, 1987. **57**:361–79.

70. Schimtz B. (1998). Forced normalization: history of a concept. In *Forced Normalization and Alternative Psychoses of Epilepsy*. Trimble M. R. and Schmitz B. (Eds.). Petersfield: Wrightson Biomedical, pp. 7–24.

71. Willmore L. J. When seizures are complicated by coma. *Geriatrics*, 1976. **31**:112–14.

72. Rolak L. A., Rutecki P., Ashizawa T., *et al.* Clinical features of Todd's post-epileptic paralysis. *J Neurol Neurosurg Psychiatry*, 1992. **55**:63–4.

73. Kanemoto K., Tsuji T., Kawasaki J. Reexamination of interictal psychosis based on DSM-IV psychosis classification and international epilepsy classification. *Epilepsia*, 2001. **42**:98–103.

74. Gibbs F. A. Ictal and nonictal psychiatric disorders in temporal lobe epilepsy. *J Nerv Ment Dis*, 1951. **113**:522–8.

75. Landolt H. (1958). Serial electroencephalographic investigations during psychotic episodes in epileptic patients and during schizophrenic attacks, In Lectures on Epilepsy. Lorentz de Haas A. M. (Ed.). Amsterdam: Elsevier, pp. 91–133.

76. Sander J. W. A. S., Hart Y. M., Trimble M. R., *et al.* Vigabatrin and psychosis. *J Neurol Neurosurg Psychiatry*, 1991. **54**:435–9.

77. Mula M., Trimble M. R. The importance of being seizure free: topiramate and psychopathology in epilepsy. *Epilepsy Behav*, 2003. **4**:430–4.

78. Mula M., Trimble M. R., Sander J. W. A. S. Psychiatric adverse effects in patients with epilepsy and learning difficulties taking levetiracetam. *Seizure*, 2004. **13**:55–7.

79. Hirsch E., Schmitz B., Carreňo M. Epilepsy, antiepileptic drugs (AEDs) and cognition. *Acta Neurol Scand*, 2003. **108**:23–32.

80. Chapman A. G., Meldrum B. S. Excitatory amino acid antagonists and epilepsy. *Biochem Soc Trans*, 1993. **21**:106–10.

81. Itil T. M., Soldatos C. Epileptogenic side effects of psychotropic drugs. *JAMA*, 1980. **244**:1460–3.

82. Alldredge B. Seizure risk associated with psychotropic drugs: clinical and pharmacokinetic considerations. *Neurology*, 1999. **53**(Suppl 2): S68–S75.

83. Pacia S. V., Devinsky O. Clozapine-related seizures: experience with 5,629 patients. *Neurology*, 1994. **44**:2247–9.

84. Physicians' Desk Reference. Montvale, NJ: Medical Economics, 1999.

85. Pauig P. M., Deluca M. A., Osterheld R. G. Thioridazine hydrochloride in the treatment of behavior disorders in epileptics. *Am J Psychiatry*, 1961. **117**:832–3.

86. Adachi N., Kato M., Sekimoto M., *et al.* Recurrent postictal psychosis after remission of interictal psychosis: further evidence of bimodal psychosis. *Epilepsia*, 2003. **44**: 1218–22.

87. Engel J. Jr. Excitation and inhibition in epilepsy. *Can J Neurol Sci*, 1996. **23**:167–74.

88. Slater E., Beard A. W., Glithero E. The schizophrenia-like psychoses of epilepsy, i–v. *Br J Psychiatry*, 1963. **109**:95–150.

89. Stevens J. R. (1991). Psychosis and the temporal lobe. In *Neurobehavioral problems in epilepsy: advances in neurology*, vol **55**. Smith D., Treiman D., and Trimble M. (Eds.). New York Raven Press, pp. 79–96.

90. Shorvon S. D. Epidemiology, classification, natural history, and genetics of epilepsy. *Lancet*, 1990. **336**:93–6.

91. Hauser W. A., Annegess J. F., Rocca W. A. Descriptive epidemiology of

epilepsy-contributions of population-based studies from Rochester, Minnesota. *Mayo Clin Proc*, 1996. **71**:576–86.

92. Qin P., Xu H., Laursen T. M., *et al.* Risk for schizophrenia and schizophrenia-like psychosis among patients with epilepsy: population based cohort study. *BMJ*, 2005. **331**(7507): 23. [Epub June 17, 2005.]

93. Gibbs F. A., Gibbs E. L. (1952). *Atlas of Electroencephalography*, vol **11**: *Epilepsy*. Cambridge, Mass: Addison-Wesley.

94. Currie S., Heathfield K. W. G., Henson R. A., *et al.* Clinical course and prognosis of temporal lobe epilepsy. *Brain*, 1971. **94**:173–90.

95. Standage K. F., Fenton G. W. Psychiatric profiles of patients with epilepsy: a controlled investigation. *Psychol Med*, 1975. **5**:152–60.

96. Onuma T., Adachi N., Ishida S., *et al.* Prevalence and annual incidence of psychoses in patients with epilepsy (Abstract). *Epilepsia*, 1995. **36**(Suppl 3):S218.

97. Krohn W. A study of epilepsy in Northern Norway: its frequency and character. *Acta Psychiatr Scand Suppl*, 1961. **150**:215–25.

98. Gudmundsson G. Epilepsy in Iceland – a clinical and epidemiological investigation. *Acta Neurol Scand Suppl*, 1966. **25**:1–124.

99. Kat W. Uber den Gegensatz Epilepsie-Schizophrenie und das kombinierte Vorkommen dieser Krankheiten (Antagonism between epilepsy and schizophrenia and simultaneous occurrence of these diseases). *Psychiatr en Neurol*, **B1** 1937. **41**:733–45.

100. Davison K., Bagley C. R. (1969). Schizophrenia-like psychoses associated with organic disorder of the central nervous system; a review of the literature. In *Current Problems in Neuropsychiatry*. British Journal of Psychiatry Special Publication 4. Herrington R. N. (Ed.). Ashford, Kent, England: Headley Brothers, pp. 1–45.

101. Betts T. A. (1981). Epilepsy and the mental hospital. In *Epilepsy and Psychiatry*. Reynolds E. H. and Trimble M. R. (Eds.). Edinburgh, Churchill: Livingstone, pp. 175–84.

102. Lindsay J., Ounstead C., Richards P. Long term outcome in children with temporal lobe seizures, III: psychiatric aspects in childhood and adult life. *Dev Med Child Neurol*, 1979. **21**:630–6.

103. Perez M. M., Trimble M. R. Epileptic psychosis-diagnostic comparison with process schizophrenia. *Br J Psychiatry*, 1980. **137**:245–9.

104. Toone B. K., Garralda M. E., Ron M. A. The psychoses of epilepsy and the functional psychoses. *Br J Psychiatry*, 1982. **141**:256–61.

105. Kraft A. M., Price T. R. P., Peltier D. Complex partial seizures and schizophrenia. *Compr Psychiatry*, 1984. **25**:113–24.

106. McKenna P. J., Kane J. M., Parrish K. Psychotic syndromes in epilepsy. *Am J Psychiatry*, 1985. **142**:895–904.

107. Perez M. M., Trimble M. R., Murray N. M. F., *et al.* Epileptic psychosis: an evaluation of PSE profiles. *Br J Psychiatry*, 1985. **146**:155–63.

108. Onuma T., Adachi N., Hisano T., *et al.* 10-year follow-up study of epilepsy with psychosis. *Jpn J Psychiatry Neurol*, 1991. **45**:360–1.

109. Roberts G. W., Done D. J., Bruton C., *et al.* A "mock up" of schizophrenia: temporal lobe epilepsy and schizophrenia-like psychosis. *Biol Psychiatry*, 1990. **28**:127–43.

110. Bruton C. J., Stevens J. R., Frith C. D. Epilepsy, psychosis, and schizophrenia: clinical and neuropathologic correlations. *Neurology*, 1994. **44**:34–42.

111. Taylor D. C. Factors influencing the occurrence of schizophrenia-like psychosis in patients with temporal lobe epilepsy. *Psychol Med*, 1975. **5**:249–54.

112. Sachdev P. Schizophrenia-like psychosis and epilepsy: the status of the association. *Am J Psychiatry*, 1998. **155**:325–36.

113. Bruens J. H. Psychoses in epilepsy. *Psychiatr Neurol Neurochir*, 1971. **74**:174–92.

114. Small J. G., Milstein V., Stevens J. R. Are psychomotor epileptics different? *Arch Neurol*, 1962. **7**:187–94.

115. Shukla G. D., Srivastava O. N., Katiyar B. C., *et al.* Psychiatric manifestations of temporal lobe epilepsy: a controlled study. *Br J Psychiatry*, 1979. **135**:411–17.

116. Hermann B. P., Dikmen S., Schwartz M. S., *et al.* Interictal psychopathology in patients with ictal fear: a quantitative investigation. *Neurology*, 1982. **32**:7–11.

117. Flor-Henry P. Psychosis and temporal lobe epilepsy. *Epilepsia*, 1969. **10**:363–95.

118. Sherwin I. Psychosis associated with epilepsy: significance of laterality of the epileptogenic lesion. *J Neurol Neurosurg Psychiatry*, 1981. **44**:83–5.

119. Jensen I., Larsen J. K. Psychoses in drug-resistant temporal lobe epilepsy. *J Neurol Neurosurg Psychiatry*, 1979. **42**:948–54.

120. Conlon P., Trimble M. R., Rogers D. A study of epileptic psychosis using magnetic resonance imaging. *Br J Psychiatry*, 1990. **156**:231–5.

121. Gallhofer B., Trimble M. R., Frackowiak R., *et al.* A study of cerebral blood flow and metabolism in epileptic psychosis using positron emission tomography and oxygen. *J Neurol Neurosurg Psychiatry*, 1985. **48**:201–06.

122. Marshall J. E., Syed G. M. B., Fenwick P. B. C., *et al.* A pilot study of schizophrenia-like psychosis in epilepsy using single-photon emission computerized tomography. *Br J Psychiatry*, 1993. **163**:32–6.

123. Fujimoto T., Takano T., Takeuch K., *et al.* Proton magnetic resonance spectroscopy of temporal lobe in epileptic psychosis and schizophrenia (abstract). *Epilepsia*, 1995. **36**(Suppl 3):S174

124. Polkey C. E. Effects of anterior temporal lobectomy apart from the relief of seizures: a study of 40 patients. *J R Soc Med*, 1983. **76**:354–8.

125. Stevens J. R. Psychiatric consequences of temporal lobectomy for intractable seizures: a 20–30 year follow-up of 14 cases. *Psychol Med*, 1990. **20**:529–45.

126. Mace C. J., Trimble M. R. Psychosis following temporal lobe surgery: a report of six cases. *J Neurol Neurosurg Psychiatry*, 1991. **54**:639–44.

127. Shaw P., Mellers J., Henderson M., *et al.* Schizophrenia-like psychosis arising de novo following a temporal lobectomy: timing and factors. *J Neurol Neurosurg Psychiatry*, 2004. **75**:1003–8.

128. Baily P., Green J. R., Amador L., *et al.* Treatment of psychomotor states by temporal lobectomy: a report of progress. *Res Publ Assoc Res Nerv Ment Dis*, 1953. **31**:341–6.

129. Taylor D. C. Mental state and temporal lobe epilepsy: a correlative account of 100 patients treated surgically. *Epilepsia*, 1972. **13**:727–65.

130. Barr W. B., Ashtari M., Bilder R. M., *et al.* Brain morphometric comparison of first-episode schizophrenia and temporal lobe epilepsy. *Br J Psychiatry*, 1997. **170**:515–9.

131. Mellers J. D., Adachi N., Yakei N., *et al.* SPET study of verbal fluency in schizophrenia and epilepsy. *Br J Psychiatry*, 1998. **173**:69–74.

132. Guarnieri R., Wichert-Ana L., Jallak J. E. C., *et al.* Interictal SPECT in patients with mesial temporal lobe epilepsy and psychosis: a case-control study. *Psychiatry Res Neuroimaging*, 2005. **138**:75–84.

133. Reith J., Benkelfat C., Sherwin A., *et al.* Elevated dopa decarboxylase activity in living brain of patients with psychosis. *Proc Natl Acad Sci USA*, 1994. **91**:11651–4.

134. Stevens J. R. (1986). Epilepsy and psychosis: neuropathological studies of six cases, In *Aspects of Epilepsy and Psychiatry*. Trimble M. R. and Bolwig T. G. (Eds.). New York: John Wiley & Sons, pp. 117–46.

135. Sato M. Long-lasting hypersensitivity to methamphetamine following amygdaloid kindling in cats: the relationship between limbic epilepsy and the psychotic state. *Biol Psychiatry*, 1983. **18**:525–36.

136. Pollock D. C. Models for understanding the antagonism between seizures and psychosis. *Prog Neuropsychopharmacol Biol Psychiatry*, 1987. **11**:483–504.

137. Levine D. N., Finklestein S. Delayed psychosis after right temporoparietal stroke and seizures or trauma: relation to epilepsy. *Neurology*, 1982. **32**:267–73.

138. Schauwecker P. E., Steward O. Genetic determinants of susceptibility to excitotoxic cell death: implications for gene targeting approaches. *Proc Natl Acad Sci USA*, 1997. **94**:4103–8.

139. Sutula T., He X. X., Cavazos J., *et al.* Synaptic reorganization in the hippocampus induced by abnormal functional activity. *Science*, 1988. **239**:1147–50.

140. Babb T. L., Kupfer W. R., Pretorius J. K. Synaptic reorganization of mossy fibers into molecular layer in human epileptic fascia dentata. *Abstracts of the Society for Neuroscience*, 1988. **88**:351.

141. Babb T. L., Brown W. J. Neuronal, dendritic, and vascular profiles of human temporal lobe epilepsy correlated with cellular physiology in vivo. *Adv Neurol*, 1986. **44**:949–66.

142. Veith G. Anatomische Studie uber die Ammonshornsklerose im Epileptikergehirn. *Dtsch Z Nervenheilkd*, 1970. **197**:293–314.

143. Meencke H. J., Janz D. Neuropathological findings in primary generalized epilepsy: a study of eight cases. *Epilepsia*, 1984. **25**:8–21.

144. Houser C. R. Granule cell dispersion in the dentate gyrus of humans with temporal lobe epilepsy. *Brain Res*, 1990. **535**:195–204.

145. Weinberger D. R., Lipska B. K. Cortical maldevelopment, anti-psychotic drugs, and schizophrenia: a search for common ground. *Schizophr Res*, 1995. **16**:87–110.

146. Scheibel A. B., Kovelman J. A. Disorientation of the hippocampal pyramidal cell and its processes in the schizophrenic patient. *Biol Psychiatry*, 1981. **16**:101–2.

147. Akbarian S., Bunney JE Jr., Potkin SG., *et al.* Altered distribution of nicotinamide-adenine dinucleotide phosphate-diaphorase cells in frontal lobe of schizophrenia implies disturbance of cortical development. *Arch Gen Psychiatry*, 1993. **50**:169–77.

148. Benes F. M. Altered glutamatergic and GABAergic mechanisms in the cingulated cortex of the schizophrenic brain. *Arch Gen Psychiatry*, 1995. **52**:1015–18.

149. Swanson T. H. The pathophysiology of human mesial temporal lobe epilepsy. *J Clin Neuropshysiol*, 1995. **12**:2–21.

150. Cherlow D. G., Dymond A. M., Crandall P. H., *et al.* Evoked

response and after-discharge thresholds to electrical stimulation in temporal lobe epileptics. *Arch Neurol*, 1977. **34**:527–31.

151. Penfield W., Jasper H. (1954). *Epilepsy and the Functional Anatomy of the Human Brain*. Boston: Little, Brown & Co.

152. Swerdlow N. R., Koob G. F. Dopamine, schizophrenia, mania, depression: toward a unified hypothesis of cortico-striatal-pallido-thalamic function. *Behav Brain Sci*, 1987. **10**:197–245.

153. Walker E. F. Developmentally moderated expressions of the neuropathology underlying schizophrenia. *Schizophr Bull*, 1994. **20**:453–80.

154. Adler L. E., Pachtman E., Franks R. D., *et al.* Neurophysiological evidence for a deficit in neuronal mechanisms involved in sensory gating in schizophrenia. *Biol Psychiatry*, 1982. **17**:639–54.

155. Daskalakis Z. J., Christensen B. K., Chen R., *et al.* Evidence for impaired cortical inhibition in schizophrenia using transcranial magnetic stimulation. *Arch Gen Psychiatry*, 2002. **59**:347–54.

156. Lewis D. A., Pierri J. N., Volk D. W., *et al.* Altered GABA neurotransmission and prefrontal cortical dysfunction in schizophrenia. *Biol Psychiatry*, 1999. **46**:616–26.

157. Tamminga C. Glutamatergic aspects of schizophrenia. *Br J Psychiatry*, 1999. (Suppl) **37**:12–15.

158. Kanemoto K., Kawasaki J., Kawai I. Postictal psychosis: a comparison with acute interictal and chronic psychoses. *Epilepsia*, 1996. **37**:551–6.

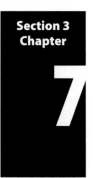

7

Understanding the pathophysiology of schizophrenia through the looking glass of forced normalization

Ennapadam S. Krishnamoorthy and Seethalakshmi Ramanathan

Facts box

- Landolt described Forced Normalization (FN) as "the phenomenon characterized by the fact that, with the occurrence of psychotic states, the EEG becomes more normal or entirely normal, as compared with previous and subsequent EEG findings."

- The terms "paradoxical normalization" and "relative normalization" have been suggested for this phenomenon.

- Although Landolt reported it to be common in psychosis of epilepsy, subsequent investigators have reported much lower figures.

- The pathophysiology of FN is incompletely understood and various mechanisms involving kindling, active inhibition, alternative propagation of epileptic discharge, neurotransmitters (dopamine, gamma-aminobutryric acid [GABA], glutamate, adenosine, opioids, and so on), apoptosis, and vascular dysfunction have been suggested.

- FN offers a good model to understand the antagonism between epilepsy and psychosis.

Introduction

Nearly a century after its conceptualization, the etiology of schizophrenia continues to remain elusive. An important reason for this uncertainty is our inability to predict the potential development of schizophrenia in an individual before the clinical onset of the illness. Induced psychotic disorders are one way of understanding neural mechanisms that play a role in the development of schizophrenia. Of these, the phenomenon of FN in epilepsy is of particular interest, in that it indicates a possible antagonism between the epileptic and psychotic processes, in line with von

Meduna's hypothesis that led to the development of electroconvulsive therapy (ECT). In this chapter, we review the phenomenon of FN and its current clinical relevance. We explore the modern understanding of putative neurobiological mechanisms that may play a role in the development of FN and the alternative psychosis of epilepsy. Finally, we discuss the lessons learned and their implications for our understanding of the psychotic process.

Forced normalization in epilepsy – evolution of a concept

The biological antagonism between epilepsy and psychopathology has been known since the nineteenth century. An increased association between epilepsy and psychiatric disorders, observed in this time, led to the suggestion that an acute onset of a psychiatric illness could be a form of epilepsy. Terms such as epileptic equivalents, larval epilepsy, and transformed epilepsy appeared in the European literature referring largely to the acute onset of behavioral problems resembling paroxysmal episodes of seizures. In the early part of the twentieth century, however, a conceptual change occurred with authors reporting a decreased incidence of comorbid epilepsy and schizophrenia [1]. Von Meduna [2] suggested that whereas epilepsy was characterized by *hyper*functioning glial cells, schizophrenia was characterized by *hypo*function. Based on the hypothesis of biological antagonism between seizures and schizophrenia, Von Meduna developed convulsive therapy. Although it was probably theoretically flawed, Von Meduna's treatment went on to witness considerable success and continued evolution.

Nearly half a century later, in 1953, Heinrich Landolt [3] observed and described the clinical and electrophysiological phenomenon of seizures and psychopathology presenting alternately in certain cases. Landolt noted three different types of psychotic states associated with epilepsy: a postparoxysmal twilight state of postictal psychosis; the nonconvulsive ictal states; and finally, productive psychotic episodes with forced normalization on electroencephalograph (EEG). Based on the observation of 107 patients with epilepsy and psychoses over 10 years, Landolt noted that 47 (44%) of these patients demonstrated "forced normalization" (*forcierte Normalisierung*) [4].

Landolt concluded that FN is "the phenomenon characterized by the fact that, with the occurrence of psychotic states, the EEG becomes more normal or entirely normal, as compared with previous and subsequent EEG findings." FN, as described by Landolt [4], was therefore an electrophysiological phenomenon with the EEG at its helm. Tellenbach's [5] description of "alternative psychosis" or the reciprocal relationship between abnormal mental states and seizures differed from Landolt's in its clinical rather than EEG description. Subsequently, this concept was refined by Wolf [6], who suggested that the term "paradoxical normalization" was more appropriate and closer to what Landolt intended, wherein both epileptic processes – subcortical and restricted – and inhibitory processes are active at the same time.

Forced normalization – clinical features and diagnosis

Clinical description

Landolt reported that 44% of people with psychoses of epilepsy manifest FN, suggesting a reasonably frequent phenomenon. Other authors [1] have reported lower frequencies of FN with no study that has screened for the phenomenon failing to identify cases. FN occurs following rapid control of seizures often with a novel antiepileptic drug (AED). Indeed, the first series of cases described by Landolt became manifest with the availability and utilization of ethosuximide, then a novel AED. Even today, drugs that have powerful antiepileptic properties and switch off seizures appear to provoke FN with normalization of the EEG, topiramate being a good example [7].

The psychiatric symptoms in FN occur in clear consciousness generally 2 to 3 days following seizure cessation. FN usually manifests after a relatively prolonged period of epilepsy and an average duration of 15.2 years has been suggested [8]. It has been observed with both generalized and focal epilepsies – temporal lobe epilepsy (TLE) perhaps being the most common

form to manifest the phenomenon. The severity and intractability of the seizure disorder and laterality of seizure focus have also been discussed as being possibly contributory. It has been suggested that following temporal lobectomy, psychosis is more common with left-sided pathology than following right-sided lobectomy [9].

As mentioned earlier, in Landolt's series of FN [4], several of the patients were on a newly introduced AED, ethosuximide. Since then, FN has been reported with nearly all AEDs: phenytoin, primidone, valproate, carbamazepine, felbamate, vigabatrin, lamotrigine, tiagabine, topiramate, zonisamide, and levetiracetam. Indeed, it is striking to note that FN has, so far, not been reported with those drugs that do not really have significant antiepileptic efficacy. Antiepileptic agents such as gabapentin are a case in point. Polytherapy, rapidity of drug introduction, and total dose prescribed appear to play a role, although the impact of drug type and its mechanism of action remain unclear. The phenomenon has also been described following temporal lobectomy [9, 10] and vagus nerve stimulation [11].

One of the largest series of FN has been described by Wolf [8]. He observed that the psychopathology could vary from hallucinations to severe anxiety and in some cases conversion disorder. The psychiatric phenomena of FN generally follow a trait phenomenon with similar symptoms occurring with every episode of FN. However, with repeated episodes of FN, the clinical presentation can vary. A recent case report [12] discusses the longitudinal course of a woman with complex partial seizures who presented serially with psychosis, depression, and later, pseudoseizures all occurring in the context of FN.

Alternative psychosis is characterized by clouding of consciousness and a pleomorphic presentation including persecutory, grandiose, referential, somatic, and religious delusions, catatonia, hallucinations, and affective symptoms, with a rather variable course. Dramatic presentations of psychopathology, including self-mutilation and suicidal behavior, have been witnessed during the course of this alternative psychosis (Michael Trimble; personal communication, 2007). Further, it is widely acknowledged that psychoses need not be the main manifestation of FN, with the term "alternative psychoses" being in itself a misnomer. Indeed, the senior author has encountered depression, anxiety, and agitation, episodic dyscontrol, and hysteria as part of the FN syndrome. Subclinical syndromes of FN are also not uncommon in clinical practice and often manifest with altered behavior and relative normalization of the EEG. Very often, the episodes terminate with a breakthrough clinical seizure followed by normal behavior.

Diagnostic criteria

Krishnamoorthy and Trimble [13] proposed diagnosed criteria for FN and elaborated on these in a subsequent paper [14]. The quantification of EEG change proposed the emergence of the concept of "relative normalization" and the integration of the FN and alternative psychosis concepts differentiate these writings from previous attempts. These diagnostic criteria are reviewed here.

Primary criteria include:

1. Established diagnosis of epilepsy based on clinical history, EEG, and imaging;
2. The presence of behavior disturbance and acute/subacute onset characterized by one or more of the following:

   a. Psychosis with thought disorder, delusions, hallucinations, and so on;

   b. Significant mood change – hypomania/mania or depression;

   c. Anxiety with depersonalization, derealization, and so on;

   d. Hysteria-motor, sensory, astasia-abasia, and so on;

3a. A reduction in the total number of spikes by more than 50%, when compared to a similar recording performed during a normal state of behavior counted in a 60-minute awake EEG recording, performed using a 16-channel machine and the standard 10–20 system of electrode placement; OR
3b. A report of complete cessation of seizures corroborated by a relative or caregiver.

Supportive criteria include:

1. A recent change (within 30 days) of the pharmacologic regimen;
2. Report of similar episodes of seizure cessation and behavioral disturbance in the past, from a close relative, caregiver, or general practitioner – or documentation of this in hospital records, with or without EEG evidence. This may or may not be linked to anticonvulsant drugs.

In order to make the diagnosis of FN, it is necessary to identify primary criteria 1, 2, and 3a, or primary criteria 1, 2, and 3b plus one supportive criterion.

Putative neurobiological mechanisms

One of the earliest explanations of FN was put forward by Wolf [6]. He suggested that in FN, epileptic processes are still active but subcortical and restricted due to the influence of active inhibitory processes. These inhibitory processes also lead to insomnia, hypervigilance, and dysphoria. These, along with other risk factors such as past psychotic experiences, premorbid personality, social competence, and general life situations, lead to the development of psychosis. Thus, according to Wolf [6], continuing epileptic status in the limbic system; propagation of epileptiform discharges along unusual pathways; a possible role of the reticular activating system (RAS) and its interactions with hippocampal structures; a role of AEDs in influencing underlying metabolic processes or increasing activation, leading to sleep withdrawal and psychoses; reactions of the healthy parts of the brain against the epileptic focus of illness and the entire psychosocial consequences of that reaction; and inability of patients with epilepsy to adjust socially to the sudden loss lead to FN. Since then a number of possible explanations have been put forward.

Limbic kindling

One of the most discussed explanations for FN is amygdaloid and limbic kindling, or occurrence of subthreshold seizures that in turn result in long-term potentiation of synapses [13, 15].

Kindling defines a mechanism by which repeated (daily) brief, high-frequency trains of electrical pulses to limbic and cortical areas produce a change in response to the stimulus, such that the latter elicits a motor convulsion that outlasts the stimulus train. Thus, when a current of low amplitude but high pulse frequency is applied to the amygdala, a region of great susceptibility, there is a gradual stepwise progression of behavioral and EEG responses that finally culminate in a full motor seizure. Kindling thus results in a progressive behavioral sequence that follows the EEG changes.

Although electrical kindling has gained acceptance as a useful model for understanding epilepsy, it has also been postulated that pharmacologic kindling and behavioral sensitization may be a used to explain psychosis in human epilepsy. A number of pharmacologic compounds have been shown to produce behavioral responses, beyond their documented pharmacologic effects. It has been postulated that the end-point for pharmacologic kindling may be a particular form of affective expression or behavior, unlike electrical kindling that terminates in a motor seizure. Stevens and Livermore [16] and later Sato and colleagues [17] developed interesting experimental models whereby they demonstrated that pharmacological kindling, with the use of various dopamine agonists, antagonists, and catecholaminergic agents can modify behaviors.

The process of kindling involves the spread of seizure activity from the site of stimulation to other areas of the CNS. It has therefore been postulated that it may be a potential mechanism by which focal epilepsy may lead to a more generalized effect on behavior and psychosis. The development of epileptiform activity in areas of the brain that receive synaptic input from the epileptic focus, the development of secondary foci, is called secondary epileptogenesis. There is no convincing hypothesis to explain how kindling might lead to secondary epileptogenesis. One mechanism that has been proposed is the phenomenon of long-term potentiation (LTP). LTP is the enhancement of synaptic activity after high-frequency stimulation of an afferent pathway. The enhancement of synaptic efficacy is specific to the input that has been tetanized (it is homosynaptic), and therefore the postsynaptic neurons respond to other stimuli normally. In the Stevens and Livermore experiment, kindling of the Ventral Tegmental Area (VTA) in cats produced electrophysiologic changes that correlated with behavioral change. They thereby postulated that because stimulation of the VTA resulted in increased dopamine release in the limbic system and neocortex, kindling in the VTA might result in potentiation of dopamine transmission. If psychosis in patients with epilepsy, at least to a significant extent, were a manifestation of enhanced dopamine transmission, then spread of seizure activity to the VTA may well explain the development of psychosis through secondary epileptogenesis. It is possible to envision a role for secondary epileptogenesis in the development of psychopathology in patients with epilepsy. If a new site of epileptic activity were to develop distant to the original focus that led to seizure expression, and if that site was one in which seizures were poorly expressed, this may well lead to inhibition of epileptic activity in the primary focus (as has been

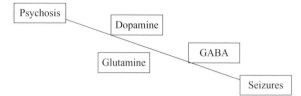

Figure 7.1 Role of various neurotransmitters in psychosis and seizures: putative relationships.

demonstrated in kindling) and a behavioral expression may then predominate [18].

Role of neurotransmitters

A number of neurotransmitters encourage this antagonism between seizure and psychosis. Dopamine remains the neurotransmitter most consistently and definitively exemplifying the antagonism between psychosis and seizures. Dopamine, being inhibitory in nature, reduces the hyperexcitability associated with seizures and is psychogenic in nature. Glutamine as a possible culpable neurotransmitter is gaining importance. Enhanced glutaminergic excitation is a potential epileptogenic mechanism, particularly with respect to the N-methyl-D-aspartate (NMDA) glutamate receptor. Both electrical kindling and LTP involve activation of the excitatory amino acid (probably glutaminergic) pathways involving NMDA receptors. In schizophrenia, on the other hand, an endogenous antagonist at the NMDA receptor, N-acetyl-aspartyl-glutamate, appears to have enhanced activity in the frontal cortex and hippocampal formation. Interestingly, this hypothesized dysfunction of glutaminergic transmission also interdigitates with the traditional dopamine hypothesis of schizophrenia. Presynaptic dopamine receptors on corticostriatal and limbic glutaminergic terminals provide a negative regulation of glutamate release. Neuroleptic blockade of these presynaptic receptors may thereby enhance glutaminergic input to the caudate and putamen and to other forebrain regions receiving dopaminergic innervation. Loss of GABA inhibition is another potential epileptogenic factor; AEDs that increase GABA levels are associated with the development of a psychopathologic state in up to 10% of patients, characterized by mood changes, agitation, and even psychotic symptoms of a paranoid nature. Catecholamines such as norepinephrine and serotonin, as well as peptides, may also play a role in FN [14]. See Figure 7.1.

An important observation, not clearly evident from the illustration, is that although epilepsy is believed to be a consequence of glutaminergic preponderance and GABAergic deficit, the converse is believed to be true for schizophrenia. Attempting to understand this impairment leads us to a neurodevelopmental affliction on the GABAergic interneurons [19]. The GABAergic neurons, unlike the usual inside-out pattern of development of the pyramidal layer, migrate tangentially outward from the thalamus [20]. This migration is affected by perinatal neurosteroids, which also affects normal lamination. These interneurons are the anatomical or functional targets for (basal forebrain) cholinergic (ACh) and/or brainstem raphe nucleus serotonergic (5-HT) neurons. The cortical GABAergic system plays an important role in cortical development and localization of different types of interneurons relative to one another, thereby influencing cortical networks and functioning. These cells provide both inhibitory and disinhibitory modulation of cortical and hippocampal circuits generating oscillatory rhythms that affect gating of sensory information within the corticolimbic system. Morphological changes in the GABAergic interneurons have been noted in postmortem studies of schizophrenic brains. Besides developmental influences, stressful conditions that modulate that dopamine system causing ingrowths of extrinsic afferents, such as the mesocortical dopamine projections, may "trigger" the appearance of a defective GABA system [21].

Cannabinoid and opioid receptor systems

Endogenous cannabinoids have been shown to have antiepileptic potential, whereas cannabis is known to cause transient psychotic states. This raises the possibility that an increase in endogenous cannabinoids in the synapse accompanying seizure cessation can result in the development of psychopathology. Cannabinoids activate the dopaminergic neurons in VTA that form the main ascending projections of the mesocorticolimbic dopamine system and modulate GABA and glutamate transmission through presynaptic CB1 receptors [22]. Both these neurotransmitter systems, that is, the mesolimbic dopaminergic and glutamatergic systems, have been implicated in the etiology of schizophrenia. Akin to endogenous cannabinoids, κ opioids have been found to have antiepileptic potentials in experimental animal models. Recurrent seizures stimulating mossy fiber development in areas

such as the hippocampus provide an important loss of inhibitory control leading to enhanced seizure activity. However, it also activates important feedback mechanisms through the κ opioids [23]. However, κ opioids can significantly reduce prepulse inhibition that has been known to induce perceptual abnormalities and thus have been identified as having psychotogenic potential.

Channelopathy

A recent hypothesis [14] gains support from evidence of abnormal ion channels in episodic neuropsychiatric disorders. Ion channels provide the basis for regulation of excitability in the central nervous system. Mutations in ion channels have been implicated in various epilepsy syndromes, including autosomal dominant nocturnal frontal lobe epilepsy (neuronal nicotinic acetylcholine receptor), benign familial neonatal convulsions (potassium channels), generalized epilepsy with febrile seizures plus (sodium channels or the GABA (A) receptor), and episodic ataxia type-1, which is associated with epilepsy in a few patients (another type of potassium channel). That ion channels are expressed in the limbic regions of the brain, with a putative role in behavior and that a number of AEDs influence ion channel functioning, leads one to speculate whether "forced normalisation of the EEG with its associated behavioral changes is the phenotype, albeit rarely expressed, of a channel disorder" [14].

Apoptosis and vascular dysfunction

Recurrent limbic seizures lead to an increased expression of messenger ribonucleic acid (RNA) for c-fos and nerve growth factor (NGF) that in turn can result in expansion of glutamatergic presynaptic mossy fibers and an increase in postsynaptic densities on granule cell dendrites [24]. Recurrent kindling on a background of this altered glutamate activity can result in programmed cell death or apoptosis [25]. Another possible explanation, encouraged by SPECT studies, is a process of slow vascular compromise, proceeding further to programmed cell death or apoptosis. With alteration in membrane dynamics because of apoptosis, channelopathies, deoxyribonucleic acid (DNA) fragmentation, and mitochondrial dysfunction can occur, resulting in chaotic release of neurotransmitters and the varied psychiatric manifestation of FN. See Figure 7.2.

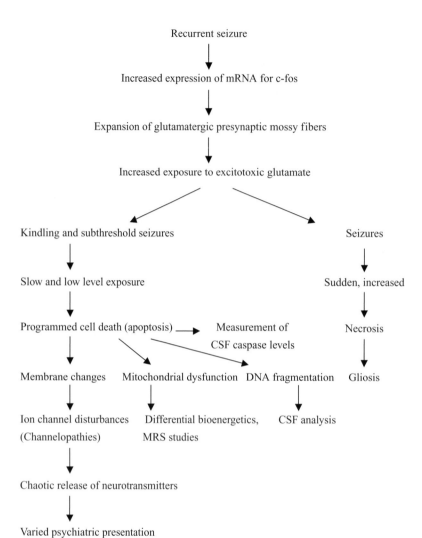

Figure 7.2 Flowchart of mechanisms linking recurrent seizures with apoptosis and diverse psychiatric phenomena.

The adenosine hypothesis

Stimulation of adenosine receptors leads to inhibition through Ca^{++} gated voltage channels, thereby inhibiting excitotoxic glutamate release resulting in suppression of seizures. Although small doses of adenosine can exert an inhibitory action on the release of excitatory neurotransmitters such as glutamine, inhibition of release of inhibitory neurotransmitters requires very high concentrations of adenosine. Cerebral adenosine levels have been found to increase substantially during seizures. It can be hypothesized that during kindling, these doses are small and sufficient to exert an inhibitory action on excitatory neurotransmitters resulting in seizure suppression. In a FN situation wherein there is a sudden cessation of seizures, the delicate balance in the distribution of adenosine may be altered, leading to imbalances in the release of neurotransmitters and the psychopathology associated with FN.

Implications for a neurobiological understanding of schizophrenia

None of these hypotheses may individually provide the neurobiological explanation for the antagonism between seizures and psychopathology in a proportion of patients. However, it seems possible, even likely, that these varied mechanisms are closely interlinked.

Various brain regions also have been implicated. For example, reduced cortical inhibition has been implicated as being responsible for the defective sensory gating observed in schizophrenia, leading to hallucinations [26, 27]. Although this "excessive neuronal noise" is primarily in the thalamus, it is noteworthy that this structure has extensive neuronal connections with other regions of the brain, including the cortex, limbic system, and the cerebellum.

There is also today a convergence of evidence pointing to the temporal lobe, especially the mesial temporal structures, as a region of interest in the genesis of schizophrenia. A substantial body of MRI literature has demonstrated mesial temporal involvement in this condition [28]. Further, we know from basic science research that the neurobiological changes that underlie this condition demonstrate to a considerable

extent a predilection for this region of interest. That patients with temporal lobe epilepsy appear to have a greater predilection for FN makes this a region of interest for neurobiological study.

FN is thus a useful clinical model for further study of the antagonism between epilepsy and psychopathology, the psychoses in particular. Those who specialize in epilepsy neuropsychiatry do not regard it as an uncommon phenomenon, rather one that has putative importance as a clinical research tool that can facilitate our understanding of psychopathology. Perhaps the antagonistic relationship that fostered a successful treatment paradigm – ECT – will also lead eventually to viable neurobiological models of psychopathology and thereby to advances in treatment.

References

1. Schmitz B. (1998). Forced normalisation: history of a concept. In *Forced Normalisation and Alternative Psychosis of Epilepsy*, Trimble M. R. and Schmitz B. (Eds.). Petersfield: Wrightson Biomedical Publishing, pp. 7–24.

2. Von Meduna L. V. Autobiography of LB Meduna. *Convuls Ther*, 1985. **1**:43–57.

3. Landolt H. Some clinical EEG correlations in epileptic psychoses (twilight states). *EEG Clin Neurophysiol*, 1953. **5**:121.

4. Landolt H. (1958). Serial EEG investigations during psychotic episodes in epileptic patients and during schizophrenic attacks. In *Lectures on Epilepsy*, Lorentz De Haas A. M. (Ed.). Amsterdam: Elsevier, pp. 91–133.

5. Tellenbach H. Epilepsy as a convulsive disorder and as a psychosis. On alternative psychoses of paranoid nature in "forced normalisation" (Landolt) of the electroencephalogram of epileptics. *Nervenarzt*, 1965. **36**:190–202.

6. Wolf P. (1991). Acute behavioral symptomatology at disappearance of epileptiform EEG abnormality: paradoxical or forced normalisation. In *Neurobehavioral Problems in Epilepsy*, Smith D., Treiman D., and Trimble M. R. (Eds.). New York: Raven Press, pp. 127–42.

7. Trimble M. R., Schmitz B. (Eds.) (1998). *Forced Normalization and Alternative Psychosis of Epilepsy*. Petersfield: Wrightson Biomedical Publishing.

8. Wolf P. (1976). The prevention of alternative psychosis in outpatients. In *Epileptology*, Janz D. (Ed.). Stuttgart: Thieme, pp. 75–9.

9. Mace C. J., Trimble M. R. Psychosis following temporal lobe surgery: a report of six cases. *J Neurol, Neurosurg, and Psychiatry*, 1991. **54**:639–44.

10. Shaw P., Mellers J., Henderson M., *et al.* Schizophrenia-like psychosis arising de novo following a temporal lobectomy: timing and risk factors. *J Neurol Neurosurg Psychiatry*, 2004. **75**(7):1003–8.

11. Gatzonis S. D., Stamboulis E., Siafakas, Angelopoulos E., *et al.* Acute psychosis and EEG normalisation after vagus nerve stimulation. *J Neurol Neurosurg Psychiatry*, 2000. **69**(2):278–9.

12. Seethalakshmi R., Krishnamoorthy E. S. The complex relationship between seizures and behaviour: an illustrative case report. *Epilepsy Behav*, 2007. **10**(1):203.

13. Krishnamoorthy E. S., Trimble M. R. Forced normalisation: clinical and therapeutic relevance. *Epilepsia*, 1999. **40**(Suppl 10): S57–64.

14. Krishnamoorthy E. S., Trimble M. R., Sander J. W. A. S., *et al.* Forced normalisation at the interface between epilepsy and psychiatry. *Epilepsy Behav*, 2002. 3:3–8.

15. Smith P. F., Darlington C. L. The development of psychosis in epilepsy: a re-examination of the kindling hypothesis. *Behav Brain Res*, 1996. **75**(1–2): 59–66.

16. Stevens J. R., Livermore A. Kindling of the mesolimbic dopamine system: animal model of psychosis. *Neurology*, 1978. **28**:36–46.

17. Sato M., Racine R. J., McIntyre D.C. Kindling: basic mechanisms and clinical validity. *Electroencephal Clin Neurophysiol*, 1990. **76**:459–72.

18. Krishnamoorthy E. S., Trimble M. R. (1998). Mechanisms of forced normalisation. In *Forced Normalisation and Alternative Psychosis of Epilepsy*, Trimble M. R. and Schmitz B. (Eds.). Petersfield: Wrightson Biomedical Publishing, pp. 193–208.

19. Grobin A. C., Heenan E. J., Lieberman J. A., *et al.* Perinatal neurosteroid levels influence GABAergic interneuron localisation in adult rat prefrontal cortex. *J Neurosci*, 2003. **23**(5):1832–9.

20. Marin O., Rubenstein J. L. A long, remarkable journey: tangential migration in the telencephalon. *Nat Rev Neurosci*, 2001. **2**: 780–90.

21. Benes F. M., Berretta S. GABAergic interneurons: implications for understanding schizophrenia and bipolar disorder. *Neuropsychopharmacology*, 2001. **25**(1):1–27.

22. Cheer J. F., Wassum K. M., Heien M. L. A. V., *et al.* Cannabinoids enhance subsecond dopamine release in the nucleus accumbens of awake rats. *J Neurosci*, 2004. **24**(18):4393–400.

23. Terman G. W., Drake C. T., Simmons M. L., *et al.* Opioid modulation of recurrent excitation in the hippocampal dentate gyrus. *J Neurosci*, 2000. **20**(12):4379–88.

24. Sutula T., He X. X., Cavazos J., *et al.* Synaptic reorganization in the hippocampus induced by abnormal functional activity. *Science*, 1988. **239**:1147–50.

25. Coyle J. T., Puttfarcken P. Oxidative stress, glutamate, and neurodegenerative disorders [Review]. *Science*, 1993. **262**:689–95.

26. Swerdlow N. R., Koob G. F. Dopamine, schizophrenia, mania, depression: toward a unified hypothesis of cortico-striatal-pallido-thalamic function. *Behav Brain Sci*, 1987. **10**:197–245.

27. Ralf-Peter Behrendt. Dysregulation of thalamic sensory "transmission" in

schizophrenia: neurochemical vulnerability to hallucinations. *J Psychopharm*, 2006. **20**(3): 356–72.

28. Nelson M. D., Saykin A. J., Flashman L. A., *et al.* Hippocampal volume reduction in schizophrenia as assessed by magnetic resonance imaging: a metaanalytic study. *Arch Gen Psychiatry*, 1998. **55**:433–40.

8 Substance-induced psychosis: an overview

Jagadisha Thirthalli, Vivek Benegal, and Bangalore N. Gangadhar

Facts box

- Although different substances consistently produce or exacerbate psychotic symptoms in patients with primary psychosis, they differ in their psychotogenic properties in "healthy" individuals.
- Individuals with substance use/dependence are five times more likely to experience clinically significant delusions and/or hallucinations than nonusers.
- Cohort studies suggest that the rate of schizophrenia is increased in chronic cannabis users.
- Alcohol use may worsen psychotic symptoms or increase risk of relapse, but it is not considered to "cause schizophrenia."
- Brief amphetamine-induced psychosis is well documented. Chronic heavy use also predisposes to psychosis.
- Schizophrenic brains may be sensitized to the effects of psychotogenic drugs.
- Evidence suggests that in some individuals, genetic vulnerability combined with drug abuse can bring about psychosis.
- Nosological status of substance-induced psychoses (SIP) and causal role of substances in causing schizophrenia remain controversial.

Introduction

On the afternoon of December 17, 1992, in an unprovoked act of violence, Christopher Clunis killed young musician Jonathan Zito on the platform of Finsbury Park subway station in London. One of the several errors identified by the inquiry into the case of Christopher Clunis was attribution of his psychotic symptoms as secondary to drug use [1].

Substance use disorders and psychotic disorders are both mental health problems of considerable public health significance. Not only do they coexist in a substantial proportion of patients, but also they may share a common neurobiological substrate. Knowledge about the conditions that influence this conjunction is of obvious clinical importance – acute management and rehabilitation depend on their accurate evaluation. Studying these conditions is also of great heuristic value because the construction of these conditions has the potential to reveal valuable clues about the etiopathogenesis of both substance use disorders and "functional" psychotic disorders. Circumstances in which there is coexistence of the two conditions vary. Traditionally, the diagnostic debate has focused on two different sequential presentations – whether a person with a primary psychotic disorder consequently abuses substances or, conversely, whether a person with primary substance abuse experiences psychotic symptoms. If the onset of the two conditions is clearly separated by a considerable time gap, then the one that occurs first may be argued as the primary, and the other, secondary. However, this is not an absolute truism. For instance, it is known that patients with schizophrenia have subtle behavioral changes several months prior to the onset of positive symptoms. This may sometimes lead to interpersonal difficulties and the breaking up of relationships. If the individual develops frank psychosis following this, it may be construed as a reaction to this "life event" even though he/she has developed psychosis as part of its natural history. In fact, in this case the life event is a *result*, rather than *cause*, of psychosis. It is clear that it is too naïve to presume causality on the basis of temporal sequence alone.

The term "substance-induced psychosis" presupposes that the substance use influences the causation of the psychosis – that is, if the person did not use the substance, then he/she would not develop the psychosis. Although there is little doubt that substance use is *associated* with a greater risk of developing either short-lasting or chronic psychoses, whether it *causes* psychosis is debatable. In this, chapter, we focus on conditions marked by coexistence of substance use and psychosis, in which substance use has preceded the onset of psychosis. This is, admittedly, only one facet of the complex phenomenon of comorbid substance abuse and psychotic disorder. A substantial body of literature details the reasons why patients with schizophrenia abuse substances more frequently than the general population, which we do not discuss in this chapter.

Definition

Lack of clarity as to what constitutes SIP has been a major hurdle for research in this area. To begin with, there is no universally accepted definition of the term "psychosis" and it is used to mean different things in different contexts. About two decades ago, any impairment that grossly interfered with day-to-day functioning would be called a "psychotic" feature. Currently, the Diagnostic and Statistical Manual of Mental Disorders-IV (DSM-IV) definition of "psychosis" requires the presence of "delusions, prominent hallucinations, disorganized speech, disorganized or catatonic behavior" and the International Classification of Disorders-10 (ICD-10) defines it as comprised of "hallucinations, delusions, or a limited number of severe abnormalities of behavior, such as gross excitement and over-activity, marked psychomotor retardation, and catatonic behavior." In the context of substance use, DSM-IV restricts the definition to the presence of delusions or only those hallucinations for which the individual lacks insight. No such distinction is made in ICD-10.

Persons using psychoactive substances experience psychotic symptoms in various contexts of substance use: intoxication, withdrawal, delirium (related to intoxication or withdrawal), substance-induced mood disorder (with psychotic symptoms), or SIP. Substance-induced psychoses are best conceptualized as those conditions where delusions and prominent hallucinations begin in the context of substance use but persist for a few days to a few weeks in the absence of continued use of the substance; relapse of psychotic symptoms upon re-exposure to the substance further supports the diagnosis [2].

DSM-IV defines SIP as those conditions in which delusions and prominent hallucinations occur within a month of substance intoxication or withdrawal. However, the psychotic symptoms must be clearly in excess of those usually associated with the intoxication or withdrawal syndrome, or the symptoms must be sufficiently severe to warrant independent clinical attention. Further, hallucinations for which the person has insight are considered to be a part of intoxication and are not considered to be psychotic. The rest of the substance-induced conditions (delirium, psychotic mood disorders) are not considered to be SIP, though they may be associated with psychotic symptoms. Diagnosis of primary psychotic disorder is encouraged when psychotic features last for more than a month with sustained abstinence. However, it does recognize that certain agents can cause longer-lasting psychotic disorders. ICD-10 criteria are largely similar but require that the onset of psychosis should occur within 48 hours of use of the substance and the disorder may last for up to 6 months, beyond which a primary psychosis would be diagnosed.

Both DSM-IV and ICD-10 offer useful criteria to diagnose SIPs, which can be operationalized for research purposes. However, most reports of SIP in existing scientific literature have used inconsistent definitions or even failed to mention the definition used. For instance, reports on amphetamine-induced psychosis [3, 4] have generally used DSM-III-R or DSM-IV diagnoses but those on cocaine-induced psychosis [5, 6] have used questionnaires specifically prepared for cocaine-related disorders, making comparisons across studies difficult.

Research directions

The question of the relationship between substances and psychosis has been approached using different but complementary lines of research. The basic questions they have tried to answer are i) whether exposure to drugs of abuse can cause psychotic symptoms and, if so, do different drugs differ in their psychotogenic properties? ii) Whether substance users are at an increased risk of developing acute or chronic psychoses? and iii) What is the construct validity of SIP?

Do drugs cause psychoses? If so, which drugs?

Many studies have administered controlled doses of substances of abuse in laboratory settings to assess the psychotogenic properties of these drugs.

Amphetamine-type stimulants worsen psychotic symptoms in patients with schizophrenia, particularly in persons with active symptoms rather than persons with psychosis in remission [7]. However, healthy volunteers rarely experience psychotic symptoms at doses sufficient to cause or exacerbate psychotic symptoms in schizophrenia patients (0.25–0.3 mg/kg dexamphetamine or 0.5 mg/kg methylphenidate). Given in sufficiently high doses, amphetamines can produce psychotic symptoms even in healthy individuals [8]. Similarly, 3,4-methylenedioxymethamphetamine (MDMA) does not provoke psychotic symptoms in healthy adults at doses used by recreational users [9, 10, 11]. Sherer (1988) [12] found a positive correlation between cumulative dose of intravenous cocaine and degree of paranoia in otherwise healthy cocaine addicts. However, there was no correlation between plasma cocaine concentration and paranoia; indeed, the person having a severe psychotic reaction had relatively low plasma cocaine. This points to a complex interaction between interindividual differences and the dose of cocaine in producing paranoia.

These experiments suggest that the brains of schizophrenia patients may be sensitized (see later) to the psychotogenic effects of stimulants in such a way that even low doses of these substances cause psychotic exacerbations. Use of much higher doses of substances, probable sensitization due to long duration of use, use in combination with other drugs, and the presence of individual vulnerability factors may explain psychoses attributed to stimulants in nonschizophrenic individuals.

In contrast, δ-9-tetrahydrocannabinol (δ-THC) produces significant psychotic symptoms even in healthy volunteers. Further, it produces not just positive symptoms but negative and cognitive symptoms as well, mimicking typical features of schizophrenia in the healthy subjects [13]. These effects are more pronounced in clinically stable, medicated schizophrenia patients than in the healthy controls [14], suggesting that schizophrenia patients are particularly prone to react adversely to cannabis, as they do to stimulants. Glutamate-N-methyl-D-aspartic acid (NMDA)-receptor antagonists like phencyclidine (PCP) have been consistently shown to produce psychotic symptoms in healthy volunteers [15, 16]. Again, similar to δ-THC and in contrast to stimulants, these symptoms include positive, negative, and cognitive symptoms resembling schizophrenia.

It is therefore evident that although different substances consistently produce or exacerbate psychotic symptoms in patients with primary diagnoses of psychosis, they differ in their psychotogenic properties in "healthy" individuals. It is interesting to speculate on the reasons that may underlie this phenomenon. First, the reason for the differential effects of substances in producing psychotic symptoms may lie in the differential susceptibility of the "healthy" subjects. Second, although all substances with reinforcing property enhance dopamine transmission, they differ widely in their ability to directly or indirectly affect other neurotransmitter systems. Different neurotransmitters interact in a complex way to cause psychosis and different substances seem to facilitate this interaction variably in healthy persons.

Epidemiological studies examining psychotic experience among substance abusers

Psychoses do not follow an "all-or-none" principle. Strauss [17] proposed that psychotic symptoms are "points on continua of function" rather than being dichotomous entities. In many ways, psychotic symptoms in patients with psychosis occur in continuity with psychosis-like experiences in the general population [18, 19]. Psychotic symptoms of varying severity are reported by a large number of individuals in the community, but only a small proportion qualify for the diagnosis of psychosis of any kind [20, 21]. Substance abuse increases the risk of experiencing psychotic symptoms. Several studies have concluded that the daily use of cannabis or cocaine, cannabis dependence, and alcohol use disorders independently increase the risk of experiencing psychotic symptoms by several folds in adults [19, 22, 23]. After controlling for confounding factors including age, sex, ethnic group, urban living, IQ, life events, neuroses, and victimization experience, the risk is substantially reduced but nevertheless remains significantly greater in substance abusers than nonabusers [22]. Although 4% of the general population experiences clinically significant delusions and hallucinations, which are not secondary to substance use [19], those with substance abuse/dependence are five times more likely to experience these symptoms. Substance use thus appears to be associated with a greater likelihood of experiencing psychotic symptoms and is not necessarily secondary to substance use.

The studies that are best positioned to test whether substance use causes psychosis are prospective cohort studies (preferably from birth) but few of these exist and those that do have focused exclusively on the link between cannabis use and psychosis [24, 25, 26, 27, 28, 29, 30, 31]. There is now a large body of literature on the relationship between cannabis and psychosis: more than 180 articles have been indexed on PubMed since 2000, with more than 100 of these appearing in the last two years. A large number of studies have reported a significant association between cannabis use and psychosis and there is abundant evidence of the link between the two in epidemiological studies involving the general population.

A study from the Netherlands [32] followed 4,045 people between 1996 and 1999. Cannabis users with no psychotic disorder at baseline were at increased risk of clinically significant psychotic symptoms at the end of follow-up (OR = 3.5–3.7). This association was independent of any comorbid nonpsychotic psychiatric disorder or use of other substances at baseline. A second Netherlands study [33] was a 14-year follow-up of 1,580 young adults in the "Zuid Holland" study. In this sample, cannabis use significantly predicted psychotic symptoms in participants who did not have psychotic symptoms before they began using cannabis (OR = 2.8). A German study [34] followed 2,437 young people aged 14 to 24 for 4 years between 1996 and 1999. Any cannabis use at baseline was reported to increase the risk of psychotic symptoms at the 4-year follow-up in a dose–response fashion, regardless of confounders. The association was much stronger for those who had been identified as being prone to psychosis at baseline. A New Zealand study [35] was a birth cohort based on 1,037 people born in Dunedin, New Zealand between 1972 and 1973. Cannabis use at ages 15 and 18 increased the risk of presenting with psychotic symptoms or schizophreniform disorder at age 26 (OR = 11.4 for those who had used cannabis before the age of 15). Like the other cohort studies, this relationship was independent of the use of other substances. Significantly, this study also assessed the presence of psychotic symptoms at age 11 and was therefore able to demonstrate that the observed association between cannabis use and increased risk of psychosis was independent from pre-existing psychotic symptoms. A second New Zealand study [36] followed 1,011 individuals taking part in the Christchurch health and development study from birth. Assessments were conducted annually until age 16 and then again at 18, 21, and 25. Those who were daily users of cannabis had rates of psychotic symptoms that were between 2.3 and 3.3 times higher than the rates for those who did not use cannabis.

Do substances differ in their association with psychotic symptoms?

Although no systematic study has been conducted comparing the psychotogenic properties of different substances of abuse, clinical observation suggests that it varies widely.

Alcohol

Studies have shown alcohol dependence, but not alcohol use in itself, to be predictive of psychotic experiences in the general population [22, 23]. Patients with psychotic symptoms are more likely to abuse alcohol than those without psychotic symptoms; alcohol abuse may worsen the symptoms of schizophrenia and psychotic symptoms may precipitate relapse (e.g. Olfson *et al.*, 2002 [37]) but it is generally accepted that alcohol use does not actually cause schizophrenia [38].

Amphetamines

Although brief amphetamine-induced psychosis is well documented, the extent to which amphetamine use contributes to schizophrenia is not known. There is a high rate of mental health problems among regular amphetamine users with more than a quarter (26.7%) of those with such mental health problems diagnosed with psychosis and the majority of these (71.4%) reportedly having received this diagnosis after commencing regular amphetamine use [39]. However, a study of amphetamine users found that users with psychosis were younger when amphetamine use was first initiated and used larger amounts of amphetamines than those without psychosis, leading to the conclusion that premorbid schizotypal personality predisposes amphetamine users to psychosis [4].

Cocaine

A number of studies [5, 39] have reported that cocaine can induce psychotic symptoms in some users but comparatively little research has been conducted to date.

Opiates

Research into the relationship between opiate use and psychosis is limited. Studies have generally shown a low comorbidity rate between opiate use and psychosis [40, 41], and there is evidence to suggest that heroin users may actually be at lower risk of psychosis than users of other substances [42].

Nicotine

Though it enhances extracellular dopamine in the nucleus accumbens, it does not cause psychosis even in heavy smokers.

Preliminary research evidence supports the observation of differential psychotogenetic properties of substances. In a study on out-of-treatment substance abusers, 86% percent of persons dependent on any of the substances reported lifetime experiences of psychotic symptoms in the context of use of, or withdrawal from, those specific substances [43]. Percentages of dependent persons reporting psychotic symptoms in the context of specific substances were 80% for cocaine, 64% for cannabis, 56% for amphetamines and 53% for opioids. When subjects dependent on more than one substance were questioned about psychotic experiences with specific drugs, the association was significantly greater for cocaine than with other substances. In terms of relative association with psychotic symptoms, cocaine was followed by cannabis and amphetamines. Hallucinogens and phencyclidine were used by only a small number of subjects and were not considered for analysis. It appears that at the dependence level, cocaine has the greatest psychotogenic property.

It is evident from the earlier review that substance use is associated with a greater risk of psychotic experience in the nonclinical population. Although this association is stronger for those who are vulnerable to develop psychosis, substances appear to have an independent association with psychotic experience. Some other risk factors for the development of psychotic symptoms in the nonclinical populations are impairments in development, including neuro-motor development, receptive language, intelligence and emotional development, urban residence, lower level of education, life events, neurosis, victimization, and lower quality of life [20, 23, 44, 45]. These are also risk factors for the development of substance-use disorders.

Validity of the construct of substance-induced psychosis

Although the term "substance-induced psychosis" (SIP) is frequently used in common psychiatric parlance, there is surprisingly little agreement on its validity. Poole and Brabbins [2] have even questioned the existence of such a syndrome and suggested that the term be discontinued from use.

Robins and Guze [46] listed five criteria for establishing the validity of psychiatric diagnoses: i) clinical description (including symptom profiles, demographic characteristics, and typical precipitants), ii) laboratory studies (including psychological tests, radiology, and postmortem findings), iii) delimitation from other disorders (by means of exclusion criteria), iv) follow-up studies (including evidence of diagnostic stability), and v) family studies.

Clinical description

The clinical descriptions of SIP are extensive and consistent, with minor differences across different substances. They generally present with an acute onset of psychotic episode in the background of heavy use of substances. They are characterized by prominent delusions and hallucinations of auditory, visual and tactile nature and prominent affective symptoms (euphoria and fear are common) but disorganization, negative symptoms, and catatonia are rare. There are occasional reports of disorientation and confusion, especially with acute cannabis and inhalant intoxication ("toxic psychoses"). Cocaine abuse is associated with prominent paranoia, especially about being caught by law-enforcing agencies. Tactile hallucinations of insects crawling under the skin ("cocaine bugs"), although relatively infrequent, are also typical of cocaine-induced psychosis. Alcohol-induced psychosis is characterized by prominent hallucinations ("alcoholic hallucinosis"); delusions generally occur secondarily in response to them. Only PCP-induced psychosis is characterized by prominent negative symptoms and catatonic behaviors. However, in contrast to acute schizophrenic episodes, passivity and thought alienation phenomena are very rare in SIPs.

Diagnostic stability, delimitation from other disorders, and family history

A recent methodologically rigorous study of 400 subjects with recent-onset psychosis in substance-using persons presenting to emergency psychiatric services

[47, 48] reported that SIPs are distinguishable from primary psychoses, have diagnostic stability, and a distinct family history. Forty-four percent of the sample was reliably diagnosed with SIP (DSM-IV criteria). These included patients with psychoses induced by cannabis, cocaine, alcohol, hallucinogens, sedatives, heroin, and stimulants. They differed from the primary nonorganic psychosis group (schizophrenia, psychotic mood disorder, psychotic disorder not otherwise specified, schizophreniform disorder, schizoaffective disorder, and delusional disorder) on several counts. They were older and more likely to be married, homeless, have poorer family support, have greater parental substance abuse, and lesser parental mental illness. They scored significantly less on positive syndrome, negative syndrome, general psychopathology, and total scores of PANSS; and had greater awareness and lesser misattribution of their symptoms and a more common incidence of visual hallucinations. Expectedly, a greater proportion of patients had substance abuse/dependence and antisocial personality disorder.

At the end of one year, 75% of patients diagnosed as SIP had retained their diagnosis; the rest were classified as primary psychotics [48]. In addition to the differences discussed earlier, the follow-up SIPs showed lesser parental mental illness than follow-up primary psychotics. Little can be commented on the generalizability of the results to other settings (e.g. community/clinics). Comparison was made between SIP and a heterogeneous group of psychotic disorders, with significant histories of substance use. How SIPs would compare with nonaffective psychotic patients without substance abuse remains to be studied. Family history was not assessed using standardized methods. Notwithstanding these caveats, the two reports from this group of researchers have contributed to validating SIPs.

An earlier report [49] of inpatients with substance abuse and psychosis compared patients with short- and long-lasting psychoses (with a 6-month cutoff duration before admission). Patients with long-lasting psychoses had more symptoms of psychosis, poorer premorbid adjustment, longer durations of drug treatment and hospital stay, and greater number of family members with schizophrenia. This suggested that at least two kinds of psychoses exist in the context of substance abuse: i) one that is brief-lasting, milder, with better premorbid functioning and without familial risk of schizophrenia; in this, the role of substance as an etiological agent is more compelling; and ii) one

that lasts longer, is more severe, and is associated with poorer premorbid and familial risk of schizophrenia – in this they resemble schizophrenic illness precipitated or exacerbated by substance use.

Very little work has been done to delineate specific SIPs from schizophrenia except for alcoholic hallucinosis. There is some evidence that there is a genetic vulnerability to develop alcoholic psychosis that is transmitted separately from the vulnerability to develop schizophrenia [50]. However, the predictive validity of alcoholic hallucinosis is very poor – only a small proportion of patients with such a diagnosis retain the diagnosis [51].

SIPs seem to fulfill most of Robins and Guze [46] criteria. As for the *laboratory evidence* supporting the diagnostic validity, SIPs and psychiatric disorders due to general medical disorders share the common platform. Laboratory evidence, namely qualitative or quantitative assays of drug metabolites in body fluids, can support the association of substance use with the psychotic state. Studies elucidating the neurobiological substrates for psychotogenic properties of substances (see later) support the plausibility of SIP as a valid construct.

Susceptibility for developing SIP

Not all people who abuse substances develop psychosis. It would appear from the available evidence that both i) substance-related and ii) individual risk factors modulate the susceptibility for SIP.

Substance-related factors

These include different indices of cumulative exposure to substances, including earlier onset of substance use, heavier use, greater lifetime consumption, more severe dependence, and greater amount of money spent on substances [4, 5, 6, 52, 53]. An interesting phenomenon associated with SIP is that of sensitization. Psychosis develops more rapidly and manifests more severely at lower doses than used in the past; this is seen even after several years of abstinence [5, 54, 55]. Interestingly, sensitization occurs only for the psychotic effects but not the other effects of cocaine [56]. Cocaine abusers who experience sensitization to the psychotogenic property of cocaine paradoxically have less naturally occurring craving and are likely to reduce their cocaine and other substance use [57].

Sensitization in animals generally occurs after repeated administration of substances. Once initiated,

117

the phenomenon lasts for several years without requiring repeated use of substances. Animals sensitized to stimulants show cross-sensitization to other substances and stress. There appears to be a genetic influence in the vulnerability to sensitization. Several molecular mechanisms underlie the development of sensitization, which result in expression of genes that play a key role in synaptogenesis and neuritogenesis [58, 59], ultimately resulting in enhanced dopamine efflux when exposed to stimulants or stress. The observation that low doses of antipsychotics blunt the behavioral response in sensitized persons [59] is in keeping with this hypothesis.

The concept of sensitization has considerable relevance to the neurobiology of schizophrenia. As has been noted earlier, stimulants consistently evoke psychotic responses in patients with schizophrenia at doses that do not provoke such responses in healthy volunteers. This suggests that the brains of schizophrenia patients may already be sensitized. Lieberman and colleagues [60] suggest that schizophrenic brains seem to have a developmental neural dysregulation. This could lead to neurochemical sensitization when exposed to stress or psychostimulants during adolescence, which in turn leads to psychotic phenomena. Indeed, there is direct evidence of the phenomenon of sensitization at a molecular level. Schizophrenia patients have been shown to have a greater decrement of D-2 binding by ^{123}I-iodobenzamide, a D-2 radioligand, following stimulant exposure than healthy controls, suggesting greater release of dopamine in these patients [61]. Similar results have been found with C-11 raclopride, another D-2 radioligand [62]. In this latter study, the effect was observed even in antipsychotic-naïve patients, suggesting that the effect was unrelated to antipsychotic activity.

Individual risk factors

Among individual risk factors, the effects of a strong family history are well documented. Although most studies have reported the presence of a stronger family history of schizophrenia among relatives of psychotic substance abusers [57, 63, 64], some have failed to find such differences [50, 53] Personality difficulties, "psychosis proneness," and lifetime history of depression have been associated with patients with SIP [3, 65] in some but not all studies [50, 53]. One cannot rule out the confounding effect of interactions among these risk factors. It is conceivable that those with a fam-

ily history of psychosis, poor premorbid adjustment, and comorbid affective illness are likely to start substance use early, use more heavily, and develop more severe dependence [66]. Gene-environment interactions have been hypothesized to underlie this differential susceptibility to SIP, with some individuals being genetically vulnerable to the effects of substances. This hypothesis was tested by Caspi and colleagues [67] in a longitudinal birth cohort study and found that a functional polymorphism of the catechol-O-methyltransferase (COMT) gene moderated the influence of adolescent cannabis use on adult psychosis: carriers of the COMT valine-158 allele were more likely to experience psychotic symptoms after cannabis consumption than carriers of the COMT methionine allele. In another study, patients with a psychotic disorder and their relatives were exposed to delta-9-tetrahydrocannabinol in a double-blind placebo-controlled design. Carriers of the valine-158 allele were most sensitive to Δ-9-THC induced psychotic experiences [68]. Significantly, this finding was conditional on pre-existing psychosis liability.

Common neural substrate

Although different substances of abuse have different mechanisms of action, a growing body of evidence suggests that neuropathological variations of certain brain circuits that regulate positive reinforcement, incentive motivation, behavioral inhibition, executive functions, emotion, and stress may contribute to a common vulnerability to addiction and of psychosis/schizophrenia (see Chambers *et al.* 2001 [69] for an extensive review).

The mesolimbic dopamine system [consisting of dopamine (DA) neurons in the ventral tegmental area (VTA) and their target neurons in forebrain regions such as the nucleus accumbens (NAc)] has been proposed as a major neural substrate for the reinforcing effects of natural rewards as well as alcohol and other drugs. All substances of abuse affect this system [70] and this is thought to mediate drug craving. Drug reward and craving is induced by stimuli that facilitate, rather than depress, DA reward systems. Both D1-like and D2-like dopamine receptors mediate the reinforcing effects of the substances [71, 72]. Animals self-administer both D1- and D2-selective agonists. D1, D2, and D3 antagonists all attenuate the rewarding effects of psychostimulant drugs [73, 74, 75, 76]. The mesolimbic DA system is also implicated in schizophrenia. Several lines of evidence suggest such a mechanism: (1) all antipsychotic drugs useful against positive symptoms of psychosis have dopamine receptor D2 blocking properties [77, 78]; (2) post-mortem studies have shown an increase in striatal D2 receptor density but whether this is due to antemortem use of D2 blocking agents is debatable; (3) several studies show elevated D2 receptor binding in the striatum in schizophrenia [79]; and (4) abusers of psychostimulants like amphetamines, which enhance dopamine neurotransmission, experienced delusions, and hallucinations typical of paranoid schizophrenia.

There has been much attention on the neural network implicated in reward, drug addiction, and in schizophrenia. Excitatory afferents to the NAc from the hippocampal formation relay contextual information relevant to reward and motivation. Excitatory afferents from the PfC relay command and inhibitory information to the NAc relevant to regulation of thought and motivation. In the NAc, glutamatergic afferents from the PfC and the hippocampal formation interact with DA afferents from the VTA to regulate motivational processes.

In both psychoses/schizophrenia and addiction, a functional disorganization of afferent excitatory communication to the NAc contributes to relative hyper-responsivity to DA input from the VTA, increasing motivational salience of drugs and drug-related stimuli. In schizophrenia, disregulation of hippocampal outputs may disrupt PfC communication to the NAc, weakening executive-inhibitory influences by reducing the impact of PfC inputs (gating), reducing excitatory drive of PfC-NAc projections, or both. It has been suggested that psychotic symptoms emerge from a functional hyperactivity of DA neurons projecting to the NAc, and functional hypoactivity of DA neurons projecting to the frontal cortex. Psychosis and thought disorder may result, in part, from a state of abnormal glutamatergic cortical activity associated with exaggerated DA release or dysregulated DA signaling in the NAc. This imbalance may contribute to improper gating of perceptual and thought processes. The disinhibition of subcortical DA systems in schizophrenia parallels theories of reduced cortico-striatal tone associated with drug addiction. Thus, the evidence of hyperactivity in NAc DA signaling relates both to psychotic symptoms and addictive behavior.

Current theories focus on neurodevelopmental abnormalities in cortical and temporal-limbic structures, particularly the hippocampal formation, amyg-dala, and the PfC. Neuroimaging and postmortem tissue studies in schizophrenic patients show abnormalities in hippocampal-amygdaloid volume, proportional to severity of symptoms. These regions normally provide excitatory input to the PfC and frontal subcortical structures. It has been hypothesized that developmental abnormalities in hippocampal and PfC projections to the NAc may contribute to an overall functional hyperresponsiveness to mesoaccumbens DA release by reducing cortical and hippocampal regulation over DA-mediated responses in schizophrenia.

Recent neuroimaging studies have revealed deficits in brain volume – hippocampal formation, amygdala, prefrontal cortex, cingulum, and thalamus in alcohol naïve offspring of alcoholics who are at higher risk of substance use disorders [80, 81, 82].

Do drugs cause chronic psychoses or schizophrenia?

In their review of literature on substance-induced chronic psychoses, Boutros and Bowers [83] identified a subgroup of people with chronic psychoses developing in the context of using commonly abused substances. In many cases, they were unable to identify any other diatheses/susceptibility factors for psychoses (e.g., family history, premorbid adjustment difficulties) apart from heavy use of substances for long periods. On the basis of fairly consistent findings of male predominance, younger age at onset of psychosis, increased family history of drug use, and better premorbid adjustment, they concluded that SIP disorders have diagnostic validity and there is "presumptive evidence" regarding the role of substances in causing them.

The issue of cannabis as a cause of schizophrenia has been researched in greater detail, and many have reported the temporal association of prior cannabis use to later development of schizophrenia. Andreasson and colleagues linked prior heavy cannabis use to later development of schizophrenia in a cohort of Swedish conscripts with a long-term (27 years) follow-up [84]. To rule out the possibility that this association was due to use of cannabis in the prodrome of schizophrenia, they studied the association of cannabis use before conscription with development of schizophrenia more than 5 years after conscription. The association was still significant. Weiser and colleagues [85] found a similar association between adolescent use of cannabis and later development of schizophrenia in

Israeli conscripts. Such an association was found neither for depression nor for drugs other than cannabis. Meta-analytic and systematic reviews [86, 87] have established a consistent, almost twofold greater risk for consequent psychosis among cannabis users. Based on the criteria of association, temporal priority, and direction, Witton and colleagues [88] opine that cannabis is a component cause of schizophrenia. Arseneault and colleagues [86] calculated that schizophrenia could be averted in about 8% of the population if cannabis use could be eliminated (population-attributable fraction = 8). The finding that a significant gene X environment interaction exists between cannabis use and schizophrenia [71] partly explains why not all those who use cannabis heavily develop schizophrenia.

The cumulative evidence from these different lines of research appears to confirm that substances do put a person at risk for developing psychosis. However, various susceptibility factors are important in modulating the risk for developing psychosis. This is in keeping with the continuum model of "cocaine psychosis," hypothesized by Post [89], wherein the risk depends on interactions between duration and dose of cocaine with genetic and experiential predispositions. At the lower end of the continuum of vulnerability to psychosis, large doses of substances abused for long periods would cause psychosis (substance is both necessary and sufficient to cause psychosis). In the middle of the continuum are conditions, where substances are necessary, but not sufficient cause for psychosis. At the other end, psychosis may develop following little or no exposure to drugs (substance use is not a necessary cause; may be coincidental). In the latter condition, there is consistent evidence that substance use brings down the age of onset [90, 91] – one of the reasons for earlier age of onset of schizophrenia in males is greater prevalence of substance use in them. Conversely, in communities where substance abuse among psychotics is much less, earlier age of onset of psychosis in males is not observed (Venkatesh et al., in press [92]).

Diagnosis and treatment

The differentiation between a primary psychotic disorder that co-occurs with substance use and an SIP is critically important for treatment. The assessment of psychotic symptoms that occur during a period of substance use requires: i) knowledge about the etiological relationship between specific substances and specific psychotic symptoms (e.g. what substances cause physiological changes resulting in hallucinations or delusions); and ii) the ability to differentiate the expected effects of intoxication and withdrawal from psychotic symptoms. Routine mental status examination should include a thorough description of presenting symptoms, description of onset of psychotic symptoms, history of current and lifetime substance use, and a probe of timing and course of the current substance use and psychosis. The sources of information that the clinician requires to consider are patient self-reports, information from family members or other reliable informants about patterns of substance use and onset of psychosis, urine toxicology screens if available, and observations of clinical staff. The differential diagnosis of patients presenting with substance use and psychosis should include delirium, intoxication, withdrawal-related psychosis, SIP, and primary psychiatric disorders associated with substance abuse.

Delirium

Substance abusers are prone to develop delirium due to intoxication or withdrawal of substances or associated medical complications, including head trauma, electrolyte imbalance, hypoglycemia, hepatic encephalopathy, infections including meningitis, septicemia, and so on. Delirium should be suspected when there is acute onset of psychosis, fluctuating consciousness, marked inattention, disorientation (particularly to time), visual hallucinations and illusions, signs of autonomic arousal, affective dysregulation (commonly fear, but may include euphoria or apathy), and abnormal motor behavior (commonly restlessness, but may include retardation or catatonic posturing). Detailed neurological examination and appropriate investigations lead to accurate diagnosis, which can be life saving.

Intoxication

Psychotic symptoms can be symptoms of intoxication with several addictive substances. Each substance produces its characteristic picture. Apart from the characteristic psychotic symptoms described earlier, hypervigilance, euphoria, choreoathetoid movements, tachycardia, hypertension, and papillary dilatation characterize intoxication with amphetamines. Psychotic agitation that rapidly shifts to intense dysphoria and then to somnolence without any sedative medications is characteristic of cocaine intoxication.

Presence of vivid visual hallucinations, time distortion, and synesthesias suggest use of hallucinogens and LSD. Intoxication with PCP produces a state of dissociation with unpredictable secondary effects, including agitation, unpredictable aggressive outbursts, and catatonic postures sometimes associated with significant autonomic arousal mimicking neuroleptic malignant syndrome.

Withdrawal

Withdrawal from alcohol, benzodiazepines, and other sedatives produces withdrawal-related psychotic symptoms with or without delirium. Auditory and visual hallucinations, paranoid delusions, and autonomic arousal associated with withdrawal from these may mimic stimulant intoxication.

Identifying SIP and primary psychosis associated with substance abuse

Identifying SIP and differentiating it from primary psychosis can be particularly challenging. SIP is diagnosed when psychotic symptoms start during intoxication or withdrawal but persist beyond periods of acute intoxication or withdrawal for a few days or weeks. It is also diagnosed during intoxication or withdrawal if the psychotic symptoms are very prominent and warrant independent clinical attention or when they are clearly in excess of what may be expected in an intoxication or withdrawal syndrome. It is of obvious importance to learn whether heavy substance consumption or psychosis started first. If there is reliable history that the psychotic syndrome had started either along with or before heavy use of the substance, then the diagnosis is one of primary psychosis. However, typically substance abusers provide a very unreliable history; sometimes they present after several years of substance use and psychosis, which makes recall difficult and unreliable. The diagnosis becomes unclear if substance abuse had begun first and there was no substantial period of abstinence. The following points are helpful in arriving at a differential diagnosis of SIP and primary psychoses:

1. *Past and family history*: Past and family history of nonsubstance induced psychosis weighs the diagnosis in favor of a primary psychosis.
2. *Age of onset*: Most primary psychoses have onset in the second and third decades of life. In persons using substances, onset of psychotic symptoms beyond the fourth decade of life should alert the clinician regarding the possibility of them being secondary to substance use.
3. *Type amount of substance*: Clinicians should take into account the likelihood that the type and amount of drug abused could cause psychotic symptoms. For instance, a small dose of cocaine is known to cause psychotic symptoms, whereas opioid drugs cause psychotic reactions, only at much higher doses.
4. *Symptoms*: Symptoms of SIP may mimic schizophrenic symptoms quite closely. However, nonauditory hallucinations, which are rare in schizophrenia, commonly occur with SIP. Conversely, passivity and thought-alienation phenomena and formal thought disorders are rare in SIP.
5. *Persistence during sustained abstinence*: Psychotic symptoms persisting beyond several weeks of sustained abstinence from substance use also strengthen evidence for the diagnosis of primary psychosis. Typically, the psychotic symptoms of SIP start decreasing in severity following abstinence even without antipsychotic medications. If they persist at the same severity despite documented abstinence, then the clinician should suspect primary psychosis and consider starting antipsychotics. However, the situation can be confusing when the psychotic symptoms are so severe that the clinician is compelled to use antipsychotics at the outset. In this situation, it may be worthwhile to stop antipsychotics and observe for re-emergence of psychotic symptoms while ensuring continued abstinence.

It is clear that differentiating SIP from nonSIP is a complex task requiring time, multiple sources of information, laboratory facilities, and expertise. This may not be possible in an emergency setting or outpatient clinics where these patients usually present. Admission for a few weeks facilitates repeated and thorough physical and mental status examination, provides time for collecting information from different sources, including family members and friends, and ensures abstinence. Many features of SIP are shared by psychotic disorders due to general medical/neurological disorders. Inpatient evaluation also helps to rule these out. Alternatively, if family members and friends can ensure abstinence and frequent visits, then outpatient evaluation is also possible.

A number of research instruments have been developed to assess substance use disorders and Axis 1 psychiatric disorders (see Caton *et al.* for review [93]). These include general-purpose diagnostic instruments: clinician-administered instruments such as Schedules for Clinical Assessment in Neuropsychiatry (SCAN), the Structured Clinical Interview for DSM-IV (SCID), and the Schedule for Affective Disorders and Schizophrenia (SADS) that leave the differentiation of "primary" or "secondary" to clinical judgment; interviews designed for lay interviewers such as the Composite International Diagnostic Interview (CIDI) or the Diagnostic Interview Schedule that rely on the subject's attribution of the etiology. Both these approaches are conducive to diagnostic unreliability as they rely on individual judgment rather than a built-in, systematic method of differentiation. The Psychiatric Research Interview for Substance and Mental Disorder (PRISM) was developed to address this lacuna and to provide an instrument that is suitable for comorbidity research and designed to assess 20 Axis 1 and 2 Axis II psychiatric disorders in heavy users of alcohol and other substances. The PRISM includes the following features: periods of drug/alcohol use and abstinence explored in detail prior to other sections of the interview, so that when the interviewer administers sections on psychotic disorders, the history of drug and alcohol use is known; interviewer instructions and guidelines to assist in differentiating substance-induced from primary symptoms and in determining the timing of the psychiatric symptoms and substance use.

Treatment

Many researchers and clinicians assert that patients who abuse substances and develop severe mental illness require a unique set of treatment interventions apart from the traditional mental health and substance abuse programs. It has been suggested that such patients do not benefit from the standard treatments and that failure to address both mental health and substance abuse problems leads to undesirable outcomes. There is also a prevailing viewpoint that such patients do better in the substance abuse service system.

Risk of violence and suicide

Special mention should be made about the risk of violence and suicide among patients with substance use and psychotic symptoms. Substance use and psychosis are both associated with impaired inhibition, of impulses, including aggressive ones. They both independently put persons in greater risk for violence, and, not surprisingly, persons having the greatest risk of violence have dual diagnoses. The likelihood of committing a violent crime is 8–25 times higher than in mentally healthy men; this is about 2–4 times greater than those with schizophrenia without substance abuse [94, 95]. Reports of suicide risks in dually diagnosed persons are, however, conflicting. Some studies report increased risk [96] and others decreased risk [97] of suicide in schizophrenia patients when they have comorbid substance abuse. Although violence and suicide risks associated with SIP per se are unknown, we believe that clinicians should be vigilant for such risks since both psychosis and substance use themselves have greater risk of suicide than mentally healthy individuals.

Future directions

Co-occurrence of substance use and psychosis is an important health problem. Although it is a challenging clinical situation, it gives ample opportunity to understand the biology of both conditions. Nosological status of SIP and the role of substances in causing schizophrenia still remain controversial and are only recently being clarified. The need for further research is felt in these fields because they have significant clinical and public health implications. Advancement in neuroimaging and genetic technology hold promise in elucidating the pathophysiology of these conditions. This should lead to improvement in clinical care of these conditions and guide public health policies regarding substances.

References

1. Ritchie J., Dick D., Lingham R. (1994). *The Report of the Inquiry into the Care and Treatment of Christopher Clunis*. London: HMSO.

2. Poole R., Brabbins C. Drug induced psychosis. *Br J Psychiatry*, 1996. **168**:135–8.

3. Iwanami A., Sugiyama A., Kuroki N., *et al.* Patients with methamphetamine psychosis admitted to a psychiatric hospital in Japan. A preliminary report. *Acta Psychiatr Scand*, 1994. **89**:428–32.

4. Chen C. K., Lin S. K., Sham P. C., *et al.* Pre-morbid characteristics and co-morbidity of methamphetamine users with and without psychosis. *Psychol Med*, 2003. **33**:1407–14.

5. Brady K. T., Lydiard R. B., Malcolm R., Ballenger J. C. Cocaine-induced psychosis. *J Clin Psychiatry*, 1991. **52**:509–12.

6. Cubells J. F., Feinn R., Pearson D., *et al.* Rating the severity and character of transient cocaine-induced delusions and hallucinations with a new instrument, the Scale for Assessment of Positive Symptoms for Cocaine-Induced Psychosis (SAPS-CIP). *Drug Alcohol Depend*, 2005. **80**:23–33.

7. Curran C., Byrappa N., McBride A. Stimulant psychosis: systematic review. *Br J Psychiatry*, 2004. **185**:196–204.

8. Angrist B. M., Gershon S. The phenomenology of experimentally induced amphetamine psychosis – preliminary observations. *Biol Psychiatry*, 1970. **2**:95–107.

9. Cami J., Farre M., Mas M., *et al.* Human pharmacology of 3,4-methylenedioxymethamphetamine ("ecstasy"): psychomotor performance and subjective effects. *J Clin Psychopharmacol*, 2000. **20**:455–66.

10. Downing J. The psychological and physiological effects of MDMA on normal volunteers. *J Psychoactive Drugs*, 1986. **18**:335–40.

11. Grob C. S., Poland R. E., Chang L., Ernst T. Psychobiologic effects of 3,4-methylenedioxymethamphetamine in humans: methodological considerations and preliminary observations. *Behav Brain Res*, 1996. **73**:103–7.

12. Sherer M. A. Intravenous cocaine: psychiatric effects, biological mechanisms. *Biol Psychiatry*, 1988. **24**:865–85.

13. D'Souza D. C., Perry E., MacDougall L., *et al.* The psychotomimetic effects of intravenous delta-9-tetrahydrocannabinol in healthy individuals: implications for psychosis. *Neuropsychopharmacology*, 2004. **29**:1558–72.

14. D'Souza D. C., Abi-Saab W. M., Madonick S., *et al.* Delta-9-tetrahydrocannabinol effects in schizophrenia: implications for cognition, psychosis, and addiction. *Biol Psychiatry*, 2005. **57**:594–608.

15. Bakker C. B., Amini F. B. Observations on the psychotomimetic effects of Sernyl. *Compr Psychiatry*, 1961. **2**:269–80.

16. Breier A., Malhotra A. K., Pinals D. A., Weisenfeld N. I., Pickar D. Association of ketamine-induced psychosis with focal activation of the prefrontal cortex in healthy volunteers. *Am J Psychiatry*, 1997. **154**:805–11.

17. Strauss J. S. Hallucinations and delusions as points on continua function. Rating scale evidence. *Arch Gen Psychiatry*, 1969. **21**:581–6.

18. Claridge G. Single indicator of risk for schizophrenia: probable fact or likely myth? *Schizophr Bull*, 1994. **20**:151–68.

19. Coleman M. J., Levy D. L., Lenzenweger M. F., Holzman P. S. Thought disorder, perceptual aberrations, and schizotypy. *J Abnorm Psychol*, 1996. **105**:469–73.

20. van Os J., Hanssen M., Bijl R. V., Ravelli A. Strauss (1969) revisited: a psychosis continuum in the general population? *Schizophr Res*, 2000. **45**:11–20.

21. Eaton W. W., Romanoski A., Anthony J. C., Nestadt G. Screening for psychosis in the general population with a self-report interview. *J Nerv Ment Dis*, 1991. **179**: 689–93.

22. Tien A. Y., Anthony J. C. Epidemiological analysis of alcohol and drug use as risk factors for psychotic experiences. *J Nerv Ment Dis*, 1990. **78**:473–80.

23. Johns L. C., Cannon M., Singleton N., *et al.* Prevalence and correlates of self-reported psychotic symptoms in the British population. *Br J Psychiatry*, 2004. **185**:298–305.

24. Degenhardt L., Hall W. The association between psychosis and problematical drug use among Australian adults: findings from the National Survey of Mental Health and Well-Being. *Psychol Med*, 2001. **31**:659–68.

25. Skosnik P. D., Spatz-Glenn L., Park S. Cannabis use is associated with schizotypy and attentional disinhibition. *Schizophr Res*, 2001. **48**:83–92.

26. Verdoux H., Sorbara F., Gindre C., Swendsen J. D., van Os J. Cannabis use and dimensions of psychosis in a nonclinical population of female subjects. *Schizophr Res*, 2002. **59**:77–84.

27. Verdoux H., Gindre C., Sorbara F., Tournier M., Swendsen J. D. Effects of cannabis and psychosis vulnerability in daily life: an experience sampling test study. *Psychol Med*, 2003. **33**:23–32.

28. Degenhardt L., Hall W. The association between psychosis and problematical drug use among Australian adults: findings from the National Survey of Mental

Health and Well-Being. *Psychol Med*, 2001. **31**:659–68.

29. Skosnik P. D., Spatz-Glenn L., Park S. Cannabis use is associated with schizotypy and attentional disinhibition. *Schizophr Res*, 2001. **48**:83–92.

30. Verdoux H., Sorbara F., Gindre C., Swendsen J. D., van Os J. Cannabis use and dimensions of psychosis in a nonclinical population of female subjects. *Schizophr Res*, 2002. **59**:77–84.

31. Verdoux H., Gindre C., Sorbara F., Tournier M., Swendsen J. D. Effects of cannabis and psychosis vulnerability in daily life: an experience sampling test study. *Psychol Med*, 2003. **33**:23–32.

32. van Os J., Bak M., Hanssen M., *et al.* Cannabis use and psychosis: a longitudinal population-based study. *Am J Epidemiol*, 2002. **156**:319–27.

33. Ferdinand R. F., Sondeijker F., Van Der Ende J., *et al.* Cannabis use predicts future psychotic symptoms, and vice versa. *Addiction*, 2005. **100**:612–18.

34. Henquet C., Krabbendam L., Spauwen J., *et al.* Prospective cohort study of cannabis use, predisposition for psychosis, and psychotic symptoms in young people. *Br Med J*, 2005. **330**:11.

35. Arseneault L., Cannon M., Poulton R., *et al.* Cannabis use in adolescence and risk for adult psychosis: longitudinal prospective study. *Br Med J*, 2002. **325**:1212–3.

36. Fergusson D. M., Horwood L. J., Ridder E. M. Tests of causal linkages between cannabis use and psychotic symptoms. *Addiction*, 2005. **100**:354–66.

37. Olfson M., Lewis-Fernandez R., Weissman M. M., *et al.* Psychotic symptoms in an urban general medicine practice. *Am J Psychiatry*, 2002. **159**:1412–19.

38. Hambrecht M., Hafner H. Do alcohol or drug abuse induce schizophrenia? *Nervenarzt*, 1996. **67**:36–45.

39. Floyd A. G., Boutros N. N., Struve F. A., Wolf E., Oliwa G. M. Risk factors for experiencing psychosis during cocaine use: a preliminary report. *J Psychiatr Res*, 2006. **40**:178–82.

40. Dalmau A., Bergman B., Brismar B. Psychotic disorders among inpatients with abuse of cannabis, amphetamine and opiates. Do dopaminergic stimulants facilitate psychiatric illness? *Eur Psychiatry*, 1999. **14**:366–71.

41. Margolese H. C., Malchy L., Negrete J. C., Tempier R., Gill K. Drug and alcohol use among patients with schizophrenia and related psychoses: levels and consequences. *Schizophr Res*, 2004. **67**:157–66.

42. Farrell M., Boys A., Bebbington P., *et al.* Psychosis and drug dependence: results from a national survey of prisoners. *Br J Psychiatry*, 2002. **181**: 393–8.

43. Smith M. J., Thirthalli J., Abdalla A. B., Murray R. M., Cottler L. B. Prevalence of psychotic symptoms in substance users: a comparison across substances. *Comprehensive Psychiatry*, 2009. **50**:245–50.

44. van Os J., Hanssen M., Bijl R. V., Vollebergh W. Prevalence of psychotic disorder and community level of psychotic symptoms: an urban-rural comparison. *Arch Gen Psychiatry*, 2001. **58**:663–8.

45. Cannon M., Caspi A., Moffitt T. E., *et al.* Evidence for early-childhood, pan-developmental impairment specific to schizophreniform disorder: results from a longitudinal birth cohort. *Arch Gen Psychiatry*, 2002. **59**:449–56.

46. Robins E., Guze S. B. Establishment of diagnostic validity in psychiatric illness: its application to schizophrenia.

Am J Psychiatry, 1970. **126**: 983–7.

47. Caton C. L., Drake R. E., Hasin D. S., *et al.* Differences between early-phase primary psychotic disorders with concurrent substance use and substance-induced psychoses. *Arch Gen Psychiatry*, 2005. **62**:137–45.

48. Caton C. L., Hasin D. S., Shrout P. E., *et al.* Stability of early-phase primary psychotic disorders with concurrent substance use and substance-induced psychosis. *Br J Psychiatry*, 2007. **190**:105–11.

49. Tsuang M. T., Simpson J. C., Kronfol Z. Subtypes of drug abuse with psychosis. Demographic characteristics, clinical features, and family history. *Arch Gen Psychiatry*, 1982. **39**:141–47.

50. Kendler K. S. A twin study of individuals with both schizophrenia and alcoholism. *Br J Psychiatry*, 1985. **147**:48–53.

51. Glass I. B. Alcoholic hallucinosis: a psychiatric enigma–2. Follow-up studies. *Br J Addict*, 1989. **84**:151–64.

52. Tsuang J. W., Irwin M. R., Smith T. L., Schuckit M. A. Characteristics of men with alcoholic hallucinosis. *Addiction*, 1994. **89**:73–8.

53. Kalayasiri R., Kranzler H. R., Weiss R., *et al.* Risk factors for cocaine-induced paranoia in cocaine-dependent sibling pairs. *Drug Alcohol Depend*, 2006. **84**:77–84.

54. Satel S. L., Southwick S. M., Gawin F. H. Clinical features of cocaine-induced paranoia. *Am J Psychiatry*, 1991. **148**:495–98.

55. Sato M., Chen C. C., Akiyama K., Otsuki S. Acute exacerbation of paranoid psychotic state after long-term abstinence in patients with previous methamphetamine psychosis. *Biol Psychiatry*, 1983. **18**:429–40.

56. Bartlett E., Hallin A., Chapman B., Angrist B. Selective sensitization to the psychosis-inducing effects of cocaine: a possible marker for addiction relapse vulnerability? *Neuropsychopharmacology*, 1997. **16**:77–82.

57. Reid M. S., Ciplet D., O'Leary S., *et al.* Sensitization to the psychosis-inducing effects of cocaine compared with measures of cocaine craving and cue reactivity. *Am J Addict*, 2004. **13**:305–15.

58. Ujike H. Stimulant-induced psychosis and schizophrenia: the role of sensitization. *Curr Psychiatry Rep*, 2002. **4**:177–84.

59. Ujike H., Takaki M., Kodama M., Kuroda S. Gene expression related to synaptogenesis, neuritogenesis, and MAP kinase in behavioral sensitization to psychostimulants. *Ann N Y Acad Sci*, 2002. **965**:55–67.

60. Lieberman J. A., Sheitman B. B., Kinon B. J. Neurochemical sensitization in the pathophysiology of schizophrenia: deficits and dysfunction in neuronal regulation and plasticity. *Neuropsychopharmacology*, 1997. **17**:205–29.

61. Laruelle M., Abi-Dargham A., van Dyck H., *et al.* Single photon emission computerized tomography imaging of amphetamine-induced dopamine release in drug-free schizophrenic subjects. *Proc Natl Acad Sci USA*, 1996. **93**: 9235–40.

62. Breier A., Su T. P., Saunders R., *et al.* Schizophrenia is associated with elevated amphetamine-induced synaptic dopamine concentrations: evidence from a novel positron emission tomography method. *Proc Natl Acad Sci USA*, 1997. **94**: 2569–74.

63. Chen C. K., Lin S. K., Sham P. C., *et al.* Morbid risk for psychiatric disorder among the relatives of methamphetamine users with and without psychosis. *Am J Med Genet B Neuropsychiatr Genet*, 2005. **136**:87–91.

64. McGuire P. K., Jones P., Harvey I., *et al.* Morbid risk of schizophrenia for relatives of patients with cannabis-associated psychosis. *Schizophr Res*, 1995. **15**:277–81.

65. Satel S. L., Edell W. S. Cocaine-induced paranoia and psychosis proneness. *Am J Psychiatry*, 1991. **148**:1708–11.

66. Thirthalli J., Benegal V. Psychosis among substance users. *Curr Opin Psychiatry*, 2006. **19**:239–45.

67. Caspi A., Moffitt T. E., Cannon M., *et al.* Moderation of the effect of adolescent-onset cannabis use on adult psychosis by a functional polymorphism in the catechol-O-methyltransferase gene: longitudinal evidence of a gene X environment interaction. *Biol Psychiatry*, 2005. **57**:1117–27.

68. Henquet C., Rosa A., Krabbendam L., *et al.* An experimental study of catechol-O-methyltransferase Val158Met moderation of delta-9-tetrahydrocannabinol-induced effects on psychosis and cognition. *Neuropsychopharmacology*, 2006. **31**(12):2748–57.

69. Chambers R. A., Krystal J. H., Self D. W. A neurobiological basis for substance abuse comorbidity in schizophrenia. *Biol Psychiatry*, 2001. **50**:71–83.

70. Koob G. F., Sanna P. P., Bloom F. E. Neuroscience of addiction. *Neuron*, 1998. **21**:467–76

71. Beninger R. J., Miller R. Dopamine D1-like receptors and reward-related incentive learning. *Neurosci Biobehav Rev*, 1998. **22**:335–45.

72. Self D. W., Nestler E. J. Molecular mechanisms of drug reinforcement and addiction. *Ann Rev Neurosci*, 1995. **18**:463–95.

73. Koob G. F., Le Moal M. Drug abuse: hedonic homeostatic dysregulation. *Science*, 1997. **278**:52–8.

74. Epping-Jordan M. P., Markou A., Koob G. F. The dopamine D-1 receptor antagonist SCH 23390 injected into the dorsolateral bed nucleus of the stria terminalis decreased cocaine reinforcement in the rat. *Brain Res*, 1998. **784**:105–15.

75. Self D. W., Stein L. The D1 agonists SKF 82958 and SKF 77434 are self-administered by rats. *Brain Res*, 1992. **582**:349–52.

76. Caine S. B., Koob G. F. Effects of dopamine D-1 and D-2 antagonists on cocaine self-administration under different schedules of reinforcement in the rat. *J Pharmacol Exp Ther*, 1994. **270**:209–18.

77. Talbot P. S., Laruelle M. The role of in vivo molecular imaging with PET and SPECT in the elucidation of psychiatric drug action and new drug development. *Eur Neuropsychopharmacol*, 2002. **12**:503–11.

78. Weinberger D. R. Implications of normal brain development for the pathogenesis of schizophrenia. *Arch Gen Psychiatry*, 1987. **44**:660–9.

79. Laruelle M. Imaging dopamine transmission in schizophrenia. A review and meta-analysis. *Q J Nucl Med*, 1998. **42**:211–21.

80. Benegal V., Antony G., Venkatasubramanian G., Jayakumar P. N. Gray matter volume abnormalities and externalizing symptoms in subjects at high risk for alcohol dependence. *Addict Biol*, 2007. **12**:122–32.

81. Selemon L. D., Goldman-Rakic P. S. The reduced neuropil hypothesis: a circuit based model of schizophrenia. *Biol Psychiatry*, 1999. **45**:17–25.

82. Volkow N. D., Fowler J. S. Addiction, a disease of compulsion and drive:

involvement of the orbitofrontal cortex. *Cereb Cortex*, 2000. **10**:318–25.

83. Boutros N. N., Bowers M. B. Jr. Chronic substance-induced psychotic disorders: state of the literature. *J Neuropsychiatry Clin Neurosci*, 1996. **8**:262–9.

84. Zammit S., Allebeck P., Andreasson S., Lundberg I., Lewis G. Self reported cannabis use as a risk factor for schizophrenia in Swedish conscripts of 1969: historical cohort study. *Br Med J*, 2002. **325**:1199.

85. Weiser M., Knobler H. Y., Noy S., Kaplan Z. Clinical characteristics of adolescents later hospitalized for schizophrenia. *Am J Med Genet*, 2002. **14**:949–55.

86. Arseneault L., Cannon M., Witton J., Murray R. M. Causal association between cannabis and psychosis: examination of the evidence. *Br J Psychiatry*, 2004. **184**:110–17.

87. Semple D. M., McIntosh A. M., Lawrie S. M. Cannabis as a risk factor for psychosis: systematic review. *J Psychopharmacol*, 2005. **19**:187–94.

88. Witton J., Arseneault L., Cannon M., Murray R. (2004). Cannabis as a causal factor for psychosis – a review of evidence. In *Search for the Causes of Schizophrenia*, vol **V**, Gattaz W. F. and Hafner H. (Eds.). Darmstaldt: Steinkopff Verlag, pp. 133–49.

89. Post R. M. Cocaine psychoses: a continuum model. *Am J Psychiatry*, 1975. **132**:225–31.

90. Barnes T. R., Mutsatsa S. H., Hutton S. B., Watt H. C., Joyce E. M. Comorbid substance use and age at onset of schizophrenia. *Br J Psychiatry*, 2006. **188**:237–42.

91. Van Mastrigt S., Addington J., Addington D. Substance misuse at presentation to an early psychosis program. *Soc Psychiatry Psychiatr Epidemiol*, 2004. **39**:69–72.

92. Venkatesh B. K., Thirthalli J., Naveen M. N., *et al*. Sex difference in age of onset of schizophrenia: findings from a community-based study in India. *World Psychiatry* 2008. 7:173–6.

93. Caton C. L. M., Samet S., Hasin D. S. When acute-stage psychosis and substance use co-occur: differentiating substance-induced and primary psychotic disorders. *J Psychiatr Pract*, 2000. **6**:256–66.

94. Rasanen P., Tiihon J., Isohanni M., *et al*. Schizophrenia, alcohol abuse, and violent behavior: a 26-year followup study of an unselected birth cohort. *Schizophr Bull*, 1998. **24**:437–41.

95. Arseneault L., Moffitt T. E., Caspi A., Taylor P. J., Silva P. A. Mental disorders and violence in a total birth cohort: results from the Dunedin Study. *Arch Gen Psychiatry*, 2000. 57:979–86.

96. Allebeck P., Varla A., Kristjansson E., Wistedt B. Risk factors for suicide among patients with schizophrenia. *Acta Psychiatr Scand*, 1987. **76**:414–19.

97. Drake R. E., Gates C., Cotton P. G., Whitaker A. Suicide among schizophrenics. Who is at risk? *J Nerv Ment Dis*, 1984. **172**:613–17.

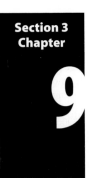

Organic syndromes of schizophrenia:
drugs and schizophrenia-like psychosis

Stimulants and psychosis

Nash N. Boutros, Matt P. Galloway, and Eric M. Pihlgren

Facts box

- Acute intoxication with psychostimulants commonly leads to the acute emergence of psychotic symptoms.
- Careful history taking and urine and blood tests are usually sufficient to alert the clinician to the possibility of a drug-related problem.
- Depending solely on the clinical presentation is not advisable given the current state of knowledge.
- A period of follow-up in the absence of continued drug use is usually helpful to confirm a diagnosis.
- First use of amphetamines or cocaine before the age of 16 years and severe cannabis or cocaine dependence may be related to an increased risk of psychosis.
- Stimulant-induced psychoses are very likely to clear within several days to about 1 month of abstinence. Only 1%–15% of patients with stimulant-induced psychoses maintain some psychotic symptoms after a month.
- Research from Japan showed that family members of patients with methamphetamine psychosis had a five times greater morbid risk for schizophrenia than users without psychosis.
- The pattern of stimulant abuse most commonly associated with the induction of psychosis is the initial use of lower doses, typically administered in an escalating manner and ultimately leading to multiple binges or runs.
- The current trend for psychostimulant-induced psychosis is for initial treatment with antipsychotics, with a

- bias toward the atypical antipsychotics as first-line treatment.
- Early treatment and retention of stimulant users in mental health care services is recommended to prevent the development of a chronic psychotic condition.

Introduction

Whether or not psychostimulant use can cause a chronic psychotic disorder in humans that is clinically similar to schizophrenia remains an open and important question *with diagnostic, therapeutic, and prognostic implications*. In this chapter, we examine the existing literature to determine if there is enough evidence to support the notion that abuse of psychostimulants can cause chronic psychotic disorders. We also investigate whether drug-induced psychotic states can be self-sustaining (i.e. autonomous) or require continued drug use. If continued drug use is necessary, what level of use is needed in order to sustain the syndrome?

Psychostimulant models of psychosis are important animal models for human schizophrenia [1, 2, 3, 4]. Angrist and Gershon [5] observed that the symptomatology of experimentally induced amphetamine psychosis closely resembles endogenous schizophrenia. Similarly, Snyder [6] considered amphetamine psychosis to be a "model" schizophrenia due to the strong similarity of its clinical features to paranoid schizophrenia.

Acute intoxication with psychostimulants (i.e., methamphetamine (MA), amphetamine, or cocaine) commonly leads to the acute emergence of psychotic symptoms [7]. Although this can contribute to diagnostic confusion in the emergency room, careful history taking and urine-and-blood tests are usually sufficient to alert the clinician to the possibility of a drug-related problem [8]. Although these authors presented evidence that some clinical differences can be discerned between cocaine users with psychotic symptoms and schizophrenia patients with and without cocaine intoxication, the evidence of reliability of such diagnostic differences remains lacking. Depending solely on the clinical presentation is not advisable given the current state of knowledge. A period of follow-up in the absence of continued drug use is also usually helpful to confirm the diagnosis [9]. Of course, the primary assumption is that drug-induced syndromes clear with continued abstinence. Although an idiopathic syndrome may show some improvement with abstinence, it is unlikely to clear altogether. This assumption is examined later. We discuss the issue of acute intoxication inasmuch as it may provide clues to the nature of the psychopathology to be seen in more protracted cases of drug-induced psychosis.

Japanese studies highlighted the difficulties of researching longer-term effects of stimulants [10, 11]. The widespread use of high-dose injected MA led to hospital admissions of individuals with chronic psychosis that persisted after substance use had ceased. The authors noted that many of these individuals qualified for a diagnosis of schizophrenia. However, genetic risks and other possible contributing factors and the presence or absence of predrug use evidence of increased risk (e.g., presence of prodromal symptoms or schizotypal traits) were not assessed. It should be noted that large series of chronic cocaine-dependent individuals with emergent psychotic disorders could not be found in the literature.

In a recent study [12], the histories of drug or alcohol use in 152 patients diagnosed with either schizophrenia or schizophreniform disorders were examined. These researchers reported that 90% of the patients with a history of any type of substance abuse reported the use of cannabis. This study highlights the inherent difficulty in assessing causality in a population largely characterized by poly drug use, increased life stressors, and possibly other factors like head injury. Poly drug use may indeed be a fundamentally different problem than use of, or addiction to, a single substance. Indeed, in another study, psychosis proneness differed between cocaine-dependent and cocaine-and-alcohol-dependent individuals, with the comorbid cocaine-and-alcohol-dependent group being significantly more likely to experience a paranoid psychosis with cocaine use [13]. Although not systematically examined in clinical populations, animal experimentation suggests that even a short duration of abuse of PCP-like agents may greatly potentiate the behavioral effects of psychostimulants [14].

Epidemiology

Yui and colleagues [2] suggested that further evidence for stimulant-induced psychosis could be found in the MA abuse epidemic in Japan shortly after World War II, when huge military stores of MA found their way to the open market in Japan, leading to widespread abuse. A significant number of MA abusers developed psychosis that did not resolve with discontinuation of drug use and many patients required years for recovery. Sato [15] reported that 10% of chronic heavy amphetamine users developed a chronic psychotic disorder lasting more than 6 months after cessation of amphetamine use.

Nakatani and Hara [16] observed that the large-scale MA abuse that occurred in Japan provides an excellent opportunity to further our understanding of these disorders. Although MA abuse became widespread shortly after World War II, it almost disappeared during the mid-1950s due to strict legal enforcement. However, beginning in the early 1970s, a new epidemic developed. Nakatani and Hara noted that some interesting differences regarding patients' profiles have been found between the first and second epidemics. Many reports during the postwar period focused on the clinical resemblance to schizophrenia and manic-depressive illness. Tatetsu [17] concluded that typical exogenous symptoms such as clouding of consciousness, amnesic syndrome, impaired intellectual functioning, and physical signs are generally not apparent in patients with MA intoxication. Although disturbance of consciousness was only sporadically reported during the first epidemic, studies focused on the more recent epidemic have found this symptom to be much more prevalent [16]. Nakatani and Hara speculate that this difference probably reflects a change in the pattern of usage, with manufactured ampoule being commonly used during the postwar era and high-density powder from the black market becoming prevalent during the more recent epidemic.

One of the most prominent effects of MA abuse on cognitive function pertains to the development of drug-related psychosis [18]. Aside from the sudden psychosis-inducing effects of high doses of MA, an enduring form of psychosis can also develop. Studies from Japan have found that between 36% and 64% of MA users who have experienced psychotic symptoms continue to present with these symptoms for more than 10 days after the discontinuation of MA use, even though MA is eliminated from the blood stream in less than 5 days [19]. Barr and colleagues note that studies in Japan show that MA users with MA psychosis are much more likely to experience psychotic symptoms again if they use MA and are also more likely to have a psychotic relapse when confronted with stressful situations, even years after cessation of MA use [18]. Another study involving female inmates in Japan found that 21% of those with MA psychosis remained in a psychotic state for more than 6 months [19]. Another 49% returned to their premorbid state but experienced "flashbacks" (i.e. spontaneous recurrence of psychotic symptoms that would fit criteria for a paranoid-schizophrenia psychotic relapse) during their 15–20 months of incarceration. Furthermore, MA users with persistent or recurrent psychotic symptoms become vulnerable to environmental stress and may benefit from antipsychotic medication in a manner similar to individuals with schizophrenia.

The relationship between psychosis and drug dependence was also examined in a large sample of prison population in England [20]. Farrell and colleagues surveyed the clinical condition and history of drug use of 503 individuals. They found that first use of amphetamines or cocaine, before the age of 16 years, and severe cannabis or cocaine dependence to be related to an increased risk of psychosis. These data agree with our recent finding regarding the significance of the age of first use as a risk factor for developing acute psychotic symptoms with cocaine use [21]. In contrast, severe dependence on heroin was associated with a reduced risk for developing a psychotic syndrome [20].

Another possible risk factor for psychosis was described by Cherland and Fitzpatrick [22] when they examined the rate of psychotic and mood-congruent psychotic side effects of stimulant medications in children treated for attention-deficit hyperactivity disorder (ADHD). These researchers conducted a chart review of all children diagnosed with ADHD in an outpatient clinic from January 1989 to March 1995. During that period, 192 children were diagnosed with ADHD, 98 (51%) of whom received treatment with stimulants. These investigators found that six children developed psychotic or mood-congruent psychotic symptoms during treatment. Cherland and Fitzpatrick concluded that awareness of the potential for psychotic side effects from stimulant medications is important when prescribing for children. Boutros and colleagues [23] also found a link between ADHD symptoms and psychotic symptoms in their examination of sensory gating and psychosis vulnerability in cocaine-dependent individuals. Their examination of 30 abstinent individuals suggested that deficient P50 sensory gating and attention deficits might be associated with increased susceptibility to developing psychotic symptoms in the context of cocaine use.

Schuckit's [24] comprehensive review of comorbidity between substance-use disorders and psychiatric conditions found psychotic symptoms to occur in about 40% of amphetamine-dependent patients, especially with higher doses. Schuckit noted that stimulant-induced psychoses are very likely to clear within several days to about 1 month of abstinence. Only 1%–15% of patients with stimulant-induced psychoses maintain some psychotic symptoms after a month. Schuckit speculated that this could reflect the fact that approximately 1% of people in any group will develop schizophrenia, or could be the consequence of the precipitation of longer-term psychotic disorders in predisposed individuals. However, it is also possible that heavy use of stimulants might cause more long-lasting, and hypothetically even permanent, neurochemical changes associated with long-term psychotic disorders in a small number of individuals, even if not so predisposed.

Clinical picture of amphetamine and cocaine-induced psychotic states

In 1958, Connell [25] published his seminal monograph on amphetamine psychosis. He reviewed 36 clinical case reports of patients developing psychosis following amphetamine use. Of these 36 patients, 9 developed a protracted psychotic syndrome persisting more than 2 months after withdrawal from amphetamines, and in 3 subjects, this prolongation of psychotic symptoms was "indefinite."

In an attempt to compare clinical pictures of amphetamine-induced psychosis and schizophrenia, Bell [26] studied 14 patients with amphetamine-induced psychosis. These patients did not have any psychotic symptoms prior to abusing drugs. Three of these patients continued to show psychotic symptoms for many months after they ceased to take amphetamines.

Ellinwood Jr. [27] interviewed 25 subjects with chronic amphetamine dependence. Of the 25 users, 8 were classifiable as no-psychosis and 10 as amphetamine-induced psychosis. Ellinwood Jr. described hyperamnesis as the acute and focused memory of the psychotic experience. Not all amphetamine users developed psychosis (although all of them were suspicious at some time), and there was no continuum of severity toward psychosis. Fear and terror were major symptoms mentioned by psychotics. Philosophical concerns increased as patients became progressively psychotic. Both auditory and visual hallucinations were noted. Gross distortion of bodily image was highly correlated with psychosis. Finally, changes in libido varied greatly but an increase in libido and polymorphous sexual activity most often preceded psychosis.

Clinical descriptions provided by Snyder [6] were similar to what has been provided in the literature except that stereotyped compulsive behavior was emphasized with patients often pacing back and forth with their mouths moving from side to side. The stereotyped compulsions seemed to be consistent in methamphetamine psychosis (MAP) [27]. The presence of tactile hallucinations was also said to differentiate MAP from schizophrenia where such hallucinations are rare.

Charles-Nicolas [28] studied the histories and clinical pictures of 25 amphetamine-abusing chronic psychotic patients. He found seven of them to have had no psychotic tendencies before the addiction. These patients were followed in his center for several years prior to the onset of psychosis.

The clinical characteristics of MAP have been well described in the Japanese population [29]. MAP involves paranoid-hallucinatory states indistinguishable from paranoid schizophrenia, with residual volitional disturbances (e.g., loss of spontaneity and idleness). Paranoid-hallucinatory states persist after the pharmacological effects of MA have worn off and readily reappear upon re-injection of MA. Additionally, individuals with a history of MAP were also observed to experience spontaneous recurrence of their paranoid-hallucinatory states in response to stress [29].

Goto [30] described 23 patients with persisting MAP who suffered from residual symptoms such as emotional blunting or manic-depressive states following a drug-free period of 4.6–9.7 years. Utena and colleagues [31] reported that 5% of patients with MAP were hospitalized for years after the cessation of MA use because of their volitional disturbances (as noted earlier).

Sato and colleagues [10] observed that MAP patients may develop acute paranoid psychotic exacerbation after long-term abstinence with minimal use (as little as a single dose) of amphetamine or alcohol. One patient in this cohort relapsed without evidence of amphetamine use. Persistent personality changes may develop in patients with chronic amphetamine use and paranoid hallucinatory state. These observations provide strong presumptive evidence that certain effects of chronic stimulant abuse can persist long after cessation of use [32]. Tomiyama [33] found postamphetamine chronic psychotic patients to have fewer negative symptoms as measured by the Scale for the Assessment of Negative Symptoms. Tomiyama suggested that these patients not be labeled as schizophrenic, and recommended the term "residual psychosis" be used in its place.

The findings of Tomiyama [33] are in contrast with Srisurapanont and colleagues [34], who showed that a substantial proportion of such patients do experience negative symptoms. This group [34] found premorbid schizoid/schizotypal traits to be a serious risk factor for developing a protracted postabstinence psychotic syndrome. They provided additional evidence implicating a premorbid vulnerability to psychosis as well as to early and heavy amphetamine use in individuals developing chronic or prolonged postabstinence psychotic syndromes [35]. Additionally, Chen and colleagues [35] showed that family members of patients with MAP had a five times greater morbid risk for schizophrenia than users without psychosis.

Disturbance of consciousness due to MA abuse was reported in two patients by Nakatani and Hara [16]. These authors noted that in both cases mental status changed, passing through three distinct stages: restlessness and insomnia, hallucinatory paranoid state, and disturbance of consciousness following a period of amphetamine use. In addition to delirium during intoxication, Askevold [36] described abstinence delirium in amphetamine abusers, reporting a latency period between the beginning of abstinence and the onset of delirium of between 3 and 10 days, followed by a period of delirium of between 4 and 18 days. Fatal delirium has also been reported in association with cocaine intoxication [37].

In a sample of 19 subjects who met DSM-IV criteria for amphetamine or cocaine-induced psychosis, Harris and Batki [7] showed that all had persecutory delusions; 95% had bizarre delusions, 53% had grandiose delusions, and 32% had somatic delusions. Of the entire sample, 95% experienced auditory hallucinations, with 32% describing voices of running commentary and 58% hearing more than one voice conversing with each other. Additionally, 68% had visual, 26%, tactile, and 26%, olfactory hallucinations. Although negative symptoms were less than what would be expected in a group of schizophrenia patients, they were detectable (particularly anergia) and correlated significantly with length of stay in the emergency room or subsequent hospitalization.

Yui and colleagues [29] observed that paranoid-hallucinatory states gradually disappear, although idleness and emotional flattening tend to increase 1 month after the cessation of MA use. Although at odds with Connell's [25] original observations that amphetamine psychosis is never prolonged after excretion of MA in the urine, suggesting that continued use of MA is essential to maintain the psychosis syndrome, some have suggested that the development of MAP may be etiologically related to persisting brain damage or changes in brain metabolism induced by MA [32]. Yui and colleagues concluded that the Japanese experience of MAP, in which psychotic symptoms can develop with the progression of MA-induced brain damage in the course of chronic MA use, therefore differs from Connell's experience. However, the authors note that, in Japan, MA is injected without any other substance, with most users re-injecting before the effects of the previous MA injection have diminished. They conclude that such exclusive and repetitive use of MA may engender enduring vulnerability to paranoid-hallucinatory states, leading to spontaneous recurrences of MAP [2].

Recent studies of amphetamine psychosis

In a recent systematic review, Curran and colleagues [38] concluded that there was clear evidence that "irrespective of the individual's mental state, a large enough dose of a stimulant drug can produce a brief psychotic reaction, usually lasting only hours and being self-limiting in the majority of individuals." The pattern of stimulant abuse most commonly associated with the induction of psychosis is the initial use of lower doses, typically administered in an escalating manner and ultimately leading to multiple binges or runs [39, 40]. Emergence of psychotic syndromes usually occurs during a binge.

Chronic psychosis, on the other hand, may emerge during a period of abstinence. Flaum and Schultz [41] presented a demonstrative case in detail exemplifying

a common clinical scenario that presents the clinician with a diagnostic dilemma:

In summary, a teenage male with no evidence of increased risk for schizophrenia (i.e. no abnormal behaviour, good school performance, good social skills, and lack of family history of psychiatric disorders except drug use) began abusing amphetamine and marijuana on a regular basis with occasional use of hallucinogens and cocaine for a period of about 10 years. Family pressure was applied and he stopped drug use. In a few weeks, he began to develop paranoid ideations that became delusions. Delusions were nonbizarre at the beginning but progressively became more bizarre and hallucinations eventually also occurred. There was no evidence of continued amphetamine use but marijuana was used occasionally. The patient also exhibited negative symptoms (withdrawal and alogia). The patient's positive symptoms responded well to haloperidol but without effect on negative symptoms.

Flaum and Schultz [41] proposed that this case suggested an etiologic role for amphetamine and polysubstance use in the development of a chronic schizophrenia-like psychotic disorder. Whether some form of genetic liability to developing a psychotic disorder existed in this case could not be positively ruled out, and brings to focus the chicken and egg nature of the question raised here. Early work by Angrist and Gershon [5] suggested that a predilection to the psychogenic effects of stimulants is an important factor contributing to the emergence of these symptoms with stimulant use.

Schuckit [24] conducted a systematic review of manuscripts published in the English language since approximately 1970 in order to investigate the comorbidity between substance-use disorders and psychiatric conditions. Results of this review generally supported the conclusion that substance-use mental disorders exist, especially regarding stimulant- or cannabinoid-induced psychoses, substance-induced mood disorders, and substance-induced anxiety conditions. Schuckit [24] concluded that "temporary schizophrenia-like conditions of hallucinations (predominantly auditory) and/or delusions (usually paranoid) developing without insight and observed in a clear sensorium can be induced by stimulants." However, Schuckit cautioned that these conditions should be distinguished from the life-long schizophrenic disorders, as they are likely to require only short-term antipsychotic medications, whereas schizophrenia often requires treatment with medications for many years.

Cocaine-induced psychosis

Post [42] reviewed the evidence for cocaine-induced psychosis and its predeterminants. He reported that with chronic cocaine use, a syndrome of insomnia, painful delusions, and apathy can develop. This phase occurs during the transition from initial euphoria to paranoid psychosis. When the cocaine-induced paranoid psychosis is fully developed, it is almost indistinguishable from paranoid schizophrenia. Post stated that with cessation of cocaine use, hallucinations usually stop, but delusions may persist.

Satel and Edell [43] showed that heavy cocaine users who experience transient paranoia while intoxicated may be at higher risk for development of psychosis than cocaine users who do not experience paranoia. However, the development of a cocaine-induced chronic psychosis seems to be rare [44]. Rounsaville and colleagues [45] found that only 4 (all male) of 298 chronic cocaine users had received the diagnosis of schizophrenia or schizoaffective disorders.

Follow-up studies

Although essential to clarify differences between drug-induced and idiopathic psychotic syndromes, follow-up studies are rare in this literature. A 6-year follow-up study provided evidence that chronic use of stimulants, but not depressants or narcotics, can lead to the development of a psychotic disorder that is not secondary to acute intoxication [46]. On the other hand, a significant number of patients who used sedatives developed serious depression. Typically, cocaine abusers develop delusions and hallucinations that tend to be related to their drug use behavior (e.g., ideas of being watched). Furthermore, first-rank Schneiderian symptoms (e.g., thought withdrawal and thought broadcast), tend to be absent in cocaine-intoxicated patients who are experiencing psychotic symptoms [47]. Retrospectively, formal thought disorder and bizarre delusions significantly predicted a diagnosis of schizophrenia, with odds ratios (OR) of 3.55:1 and 6.09:1, respectively. Suicidal ideation (OR = 0.32:1), intravenous cocaine abuse (OR = 0.18:1), and a history of drug detoxification (OR = 0.26:1) or methadone maintenance (OR = 0.18:1) demonstrate inverse relationships with a schizophrenia diagnosis [48].

In the absence of long-term follow up of large cohorts of patients with cocaine-induced psychosis, it is not known whether these differences from idiopathic schizophrenia would persist. Of interest is the observation that although cocaine-induced psychosis shows sensitization (i.e., psychosis becomes more severe and occurs earlier with repeated cocaine use), this occurs only with psychosis and not with other effects of cocaine [49]. Moreover, cocaine abusers who exhibit sensitization to the psychogenic effects of cocaine seem to have less naturally occurring craving and are likely to reduce their cocaine and other substance use [50]. Some researchers found cocaine-induced psychosis and schizophrenia to be distinct enough as to question the concept of cocaine psychosis as a model for schizophrenia [51]. These investigators highlighted that increased intensity of colors, change of light intensity, objects appearing more vivid, and macropsia and micropsia were reported by the cocaine-intoxicated individuals. They also stated that even if paranoia is present, it tends to be rather transitory.

Biological studies

Given the dearth of well-defined cohorts of stimulant-induced psychosis patients, it is not surprising that genetic, pharmacological, neuropsychological, electrophysiological, or imaging studies specifically addressing this population are few.

In one study, patients with a history of MAP exhibited impairment of selective attention, although with less cognitive deficit than schizophrenic patients [29]. Similarly, in mild to moderate drug use in humans, no differences were found between the effects of cocaine and amphetamine on cognition [52].

Information processing studies utilized the event-related potential (ERP) technique to assess deficits in these populations. Iwanami and colleagues [53] found that methamphetamine dependence correlated with a reduction in P3a amplitude, a marker of detection of novelty. Methamphetamine psychosis was associated with reduced mismatch negativity (MMN), an indicator of preattentive ability to detect change in ongoing sensory input, and not P300. Earlier, the same group reported MAP subjects to have reduced P300 anteriorly, whereas schizophrenia patients reduced more posteriorly, suggesting differences in the orientation of the cerebral sources of the activity [54]. The same group also investigated the auditory ERPs during a dichotic syllable discrimination task in 16 unmedicated subjects in residual states following the remission of MA-induced paranoid-hallucinatory states [55]. Extrapolation from these findings suggests some similarity in susceptibility to paranoid-hallucinatory states between MAP and schizophrenia.

In a separate line of investigations, evoked responses were used to examine the inhibitory function of the brain when repetitive identical stimuli are presented, that is, habituation and sensory gating. Most notably, a deficit in inhibiting irrelevant incoming sensory input was observed in abstinent cocaine-dependent individuals [56]. The finding was later replicated in a more racially mixed group [57]. More recently, our group provided further evidence of a deleterious effect of chronic cocaine on gating of the P50 evoked response [23].

Transcranial magnetic stimulation (TMS) was also used to examine cortical inhibition and excitability in this group of abstinent cocaine-dependent individuals. The initial TMS studies provided evidence of increased cortical inhibition [58]. This finding was replicated in a larger sample and was interpreted as a compensatory protective mechanism against the epileptogenic properties of cocaine [59].

Electrophysiological studies in cocaine-dependent individuals suggest a complex mechanism for the development of psychosis in these subjects. Deficits in the inhibition of incoming irrelevant sensory input (i.e. sensory gating) have been repeatedly demonstrated in schizophrenia patients [60]. As mentioned earlier, a similar decrease in inhibitory capacity was demonstrated in abstinent cocaine users [23, 56]. This decreased inhibition was correlated with psychosis proneness in this population [23]. The findings of increased inhibition demonstrated via TMS and decreased inhibition demonstrated via evoked responses presented a dilemma for interpretation. A recent study utilizing additional TMS-based measures of cortical excitability, namely paired-stimulus facilitation and inhibition, provided evidence consistent with increased excitability or decreased inhibition [61]. Given that the paired-stimulus TMS technique has been rather strongly linked with cortical inhibitory-excitatory mechanisms, and that it is likely that sensory gating may be strongly influenced by subcortical mechanisms, we postulate that some form of a cortical-subcortical imbalance in the excitatory-inhibitory balance may be important for the development of psychotic symptoms in cocaine users.

Finally, structural imaging studies comparing groups of idiopathic and presumably chronic psychostimulant-induced psychotic patients are virtually nonexistent. One CT study found no differences between drug-induced and idiopathic schizophrenia [62]. On the other hand, the few functional imaging studies examining the effects of prolonged or repeated psychostimulant use or administration focused on probing the mechanisms underlying the sensitization of the effects of these chemicals on the brain. These studies are discussed in subsection Mechanisms.

Mechanisms

Among a number of proposed mechanisms by which repeated use or administration of psychostimulants could result in a longer lasting increase in the susceptibility to psychosis, sensitization holds a prominent position.

Repeated treatment with psychostimulants produces changes in both brain and behavior that far outlast their initial pharmacological actions [63]. Exploration of sensitization mechanisms and effects of repeated exposure to psychostimulants in animals has been extensive. Discussion of this extensive literature is beyond the scope of this chapter, however the interested reader is referred to a number of authoritative reviews [64, 65, 66, 67]. It is interesting to note that the changes observed with chronic amphetamine and cocaine administration in rats, although similar, are not identical, possibly contributing to the differences in clinical effects of the two drugs.

Lieberman and colleagues [1] suggested that the initial aggravating event by which stimulant abuse could produce a chronic schizophrenic syndrome is enhanced dopaminergic activity that manifests as positive schizophrenic symptoms. Continued prolonged excessive dopaminergic activation is believed to induce neuronal degeneration in dopamine systems, leading to a hypodopaminergic state and negative symptoms [2]. In fact, chronic amphetamine treatment in rats is well documented to be toxic to dopamine nerve terminals [55]. Yui and colleagues [2] speculated that a reduction in dopamine could result in postsynaptic receptor supersensitivity, helping to explain the re-emergence of positive symptoms after transiently increased dopamine availability, as has been observed during stress or exposure to dopaminergic drugs.

Evidence for sensitization in humans is found in a small number of studies [68, 69]. Strakowski and colleagues [68] demonstrated that when two doses of a stimulant were given to volunteers free from psychosis, the second dose produced a greater "sensitized" response. Stimulant users studied by Brady and colleagues [70] reported psychotic symptoms occurring with lower doses over time. Yui and colleagues [29] concluded that the development of MAP may therefore be related to persisting brain damage or changes in brain metabolism induced by repeated MA use, and studies of the clinical course and neurological basis of MAP psychosis may provide insights into the pathophysiology of schizophrenia. Boileau and colleagues [71] investigated sensitization to stimulants in humans with an [^{11}C] raclopride/Positron Emission Tomography (PET) study to determine whether behavioral and neurochemical sensitization occur in healthy individuals after limited exposure to amphetamine in a laboratory setting. These researchers conducted an open-label, 1-year follow-up of repeated amphetamine administration in healthy volunteers. Ten healthy men (mean ± SD age, 25.8 ± 1.8 years) were administered 3 single doses of amphetamine (dextroamphetamine sulfate, 0.3 mg/kg by mouth) on 3 separate days. Using, positron emission tomography (PET) and [^{11}C] raclopride, these researchers measured dopamine release in response to amphetamine on the first exposure (day 1) and 14 days, and 1 year after the third exposure. Boileau and colleagues reported that the initial dose of amphetamine caused dopamine release in the ventral striatum (a reduction in [^{11}C] raclopride binding). The authors concluded that, "consistent with a sensitisation-like phenomenon, on 14 and 365 days after the third dose of amphetamine there was a greater psychomotor response and increased dopamine release (a greater reduction in [^{11}C] raclopride binding), relative to the initial dose, in the ventral striatum, progressively extending to the dorsal caudate and putamen." The authors also noted that proneness to sensitization was predicted by a high novelty-seeking personality trait and self-rating assessments indicating impulsivity. Boileau and colleagues concluded that sensitization to stimulants can be achieved in healthy men in the laboratory, and that this phenomenon is associated with increased dopamine release and persists for at least 1 year.

The role of sensitization was also examined by Ujike and colleagues [3]. They found that three different conditions – psychostimulant-induced behavioral sensitization in rodents, psychostimulant-induced psychoses in human, and chronic schizophrenia – demonstrated similar longitudinal alternations, progressively enhanced susceptibility to abnormal behaviors, psychotic state, and relapse. These researchers concluded that sensitisation phenomena to the drugs or endogenous dopamine should be involved in the mechanisms underlying the development of such susceptibility. Consequently, common molecular mechanisms of sensitization phenomena may develop in the three conditions they studied.

Laruelle [72] described the role of endogenous sensitization in the pathophysiology of schizophrenia in a review of brain imaging studies. He observed that sensitization of mesolimbic dopamine systems had been postulated by several authors to underlie the development of dopaminergic abnormalities associated with schizophrenia. Laruelle noted that results of recent brain imaging studies indicated that schizophrenia was associated with increased amphetamine-induced dopamine release, and that this exaggerated response was detected in patients experiencing an episode of clinical deterioration but not in clinically stable patients. Laruelle asserted that because increased stimulant-induced dopamine release was a hallmark of sensitization, these results supported the view that schizophrenia was associated with a process of endogenous sensitization. He further postulated that amphetamine-induced hyperactivity of the dopaminergic system sustained over a certain period of time is in itself sufficient to induce a psychotic state in otherwise healthy humans, although the role of an underlying vulnerability to this effect cannot be entirely ruled out. Based on the preclinical evidence that dopamine projection to the prefrontal cortex acts as a buffer that opposes the development of sensitization in subcortical dopamine projections, Laruelle proposed that, in schizophrenia, neurodevelopmental abnormalities of prefrontal dopaminergic systems might result in a state of enhanced vulnerability to sensitization during late adolescence and early adulthood. It is also proposed that D2 receptor blockade, if sustained, might allow for an extinction of this sensitization process, with possible re-emergence upon treatment discontinuation. Laruelle concluded that a better understanding of the neurocircuitry associated with endogenous sensitization and its consequence in schizophrenia might be important for the development of better treatment and relapse prevention strategies.

Finally, aside from genes and psychostimulants, there are other factors that are associated with psychosis or schizophrenia, such as prenatal influenza [73], prenatal drug treatment (e.g. reserpine), and obstetrical complications [74], most of which are known to induce dopamine supersensitivity and elevated $D2^{High}$ receptors [73].

Although clear and persisting neurotoxicity to dopaminergic projection fields can be produced by continuous amphetamine or methamphetamine use, continuous cocaine administration apparently does not induce a similar neurotoxicity and this makes DA neurotoxicity a poor candidate for an underpinning of stimulant psychoses. However, both continuous amphetamine and cocaine exposure induce a strong pattern of degeneration that is confined to the lateral habenula and its principal output pathway, fasciculus retroflexus [75]. This finding has led to a reconsideration of the role of these structures in psychoses. The habenula, as the chief relay nucleus of the descending dorsal diencephalic system (consisting of stria medullaris, habenula, and fasciculus retroflexus), is an important link between limbic and striatal forebrain and lower diencephalic and mesencephalic centres. Studies of glucose utilization have consistently shown the habenula to be highly sensitive to dopamine agonists and antagonists. Lesions of habenula produce a wide variety of behavioral alterations. The dorsal diencephalic system has major and predominantly inhibitory connections onto dopamine-containing cells and it mediates part of the negative feedback from dopamine receptors onto dopamine cell bodies. It represents one of the major inputs in brain to the raphe nuclei and has anatomical and functional connections to modulate important functions such as sensory gating through thalamus, pain gating through central grey and raphe and motor stereotypies and reward mechanisms through substantia nigra and the ventral tegmental area. Alterations in these pathways are ideal candidates for producing the behaviors that occur during psychosis and that future considerations of the circuitry underlying psychoses need to include this important but less examined system.

Available insights into the management of stimulant-induced psychotic conditions

There is indeed a paucity of data regarding treatment for MAP, with a complete lack of controlled treatment trials, including head-to-head comparison to nondrug induced psychotic patients [18]. The currently prevailing standard of care in this area parallels the management of acute psychosis from other etiologies, such as schizophrenia [18]. The current trend is for initial treatment with antipsychotics, with a bias toward the atypical antipsychotics as first-line treatment. To date, there has been no evidence that typical antipsychotics have efficacy in decreasing craving among substance abusing psychotic patients. Evidence for atypical antipsychotic use suggests some measure of efficacy, but remains limited to case reports and small open-label patient series. The length of appropriate pharmacological intervention is unknown and no consistent guidelines exist in the literature. Barr and colleagues reported a small case series that indicated that antipsychotic treatment beyond the acute psychotic episode may protect against future psychotic episodes, even at very low doses [18].

A small series of 10 patients with comorbid schizophrenia and drug use were treated with aripiprazole for 8 weeks in an open-label design [76]. In those who completed the trial (60%), positive urine drug tests dropped significantly after 2 weeks. Both mean cocaine and alcohol craving scores also dropped significantly with a positive correlation between dropping psychosis and dropping craving scores. Green and colleagues [77] examined the acute response to haloperidol and olanzapine in 97 first episode psychosis patients with comorbid substance abuse. They found no difference between typical and atypical medications but an overall less likelihood of responding when compared to patients without drug use comorbidity. These findings are in contrast to a report by Brown and colleagues [78] of 24 dually diagnosed patients who were on typical antipsychotics and were randomized to either continue or discontinue the drug. Quetiapine was substituted when necessary in those who discontinued the typical antipsychotic. They report that those discontinuing a typical antipsychotic had a significant reduction in drug craving as compared to the other patients. Brown and colleagues further reported that typical antipsychotic discontinuation combined with a quetiapine switch was associated with reduced drug craving. Finally, animal work suggests a possible role for serotonin in treating this condition. When cocaine and risperidone were coadministered to rats, the effects of cocaine seemed to have been blocked [79].

Current research indicates that people presenting with co-occurring disorders, such as MAP, warrant specific treatments that deal with both the psychosis and addiction issues [18]. In fact, the best outcomes stem from programs that are considered evidence based and that integrate mental health and substance abuse treatment. Barr and colleagues noted that most MA treatments investigated so far have used only an "addiction" treatment model for stimulant dependence and have excluded people with comorbid mental health problems, such as persistent or recurrent psychotic symptoms. Further research is required to develop a more thorough understanding of the profiles of people who suffer from persistent or recurrent MAP.

If sensitization is indeed the underlying mechanism for psychostimulants-induced psychosis, then early treatment and retention of stimulant users in mental health care services would appear to be desirable to prevent the development of a chronic psychotic condition. There is indeed a lack of good quality evidence as to whether this approach can be effective. A review by Cochrane found no relevant trials [80]. A potentially important finding in rats, without parallel human studies as yet, is the demonstration that low-dose clozapine or haloperidol can block the induction of behavioral sensitization to amphetamine in rats [81]. This finding has potential implication for future preventive use of such drugs in individuals with evidence of increased susceptibility to developing a psychotic disorder.

Conclusion

Based on the earlier review, it can be proposed that there is enough suggestive evidence that abuse of psychostimulants can result in or increase the susceptibility for a state of chronic psychosis. It can also be concluded that abuse of amphetamines, as the sole drug of abuse, can result in a chronic psychotic disorder. On the other hand, the evidence for a cocaine-induced chronic psychosis is less compelling. The exact relationships between premorbid vulnerability and the persistence of symptoms in the absence of continued drug use or the degree of use needed to sustain a psychotic syndrome are also not yet well characterized.

Based on a stress-diathesis model, we propose that the eventual development of a chronic psychotic disorder in an individual with a history of drug use is likely to be multifactorial with the specific substances used, the pattern of use (including duration and age of onset of regular use, dose and pattern of episodes of use), and environmental stress interacting with the individual's own degree of psychosis proneness to generate different degrees of severity of psychotic processes [82]. It is quite possible that the combination of drugs used, possibly with the exceptions of MA and hallucinogens that seem to be capable of producing chronic psychotic syndromes on their own, is a crucial factor in the nature of the emergent pathology.

A number of factors may contribute to the eventual development of a psychotic state. The fact that some evidence of abnormality may be evident up to 10 years prior to onset of frank symptoms makes the task of disentangling these factors extremely challenging [83]. Despite this chicken-and-egg problem, work by Hafner and colleagues [83] showed that a rather accurate determination of the onset of behavioral change can be determined. This allows the close examination of the chronological associations of drug use and the development of psychotic or even prodromal schizophrenia symptoms.

It is clear that much research is necessary in order to answer the many remaining unanswered questions. The most obvious need is for the development of cohorts of well-characterized patients that can be followed longitudinally from the time of first contact. Although obviously not an easy task, it is necessary to establish the natural course of these syndromes particularly in the absence of continued drug use. Many crucial factors must be characterized in these individuals, including an estimate of genetic risk (i.e. family history) and other risk factors (e.g. head injury, child abuse, ADD/ADHD). Once well-defined cohorts are established, other neuro-investigative (neuropsychological, electrophysiological, or imaging) as well as treatment studies can be more easily performed.

References

1. Lieberman J. A., Kinon B. J., Loebel A. D., Dopaminergic mechanisms in idiopathic and drug-induced psychoses. *Schizophr Bull*, 1990. **16**(1):97–110.

2. Yui K., Goto K., Ikemoto S., *et al.* Neurobiological basis of relapse prediction in stimulant-induced psychosis and schizophrenia: the role of sensitisation. *Mol, Psychiatry*, 1999 Nov. **4**(6): 512–23.

3. Ujike H. Stimulant-induced psychosis and schizophrenia: the role of sensitisation. *Curr Psychiatry Rep*, 2002. **4**(3): 177–84.

4. Tenn C. C., Fletcher P. J., Kapur S. A putative animal model of the "prodromal" state of schizophrenia. *Biol Psychiatry*, 2005. **57**(6):586–93.

5. Angrist B. M., Gershon S. The phenomenology of experimentally induced amphetamine psychosis– preliminary observations. *Biol Psychiatry*, 1970. **2**(2):95–107.

6. Snyder S. H. Amphetamine psychosis: a "model" schizophrenia mediated by catecholamines. *Am J Psychiatry*, 1973. **130**(1):61–7.

7. Harris D., Batki S. L. Stimulant psychosis: symptom profile and acute clinical course. *Am J Addict*, 2000. **9**(1):28–37.

8. Serper M. R., Chou J. C., Allen M. H., *et al.* Symptomatic overlap of cocaine intoxication and acute schizophrenia at emergency presentation. *Schizophr Bull*, 1999. **25**(2):387–94.

9. Shaner A., Roberts L. J., Eckman T. A., *et al.* Sources of diagnostic uncertainty for chronically psychotic cocaine abusers. *Psychiatr Serv*, 1998. **49**(5):684–90.

10. Sato M., Chen C. C., Akiyama K., Otsuki S. Acute exacerbation of paranoid psychotic state after long-term abstinence in patients with previous methamphetamine psychosis. *Biol Psychiatry*, 1983. **18**(4):429–40.

11. Iwanami A., Sugiyama A., Kuroki N., *et al.* Patients with methamphetamine psychosis admitted to a psychiatric hospital in Japan. A preliminary report. *Acta Psychiatr Scand*, 1994. **89**(6):428–32.

12. Barnes, T. R., Mutsatsa S. H., Hutton S. B., Watt H. C., Joyce E. M. Comorbid substance use and age at onset of schizophrenia. *Br J Psychiatry*, 2006. **188**: 237–42.

13. Brady K. T., Sonne S., Randall C. L., Adinoff B., Malcolm R. Features of cocaine dependence with concurrent alcohol abuse. *Drug Alcohol Depend*, 1995. **39**(1):69–71.

14. Balla A., Sershen H., Serra M., Koneru R., Javitt D. C. Subchronic continuous phencyclidine administration potentiates amphetamine-induced frontal cortex dopamine release. *Neuropsychopharmacology*, 2003. **28**(1):34–44.

15. Sato M. A. lasting vulnerability to psychosis in patients with previous methamphetamine psychosis. *Ann NY Acad Sci.*, 1992. **654**:160–70.

16. Nakatani Y., Hara T. Disturbance of consciousness due to methamphetamine abuse. A study of 2 patients. *Psychopathology*, 1998. **31**(3):131–7.

17. Tatetsu S. Methamphetamine psychosis. *Folia Psychiatr Neurol Jpn Suppl*, 1963. **7**:377–80.

18. Barr A. M., Panenka W. J., MacEwan G. W., *et al.* The need for speed: an update on methamphetamine addiction. *J Psychiatry Neurosci*, 2006. **31**(5):301–13.

19. Iyo M., Namba H., Yanagisawa M., *et al.* Abnormal cerebral perfusion in chronic methamphetamine abusers: a study using 99MTc-HMPAO and SPECT. *Prog Neuropsychopharmacol Biol Psychiatry*, 1997. **21**(5):789–96.

20. Farrell M., Boys A., Bebbington P., *et al.* Psychosis and drug dependence: results from a national survey of prisoners. *Br J Psychiatry*, 2002. **181**:393–8.

21. Floyd A. G., Boutros N. N., Struve F. A., Wolf E., Oliwa G. M. Risk factors for experiencing psychosis during cocaine use: a preliminary report. *J Psychiatr Res*, 2006. **40**(2):178–82. [Epub Jul 26, 2005.]

22. Cherland E., Fitzpatrick R. Psychotic side effects of psychostimulants: a 5-year review. *Can J Psychiatry*, 1999. **44**(8): 811–3.

23. Boutros N. N., Gelernter J., Gooding C. D., *et al.* Sensory gating and psychosis vulnerability in cocaine-dependent individuals: preliminary data. *Biol Psychiatry*, 2002. **51**(8):683–6.

24. Schuckit M. A. Comorbidity between substance use disorders and psychiatric conditions. *Addiction*, 2006. **101**(Suppl 1): 76–88.

25. Connell P. H. (1958). Amphetamine Psychosis. Maudsley Monographs No. 5. New York: Oxford University Press, pp. 15–36.

26. Bell D. S. Comparison of amphetamine psychosis and schizophrenia. *Br J Psychiatry*, 1965. **111**:701–7.

27. Ellinwood E. H., Jr. Amphetamine psychosis: I. Description of the individuals and process. *J Nervous Mental Disease*, 1967. **144**: 273–83.

28. Charles-Nicolas A. J. [Does chronic psychosis due to amphetamines abuse exist? Study of 25 drug addicts.] *Nouv Presse Med*, 1976. **5**(37):2447–50. French.

29. Yui K., Ikemoto S., Ishiguro T., Goto K. Studies of amphetamine or methamphetamine psychosis in Japan: relation of methamphetamine psychosis to schizophrenia.] *Ann NY Acad Sci*, 2000. **914**:1–12.

30. Goto, T. [Clinical pictures shown by long hospitalized cases of chronic methamphetamine psychosis: a comparative study with schizophrenia.] *Psychiatr Neurol Jpn*, 1960. **62**:163–76. Japanese.

31. Utena, H., Takano S., Yuasa S., Shimizu T., Kato T. Behavioral abnormalities in animals and metabolic changes in the brain. *No To Shinkei*, 1961. **13**: 687–95.

32. Utena H. Behavioral aberrations in methamphetamine-intoxicated animals and chemical correlates in the brain. *Prog Brain Res*, 1966. **21**:192–207.

33. Tomiyama C. Chronic schizophrenia-like states in methamphetamine psychosis. *Jpn J Psychiatr Neurol*, 1990. **44**(3):531–9.

34. Srisurapanont M., Ali R., Marsden J. *et al*. Psychotic symptoms in methamphetamine psychotic in-patients. *Int J Neuropsycho-pharmacol*, 2003. **6**(4):347–52.

35. Chen C. K., Lin S. K., Sham P. C., *et al*. Morbid risk for psychiatric disorder among the relatives of methamphetamine users with and without psychosis. *Am J Med Genet B Neuropsychiatr Genet*, 2005. **136**(1):87–91.

36. Askevold F. The occurrence of paranoid incidents and abstinence delirium in abusers of amphetamine. *Acta Psychiatr Scand*, 1959. **34**:145–64.

37. Wetli C. V., Fishbain D. A. Cocaine-induced psychosis and sudden death in recreational cocaine users. *J Forensic Sci*, 1985. **30**(3):873–80.

38. Curran C., Byrappa N., McBride A. Stimulant psychosis: systematic review. *Br J Psychiatry*, 2004. **185**:196–204.

39. Gawin F. H. Cocaine addiction: psychology and neurophysiology. *Science*, 1991. **251**(5001): 1580–6.

40. Segal D. S., Kuczenski R. Behavioral alterations induced by an escalating dose-binge pattern of cocaine administration. *Behav Brain Res*, 1997. **88**(2):251–60.

41. Flaum M., Schultz S.K. When does amphetamine-induced psychosis become schizophrenia? *Am J Psychiatry*, 1996. **153**(6): 812–5.

42. Post R. Cocaine psychoses: a continuum model. *Am J Psychiatry*, 1975. **132**(3): 225–31.

43. Satel S. L., Edell W. S. Cocaine-induced paranoia and psychosis proneness. *Am J Psychiatry*, 1991. **148**(12): 1708–11.

44. Thirthalli J., Benegal V. Psychosis among substance users. *Curr Opin Psychiatry*, 2006. **19**(3): 239–45.

45. Rounsaville B. J., Anton S. F., Carroll K., *et al*. Psychiatric diagnoses of treatment-seeking cocaine abusers. *Arch Gen Psychiatry*, 1991. **48**(1): 43–51.

46. McLellan A. T., Woody C. E., O'Brien C. P. Development of psychiatric illness in drug abusers: possible role of drug preference. *N Eng J Med*, 1979. **301**:1310–14.

47. Rosse R. B., Collins Jr, Fay-McCarthy M., *et al*. Phenomenologic comparison of the idiopathic psychosis of schizophrenia and drug-induced cocaine and phencyclidine psychoses: a retrospective study. *Clin Neuropharmacol*, 1994. **17**(4):359–69.

48. Rosenthal R. N., Miner C. R. Differential diagnosis of substance-induced psychosis and schizophrenia in patients with substance use disorders. *Schizophr Bull*, 1997. **23**(2):187–93.

49. Bartlett E., Hallin A., Chapman B., Angrist B. Selective sensitisation to the psychosis inducing effects of cocaine: a possible marker for addiction relapse vulnerability? *Neuropsychopharmacology*, 1997. **16**(1):77–82.

50. Reid M. S., Ciplet D., O'Leary S., Branchey M., Buydens-Branchey L. Sensitisation to the psychosis-inducing effects of cocaine compared with measures of cocaine craving and cue reactivity. *Am J Addict*, 2004. **13**(3): 305–15.

51. Unnithan S. B., Cutting J. C. The cocaine experience: refuting the concept of a model psychosis? *Psychopathology*, 1992. **25**(2): 71–8.

52. Pencer A., Addington J. Substance use and cognition in early psychosis. *J Psychiatr Neurosci*, 2003. **28**(1):48–54.

53. Iwanami A., Kuroki N., Iritani S., *et al*. P3a of event-related potential in chronic methamphetamine dependence. *J Nerv Ment Dis*, 1998. **186**(12): 746–51.

54. Iwanami A., Suga I., Kaneko T., Sugiyama A., Nakatani Y. P300 component of event-related potentials in methamphetamine psychosis and schizophrenia. *Prog Neuropsychopharmacol Biol Psychiatry*, 1994. **18**(3): 465–75.

55. Iwanami, S. A., Kanamori, R. Suga, I. Kaneko, T., Kamijima, K. Reduced attention-related negative potentials in methamphetamine psychosis. *J Nerv Ment Dis*, 1995. **183**(11): 693–7.

56. Fein G., Biggins C., MacKay S. Cocaine abusers have reduced auditory P50 amplitude and suppression compared to both normal controls and alcoholics. *Biol Psychiatry*, 1996. **39**(11): 955–65.

57. Adler L. E., Olincy A., Cawthra R. N., *et al.* Reversal of diminished inhibitory sensory gating in cocaine addicts by a nicotinic cholinergic mechanism. *Neuropsychopharmacology*, 2001. **24**(6):671–9.

58. Boutros N. N., Lisanby H. S., Tokuno H., *et al.* Elevated motor threshold in drug-free, cocaine-dependent patients assessed with transcranial magnetic stimulation. *Biol Psychiatry*, 2001. **49**(4): 369–73.

59. Boutros N. N., Lisanby S. H., McClain-Furmanski D., *et al.* Cortical excitability in cocaine-dependent patients: a replication and extension of TMS findings. *J Psychiatr Res*, 2005. **39**(3):295–302.

60. Bramon E., Rabe-Hesketh S., Sham P., Murray R. M., Frangou S. Meta-analysis of the P300 and P50 waveforms in schizophrenia. *Schizophr Res*, 2004. **70**(2–3): 315–29.

61. Sundaresan K., Ziemann U., Stanley J., Boutros N. N. Cortical inhibition and excitation in abstinent cocaine-dependent patients: a transcranial magnetic stimulation study. Neuro Report. (In Press.)

62. Wiesbeck G. A., Taeschner K. L. A cerebral computed tomography study of patients with drug-induced psychoses. *Eur Arch Psychiatry Clin Neurosci*, 1991. **241**(2):88–90.

63. Robinson T. E., Kolb B. Alterations in the morphology of dendrites and dendritic spines in the nucleus accumbens and prefrontal cortex following repeated treatment with amphetamine or cocaine. *Eur J Neurosci*, 1999. **11**(5):1598–604.

64. Wolf M. E. The role of excitatory amino acids in behavioral sensitisation to psychomotor stimulants. *Prog Neurobiol*, 1998. **54**(6):679–720.

65. White F. J., Kalivas P. W. Neuroadaptations involved in amphetamine and cocaine addiction. *Drug Alcohol Depend*, 1998. **51**(1–2):141–53.

66. Robinson T. E., Kolb B. Structural plasticity associated with exposure to drugs of abuse. *Neuropharmacology*, 2004. **47** Suppl 1:33–46.

67. Kalivas P. W., Hu X. T. Exciting inhibition in psychostimulant addiction. *Trends Neurosci*, 2006. **29**(11):610–6. [Epub Sept. 7, 2006.]

68. Strakowski S. M., Sax K. W., Setters M. J., Stanton S. P., Keck P. E. Jr. Lack of enhanced response to repeated d-amphetamine challenge in first-episode psychosis: implications for a sensitisation model of psychosis in humans. *Biol Psychiatry*, 1997. **42**(9):749–55.

69. Boileau I., Dagher A., Leyton M., *et al.* Modeling sensitisation to stimulants in humans: an [11C]raclopride/positron emission tomography study in healthy men. *Arch Gen Psychiatry*, 2006. **63**(12):1386–95.

70. Brady K. T., Lydiard R. B., Malcolm R., Cocaine-induced psychosis. *J Clin Psychiatry*, 1991. **52**(12):509–12.

71. Boileau I., Dagher A., Leyton M., *et al.* Modeling sensitisation to stimulants in humans: an [11C]raclopride/positron emission tomography study in healthy men. *Arch Gen Psychiatry*, 2006. **63**(12):1386–95.

72. Laruelle M. The role of endogenous sensitisation in the pathophysiology of schizophrenia: implications from recent brain imaging studies. *Brain Res Rev*, 2000. **31**(2–3):371–84.

73. Beraki S., Aronsson F., Karlsson H., Ogren S. O., Kristensson K. Influenza A virus infection causes alterations in expression of synaptic regulatory genes combined with changes in cognitive and emotional behaviors in mice. *Mol Psychiatry*, 2005. **10**(3):299–308.

74. McNeil T. F., Cantor-Graae E., Ismail B. Obstetric complications and congenital malformation in schizophrenia. *Brain Res Brain Res Rev*, 2000. 31(2–3):166–78.

75. Ellison G. Stimulant-induced psychosis, the dopamine theory of schizophrenia, and the habenula. *Brain Res Brain Res Rev*, 1994. **19**(2):223–39.

76. Beresford T. P., Clapp L. Martin B., *et al.* Aripiprazole in schizophrenia with cocaine dependence: a pilot study. *J Clin Psychopharmacol*, 2005. **25**(4):363–6.

77. Green A. I., Tohen M. F., Hamer R. M., *et al.* First episode schizophrenia-related psychosis and substance use disorders: acute response to olanzapine and haloperidol. *Schizophr Res*, 2004. **66**(2–3):125–35.

78. Brown E. S., Nejtek V. A., Perantie D.C., Rajan Thomas N., Rush A. J. Cocaine and amphetamine use in patients with psychiatric illness: a randomized trial of typical antipsychotic continuation or discontinuation. *J Clin Psychopharmacol*, 2003. **23**(4):384–8.

79. Broderick P.A., Rahni D. N., Zhou Y. Acute and subacute effects of risperidone and cocaine on accumbens dopamine and serotonin release using in vivo microvoltammetry on line with open-field behavior. *Prog Neuropsychopharmacol Biol Psychiatry*, 2003. 27(6): 1037–54.

80. Srisurapanont M., Kittiratanapaiboon P., Jarusuraisin N. Treatment for amphetamine psychosis. *Cochrane Database Syst Rev*, 2001. 4:CD003026.

81. van Os J., Hanssen M., Bijl R. V., Ravelli A. Strauss (1969) revisited: a psychosis continuum in the

139

general population? *Schizophr Res*, 2000. **45**(1–2): 11–20.

82. Jones P. B., Bebbington P., Foerster A., *et al.* Premorbid social underachievement in schizophrenia. Results from the Camberwell Collaborative Psychosis Study. *Br J Psychiatry* 1993. **162**:65–71.

83. Hafner H., Maurer K., Loffler W., Riecher-Rossler A. The influence of age and sex on the onset and early course of schizophrenia. *Br J Psychiatry*, 1993. **162**:80–6.

Organic syndromes of schizophrenia:
drugs and schizophrenia-like psychosis

10

Psychotomimetic effects of PCP, LSD, and Ecstasy: pharmacological models of schizophrenia?

Vibeke S. Catts and Stanley V. Catts

Facts box

- Phencyclidine (PCP), ketamine, D-lysergic acid diethylamide (LSD) and 3,4-methylenedioxy-methamphetamine (MDMA) have been variously referred to as schizophrenomimetics, psychotogens, or psychotomimetics.

- There have been many reports that these drugs can induce psychotic symptoms (hallucinations, delusions, formal thought disorder, or catatonia-like abnormalities) in the absence of delirium.

- There is abundant evidence that PCP induces psychotic disorder beyond the acute symptoms of intoxication.

- There is no clear evidence that either LSD or MDMA induces psychotic disorder, let alone schizophrenia, in individuals who did not have vulnerability to schizophrenia premorbidly.

- PCP and ketamine are noncompetitive antagonists of the *N*-methyl-D-aspartate (NMDA) glutamatergic receptor that bind at the intrachannel site of the receptor to prevent calcium ion flux into the cell.

- LSD is a serotonin-like hallucinogenic indoleamine that acts as an agonist at the serotonin-subtype-2A (5HT2A) receptor, and MDMA is an indirect serotonin agonist.

- Rodent and primate models induced by PCP and analogues have been presented as models of human schizophrenia, with construct validity, showing homologous behavior, cognitive deficits, alterations in regional brain activation, and underlying neuronal dysfunction, to PCP-induced psychotomimetic effects in healthy volunteers and patients with schizophrenia.

- Ketamine is considered to be a safe and valid model of PCP psychosis and applicable to preclinical human studies.

- More translational science is needed to relate animal findings to humans and vice versa.

In this chapter, the potential role of glutamatergic and serotonergic neurotransmitter systems in the pathophysiology of schizophrenia is examined from the perspective of the psychotomimetic effects of i) phencyclidine (PCP) and ketamine, noncompetitive antagonists of the *N*-methyl-D-aspartate (NMDA) glutamatergic receptor that bind at the intrachannel site of the receptor to prevent calcium ion flux into the cell; ii) D-lysergic acid diethylamide (LSD), a serotonin-like hallucinogenic indoleamine that acts as an agonist at the serotonin-subtype-2A (5HT2A) receptor; and iii) 3,4-methylenedioxy-methamphetamine (MDMA), an indirect serotonin agonist. These drugs, variously called hallucinogens, schizophrenomimetics, psychotogens, or psychotomimetics, have shown in common reports that they can induce psychotic symptoms (hallucinations, delusions, formal thought disorder, or catatonia-like abnormalities) in the absence of delirium. The primary question addressed herein, whether PCP-induced psychosis is a valid model of schizophrenia, gives rise to additional questions about the validity of ketamine challenge at subanesthetic doses in humans as a model of PCP psychosis, and in turn, questions about the validity of drug-induced changes in nonhuman animals (rodents, monkeys) treated with PCP and its analogues (ketamine or dizocilpine [MK-801]) as models of PCP-induced psychosis.

Human studies

For each drug of interest, this chapter reviews the evidence for psychotomimetic effects in humans, in terms of induced transient symptoms with acute dosing, and the epidemiological association between formal psychotic disorder and chronic abuse. The phenomenological similarity of drug-induced symptoms and the clinical features of schizophrenia are closely examined. Wherever available, human neuroimaging and clinical biomarker studies are considered for comparison of drug-induced effects and deficits seen in schizophrenia. Ketamine is included in the review because most experimental evidence supporting the validity of the PCP model arose from studies using ketamine in humans. The literature on LSD and MDMA is briefly reviewed for comparative purposes.

Phencyclidine

Phencyclidine [1-(1-phenylcyclohexyl)piperidine hydrochloride] was synthesized in 1956 [1]. Preclinical testing indicated that PCP might be a safe intravenous (IV) anesthetic because it induced analgesia and anesthesia without circulatory or respiratory depression [1]. The term "dissociative anaesthetic" was coined because PCP induced a state of detachment and dissociation from painful and environmental stimuli, without causing unconsciousness. During anesthesia the patient remained immobile with fixed sightless staring, absent facial expression, and open mouth [2]. PCP is a highly lipid soluble and readily crosses the blood-brain barrier, inducing CNS effects within minutes of IV injection. The serum half-life of PCP was reported to vary between 4 to 72 hours [3].

Early clinical use revealed that many patients experienced psychotic symptoms as they emerged from PCP anesthesia [2, 4, 5, 6]. Emergence phenomena included agitation, bizarre behavior, paranoia, formal thought disorder, hallucinations, and delusions, typically lasting for 12–72 hours but occasionally persisting for up to 10 days [4, 6]. Symptoms were schizophrenia-like, especially the motor changes [5]. Flat facies, fixed staring, manneristic grimacing, generalized rigidity, and plastic stiffness very similar to "cerea flexibilitas" occurred. Stereotypic verbalizations of select phrases were uttered. PCP-induced agitation was associated with atypical movements: head rolling or shaking the head from side to side was common. Attempts to prevent emergence reactions by pretreatment with haloperidol or diazepam were relatively

unsuccessful: diazepam [7] appeared to be as effective as haloperidol [8]. Phencyclidine was withdrawn from the market for human use in 1965. A veterinarian formulation was introduced in 1967 but because of a growing abuse problem, all legal manufacture of the drug was ceased in 1979.

Despite its propensity to cause adverse reactions, PCP abuse became widespread. It was relatively inexpensive to manufacture and the starting materials, used in many industrial processes, were readily available [9]. Illicit PCP use first appeared in 1965 on the West Coast of the United States [10]. Initially the drug was ingested orally (called the "PeaCe Pill"). Slow oral absorption resulted in inadvertent high dosing and frequent adverse reactions, limiting its appeal [9]. Once street users discovered that the dose could be lowered and self-titrated by smoking PCP added to cigarettes, illicit use escalated. National surveys in the United States indicate that peak use of PCP occurred between 1977 and 1979 [11, 12]. Between 1976 and 1977 the National Institute of Drug Abuse (NIDA) reported a doubling (from 3%–5.8%) of the number of 12- to 17-year-old users of PCP, and a 50% increase (from 9.5%–13.9%) in 18- to 25-year-old users [9]. A survey of 319 adult users reported negative events on 100% of use occasions [13], including speech difficulties (80%), perceptual disturbances (75%), restlessness (76%), disorientation (63%), anxiety (61%), paranoia (34%), hyperxcitability (27%), irritability (22%) and mental confusion (22%). The extent to which PCP posed serious problems at that time was indicated by the US. Drug Abuse Warning Network (DAWN), a national reporting system for drug-related deaths and hospital emergencies. Data from the 662 participating emergency centers showed 111 events in October 1976 versus 54 events in October 1974; and reports of PCP-related deaths increased over roughly the same period from 17 in April 1976 to 30 in March 1977 [9]. Undesirable psychological reactions were frequent.

Although a strong relationship between PCP abuse and psychotic disorder was evident, the face validity of PCP-induced psychosis as a model for schizophrenia also requires close phenomenological similarity between the two disorders. To make this comparison, three types of PCP-related conditions need to be distinguished: acute intoxication without delirium (a "'bad trip"), acute intoxication with delirium; and the more persistent drug-induced psychotic disorder [14]. Duration of acute PCP intoxication parallels the half-life of the drug. Symptom severity is dose dependent. Acute intoxication without delirium lasts about 3–8 hours and presents with restlessness, agitation, hallucinations, delusions, nystagmus, hypertension, tachycardia, ataxia, slurred speech, and hyperreflexia [14, 15, 16]. PCP-induced delirium represents a more profound degree of toxicity, which can persist for a week. Dose-dependent clinical features include clouding of consciousness, disorientation, toxic psychosis, vomiting, hypersalivation, spasticity, EEG slowing or seizures, and respiratory depression [14, 15, 17, 18, 19].

In addition to acute intoxication syndromes, PCP induces psychotic disorder that is very similar to schizophrenia or schizoaffective disorder in the absence of delirium [9, 14, 20, 21, 22, 23, 24, 25, 26, 27, 28, 29]. The duration of PCP-related psychosis bears no relationship to ingested dose or drug half-life. It characteristically shows sudden resolution within 2 to 4 weeks [22, 29], although on occasion persists for months. Patients with PCP-related psychosis could not be distinguished from schizophrenia patients on the basis of presenting symptoms [17, 23]. All domains of schizophrenic symptomatology seemed to be represented. Prominent positive symptoms were reported: paranoia; and persecutory and grandiose delusions [23, 25, 26, 27, 30], often with bizarre Schneiderian qualities [17, 28, 31]; and hallucinations in all modalities [17, 19, 23, 25, 26, 27, 30, 32]. Formal thought disorder with loosening of associations, cognitive disorganization, perseveration, or thought blocking occurred [14, 17, 20, 25, 26, 27, 30]. Catatonic behavior in a variety of forms was almost universally present with PCP psychosis: inappropriate and unpredictable behavior; excitement and violence; nudism; mannerisms and stereotypies; and catatonic posturing and mutism [10, 14, 17, 18, 19, 23, 25, 26, 27, 29, 30, 32]. Features resembling negative symptoms also occurred: blunted affect [19]; apathy and emotional disengagement [14]; social withdrawal and autistic behavior [20, 23, 27]; and amotivation [14, 20, 23, 27].

Despite marked similarities between PCP psychosis and schizophrenia, cross-sectionally, there were atypical features: a predominance of visual or haptic hallucinations over auditory hallucinations; distortion of time appreciation and body image disturbance; and prominent somatosensory deficits, especially diminished proprioception and pain perception [6, 31]. In addition, there were differences in psychiatric history with a relatively high proportion of patients not having a family history or personal history of schizophrenia and an absence of previous psychiatric history or evidence of prodromal psychosocial deterioration [9, 14, 21, 22]. Although most cases of PCP-psychosis resolved within 2 weeks without sequel [22], about 25% of patients went on to have a typical history of schizophrenia [27]. This subgroup of patients took months rather than weeks to recover from the first PCP-related psychotic episode, tended to have a family history of schizophrenia and a personal history of other psychiatric disorder [22, 23, 30].

A point of disagreement in the clinical literature concerns the effectiveness of dopamine D2 receptor (D2R) antagonist antipsychotics in the treatment of acute PCP psychosis. Some studies concluded benzodiazepines were preferable to haloperidol or chlorpromazine in PCP intoxication whereas others favored haloperidol [32, 33, 34, 35]. Apart from one group [33, 35], most agreed that antipsychotic and sedatives may reduce agitation; however, no pharmacological treatments appeared to shorten the course of the psychotic illness [10, 25]. Luisada and Brown [27] noted that in the cases subsequently rediagnosed with schizophrenia, acute response to antipsychotic drugs was faster and superior after rediagnosis than during the first PCP-induced episode of psychosis. The equivocal response of PCP psychosis to D2R antagonists was the first clue that PCP psychosis may not be primarily linked to dopamine dysregulation.

Experimental studies using PCP in hospitalized patients with chronic schizophrenia supported the view that the psychotomimetic effect of PCP was directly related to mechanisms producing the symptoms of schizophrenia [36, 38]. Luby and colleagues [36] reported that immediately after IV PCP, patients showed an acute intensification of thought disorder and inappropriate affect: "it was as though … the acute phase of their illness had been reinstated." Chronic patients frequently manifested symptom relapses persisting for more than a month after a single IV dose of PCP, indicating that PCP may act on a fundamental disease process. That is, PCP exaggerated pre-existing, or precipitated an acute relapse of previously experienced, phenomenology rather than added qualitatively different psychotic symptoms. Response to PCP in patients was distinctly different to that with LSD or mescaline that produced a milder and brief change in the level of symptoms, mainly by adding qualitatively different symptoms such as kaleidoscopic visual hallucinations [36, 37, 39, 40]. Providing the first

143

suggestion that prefrontal mechanisms were directly related to PCP effects, Itil and colleagues [38] found that leucotomized patients with schizophrenia did not show as marked a response to PCP compared to unleucotomized patients.

Experimental studies using PCP in human volunteers (healthy volunteers) also supported the view that PCP comprehensively induced symptoms resembling schizophrenia [36, 41, 42, 43, 44]. Luby and colleagues [36] gave 9 healthy volunteers PCP in a subanesthetic dose (0.1 mg/kg IV). All subjects experienced "body image changes" (impaired ability to distinguish between self and nonself stimuli, feelings of depersonalization, and a sense of unreality), "estrangement" (profound sense of aloneness or isolation, of being detached from the environment), and "disorganization of thought" (inability to maintain a set, frequent loss of goal ideas, impairment of abstract attitude, blocking, neologisms, jumbled wording and echolalia). Most subjects experienced negativism, and hostility (child-like oppositional behavior and catatonia-like reactions); about one third showed repetitive motor behaviors (rhythmic body movements, including rocking, head-rolling, and grimacing). In another study of 12 healthy volunteers, PCP (0.075–0.1 mg/kg IV) induced positive symptoms (auditory hallucinations and thought disorder), negative symptoms (blunting, apathy, and amotivation), catatonic features (psychomotor retardation, negativism, and catatonic immobility), and cognitive deficits (associative learning and abstract reasoning deficits) [42]. In contrast to LSD or mescaline, PCP in healthy volunteers induced perseveration and concreteness and nystagmus: in common with LSD and mescaline, PCP induced body image disturbance, depersonalization, and disturbances in time appreciation [42]. One study of 7 healthy volunteers given 12 mg PCP by slow IV injection provided detailed descriptions of phenomenology [44].

After a brief period of disorientation cleared, PCP caused marked cognitive deficits affecting "the function that combines, unifies, and integrates all available information into a field that is meaningful" and preventing "goal-directed behavior." Formal thought disorder (both loosening *and* concreteness) was apparent, including "catatonic-like perseveration." Sensory filtering deficits occurred so that the subject "was unable to focus actively on particular areas of his perceptual field [and] had become a victim of all inflowing stimuli but could not screen out the irrelevancies." Also, sensory distortions were experienced, like hearing your voice "seem to come from a distance – as if someone else were speaking," and yet intellectually knowing that it was yourself speaking. Feelings of passivity emerged so that "the subject saw his arms and legs move and yet did not have the feeling that he himself was making these movements." A profound sense of apathy and amotivation accompanied the PCP-induced psychotomimetic effects. Bakker and Amini [44] hypothesized that PCP produced a converse psychic state to that induced by LSD and psilocybin; PCP appeared to be a "negative" state with "decreased" functions whereas LSD and psilocybin appeared to be "stimulating" of activity.

Moreover, early neurocognitive studies in healthy volunteers demonstrated PCP-induced deficits resembling those seen in schizophrenia. Rosenbaum and colleagues [41] compared three groups of healthy volunteers, 10 receiving PCP (0.1 mg/kg IV), 10 receiving LSD orally (1 µg/kg), and 5 receiving 500 mg amobarbital sodium IV (amphetamine 15 mg added to counter drowsiness associated with the barbiturate). Using a crude measure of attention, only PCP (i.e., not LSD or barbiturate) produced a deficit equivalent to that observed on the same test in patients with schizophrenia. On a motor learning task, the performance of only the PCP-treated healthy volunteers dropped to the level of patients with schizophrenia. Cohen and colleagues [43] compared the effects of PCP, LSD, and amobarbital sodium (amphetamine 15 mg added) in three groups of healthy volunteers. In a test of symbolic thinking (proverb interpretation), only PCP subjects (i.e., not LSD or barbiturate) showed deficits in symbolic thinking quantitatively equivalent to those seen in groups of patients with schizophrenia. Similar findings were made in relation to a test of sustained attention (serial sevens).

In summary, the psychotomimetic effects of PCP were first recognized as emergence phenomena when it was used as an anesthetic. During a PCP abuse epidemic in the United States, it became evident that PCP induced formal psychotic disorder, even in individuals without evidence of predisposition to schizophrenia. The phenomenology of the psychotomimetic effects of PCP was schizophrenia-like in range and quality, whether observed as anesthetic emergence phenomena, presenting symptoms of PCP-induced psychotic disorder, or behavioral change induced by experimental use of PCP in patients with schizophrenia or healthy volunteers. Clinicians who observed PCP-induced symptoms recognized signs that Bleuler ("loosening" *plus* "concreteness") and Kraepelin ("weakening…volition" *plus* "loss of inner unity of the activities of intellect, emotion and volition") deemed primary to – and processes (e.g., sensorimotor gating [45]) that psychologists considered characteristic of – schizophrenia. Because PCP was made illegal for use in human research in 1965, no studies measuring the effect of PCP on putative biomarkers of schizophrenia (e.g. prepulse inhibition [PPI], smooth pursuit eye movement [SPEM], P50 suppression or mismatch negativity [MMN]) or functional neuroimaging measures were carried out in patients with schizophrenia or healthy volunteers. This type of human research had to await the introduction of ketamine, a safer and less potent psychotomimetic analogue of PCP.

Ketamine

Analogues of PCP were researched as alternative dissociative anesthetic agents that might have fewer adverse reactions than PCP, the most important being ketamine [2-(2-chlorophenyl)-2-(methylamino)-cyclohexanone]. Ketamine was first synthesized in 1961, first tested in human volunteers in 1964 [46], and first approved for general clinical use in 1970. It is used intravenously (analgesic dose, 1–2 mg/kg; anesthetic dose, 5–10 mg/kg), intramuscularly (analgesic dose, 1.5–2 mg/kg; anesthetic dose, 4.0–6.0 mg/kg), and less frequently as an oral (100–300 mg/kg) anesthetic [47, 48]. Ketamine is a highly lipid soluble and readily crosses the blood-brain barrier, inducing CNS effects within seconds of IV injection. The plasma half-life of ketamine has been reported to be 1–2 hours [49]. When ketamine is used intravenously, duration of anesthesia is dose dependent and may be as brief as 30 minutes [50, 51] with complete recovery taking several hours. Because ketamine does not depress respiratory or cardiovascular systems, it was widely used as a field anesthetic by the U.S. army during the Vietnam War and continues to be marketed as a valuable anesthetic for human procedures, especially in children and in veterinarian practice.

Although ketamine anesthesia can produce emergence phenomena in up to 30% of anesthetized adults, the symptoms are not as severe as those produced by PCP [52]. Emergence symptoms include alterations in mood state and body image, dissociative and out-of-body experiences, floating sensations, vivid dreams or illusions, "weird trips," and occasionally delirium [48]. Between 10%–15% of postperative patients show hallucinatory reactions [53, 54]. Ketamine emergence phenomena are dose dependent and age related, with an incidence of less than 10% in patients less than 16 years old [48]. Compared to standard anesthesia (halothane/nitrous oxide), ketamine does not cause an excess of emergence reactions in children [55]. In adults, pretreatment with droperidol or haloperidol is inferior to benzodiazepines in preventing vivid emergence reactions and delirium following ketamine (reviewed in [48]). In summary, when used as an anesthetic ketamine induces emergent psychotomimetic effects qualitatively similar to PCP but quantitatively substantially less intense, in line with its more than 10-fold lower PCP-like activity [56] and about 30-fold lower NMDA receptor complex binding affinity [57, 58].

Despite warnings about its abuse potential [59], ketamine eventually appeared on the streets (known as "'Special K, "Vitamin K," or "K") in the early 1970s [13, 60] in the same way that PCP did in the 1960s. In 1978 ketamine was authoritatively described as the "ultimate psychedelic" [61]. Ketamine is typically inhaled or injected intramuscularly. Ketamine users try to achieve or "fall into" a "k-hole" of social detachment lasting up to an hour. This experience includes a distorted sense of space, so that a small room appears the size of a football field, and an indistinct awareness of time, so that a few minutes seems like an hour [62]. Physical immobilization and disengagement from time and space are associated with psychedelic experiences such as spiritual journeys, interaction with famous or fictitious people, and hallucinatory visions. The k-hole ends abruptly but can quickly be re-entered with another injection of ketamine.

Because there have been no regionally or temporally circumscribed epidemics of illicit ketamine use, it has been difficult to establish the psychiatric consequences of its abuse. The main evidence for a link between ketamine abuse and psychotic disorder is based on the occasional psychiatric case series report [63, 64]; survey data of ketamine users who reported auditory hallucinations, paranoia, loose associations, and unusual thought content among the behavioral effects of ketamine [65]; and psychometric data on small groups of ketamine users [66, 67, 68, 69]. Chronic ketamine abusers had higher scores on tests of delusional ideation and schizotypal symptomatology, which increased with acute dosing of ketamine [66, 67, 68, 69], but also remained elevated at short-term follow-up [67, 68]. The very limited literature on the neurocognitive effects of ketamine abuse suggests acute induction of impairments of working, episodic, and semantic memory [68], and with chronic ketamine use, induction of chronic impairments in episodic memory [69]. In summary, there is evidence of an association between ketamine abuse and increased proneness to quasipsychotic symptoms and neurocognitive deficits, and psychotic disorder resembling schizophrenia; however, the research supporting these associations is underdeveloped and does not define the strength of these associations.

In contrast to patient studies using PCP, experimental use of ketamine in hospitalized patients with chronic schizophrenia is considered ethically acceptable [70]. This is partly based on experience using ketamine as an anesthetic for surgery in patients with schizophrenia stabilized on antipsychotic medication, which was associated with only brief mild postperative disturbance and not major psychotic relapse [71]. Lahti and colleagues [72] gave subanesthetic doses of ketamine (0.1, 0.3, and 0.5 mg/kg IV) to 9 hospitalized patients with schizophrenia stabilized on haloperidol (0.3 mg/kg/day for at least 12 weeks). Six of the 9 patients were withdrawn from haloperidol for more than 4 weeks before being rechallenged with ketamine. In patients on haloperidol, ketamine induced 20 minutes postinjection about a 3-fold increase (dose-related) in Brief Psychiatric Rating Scale (BPRS) psychosis scores, which returned to baseline within 90 minutes, although 4 out of the 9 patients reported delayed recurrence of psychotic symptoms for 24 hours after ketamine. In patients off haloperidol, ketamine induced dose-dependent increases in BPRS psychosis scores. Although ketamine-induced BPRS psychosis scores were slightly higher in patients off haloperidol compared with the same patients on haloperidol, it was clear that haloperidol provided little protection against the psychotomimetic effects of ketamine. Qualitatively, there was remarkable similarity between the themes and content of psychotic symptoms induced by ketamine and symptoms associated with the patients' schizophrenic illness [72]. In a replication study, Malhotra *et al.* (73) gave ketamine (0.77 mg/kg IV over one hour) to 13 hospitalized patients with schizophrenia and neuroleptic free for at least 2 weeks, and 16 healthy volunteers. In both unmedicated patients and healthy volunteers, ketamine produced significant increases in total BPRS scores, reflecting increased thought disorder and increased negative symptoms (withdrawal-retardation). Neurocognitive testing showed unmedicated patients and healthy volunteers both had significant ketamine-induced impairments in verbal recall and recognition memory, patients performing worse than healthy volunteers. When rechallenged with ketamine, patients subsequently stabilized on clozapine showed significantly blunted ketamine-induced increases in BPRS psychosis ratings [74]. In summary, unlike PCP the reaction to ketamine was mild and very brief in medicated patients, and more pronounced although still brief in unmedicated patients.

Experimental studies of the effects of ketamine in healthy volunteers confirm that ketamine-induced neurocognitive deficits show striking resemblance to those seen in schizophrenia [75]. Deficits in episodic memory are induced by ketamine consistently in healthy volunteers [76, 77, 78, 79], a result not seen with acute amphetamine challenge [80]. A substantial literature indicates selective deficits at the level of encoding (or recognition memory) rather than at the level of retrieval [77, 78, 79, 81, 82, 83, 84], a selective effect consistent with differential system dysfunction [85]. Ketamine also induces deficits in working memory in healthy volunteers [79, 80, 83, 86, 87], with greater impact on manipulation compared with maintenance of information in working memory [75], a distinction reviewed elsewhere [85]. Deficits in working memory are not observed in acute amphetamine challenge [80]. Ketamine induces deficits in other prefrontal functions including: abstraction deficits in relation to proverb interpretation [88, 89], perseverative errors in sorting tasks [77, 88, 89], impaired response inhibition [90], and impaired vigilance [80, 89] – the latter not seen with acute amphetamine challenge [80]. Most studies, although not all [79, 80], show that ketamine induces deficits in selective attention [77, 78, 88]. Although only some studies report verbal fluency deficits [77, 81, 86, 89] and others do not [79, 88], verbal fluency deficits have been found in chronic ketamine recreational users [67, 68]. Psychomotor speed is also slowed by ketamine [83, 91]. In summary, the pattern of neurocognitive deficits induced by ketamine resembles that seen in schizophrenia, and implicate dysfunction in the same systems affected by schizophrenia, namely, the prefrontal cortex and medial temporal lobe.

More proximal evidence that ketamine induces dysfunction in brain systems affected by schizophrenia has been provided by regional activation studies in healthy volunteers. Ketamine-induced regional brain activation changes have been directly assessed using functional Magnetic Resonance Imaging (fMRI) to measure the blood oxygen level-dependent (BOLD) effect, an index of regional cerebral blood flow (rCBF) change, and Positron Emission Tomography (PET) to measure changes in regional metabolic rate, either in terms of oxygen ($[^{15}O]$water) or glucose ($[^{18}F]$flurodeoxyglucose: FDG) uptake. As functional imaging studies of schizophrenia have more often than not found *reduced* activation prefrontally [92, 93, 94], in the cingulate cortex [95], and medial temporal lobe [93, 96], it was predicted that ketamine would induce *decreases* in regional brain activation in the same areas in healthy volunteers. However, contrary to hypothesis, acute ketamine dosing *increased* activation prefrontally [97, 98, 99, 100, 101, 102, 103], and in the cingulate cortex [97, 98, 103] and thalamus [97, 102, 103, 104]. No studies reported changes in the hippocampus or medial temporal lobe. Two functional imaging studies of the effects of ketamine in patients with schizophrenia have been reported: one found ketamine-induced blood flow increases in frontal and cingulate regions [98]; the other found ketamine-induced increases in rCBF in anterior cingulate and reduced rCBF in hippocampus [72].

Clinical biomarkers known to be abnormal in schizophrenia have also been assessed in experimental studies of ketamine in healthy volunteers. Contrary to expectation, deficits in prepulse inhibition (PPI) analogous to those seen in schizophrenia have not been observed [105, 106]. Indeed, three independent studies showed PPI augmentation after ketamine administration to healthy volunteers [107, 108, 109]. A single study of schizophrenia-like oculomotor abnormalities in healthy volunteers administered ketamine showed ketamine-induced smooth pursuit eye-tracking deficits. Ketamine does not significantly reduce P50 suppression [105, 106]. Deficits in MMN analogous to those observed in schizophrenia have been reported in healthy volunteers administered ketamine [110, 111].

To conclude, ketamine produces less potent PCP-like psychotomimetic effects commensurate with its more than 30-fold lower NMDA receptor complex binding activity [57] compared with PCP. Qualitatively, however, the two analogues induce equivalent psychotomimetic phenomena at the level of symptoms, neurocognition, and regional brain activation. It can be concluded therefore, that ketamine challenge studies in healthy volunteers have face and construct validity as preclinical models of PCP psychosis, and in turn as models of schizophrenia. Additional support for PCP-related models may be offered, comparing them with serotonergic models to examine evidence for discriminant validity. This will be sought by reviewing the psychotomimetic effects of the 5HT2A agonist, LSD, and the indirect serotonergic agonist, MDMA.

Lysergic acid diethylamide (LSD)

LSD (D-lysergic acid diethyamide) was originally synthesized in 1938 but its psychotomimetic effects were not discovered until 1943 when one of its codiscoverers experienced "fantastic visions of extraordinary vividness accompanied by a kaleidoscopic play of intense coloration" following inadvertent ingestion [112]. LSD acts primarily as a functional agonist at the 5HT2A receptor [113]. LSD quickly distributes to the brain and other body compartments and is metabolized in the liver and kidneys. Effects of LSD are felt within an hour after ingestion and can last from 6 to 12 hours. LSD is one of the most potent psychotomimetic drugs known. Oral psychotomimetic dosages are in the 25–150 μg range. Sensory perceptions are altered and intensified so that colors appear brighter and sounds become magnified or perceived as patterns; there is a merging of senses (synesthesia) so that sounds become whirling patterns of vivid color; perceptions of time and space are distorted, so that seconds may seems like an eternity, and objects become fluid and shifting. Depersonalization; experience of feeling merged with another object or another person; hallucinations and visions; and religious revelations and spiritual insights have been reported [114, 115, 116]. That is, LSD intensifies emotional experience as much as perceptual experience [117]. Physical effects are few and the lethal dose of LSD is so high that it has not been estimated. Psychological dependence is very uncommon [118]. Physical dependence does not develop with LSD [119] but if used daily, tolerance to the psychotomimetic effects of LSD develops rapidly but disappears after a few days of abstinence [114, 115].

No epidemiological study has determined the relationship between LSD use and the incidence of psychotic disorder. Initially, LSD was considered to have therapeutic value and reviews of its use with psychiatric supervision concluded that prolonged psychosis following LSD was rare [120, 121]. LSD therapy was initially applied to patients with an established history of schizophrenia with only a small risk of causing relapse [122, 123]. However, following broader illicit use of LSD in the late 1960s, a number of case series reports of psychosis in patients using LSD were published (see [124, 125] for reviews). Patients with psychotic disorder who had used LSD were said to present with phenomenologically similar symptoms and outcome to those with schizophrenia who did not take LSD [126, 127, 128, 129, 130, 131]. However, in contrast to many patients with PCP-induced psychosis, most individuals presenting with psychosis in the setting of LSD abuse showed poor premorbid adjustment, associated with prior psychiatric admissions [126, 127, 128, 129, 130, 131] or family history of psychotic or other serious psychiatric illness [130, 132]. Contemporary clinicians could not determine whether psychosis in the setting of LSD abuse was a separate diagnostic entity or simply represented a subgroup of patients with schizophrenia who used LSD. An important area of agreement in the clinical literature was the view that the symptoms of acute LSD intoxication were phenomenologically different to the symptoms of schizophrenia [133, 134, 135, 136]. LSD-induced perceptual disorders are visual rather than auditory; the visual distortions are not frank hallucinations but have the character of illusions; delusional ideation is not stable and usually insight is retained; negative symptoms are at most mild; and LSD-induced phenomenology is often distinguishable by patients with schizophrenia from their primary symptoms ([133, 134, 135, 136]. In marked contrast to both schizophrenia and PCP psychosis, the hallucinogenic effects of acute LSD intoxication subside rapidly with benzodiazepines [16] unless delirium is evident. Other dissimilarities with schizophrenia were reported in LSD-related (N,N-dimethyltryptamine [DMT] or psilocybin) challenge studies in healthy volunteers measuring PPI [107, 137] or MMN [138, 139] that did not find deficits, although deficits in attention [140] and P50 suppression [137] with DMT were reported.

In conclusion, although LSD has obvious hallucinogenic effects, it is debatable whether it should be considered psychotogenic. Despite periods of relatively high and low rates of use of LSD in communities, no formal or informal epidemiological data have linked fluctuations in community use to variations in the incidence of psychotic disorder. In fact, only a total of 75 individual case reports of putative LSD psychosis were found in a recent worldwide review [127]. The occurrence of psychosis in the setting of LSD abuse appears to be more related to individual vulnerabilities than specific drug actions. This does not mean that adverse events with LSD do not occur [125]. Acute LSD intoxication is associated with panic attacks and harm from misadventure, and a long-term consequence, Hallucinogen Persisting Perception Disorder (HPPD) or "flashbacks," has diagnostic validity [141]. Nonetheless, models based on LSD-related drugs are not irrelevant to the study of schizophrenia, especially to investigate disturbances in serotonergic regulation [142, 143], because of the 5HT2A receptor antagonist actions of atypical antipsychotics [136, 144, 145], and the potential relevance of interactions between glutamatergic and serotonergic systems in the pathogenesis of schizophrenia [113, 140, 146, 147, 148, 149]. For the purposes of this review, however, at this stage we conclude our formal consideration of LSD-induced psychotomimetic effects as a model of schizophrenia.

Ecstasy

MDMA (3,4-methylenedioxy-methamphetamine) is a ring-substituted amphetamine derivative. It was patented in 1914 but never made commercially available. MDMA was classified a restricted drug in the United Kingdom in 1977 and in the United States in 1985. MDMA is almost always consumed orally, the psychoactive dose being about 100 mg. The primary effect of MDMA is to produce a positive mood state with feelings of euphoria, intimacy, and closeness to other people, an effect that distinguishes it from amphetamine or hallucinogens [150]. MDMA also has stimulant effects as well as mild psychedelic effects on insight and perceptual and sensual enhancement. The peak psychoactive effects last on average 4–6 hours, although the half-life of MDMA is approximately 9 hours in humans [151]. Tolerance to the psychoactive effects develops rapidly [153]. No physical withdrawal syndrome has been described [153], but psychological dependence is common [118]. Illicit Ecstasy tablets often contain compounds related to MDMA, such as MDE (3,4-methylenedioxy-methamphetamine). The generic term "Ecstasy" is now preferred because it may refer to MDMA, analogues of MDMA, or combination of these [154]. Ecstasy use by young people has worldwide popularity ([155, 156]. In the United Kingdom during the mid-1980s, all-night dance parties called "raves" became popular. The drug of choice for people attending raves was Ecstasy and the popularity of this youth culture resulted in an explosion in recreational use. Among US college students there was a steady increase in Ecstasy use from 2.0% in 1991 to 13.1% in 2000 [157]. Similarly, in the Australian general population, there is a steady increase in the proportion of people who have ever tried Ecstasy from 4.8% in 1998, 6.1% in 2001, to 7.5% in 2004 [158, 159]. Amongst dance or rave party attendees, the use of Ecstasy is far more common (up to 80% prevalence) than the use of ketamine and PCP [160, 161, 162]; however, polysubstance abuse (especially methamphetamine, cannabis, and hallucinogens) among Ecstasy users is the norm [62].

Public alarm concerning the dangers of Ecstasy use initially arose from reports of sudden death in young healthy users, especially when ingestion occurred at dance parties that were typically hot, crowded, venues with loud repetitive music and light shows [163, 164]. Cause of death was either cardiac arrhythmia or malignant hyperthermia, and usually related to polysubstance ingestion [165]. However, a direct link between the fatalities and Ecstasy use is supported by a strong correlation between rates of Ecstasy use and rates of fatalities [166]. Milder effects of intoxication include nausea, loss of appetite, tachycardia, hypertension, jaw tension, bruxism, and sweating [167]. Chronic adverse events associated with Ecstasy use include extensive polydrug use, high rates of intravenous drug use, and financial, relationship, and occupational problems [168].

Although there are many studies reporting an association between Ecstasy use and mental disorder, especially depression and anxiety, it is impossible to determine in cross-sectional studies whether this relationship is due to Ecstasy, associated polysubstance abuse [155], or whether it pre- or postdates Ecstasy use. In prospective [169] or retrospective [170] comparisons of the age-of-onset of mental disorder and age-of-onset of Ecstasy use, psychiatric disorder appeared to precede Ecstasy consumption. A meta-analysis showed that the strength of the association between Ecstasy use and depressive symptomatology was weak and unlikely to be clinically relevant [171].

Psychotic disorder as an adverse reaction to Ecstasy use appears to be rare and idiosyncratic, mainly determined by user-related variables (familial predisposition; previous psychotic episodes; very high dose exposure; and polysubstance abuse) rather than drug related. Soar and colleagues [172] reviewed published psychiatric case studies from the previous 10 years involving MDMA. Of the 38 cases, 22 had a psychotic disorder or symptoms. Two of this subgroup had a family history of psychosis, an observed rate that is precisely comparable to the expected rate with schizophrenia itself. In addition, in the psychotic patients confounding arose from greater Ecstasy use being associated with heavier polysubstance use. In an Italian series [173] of 32 cases of psychotic disorder in Ecstasy users (patients with self-reported polysubstance abuse excluded), symptomatology was not phenomenologically distinctive, and many cases had a family history of psychiatric disorder or past personal history of nonpsychotic psychiatric disorder, making it impossible to determine whether or not Ecstasy was the primary cause of psychosis. In a community sample, the occurrence of schizophrenia was not related to heavy Ecstasy exposure [170]. There is only a single case report in which experimental MDMA intoxication produced an acute toxic hallucinosis lasting 2.5 hours [174], emphasising the rarity and idiosyncratic nature of this adverse event. The lack of evidence of an association between psychotic disorder and Ecstasy use described earlier has not prevented the medical opinion that Ecstasy "has a special risk for persistent organic psychoses" from being published [175]. Clinical biomarker studies have not supported MDMA challenge as a model of schizophrenia. Unexpected increases (i.e. not deficits) in PPI have been observed after administration of MDMA in healthy volunteers [176, 177] and in chronic Ecstasy abusers [178]. Therefore, for the purposes of this review, MDMA-induced psychotomimetic effects do not emerge as a model of schizophrenia.

Animal studies

This subsection reviews animal models induced by PCP and analogues to further assess the construct and predictive validity of the PCP model of schizophrenia. We examine how closely these animal models replicate pathophysiological and theoretical processes hypothesized to underlie schizophrenia. Evidence of predictive validity is presented by comparing the potency of novel compounds in reversing PCP-related psychotomimetic effects in the model with their antipsychotic effect in patients with schizophrenia. First, principles and constraints concerning disease modeling in animals are noted and illustrated by considering the amphetamine-induced model of psychosis.

Animal modeling: principles and constraints

Attempts at modeling psychiatric diseases in their entirety are futile because rodents have much simpler brain structure than humans, making it impossible for rodents to display the same kinds of complex symptoms as humans. It is therefore unrealistic to expect homology on *all* aspects of a disorder across two species [179]. A more feasible approach is to model specific signs or symptoms of the disease, or neurobiological correlates, for which there are relatively equivalent behaviors or measures in both humans and rodents. This approach is illustrated by the dominant animal model for schizophrenia, amphetamine-induced hyperlocomotion in rodents, a model that currently serves as the "'gold standard" in evaluating other models, especially the PCP model.

Amphetamine-induced hyperlocomotion in animals has face validity because the stereotypic hyperactivation of the model bears "'symptom similarity" to the agitation seen in patients with acute schizophrenia, and in turn because amphetamine abuse is associated with psychotic disorder resembling schizophrenia in humans (see Boutros *et al.*, Chapter 9). The model also has high predictive validity because currently available antipsychotic drugs attenuate amphetamine-induced hyperlocomotion in rodents. The limitation of using hyperlocomotion as the measure of the model is that this behavior is also reversed by compounds that have no antipsychotic effect clinically, and the compound with superior antipsychotic effect, clozapine, is no more effective in reversing hyperlocomotion than the conventional D2R antagonist, haloperidol [180]. The dangers of basing animal models on symptom similarity using analogous behavioral measurement have been long recognized [181]. A limitation with using a model that has high predictive validity for a single class of drugs is "'pharmacological isomorphism," the utility of the model being limited to identifying only one class of ("me-too") drugs and not supporting the discovery of drugs of a genuinely new class [182]. The construct validity of amphetamine-induced animal models of schizophrenia has been augmented by measurement of disease markers, such as deficits in PPI. PPI is an example of reliable measurement of an indicator of human disease (also putatively indexing a theoretical process, "sensorimotor gating" [45]), that has an equivalent measureable in the animal model ("homologous" measurement). However, the disease nonspecificity of PPI and hyperlocomotion constrains their utility in animal studies of the pathophysiology of schizophrenia.

This constraint has been addressed in amphetamine-induced animal models by measuring brain system/neuronal dysfunction, in addition to assessing behavioral change. A step in this direction was based on findings in rodents and primates that induction of hyperlocomotion by dopamine agonist (e.g., amphetamine) is related to increased subcortical dopamine release in ventral striatum [183]. Notably, these preclinical findings informed research that produced the first direct evidence in living patients of significant dysregulation of subcortical dopamine neurotransmission in schizophrenia using an *in vivo* receptor binding method, a consistently confirmed finding [184]. Patients show amphetamine-induced sensitivity to presynaptic dopamine release, resulting from inhibition of the dopamine transport (DAT) and the vesicular monoamine transporter (VMAT). Increases in positive (but not negative) symptoms in patients following amphetamine challenge were found to correlate with *in vivo* dopamine release [185]. That is, a neurobiological correlate of the animal model correctly predicted the nature of the dopaminergic dysregulation later found in patients with schizophrenia.

Recent research on amphetamine-induced animal models has revealed abnormalities at the neuronal level in prefrontal cortex [186]. Homayoun and Moghaddam [186] investigated PFC neuronal activation in rats after amphetamine sensitization (5 days repeated daily dosing). Emphasizing the importance of specifying pharmacological models in terms of exposure to single (acute) or repeated (subchronic or chronic) dosing, this group reported that the electrophysiological responses of PFC neurons begin to change after a few doses of amphetamine. Repeated amphetamine exposure had opposite effects in two regions of prefrontal cortex – a progressive hyperactivation of orbitofrontal cortex and hypoactivation of medial prefrontal cortex. These alterations were present irrespective of whether the rats were behaving spontaneously or performing an operant responding task, indicating they were not secondary to hyperlocomotion. The pattern of prefrontal findings is homologous to prefrontal findings reported in human in vivo neuroimaging studies of schizophrenia (hypoactivation of dorsolateral PFC [187]) and substance addiction (hyperactivation of orbitofrontal cortex [188]), another example of the animal model informing human disease research. As only subchronic or chronic amphetamine dosing, and not single dosing, induces psychosis in healthy or substance-abusing volunteers, prefrontal neuronal dysfunction demonstrated in the repeat-dosing amphetamine model [186] may be of pathophysiological importance to schizophrenia, providing a marker for identifying novel and more specific pharmacotherapies, as well as sign-posting future research into prefrontal neuronal dysfunction in patients with schizophrenia. Linking the repeat-dosing amphetamine model back to the PCP model of schizophrenia are studies showing that psychostimulant sensitization (both behavioral and neurochemical) is mediated by NMDA and non-NMDA glutamate-dependent processes secondary to increased stimulant-induced dopamine release.

In summary, lessons from the extensive characterization of the amphetamine-induced model of schizophrenia are relevant to evaluating other animal models. For example PCP-related models are also sensitive to dosing schedule, with chronic (repeated daily) dosing inducing hypoactivation [189], not hyperactivation as seen in acute (single) dosing models. An issue of utmost importance is characterizing an animal model at the neuronal and brain tissue level [190, 191]. This level of information is the basis of a model's capacity to generate predictions about human pathophysiology and likely clinical effectiveness of novel pharmacotherapies [192, 193]. These issues are as relevant to the burgeoning literature on genetically modified models [179, 192, 194], as they are to the evaluation of PCP-related animal models, the subject to which we now proceed.

Animal models and controversy about the pharmacology of phencyclidine and its analogues

Animal studies use a range of PCP analogues, all of which are considered to have their primary pharmacological action at a binding site located within the ion channel formed by the NMDA glutamatergic receptor (called "the PCP binding site"). PCP inhibits NMDA receptor-mediated neurotransmitter release and therefore functions as an NMDA receptor antagonist. As PCP binds to a site of the NMDA receptor complex that is distinct from the recognition site for the neurotransmitter glutamate, its inhibitory effects are noncompetitive in that they cannot be overcome by increased neurotransmitter concentrations. PCP analogues, ketamine, and MK-801 (dizocilpine), also have high affinity for the PCP binding site and are NMDA antagonists. Compared to PCP, ketamine has lower affinity and MK-801 higher affinity for the PCP binding site. Although PCP and ketamine interact with catecholamine re-uptake transporters at anesthetic doses, psychotomimetic effects occur at lower serum levels where these agents have appreciable affinity only at the NMDA receptor complex [56].

A leading research group has argued that the psychotomimetic effects of PCP and ketamine are primarily mediated by direct actions on dopaminergic transmission [195]. They propose that all psychotomimetic drugs exert this effect via D2R-related action [196]. This group presented *in vitro* experimental evidence that PCP and ketamine are potent ligands at striatal D2R in the high-affinity state [197]. No other group has replicated these findings, which have been contradicted [198] or refuted either in a functional assay [199] or other experiments [200, 201]. Another source of evidence that is in complete disagreement with the hypothesis that the psychotomimetic effects of PCP analogues are directly caused by an amphetamine-like striatal dopaminergic dysregulation are the negative results reported in the substantial *in vivo* ligand binding imaging literature (reviewed in [202]). In contrast to PCP and ketamine, MK-801 is highly selective for the PCP site even at very high concentrations, yet it has strong psychotomimetic effects as does the highly selective competitive NMDA antagonist, CGS 19755 [203]. Moreover, drug discrimination studies in which animals are trained to recognize drugs with a common pharmacological effect demonstrate that MK-801 and ketamine have PCP-like effects directly proportional to their binding affinity potency at the PCP site. The PCP-like effects are not related to the differential affinity of these drugs to catecholamine transporters, which are only evident at anesthetic doses [56]. It can therefore be confidently concluded that the primary pharmacological action responsible for the psychotomimetic effects of PCP and analogues is noncompetitive antagonism of the NMDA receptor complex, and any disturbance of dopaminergic systems is secondary to and downstream from, glutamatergic antagonism.

Changes in behavior and clinical biomarkers in PCP-related models

As discussed earlier, amphetamine-induced hyper-locomotion in animal models represents analogous measurement of the psychotomimetic effects of amphetamine seen in humans. It is assumed that hyperlocomotion in animal models of psychosis is analogous to the positive symptoms of schizophrenia, an assumption supported by antipsychotic-induced attenuation of hyperlocomotion in animal models, and positive symptoms in patients. However, analogous measurement in models may have no relationship to disease pathophysiology [182]. PCP [204], ketamine [205], and MK-801 [191] also induce hyperlocomotion in animals, illustrating that two different pharmacological models show the same analogous behavior. However, if a characteristic sign of the human disease, such as a distinctive catatonia-like stereotopy, impairment in working memory, or a deficit in sensorimotor gating, is assessed across species using homologous measurement, it is more likely that aspects of construct validity will be measured. PCP induces characteristic stereotypic head movements in humans (discussed earlier), which are replicated in animal models treated with PCP [204], ketamine [205], or MK-801 [191]. That is, hyperloco-motion is common to both PCP and amphetamine models, whereas only PCP and analogues induce head movements that are identical to PCP-induced stereo-types in humans and similar to catatonia-like motor changes in schizophrenia. Additional face validity for PCP-induced animal models for schizophrenia relates to measurement of PCP-induced "negative" symptoms. In contrast to acute amphetamine-induced models that do not show homologous behavior to negative symptoms [206, 207], animal models induced by PCP [206] and MK-801 [207] show deficits in social interaction, considered to be homologous to negative symptoms.

Increased regional brain activation in acute PCP-related animal models

Animal models induced by MK-801 [208] or ketamine [208, 209, 210] show altered 2-Deoxy-D-glucose (2DG) activation in: frontal regions, especially medial prefrontal and retrosplenial (cingulate) cortex; medial temporal regions, especially the hippocampal formation; anterior ventral thalamic nucleus; and subcortical limbic centers. Areas of altered BOLD contrast in ketamine-induced animal models included frontal regions and the hippocampal formation [211]. Against prediction, regional activation indexed by either BOLD contrast or 2DG autoradiography is *increased* in animal models induced by MK-801 and ketamine in acute (single) doses [208, 209, 210]. In summary, distribution of hyperactivation in PCP-related animal models shows regional homology with activation abnormalities reported in studies of patients with schizophrenia, implicating four specific brain regions, namely: prefrontal cortex, hippocampal formation subcortical limbic nuclei, and thalamic nuclei.

Paradoxical *hyperactivation* seen in PCP-related animal models, compared to the *hypoactivation* usually reported in studies of patients, is of special interest. Possible causes of animal model-human disease discrepancies include mismatch in a number of areas: (i) use of acute pharmacological challenges to model chronic brain disease, (ii) use of neurochemical challenges to model neurodevelopmental disorder, (iii) modeling a different stage of the human disease in an animal, compared to the disease stage in which human findings were made (e.g. early-stage model versus late-stage disease), and (iv) modeling different phases of the disease (e.g. acute relapse versus interepisode residua). Two lines of evidence suggest that the direction-of-activation discrepancy may be due to administration of an acute (single) dose of PCP or analogue to model chronic disease findings. First, PET studies in humans show that a single dose of ketamine induced *increased* brain activation [102], whereas PET studies of subjects who chronically abused PCP showed *reduced* brain activation [212]. Second, in the only repeat-dosing animal model to study regional brain activation (using 2DG), *reduced* prefrontal and thalamic reticulate nucleus activation was found [213]. Although these findings suggest that there is not a real discrepancy between the clinical and preclinical models, the intriguing question as to why NMDA antagonists should induce brain hyperactivation remains.

Increased prefrontal glutamate in PCP-related animal models

Using microdialysis in rats, Moghaddam and Adams [204, 214] showed that PCP induces presynaptic release of glutamate and dopamine, both showing increased extracellular levels in prefrontal cortex and nucleus accumbens. In this landmark study (see commentary in [214]) a single dose of PCP (5 mg/kg IP) elicited marked motor activity, stereotopy with head rolling, and spatial working memory impairments. By manipulating the level of extracellular glutamate (and not altering dopamine levels) with a metabotropic glutamate receptor (mGluR) agonist (see the next subsection), these authors demonstrated that psychotomimetic behavior of the model (hyperlocomotion and stereotopy) was related to glutamate levels, not dopamine levels. Increased prefrontal/hippocampal/subcortical glutamate efflux is a consistent effect replicated with a range of NMDA antagonists, including ketamine [216], PCP [216], and a competitive antagonist [217]. Taken together, the work of Moghaddam and colleagues has characterized a key element of the neuronal dysfunction underlying psychotomimetic behavior in this animal model – increased levels of extracellular glutamate and dopamine. But is glutamate efflux related to prefrontal hyperactivation at the neuronal level?

Increased prefrontal neuronal firing in PCP-related animal models

Another cornerstone in our understanding of the cellular mechanism of the PCP-induced animal model concerns the firing rate of prefrontal neurons. Jackson and colleagues [191] administered single systemic doses of MK801 (0.01, 0.05, 0.1, and 0.3 mg/kg) to rats. At the two highest doses of MK801 sustained and substantial increases in prefrontal neuron firing occurred, firing rates highly correlated with stereotopy counts. MK801 also induced spatial working memory deficits. These important in vivo findings, demonstrating that MK-801-induced increases in firing rate in prefrontal neurons are directly related to behavioral measures of the animal model, have been replicated [218, 219, 220]. Two other studies from the Fukushima Medical University, one of which represented the first demonstration of the effect of PCP on prefrontal neuron firing rate [221], add important detail to the description of the PCP-induced cellular dysfunction. Suzuki et al. [221] found a differential effect on prefrontal neuronal firing between systemic and locally (prefrontally) administered PCP, indicating that afferents (presumably nonNMDA glutamate) from other brain regions partly drive the prefrontal neuronal fir-

ing. This hypothesis was supported by a subsequent study showing that PCP applied locally to the ventral hippocampus led to increased prefrontal neuronal firing [222], apparently mediated by AMPA/kainate glutamate receptors [223]. The thalamocortical circuit may also be a major driver of pathological prefrontal activation and increased cortical glutamate release. MK-801 injections into the anterior nucleus of the thalamus induced cortical degeneration in a pattern indistinguishable from systemic administration, whereas injection directly into cortical regions did not lead to degenerative change [224]. As glutamatergic systems are the major energy users in the brain, and pyramidal cells are the major excitatory cell type, it is likely that PCP-induced regional hyperactivation indexed by BOLD or 2DG uptake is related to increases in pyramidal cell firing. The question as to how NMDA antagonism induces increased extracellular glutamate and dopamine, and increased prefrontal neuronal firing, remains to be considered.

GABAergic interneuron deficits in PCP-related animal models

A long held assumption about the PCP model of psychosis is that deficits in GABAergic interneuron transmission, presumed to be related to PCP-induced dysfunction of the NMDA receptor complex on GABAergic neurons, results in disinhibition of pyramidal cells [113, 224, 225]. There is now a wealth of evidence to support this assumption. Parvalbumin (PV) is a calcium binding protein located within a subpopulation of GABAergic interneurons. PV interneurons receive the largest glutamatergic input among all GABA-releasing neurons in cortex [226] and are highly sensitive to NMDA antagonists [227], a property related to the role played by NMDA receptors in control of basal synaptic activation of these interneurons [228]. In an acute PCP dosing rat study, expression of PV was decreased in the reticular nucleus of the thalamus and substantia nigra pars reticulate [229]. In repeat-dosing rat models, the density or number of hippocampal GABAergic interneurons expressing PV was decreased with PCP [230, 231] and with ketamine [232]. In a repeat-dosing PCP monkey model, the density of prefrontal PV containing axo-axonic structures was decreased [233]. Also, ketamine induced dose-dependent decreases in PV and GAD67 immunoreactivity in cultured PV interneurons specifically [234.] Because PV interneurons are involved in the

153

generation of gamma oscillations responsible for temporal encoding and storage or recall of information required for working memory [235], alterations in gamma frequencies have been used to index functional deficits in GABAergic interneurons induced by ketamine [236]. Juvenile rats given MK-801 for 14 days that showed increased firing of pyramidal cells and deficits in spatial memory premortem, also showed decreased numbers of PV interneurons postmortem [230]. A recent study provided the first direct evidence of an inverse relationship between MK-801-induced increases in prefrontal pyramidal cell firing rate and decreased activity in GABAergic interneurons [219]. This important study [219] demonstrated that NMDA receptors preferentially drive the activity of cortical inhibitory interneurons, and that NMDA receptor antagonism causes cortical excitation by disinhibition of prefrontal pyramidal neurons.

The significance of the cellular dysfunctions affecting GABAergic interneurons in PCP-related animal models pertains to reports of homologous changes in prefrontal PV interneurons in postmortem studies of schizophrenia [237, 238, 239, 240, 241]. Moreover, disturbances in the gamma frequency band of scalp-recorded EEG, considered to reflect gamma oscillations arising from PV interneuron cortical synchronization, are evident in schizophrenia and correlated with prefrontal-related cognitive deficits in patients [242, 243, 244, 245]. That is, the PCP model of schizophrenia offers sufficient construct validity at the level of cellular dysfunction to inform hypotheses about the pathophysiology of schizophrenia that can be tested in the model. An example of such a hypothesis concerns the possibility that reduced nicotinamide adenine dinucleotide phosphate (NADPH) oxidase activation may be involved in the loss of PV expression in prefrontal cortex in schizophrenia [246]. This hypothesis arose directly from a study of the animal model and awaits investigation in studies of the human disease itself.

Secondary monoaminergic system disturbances in PCP-related animal models

Another component of the cellular dysfunction related to the PCP model concerns secondary effects of NMDA antagonism on catecholaminergic and serotonergic pathways. As noted earlier, there is little evidence of direct action on these neurotransmitter systems. However, there is a wealth of evidence that glutamatergic systems closely interact with dopaminergic [247] and serotonergic [113] pathways. In a series of ground-breaking studies, Jentsch and colleagues showed that acute PCP dosing induces marked increases in prefrontal dopamine turnover [247], whereas daily chronic (14 days) dosing causes significantly reduced prefrontal dopamine utilization [248] that persists up to four weeks after ceasing PCP administration [249]. This laboratory showed that chronic PCP-induced decreased dopamine utilization was associated with deficits in spatial learning memory in rats [248], and with deficits in perseverative learning in monkeys [249]. These findings illustrate the importance of specifying acute or chronic exposure to PCP and analogues in describing the animal model [189]. Glutamatergic-serotonergic system interactions are also of relevance, increased prefrontal glutamate efflux being induced by 5HT2A receptor activation presynaptically [140].

The PCP model of schizophrenia is now supported by an extensive literature describing model-induced animal behavior and neurocognitive deficits, regional brain activation patterns, and a comprehensive range of cellular dysfunctions. Advanced *in vitro* and *in vivo* assays applied to this animal model permit a high level of homologous measurement. Novel hypotheses about pathogenesis and pathophysiology have been generated based on the model, which now go well beyond generalizations about hypoglutamatergic function in schizophrenia [250, 251, 252, 253, 254]. Ultimately however, the most important form of validity is whether the model can predict antipsychotic efficacy in the development of new medications for schizophrenia.

Drug development using PCP-related animal models

Several studies demonstrate a differential response to clozapine as compared to other antipsychotic agents using the PCP animal model. To illustrate, in an acute ketamine-induced model, clozapine completely blocked all ketamine-induced regional brain activation (indexed by 2DG uptake), an effect not seen with haloperidol [209]; and in a PCP repeat-dosing model, clozapine but not haloperidol reversed PCP-induced prelimbic reductions in PV staining [213]. The reader is reminded that amphetamine-induced models did not behaviorally differentiate the effect of clozapine and haloperidol [180]. Of greater importance however, is the predictive validity of the model in relation to novel drug development, drugs that are not simply variations of those based on D2R antagonism.

The first indication that the PCP-induced model might have predictive validity for agents with novel modes of action concerns the anticonvulsant, lamotrigine. Lamotrigine inhibits glutamate release via blockade of sodium channels. When tested in a ketamine-induced mouse model, lamotrigine reversed ketamine-induced PPI deficits, an effect it did not have on amphetamine-induced PPI deficits [255]. Moreover, lamotrigine reduced ketamine-induced perceptual abnormalities in healthy volunteers [256]. Although lamotrigine is not effective as monotherapy in patients with schizophrenia, when used to augment atypical antipsychotics [257, 258, 259] or clozapine [260, 261, 262] in treatment-resistant patients, lamotrigine does have modest beneficial effect. Carbamazapine, which does not appreciably reduce glutamate release despite its similar action to lamotrigine in blocking sodium channels [263], is ineffective as an augmenting agent in treatment-resistant schizophrenia.

Of greater interest is the predictive validity of the PCP animal model in relation to new drugs that act directly on glutamate. Based on the PCP model, researchers have now identified and tested a range of new and promising compounds. Among these is sarcosine, a glycine transport 1 (Glyt-1) inhibitor, which increases glycine at the NMDA receptor complex, thereby facilitating NMDA transmission. Preclinical testing on PCP-induced models showed reversal of PCP effects [264], not as apparent in the amphetamine-induced model. Subsequent clinical testing revealed that sarcosine was ineffective as monotherapy [265], but that it shows a significant beneficial effect when used as an augmenting agent with conventional antipsychotic treatment [266]. Sarcosine did not offer additional benefit as an adjunct treatment with clozapine [267], suggesting that clozapine may have direct glutamatergic actions. Another example of drug development based on the PCP model is the preclinical testing of N-acetylaspartylglutamate (NAAG) peptidase inhibitors. These compounds are selective group II mGluR agonists, which inhibit presynaptic glutamate release [268]. Preclinical testing of the NAAG peptidase inhibitor, ZJ43, showed that it reduced MK-801-induced hyperlocomotion and PCP-induced stereotypic movements [269], effects due to the mGluR3 agonist action of ZJ43 [270]. The field

awaits the results of clinical trials of this class of agents.

The most important example of predictive validity of the PCP model concerns the development of the mGluR3 agonist, LY354740, which acts to reduce release of presynaptic glutamate [271]. Preclinical testing on an acute PCP-induced model demonstrated that LY354740 reduced PCP-induced stereotypic movement, hyperlocomotion, and spatial working memory deficits. Significantly, these effects were associated with reversal of increased glutamate and dopamine effluxes prefrontally [204]. Interestingly, preclinical testing of LY354740 in healthy volunteers did not significantly improve ketamine-induced psychosis ratings, although it improved ketamine-induced working memory deficits [272]. Based on these results, LY354740 has been subjected to clinical trial in patients with schizophrenia. In a landmark study, acute ill patients were randomized to LY2140023 (an orally absorbable analogue of LY354740), olanzapine, or placebo. This study demonstrated that LY2140023 was effective against the positive and negative symptoms of schizophrenia and had few side effects [273]. Hence, the PCP model showed accurate predictive validity in the case of the first effective novel antipsychotic since the introduction of chlorpromazine.

The PCP model of schizophrenia: an integration

When the psychotomimetic effect of PCP was first proposed as a model of schizophrenia, the pharmacological actions of PCP were unknown. Although an early report hypothesized impaired function of glutamatergic neurons as a model of schizophrenia [274], it was not until the PCP binding site was localized to the NMDA receptor complex that the NMDA receptor hypofunction could be incorporated into the PCP model [253, 254]. A "thalamic filter dysfunction" was proposed [253] and pathological activation of the cortico-striato-thalamo-cortical feedback loop was hypothesized to cause information overload in the cortex (reviewed in [275]). Strengthening evidence that the psychotomimetic effects of PCP were directly related to NMDA receptor complex antagonism challenged the highly influential dopamine hypothesis of schizophrenia [56]. An important element of the PCP model, glutamatergic neuronal disinhibition due to functional antagonism of NMDA receptors on GABAergic interneurons that normally

A

B

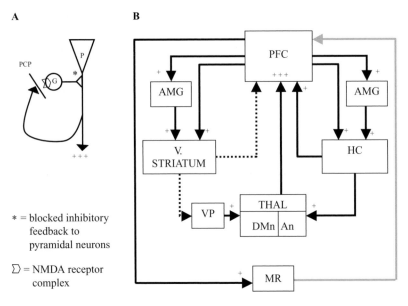

* = blocked inhibitory
  feedback to
  pyramidal neurons

$\sum$ = NMDA receptor
  complex

Figure 10.1 Panel A: Site of action of PCP. G: GABAergic interneuron; P: pyramidal neuron. Panel B: Circuits of the brain relevant to the PCP model of schizophrenia. Black unbroken lines indicate glutamatergic neurotransmission, the strength of which is indicated by the number of + signs. Black dotted lines indicate dopaminergic neurotransmission. Grey unbroken lines indicate serotonergic neurotransmission. PFC: prefrontal cortex; AMG: amygdala; V. STRIATUM: ventral striatum; VP: ventral pallidum; THAL: thalamus; DMn: dorsomedial nucleus of thalamus; An: anterior nucleus of thalamus; HC: hippocampus; MR: median raphe.

place excitatory pyramidal neurons under inhibitory control, was added more recently [276]. The putative role of cortical pruning [277] and evidence of reduced prefrontal neuropil [278] in schizophrenia have also been incorporated into the model [252].

A number of neuropharmacological descriptions of the PCP model (hypoglutamatergic model) of schizophrenia have been published [224, 279, 280, 281, 282, 283]. Central to these models is a PCP-induced deficit of GABAergic interneurons, which results in disinhibition of glutamatergic pyramidal cells (Figure 10.1, Panel A). Although this disinhibition is assumed to be widespread throughout grey matter, models emphasize its impact on prefrontal cortex in accounting for psychotomimetic effects. Increased levels of extracellular glutamate in acute PCP models are thought to result from local collateral feedback by disinhibited pyramidal neurons onto presynaptic terminals, and increased nonNMDA glutamatergic efferent feedback from the thalamus, other subcortical centers, and the hippocampal formation (Figure 10.1, Panel B). Completing the PCP model are descriptions of increased dopamine efflux in the prefrontal cortex and ventral pallidum, resulting from greater cortical drive to striatal/limbic subcortical centers. Increased cortical drive to the median raphe results in increased prefrontal serotonin concentrations, which augment glutamate efflux via presynaptic 5HT2A receptor activation. Importantly, ventral pallidal stimulation of the dorsomedial thalamic

nucleus, and hippocampal-hippocampal-limbic stimulation of the anterior nucleus of the thalamus, provides an explanation for excessive subcortical-cortical glutamatergic feedback drive to the prefrontal cortex (Figure 10.1, Panel B).

The acute model has been supplemented by a chronic PCP model, which includes reduced prefrontal extracellular glutamate and dopamine [249]. A number of cellular mechanisms have been advanced to link these surface receptor-focused models to intracellular final common pathway models. Svenningson and colleagues [200] have implicated a common signaling pathway in the mediation of the psychotomimetic effects of glutamatergic antagonists (such as PCP), serotonergic agonists (such as LSD), and dopaminergic agonists (such as amphetamine). In this pathway, phosphorylation status of Dopamine- and an Adenosine 3′,5′monophosphate (cAMP)-Regulated Phospho-Protein of 32 kilodaltons (DARPP-32) regulates downstream effector proteins, glycogen synthesis kinase-3 (GSK-3), cAMP response element-binding proteins (CREP) and c-Fos, thereby influencing electrophysiological, transcriptional, and behavioral responses. An alternative mechanism for linking the PCP model to intracellular signaling pathways is via glutamate-mediated excitotoxicity, which has been found to induce apoptotic loss of dendrites and synapses without cell body death or gliosis (reviewed in [283]). Postmortem studies have reported elevated Bax:Bcl-2 ratio (a marker of increased propensity for apoptosis) in the temporal cortex [284], comparable to functional findings in cultured fibroblasts from patients with schizophrenia [285]. Taken together, these proposals provide a rich source of hypotheses for testing in studies of the pathogenesis of schizophrenia.

Summary and conclusion

It is concluded that although PCP, LSD, and MDMA have well-documented psychotomimetic effects, only for PCP is there abundant evidence that it induced psychotic disorder beyond the acute symptoms of intoxication. In fact, there is no clear evidence that either LSD or MDMA induces psychotic disorder, let alone schizophrenia, in individuals who did not have vulnerability to schizophrenia premorbidly. Although inducing quantitatively less intense psychotomimetic effects, ketamine is considered a safe and valid model of PCP psychosis and applicable to preclinical human studies. We also concluded that rodent and primate models induced by PCP and analogues have construct validity, showing homologous behavior, cognitive deficits, alteration in regional brain activation, and underlying neuronal dysfunction, to PCP-induced psychotomimetic effects in healthy volunteers and patients with schizophrenia. Most importantly, animal models demonstrated predictive validity at the level of hypothesis generation about human pathophysiology and efficacy of novel drug therapies. Indeed, it could be said that PCP-related animal models have been instrumental in the discovery of the first novel class of antipsychotic drug treatments (i.e., mGluR2/3 agonists) without D2R antagonist action since the introduction of chlorpromazine. The relative merits of PCP-related and amphetamine-induced models of schizophrenia have been discussed elsewhere [223]. We considered both models to have high validity when descriptions and measurement are carried out at the level of neuronal dysfunction. A notable limitation of neurochemical models is that they usually do not incorporate a neurodevelopmental perspective [286, 287]. This implies that alternative models may be required to complement pharmacological models (reviewed in [192]), preferably etiologically linked to the occurrence of schizophrenia and based on a specific genetic alteration, exemplified by mouse models of velo-cardio-facial syndrome [288].

In a more general sense, this review reminds us of our field's historic dependence on research using patients. Preclinical models, especially in animals, release research from the inevitable confounding factors related to illness experience and treatment. Most importantly, animal models allow direct observation of neuronal dysfunction that models the human pathophysiology. Without this opportunity, major improvements in the drug treatment of schizophrenia will not be possible. This review also reminded us of our dependence on clinical observation and measurement in developing adequately valid animal models, which rely on the clinical insights of well-trained clinicians who are interested in the neurobiology of psychiatric disorder. Communication from the clinic to the preclinical behavioral laboratory will enable the refinement of established models and the creation of new ones [179]. The absence of well-validated, objective, and reliable measures of psychopathology is a barrier to the development of homologous measurement in animal models. Insufficient validation of an animal model can be only as good as the information available in the relevant preclinical human research and the clinical literature. Clinical studies need to be informed by results from animal studies as much as the reverse is true. More translational science is needed to relate animal findings to humans and vice versa [179].

Note

Supplementary information related to this chapter may be found at www.qsrf.com.au.

References

1. Maddox V. H. (1981). The historical development of phencyclidine. In *PCP (Phencyclidine): Historical and Current Perspectives*, Domino E. F. (Ed.). Ann Arbor, Michigan: NPP Books, pp. 1–8.

2. Johnstone M., Evans V., Baigel S. Sernyl (Cl-395) in clinical anaesthesia. *B J Anaesth*, 1959. **31**(10):433–9.

3. Cook C. E., Brine D. R., Jeffcoat A. R., *et al*. Phencyclidine disposition after intravenous and oral doses. *Clin Pharm Therapeutics*, 1982. **31**(5):625–34.

4. Griefenstein F. E., Yoshitake J., Devault M., *et al*. A study of a 1-Aryl cyclo hexyl amine for anesthesia. *Anesth Analg*, 1958. **37**(5):283–94.

5. Collins V. J., Gorospe C. A., Rovenstine E. A. Intravenous nonbarbiturate, nonnarcotic analgesics: preliminary studies. Cyclohexylamines. *Anesth Analg*, 1960. **39**:302–6.

6. Meyer J. S., Greifenstein F., Devault M. A new drug causing symptoms of sensory deprivation – neurological, electroencephalographic and pharmalogical effects of sernyl. *J Nerv Ment Dis*, 1959. **129**(1):54–61.

7. Kothary S. P., Zsigmond E. K. A double-blind study of the effective antihallucinatory doses of diazepam prior to ketamine anesthesia. *Clin Pharmacol Therapeutics*, 1977. **21**:108–9.

8. Helrich M., Atwood J. M. Modification of sernyl anesthesia with haloperidol. *Anesth Analg*, 1964. **43**(5):471–4

9. Petersen R. C., Stillman R. C. (1978). Phencyclidine: an overview. In *Phencyclidine (PCP) Abuse: An Appraisal*, vol Monograph 21. Petersen R. C. and Stillman R. C. (Eds.). Rockville, Maryland: National Institute on Drug Abuse, pp. 1–17.

10. Sioris L. J., Krenzelok E. P. Phencyclidine intoxication – literature review. *Am J Hosp Pharm*, 1978. **35**(11):1362–7.

11. Newmeyer J. A. The epidemiology of PCP use in the late 1970s. *J Psych Drugs*, 1980. **12**(3–4): 211–15.

12. Stillman R., Petersen R. C. Paradox of phencyclidine (PCP) abuse. *Annals of Intern Med*, 1979. **90**(3):428–30.

13. Siegel R. K. (1978). Phencyclidine and ketamine intoxication: a study of four populations of recreational users. In *Phencyclidine (PCP) Abuse: An Appraisal*, vol Monograph 21, Petersen R. C. and Stillman R. C. (Eds.). Rockville, Maryland: National Institute on Drug Abuse, pp. 119–47.

14. Pearlson G. D. Psychiatric and medical syndromes associated with phencyclidine (PCP) abuse. *Johns Hopkins Med J*, 1981. **148**(1):25–33.

15. Lerner S. E., Burns R. S. (1978). Phencyclidine use among youth: history, epidemiology, and acute and chronic intoxication. In *Phencyclidine (PCP) abuse: An appraisal*, vol Monograph 21, Petersen R. C. and Stillman R. C. (Eds.). Rockville, Maryland: National Institute on Drug Abuse, pp. 66–118.

16. Kay J., Tasman A. (2006). *Essentials of Psychiatry*. West Sussex: John Wiley and Sons.

17. Yesavage J. A., Freman A. M. Acute phencyclidine (PCP) intoxication – psychopathology and prognosis. *J Clin Psychol*, 1978. **39**(8):664–66.

18. Liden C. B., Lovejoy F. H., Costello C. E. Phencyclidine – 9 cases of poisoning. *JAMA*, 1975. **234**(5):513–16.

19. Burns R. S., Lerner S. E., Corrado R., *et al*. Phencyclidine – states of acute intoxication and fatalities. *West J Med*, 1975. **123**(5):345–9.

20. Fauman B., Baker F., Coppleson L. W., *et al*. Psychosis induced by phencyclidine. *Concepts, Comp and Config*, 1975. **4**(3):223–5.

21. Fauman M. A., Fauman B. (1978). The psychiatric aspects of chronic phencyclidine use: a study of chronic PCP users. In *Phencyclidine (PCP) Abuse: An Appraisal*, vol Monograph 21, Petersen R. C. and Stillman R. C. (Eds.). Rockville, Maryland: National Institute on Drug Abuse, pp. 183–200.

22. Luisada P. V. (1978). The phencyclidine psychosis: phenomenology and treatment. In *Phencyclidine (PCP) Abuse: An Appraisal*, vol Monograph 21, Petersen R. C. and Stillman R. C. (Eds.). Rockville, Maryland: National Institute on Drug Abuse, pp. 241–53.

23. Erard R., Luisada P. V., Peele R. The PCP psychosis – prolonged intoxication or drug-precipitated functional illness. *J Psychedelic Drugs*, 1980. **12**(3–4):235–51.

24. Yago K. B., Pitts F. N., Burgoyne R. W., *et al*. The urban epidemic of phencyclidine (PCP) use – clinical and laboratory evidence from a public psychiatric-hospital emergency service. *J Clin Psychiatry*, 1981. **42**(5):193–6.

25. Allen R. M., Young S. J. Phencyclidine-induced psychosis. *Am J Psychiatry*, 1978. **135**(9): 1081–4.

26. McCarron M. M., Schulze B. W., Thompson G. A., *et al*. Acute phencyclidine intoxication – incidence of clinical findings in 1,000 cases. *Annals of Emerg Med*, 1981. **10**(5):237–42.

27. Luisada P. V., Brown B. I. Clinical management of phencyclidine psychosis. *Clin Toxicol*, 1976. **9**(4):539–45.

28. Burns R. S., Lerner S. E. Perspectives – acute phencyclidine intoxication. *Clin Toxicol*, 1976. **9**(4):477–501.

29. Rainey J. M., Crowder M. K. Prevalence of phencyclidine in

street drug preparations. *N Engl J Med*, 1974. **290**(8):466–7.

30. Wright H. H., Cole E. A., Batey S. R., *et al.* Phencyclidine-induced psychosis – 8-year follow-up of 10 cases. *South Med J*, 1988. **81**(5):565–7.

31. Rosse R. B., Collins J. P., Faymccarthy M., *et al.* Phenomenological comparison of the idiopathic psychosis of schizophrenia and drug-induced cocaine and phencyclidine psychoses – a retrospective study. *Clin Neuropharm*, 1994. **17**(4):359–69.

32. Gwirtsman H. E., Wittkop W., Gorelick D., *et al.* Phencyclidine intoxication – incidence, clinical-patterns and course of treatment. *Res Comm in Psych Psych and Behav*, 1984. **9**(4):405–10.

33. Giannini A. J., Eighan M. S., Loiselle R. H., *et al.* Comparison of haloperidol and chlorpromazine in the treatment of phencyclidine psychosis. *J Clin Pharmacol*, 1984. **24**(4):202–4.

34. Carls K. A., Ruehter V. L. An evaluation of phencyclidine (PCP) psychosis: a retrospective analysis at a state facility. *Am J Drug Alcohol Abuse*, 2006. **32**(4):673–8.

35. Giannini A. J., Nageotte C., Loiselle R. H., *et al.* Comparison of chlorpromazine, haloperidol and pimozide in the treatment of phencyclidine psychosis – D2 receptor specificity. *J Toxicol Clin Toxicol*, 1984. **22**(6):573–9.

36. Luby E. D., Cohen B. D., Rosenbaum G., *et al.* Study of a new schizophrenomimetic drug – sernyl. *Arch Neurol Psychiatry*, 1959. **81**(3):363–9.

37. Levy L., Cameron D. E., Aitken R. C. B. Observation on 2 psychotomimetic drugs of piperidine derivation-Ci-395 (sernyl) and Ci-400. *Am J Psychiatry*, 1960. **116**(9):843–4.

38. Itil T., Keskiner A., Kiremitci N., *et al.* Effect of phencyclidine in

chronic schizophrenics. *Can Psychiatr Assoc J*, 1967. **12**(2):209–12.

39. Domino E. F., Luby E. D. (1981). Abnormal mental states induced by phencyclidine as a model of schizophrenia. In *PCP (Phencyclidine): Historical and Current Perspectives*, Domino E. F. (Ed.). Ann Arbor, Michigan: NPP Books, pp. 401–19.

40. Ban T. A., Lohrenz J. J., Lehmann H. E. Observations on the action of sernyl – a new psychotropic drug. *Can Psychiatr Assoc J.*, 1961. **6**(3):150–7.

41. Rosenbaum G., Cohen B. D., Luby E. D., *et al.* Comparison of sernyl with other drugs – simulation of schizophrenic performance with sernyl, Lsd-25, and amobarbital (amytal) sodium. 1. Attention, motor function, and proprioception. *Arch of Gen Psychiatry*, 1959. **1**(6):651–6.

42. Davies B. M., Beech H. R. The effect of 1-arylcyclohexylamine (sernyl) on 12 normal volunteers. *J Ment Sci*, 1960. **106**(444):912–24.

43. Cohen B. D., Rosenbaum G., Gottlieb J. S., *et al.* Comparison of phencyclidine hydrochloride (sernyl) with other drugs – simulation of schizophrenic performance with phencyclidine hydrochloride (sernyl), lysergic-acid diethylamide (Lsd-25), and amobarbital (amytal) sodium. 2. Symbolic and sequential thinking. *Arch of Gen Psychiatry*, 1962. **6**(5):395–401.

44. Bakker C. B., Amini F. B. Observations on the psychotomimetic effects of sernyl. *Compr Psychiatry*, 1961. **2**:269–80.

45. Braff D. L., Geyer M. A., Swerdlow N. R. Human studies of prepulse inhibition of startle: normal subjects, patient groups, and pharmacological studies. *Psychopharmacology*, 2001. **156**(2–3):234–58.

46. Domino E. F., Chodoff P., Corssen G. Pharmacologic effects of

Cl-581 a new dissociative anesthetic in man. *Clin Pharmacol Therapeutics*, 1965. **6**(3):279–90

47. Wolff K., Winstock A. R. Ketamine – from medicine to misuse. *CNS Drugs*, 2006. **20**(3):199–218.

48. White P. F., Way W. L., Trevor A. J. Ketamine – its pharmacology and therapeutic uses. *Anesthesiology*, 1982. **56**(2):119–36.

49. Idvall J., Ahlgren I., Aronsen K. F., *et al.* Ketamine infusions – pharmacokinetics and clinical effects. *Br J Anaesth*, 1979. **51**(12):1167–73.

50. Bennett J. A., Bullimore J. A. Use of ketamine hydrochloride anesthesia for radiotherapy young children. *Br J Anaesth*, 1973. **45**(2):197–201.

51. Slogoff S., Allen G. W., Wessels J. V., *et al.* Clinical experience with subanesthetic ketamine. *Anesth Analg*, 1974. **53**(3):354–8.

52. White J. M., Ryan C. F. Pharmacological properties of ketamine. *Drug Alcohol Rev*, 1996. **15**(2):145–55.

53. Reier C. E. Ketamine – dissociative agent or hallucinogen. *N Engl J Med*, 1971. **284**(14):791–2

54. Collier B. B. Ketamine and conscious mind. *Anaesthesia*, 1972. **27**(2):120–34

55. Modvig K. M., Nielsen S. F. Psychological changes in children after anesthesia – comparison between halothane and ketamine. *Acta Anaesthesiol Scand*, 1977. **21**(6):541–4.

56. Javitt D. C., Zukin S. R. Recent advances in the phencyclidine model of schizophrenia. *Am J Psychiatry*, 1991. **148**(10):1301–8.

57. Vincent J. P., Kartalovski B., Geneste P., *et al.* Interaction of phencyclidine (angel dust) with a specific receptor in rat-brain membranes. *Proc Natl Acad Sci USA*, 1979. **76**(9):4678–82.

58. Hampton R. Y., Medzihradsky F., Woods J. H., *et al.* Stereospecific

binding of H-3-labeled phencyclidine in brain membranes. *Life Sci*, 1982. **30**(25):2147–54.

59. FDA Drug Bulletin: Ketamine abuse. *FDA Drug Bulletin*, 1979. **9**(4):24.

60. Dotson J. W., Ackerman D. L., West L. J. Ketamine abuse. *J Drug Issues*, 1995. **25**(4):751–7.

61. Stafford P. (1992). *Psychedelics Encyclopedia*. Berkeley, California: Ronin Publishing.

62. Maxwell J. C. Party drugs: properties, prevalence, patterns, and problems. *Subst Use Misuse*, 2005. **40**(9–10):1203–40.

63. Jansen K. L. R. A review of the nonmedical use of ketamine: use, users and consequences. *J Psychoactive Drugs*, 2000. **32**(4):419–33.

64. Weiner A. L., Vieira L., McKay C. A., *et al.* Ketamine abusers presenting to the emergency department: a case series. *J Emerg Med*, 2000. **18**(4):447–51.

65. Dillon P., Copeland J., Jansen K. Patterns of use and harms associated with non-medical ketamine use. *Drug Alcohol Depend*, 2003. **69**(1):23–8.

66. Uhlhaas P. J., Millard I., Muetzelfeldt L., *et al.* Perceptual organization in ketamine users: preliminary evidence of deficits on night of drug use but not 3 days later. *J Psychopharmacol*, 2007. **21**(3):347–52.

67. Curran H. V., Monaghan L. In and out of the K-hole: a comparison of the acute and residual effects of ketamine in frequent and infrequent ketamine users. *Addiction*, 2001. **96**(5):749–60.

68. Curran H. V., Morgan C. Cognitive, dissociative and psychotogenic effects of ketamine in recreational users on the night of drug use and 3 days later. *Addiction*, 2000. **95**(4):575–90.

69. Morgan C. J. A., Riccelli M., Maitland C. H., *et al.* Long-term effects of ketamine: evidence for a persisting impairment of source memory in recreational users. *Drug Alcohol Depend*, 2004. **75**(3):301–8.

70. Carpenter W. T. The schizophrenia ketamine challenge study debate. *Biol Psychiatry*, 1999. **46**(8):1081–91.

71. Kudoh A., Katagai H., Takazawa T. Anesthesia with ketamine, propofol, and fentanyl decreases the frequency of postoperative psychosis emergence and confusion in schizophrenic patients. *J Clin Anesth*, 2002. **14**(2):107–10.

72. Lahti A. C., Holcomb H. H., Medoff D. R., *et al.* Ketamine activates psychosis and alters limbic blood-flow in schizophrenia. *Neuroreport*, 1995. **6**(6):869–72.

73. Malhotra A. K., Pinals D. A., Adler C. M., *et al.* Ketamine-induced exacerbation of psychotic symptoms and cognitive impairment in neuroleptic-free schizophrenics. *Neuropsychopharmacology*, 1997. **17**(3):141–50.

74. Malhotra A. K., Adler C. M., Kennison S. D., *et al.* Clozapine blunts N-methyl-D-aspartate antagonist-induced psychosis: a study with ketamine. *Biol Psychiatry*, 1997. **42**(8):664–8.

75. Morgan C. J. A., Curran H. V. Acute and chronic effects of ketamine upon human memory: a review. *Psychopharmacology*, 2006. **188**(4):408–24.

76. Ghoneim M. M., Hinrichs J. V., Mewaldt S. P., *et al.* Ketamine – behavioral effects of subanesthetic doses. *J Clin Psychopharmacol*, 1985. **5**(2):70–7.

77. Krystal J. H., Karper L. P., Seibyl J. P., *et al.* Subanesthetic effects of the noncompetitive NMDA antagonist, ketamine, in humans. Psychotomimetic, perceptual, cognitive, and neuroendocrine responses. *Arch Gen Psychiatry*, 1994. **51**(3):199–214.

78. Malhotra A. K., Pinals D. A., Weingartner H., *et al.* NMDA receptor function and human cognition: the effects of ketamine in healthy volunteers. *Neuropsychopharmacology*, 1996. **14**(5):301–7.

79. Newcomer J. W., Farber N. B., Jevtovic-Todorovic V., *et al.* Ketamine-induced NMDA receptor hypofunction as a model of memory impairment and psychosis. *Neuropsycho-pharmacology*, 1999. **20**(2): 106–18.

80. Krystal J. H., Perry E. B., Gueorguieva R., *et al.* Comparative and interactive human psychopharmacologic effects of ketamine and amphetamine. Implications for glutamatergic and dopaminergic model psychoses and cognitive function. *Arch Gen Psychiatry*, 2005. **62**(9):985–95.

81. Radant A. D., Bowdle T. A., Cowley D. S., *et al.* Does ketamine-mediated N-methyl-D-aspartate receptor antagonism cause schizophrenia-like oculomotor abnormalities? *Neuropsychopharmacology*, 1998. **19**(5):434–44.

82. Hetem L. A. B., Danion J. M., Diemunsch P., *et al.* Effect of a subanesthetic dose of ketamine on memory and conscious awareness in healthy volunteers. *Psychopharmacology*, 2000. **152**(3):283–8.

83. Lofwall M. R., Griffiths R. R., Mintzer M. Z. Cognitive and subjective acute dose effects of intramuscular ketamine in healthy adults. *Clin Psychopharmacol*, 2006. **14**(4):439–49.

84. Honey G. D., O'Loughlin C., Turner D. C., *et al.* The effects of a subpsychotic dose of ketamine on recognition and source memory for agency: implications for

pharmacological modelling of core symptoms of schizophrenia. *Neuropsychopharmacology*, 2006. **31**(2):413–23.

85. Fletcher P. C., Honey G. D. Schizophrenia, ketamine and cannabis: evidence of overlapping memory deficits. *Trends a Cogn Sci*, 2006. **10**(4):167–74.

86. Adler C. M., Goldberg T. E., Malhotra A. K., *et al.* Effects of ketamine on thought disorder, working memory, and semantic memory in healthy volunteers. *Biol Psychiatry*, 1998. **43**(11):811–16.

87. Honey R. A. E., Turner D. C., Honey G. D., *et al.* Subdissociative dose ketamine produces a deficit in manipulation but not maintenance of the contents of working memory. *Neuropsychopharmacology*, 2003. **28**(11):2037–44.

88. Krystal J. H., D'Souza D. C., Karper L. P., *et al.* Interactive effects of subanesthetic ketamine and haloperidol in healthy humans. *Psychopharmacology*, 1999. **145**(2):193–204.

89. Krystal J. H., Karper L. P., Bennett A., *et al.* Interactive effects of subanesthetic ketamine and subhypnotic lorazepam in humans. *Psychopharmacology*, 1998. **135**(3):213–29.

90. Morgan C. J. A., Mofeez A., Brandner B., *et al.* Ketamine impairs response inhibition and is positively reinforcing in healthy volunteers: a dose-response study. *Psychopharmacology*, 2004. **172**(3):298–308.

91. Harborne G. C., Watson F. L., Healy D. T., *et al.* The effects of sub-anaesthetic doses of ketamine on memory, cognitive performance and subjective experience in healthy volunteers. *J Psychopharmacol*, 1996. **10**(2):134–40.

92. Ragland J. D., Gur R. C., Valdez J., *et al.* Event-related fMRI of frontotemporal activity during word encoding and recognition in schizophrenia. *Am J Psychiatry*, 2004. **161**(6):1004–15.

93. Hofer A., Weiss E. M., Golaszewski S. M., *et al.* Neural correlates of episodic encoding and recognition of words in unmedicated patients during an acute episode of schizophrenia: a functional MRI study. *Am J Psychiatry*, 2003. **160**(10):1802–8.

94. Glahn D. C., Ragland J. D., Abramoff A., *et al.* Beyond hypofrontality: a quantitative meta-analysis of functional neuroimaging studies of working memory in schizophrenia. *Hum Brain Mapp*, 2005. **25**(1):60–9.

95. Tamminga C. A., Thaker G. K., Buchanan R., *et al.* Limbic system abnormalities identified in schizophrenia using positron emission tomography with fluorodeoxyglucose and neocortical alterations with deficit syndrome. *Arch Gen Psychiatry*, 1992. **49**(7):522–30.

96. Jessen F., Scheef L., Germeshausen L., *et al.* Reduced hippocampal activation during encoding and recognition of words in schizophrenia patients. *Am J Psychiatry*, 2003. **160**(7):1305–12.

97. Vollenweider F. X., Leenders K. L., Oye I., *et al.* Differential psychopathology and patterns of cerebral glucose utilisation produced by (S)- and (R)-ketamine in healthy volunteers using positron emission tomography (PET). *Eur Neuropsychopharmacol*, 1997. **7**(1):25–38.

98. Holcomb H. H., Lahti A. C., Medoff D. R., *et al.* Effects of noncompetitive NMDA receptor blockade on anterior cingulate cerebral blood flow in volunteers with schizophrenia. *Neuropsychopharmacology*, 2005. **30**(12):2275–82.

99. Honey G. D., Honey R. A. E., O'Loughlin C., *et al.* Ketamine disrupts frontal and hippocampal contribution to encoding and retrieval of episodic memory: an fMRI study. *Cereb Cortex*, 2005. **15**(6):749–59.

100. Honey R. A. E., Honey G. D., O'Loughlin C., *et al.* Acute ketamine administration alters the brain responses to executive demands in a verbal working memory task: an fMRI study. *Neuropsychopharmacology*, 2004. **29**(6):1203–14.

101. Fu C. H. Y., Abel K. M., Allin M. P. G., *et al.* Effects of ketamine on prefrontal and striatal regions in an overt verbal fluency task: a functional magnetic resonance imaging study. *Psychopharmacology*, 2005. **183**(1):92–102.

102. Langsjo J. W., Salmi E., Kaisti K. K., *et al.* Effects of subanesthetic ketamine on regional cerebral glucose metabolism in humans. *Anesthesiology*, 2004. **100**(5):1065–71.

103. Langsjo J. W., Kaisti K. K., Aalto S., *et al.* Effects of subanesthetic doses of ketamine on regional cerebral blood flow, oxygen consumption, and blood volume in humans. *Anesthesiology*, 2003. **99**(3):614–23.

104. Stone J. M., Erlandsson K., Arstad E., *et al.* Ketamine displaces the novel NMDA receptor SPET probe [I-123]CNS-1261 in humans in vivo. *Nucl Med Biol*, 2006. **33**(2):239–43.

105. van Berckel B. N. M., Oranje B., van Ree J. M., *et al.* The effects of low dose ketamine on sensory gating, neuroendocrine secretion and behavior in healthy human subjects. *Psychopharmacology*, 1998. **137**(3):271–81.

106. Oranje B., Gispen-de Wied C. C., Verbaten M. N., *et al.* Modulating sensory gating in healthy volunteers: the effects of ketamine and haloperidol. *Biol Psychiatry*, 2002. **52**(9):887–95.

107. Heekeren K., Neukirch A., Daumann J., *et al.* Prepulse inhibition of the startle reflex and

its attentional modulation in the human S-ketamine and N,N-dimethyltryptamine (DMT) models of psychosis. *J Psychopharmacol*, 2007. **21**(3):312–20.

108. Abel K. M., Allin M. P. G., Hemsley D. R., *et al.* Low dose ketamine increases prepulse inhibition in healthy men. *Neuropharmacology*, 2003. **44**(6):729–37.

109. Duncan E. J., Madonick S. H., Parwani A., *et al.* Clinical and sensorimotor gating effects of ketamine in normals. *Neuropsychopharmacology*, 2001. **25**(1):72–83.

110. Umbricht D., Schmid L., Koller R., *et al.* Ketamine-induced deficits in auditory and visual context-dependent processing in healthy volunteers – Implications for models of cognitive deficits in schizophrenia. *Arch Gen Psychiatry*, 2000. **57**(12):1139–47.

111. Sauer H., Kreitschmann-Andermahr I., Gaser E., *et al.* Ketamine reduces the neuromagnetic mismatch reaction. *Schizophr Res*, 2000. **41**(1):148–.

112. O'Brien R., Cohen S. (1984). *Encyclopedia of Drug Abuse.* New York: Facts on File.

113. Aghajanian G. K., Marek G. J. Serotonin model of schizophrenia: emerging role of glutamate mechanisms. *Brain Res Rev*, 2000. **31**(2–3):302–12.

114. Henderson L. A., Glass W. J. (1998). LSD: *Still with Us After All These Years.* San Francisco: Jossey-Bass Publishers.

115. Grinspoon L., Bakalar J. B. (1998). *Psychedelic Drugs Reconsidered.* New York: The Lindesmith Center.

116. Houston J. (1969). Phenomeno-logy of the psychedelic experience. In *Psychedelic Drugs*, Hicks R. E. and Fink P. J. (Eds.). New York: Grune & Stratton, pp. 1–7.

117. Katz M. M., Waskow I. E., Olsson J. Characterizing psychological state produced *by LSD. J Abnorm Psychol*, 1968. **73**(1):1–14

118. Stone A. L., O'Brien M. S., De la Torre A., *et al.* Who is becoming hallucinogen dependent soon after hallucinogen use starts? *Drug Alcohol Depend*, 2007. **87**(2–3):153–63.

119. Siegel R. K., West L. J. (1975). Hallucinations: *Behavior, experience, and theory.* New York: John Wiley & Sons.

120. Halpern J. H. The use of hallucinogens in the treatment of addiction. *Addict Res*, 1996. **4**(2):177–89.

121. Cohen S. Lysergic-acid diethylamide – side-effects and complications. *J Nerv Ment Dis*, 1960. **130**(1):30–40.

122. Cholden L. S., Kurland A., Savage C. Clinical reactions and tolerance to LSD in chronic schizophrenia. *J Nerv Ment Dis*, 1955. **122**(3):211–21.

123. Fink M., Simeon J., Haque W., *et al.* Prolonged adverse reactions to LSD in psychotic subjects. *Arch Gen Psychiatry*, 1966. **15**(5):450.

124. Abraham H. D., Aldridge A. M. Adverse consequences of lysergic-acid diethylamide. *Addiction*, 1993. **88**(10):1327–34.

125. Strassman R. J. Adverse reactions to psychedelic drugs – a review of the literature. *J Nerv Ment Dis*, 1984. **172**(10):577–95.

126. Glass G. S., Bowers M. B. Chronic psychosis associated with long-term psychotomimetic drug abuse. *Arch Gen Psychiatry*, 1970. **23**(2):97.

127. Abraham H. D., Aldridge A. M., Gogia P. The psychopharmaco-logy of hallucinogens. *Neuro-psychopharmacology*, 1996. **14**(4):285–98.

128. Hays P., Tilley J. R. Differences between LSD psychosis and schizophrenia. *Can Psychiatr Assoc J*, 1973. **18**(4):331–3.

129. Sedman G., Kenna J. C. The use of LSD-25 as a diagnostic aid in doubtful cases of schizophrenia. *Br J Psychiatry*, 1965. **111**(470):96–100.

130. Vardy M. M., Kay S. R. LSD psychosis or LSD-induced schizophrenia – a multimethod inquiry. *Arch Gen Psychiatry*, 1983. **40**(8):877–83.

131. Ungerleider J.T., Fisher D. D., Fuller M. Dangers of LSD. Analysis of 7 months' experience in a university hospital's psychiatric service. *JAMA*, 1966. **197**(6):389–92

132. Bowers M. B., Swigar M. E. Vulnerability to psychosis associated with hallucinogen use. *Psychiatr Res*, 1983. **9**(2):91–7.

133. Potvin S., Stip E., Roy J-Y. Toxic psychoses as pharmacological models of schizophrenia. *Curr Psychiatr Rev*, 2005. **1**:23–32.

134. Langs R. J., Barr H. L. Lysergic acid diethylamide (Lsd-25) and schizophrenic reactions – a comparative study. *J Nerv Ment Dis*, 1968. **147**(2):163.

135. Hollister L. E. Clinical syndrome from LSD-25 compared with epinephrine. *Dis Nerv Syst*, 1964. **25**(7):427.

136. Breier A. Serotonin, schizophrenia and antipsychotic drug-action. *Schizophr Res*, 1995. **14**(3):187–202.

137. Riba J., Rodriguez-Fornells A., Barbanoj M. J. Effects of ayahuasca on sensory and sensorimotor gating in humans as measured by P50 suppression and prepulse inhibition of the startle reflex, respectively. *Psychopharmacology*, 2002. **165**(1):18–28.

138. Umbricht D., Koller R., Vollenweider F. X., *et al.* Mismatch negativity predicts psychotic experiences induced by NMDA receptor antagonist in healthy volunteers. *Biol Psychiatry*, 2002. **51**(5):400–6.

139. Umbricht D., Vollenweider F. X., Schmid L., *et al.* Effects of the 5-HT2A agonist psilocybin on mismatch negativity generation and AX-continuous performance task: implications for the neuropharmacology of cognitive deficits in schizophrenia. *Neuropsychopharmacology*, 2003. **28**(1):170–81.

140. Gouzoulis-Mayfrank E., Heekeren K., Neukirch A., *et al.* Inhibition of return in the human 5HT(2A) agonist and NMDA antagonist model of psychosis. *Neuropsychopharmacology*, 2006. **31**(2):431–41.

141. Halpern J. H., Pope H. G. Hallucinogen persisting perception disorder: what do we know after 50 years? *Drug Alcohol Depend*, 2003. **69**(2):109–19.

142. AbiDargham A., Laruelle M., Charney D., *et al.* Serotonin and schizophrenia: a review. *Drugs Today*, 1996. **32**(2):171–85.

143. Iqbal N., van Praag H. M. The role of serotonin in schizophrenia. *Eur Neuropsychopharmacol.*, 1995. **5**:11–23.

144. Amargos-Bosch M., Lopez-Gil X., Artigas F., *et al.* Clozapine and olanzapine, but not haloperidol, suppress serotonin efflux in the medial prefrontal cortex elicited by phencyclidine and ketamine. *Intl J Neuropsychopharmacol*, 2006. **9**(5):565–73.

145. Lopez-Gil X., Babot Z., Amargos-Bosch M., *et al.* Clozapine and haloperidol differently suppress the MK-801-increased glutamatergic and serotonergic transmission in the medial prefrontal cortex of the rat. *Neuropsychopharmacology*, 2007. **32**(10):2087–97.

146. Breese G. R., Knapp D. J., Moy S. S. Integrative role for serotonergic and glutamatergic receptor mechanisms in the action of NMDA antagonists: potential relationships to antipsychotic drug actions on NMDA antagonist responsiveness. *Neurosci Biobehav Rev*, 2002. **26**(4):441–55.

147. Noda Y., Kamei H., Mamiya T., *et al.* Repeated phencyclidine treatment induces negative symptom-like behavior in forced swimming test in mice: imbalance of prefrontal serotonergic and dopaminergic functions. *Neuropsychopharmacology*, 2000. **23**(4):375–87.

148. Martin P., Carlsson M. L., Hjorth S. Systemic PCP treatment elevates brain extracellular 5-HT: a microdialysis study in awake rats. *Neuroreport*, 1998. **9**(13):2985–8.

149. Nichols C. D., Sanders-Bush E. A single dose of lysergic acid diethylamide influences gene expression patterns within the mammalian brain. *Neuropsychopharmacology*, 2002. **26**(5):634–42.

150. Solowij N. Ecstasy (3,4-methylenedioxymethamphetamine). *Curr Opin Psychiatry*, 1993. **6**:411–15.

151. Gamma A., Buck A., Berthold T., *et al.* 3,4-methylenedioxymeth-amphetamine (MDMA) modulates cortical and limbic brain activity as measured by [(H2O)-O-15]-PET in healthy humans. *Neuropsychophar-macology*, 2000. **23**(4): 388–95.

152. Parrott A. C. Human psychopharmacology of Ecstasy (MDMA): a review of 15 years of empirical research. *Hum Psychopharmacol*, 2001. **16**(8):557–77.

153. Bialer P. A. Designer drugs in the general hospital. *Psychiatr Clin North Am*, 2002. **25**(1):231–43.

154. World Health Organization. (1996). Amphetamine Like Stimulants. Report from the WHO meeting on amphetamines, MDMA and other psychostimulants. Geneva: WHO.

155. Cole J. C., Sumnall H. R. Altered states: the clinical effects of ecstasy. *Pharmacol Therapeutics*, 2003. **98**(1):35–58.

156. Green A. R., Mechan A. O., Elliott J. M., *et al.* The pharmacology and clinical pharmacology of 3,4-methylenedioxymethamphetamine (MDMA, "ecstasy"). *Pharmacol Rev*, 2003. **55**:463–508.

157. Landry M. J. MDMA: a review of epidemiologic data. *J Psychoactive Drugs*, 2002. **34**(2):163–9.

158. Australian Institute of Health and Welfare. (2005). *2004 National Drug Strategy Household Survey: Detailed Findings.* AIHW cat. no. PHE 66. Canberra: AIHW.

159. Australian Institute of Health and Welfare. (2002). *2001 National Drug Strategy Household Survey; First Results.* AIHW cat. no. PHE 35. Canberra: AIHW.

160. Degenhardt L., Copeland J., Dillon P. Recent trends in the use of "club drugs": an Australian review. *Subst Use Misuse*, 2005. **40**(9–10):1241–56.

161. Lenton S., Boys A., Norcross K. Raves, drugs and experience: drug use by a sample of people who attend raves in Western Australia. *Addiction*, 1997. **92**(10):1327–37.

162. Riley S. C. E., James C., Gregory D., *et al.* Patterns of recreational drug use at dance events in Edinburgh, Scotland. *Addiction*, 2001. **96**(7):1035–47.

163. Schifano F. A bitter pill. Overview of ecstasy (MDMA, MDA) related fatalities. *Psychopharmacology*, 2004. **173**(3–4):242–8.

164. Henry J. A., Jeffreys K. J., Dawling S. Toxicity and deaths from 3,4-methylenedioxymethamphetamine (Ecstasy). *Lancet*, 1992. **340**(8816):384–7.

165. Schifano F., Oyefeso A., Corkery J., *et al.* Death rates from ecstasy (MDMA, MDA) and polydrug use in England and Wales 1996–2002. *Hum Psychopharmacol*, 2003. **18**(7):519–24.

166. Schifano F., Corkery J., Deluca P., *et al.* Ecstasy (MDMA, MDA, MDEA, MBDB) consumption, seizures, related offences, prices, dosage levels and deaths in the UK (1994–2003). *J Psychopharmacol*, 2006. **20**(3):456–63.

167. Solowij N., Hall W., Lee N. Recreational MDMA use in Sydney – a profile of ecstasy users and their experiences with the drug. *Br J Addict*, 1992. **87**(8):1161–72.

168. Topp L., Hando J., Dillon P., *et al.* Ecstasy use in Australia: patterns of use and associated harm. *Drug Alcohol Depend*, 1999. **55**(1–2):105–15.

169. Lieb R., Schuetz C. G., Pfister H., *et al.* Mental disorders in ecstasy users: a prospective-longitudinal investigation. *Drug Alcohol Depend*, 2002. **68**(2):195–207.

170. Falck R. S., Carlson R. G., Wang J. C., *et al.* Psychiatric disorders and their correlates among young adult MDMA users in Ohio. *J Psychoactive Drugs*, 2006. **38**(1):19–29.

171. Sumnell H. R., Cole J. C. Self-reported depressive symptomatology in community samples of polysubstance misusers who report Ecstasy use: a meta-analysis. *J Psychopharmacol*, 2005. **19**(1):84–92.

172. Soar K., Turner J. J. D., Parrott A. C. Psychiatric disorders in Ecstasy (MDMA) users: a literature review focusing on personal predisposition and drug history. *Hum Psychopharmacol*, 2001. **16**(8):641–5.

173. Landabaso M. A., Iraurgi I., Jimenez-Lerma J. M., *et al.* Ecstasy-induced psychotic disorder: six-month follow-up study. *Eur Addiction Res*, 2002. **8**(3):133–40.

174. Gouzoulis E., Borchardt D., Hermle L. A case of toxic psychosis induced by Eve (3,4-Methylene-Dioxyethylam-Phetamine). *Arch Gen Psychiatry*, 1993. **50**(1):75.

175. Schuler S. Early recognition and early intervention in drug-induced psychoses. *Neurol Psychiatr Brain Res*, 1998. **5**(4):197–204.

176. Liechti M. E., Geyer M. A., Hell D., *et al.* Effects of MDMA (ecstasy) on prepulse inhibition and habituation of startle in humans after pretreatment with citalopram, haloperidol, or ketanserin. *Neuropsychopharmacology*, 2001. **24**(3):240–52.

177. Vollenweider F. X., Remensberger S., Hell D., *et al.* Opposite effects of 3,4-methylenedioxymethamphetamine (MDMA) on sensorimotor gating in rats versus healthy humans. *Psychopharmacology*, 1999. **143**(4):365–72.

178. Quednow B. B., Kuhn K. U., Hoenig K., *et al.* Prepulse inhibition and habituation of acoustic tartle response in male MDMA ('ecstasy') users, cannabis users, and healthy controls. *Neuropsychopharmacology*, 2004. **29**(5):982–90.

179. Geyer M. A., Markou A. (2002). The role of preclinical models in the development of psychotropic drugs. In *Neuropsychopharmacology: The Fifth Generation of Progress*. Davis K. L., Charney D., Coyle J. T., and Nemeroff C. (Eds.). Philadelphia: Lippincott Williams & Wilkins, pp. 445–55.

180. O'Neill M. F., Shaw G. Comparison of dopamine receptor antagonists on hyperlocomotion induced by cocaine, amphetamine, MK-801 and the dopamine D-1 agonist C-APB in mice. *Psychopharmacology (Berl)*, 1999. **145**:237–25.

181. Russell R. W. (1964). Extrapolation from animals to man. In *Animal Behavior and Drug Action*. Steinberg H.

(Ed.). Boston: Little, Brown, pp. 410–18.

182. Mathysse S. (1986). Animal models in psychiatric reasearch. In *Progress in Brain Research*, vol **65**, van Ree J. M. and Mathysse S. (Eds.). Amsterdam: Elsevier Science, pp. 259–70.

183. Creese I., Iversen S. D. Pharmacological and anatomical substrates of amphetamine response in rat. *Brain Res*, 1975. **83**(3):419–36.

184. Breier A., Malhotra A. K., Pinals D. A., *et al.* Association of ketamine-induced psychosis with focal activation of the prefrontal cortex in healthy volunteers. *Am J Psychiatry*, 1997; **154**(6):805–11.

185. Abi-Dargham A., Gil R., Krystal J., *et al.* Increased striatal dopamine transmission in schizophrenia: confirmation in a second cohort. *Am J Psychiatry*, 1998. **155**:761–7.

186. Homayoun H., Moghaddam B. Progression of cellular adaptations in medial prefrontal and orbitofrontal cortex in response to repeated amphetamine. *J Neurosci*, 2006; **26**(31):8025–39.

187. Hill K., Mann L., Laws K. R., *et al.* Hypofrontality in schizophrenia: a meta-analysis of functional imaging studies. *Acta Psychiat Scand*, 2004. **110**:243–56.

188. Dom G., Sabbe B., Hulstijn W., van den Brink W. Substance use disorders and the orbitofrontal cortex. *Br J Psychiat*, 2005. **187**:209–20.

189. Jentsch J. D., Roth R. H. The neuropsychopharmacology of phencyclidine: from NMDA receptor hypofunction to the dopamine hypothesis of schizophrenia. *Neuropsychopharmacology*, 1999. **20**(3):201–25.

190. Sams-Dodd F. Strategies to optimize the validity of disease models in the drug discovery

process. *Drug Discov Today*, 2006. **11**(7–8):355–63.

191. Jackson M. E., Homayoun H., Moghaddam B. NMDA receptor hypofunction produces concomitant firing rate potentiation and burst activity reduction in the prefrontal cortex. *Proc Natl Acad Sci USA* 2004. **101**(22):8467–72.

192. Carpenter W. T., Koenig J. I. The evolution of drug development in schizophrenia: past issues and future opportunities. *Neuropsychopharmacology*, 2008. **33**:2061–79. [Epub Nov 28, 2007.]

193. Agid Y., Buzsaki G., Diamond D. M., *et al.* Viewpoint – How can drug discovery for psychiatric disorders be improved? *Nat Rev Drug Discov*, 2007. **6**(3):189–201.

194. Robbins T. W. (2004). Animal models of psychosis. In *Neurobiology of Mental Illness.* Charney D. S., Nestler E. J. (Eds.). New York: Oxford University Press, pp. 263–86.

195. Kapur S., Seeman P. Ketamine has equal affinity for NMDA receptors and the high-affinity state of the dopamine D-2 recep. *Biol Psychiatr*, 2001. **49**(11):954–5.

196. Seeman P., Schwarz J., Chen J. F., *et al.* Psychosis pathways converge via D2(High) dopamine receptors. *Synapse*, 2006. **60**(4):319–46.

197. Kapur S., Seeman P. NMDA receptor antagonists ketamine and PCP have direct effects on the dopamine D-2 and serotonin 5-HT2 receptors – implications for models of schizophrenia. *Mol Psychiatry*, 2002. **7**(8):837–44.

198. Svenningsson P., Nomikos G. G., Greengard P. Response to comment on "Diverse psychotomimetics act through a common signaling pathway." *Science*, 2004; **305**(5681):180.

199. Jordan S., Chen R., Fernalld R., *et al.* In vitro biochemical evidence that the psychotomimetics phencyclidine, ketamine and dizocilpine (MK-801) are inactive

at cloned human and rat dopamine D-2 receptors. *Eur J Pharmacol*, 2006. **540**(1–3):53–6.

200. Svenningsson P., Nishi A., Fisone G., *et al.* DARPP-32: an integrator of neurotransmission. *Ann Rev Pharmacol Toxicol*, 2004. **44**:269–96.

201. Svenningsson P., Tzavara E. T., Carruthers R., *et al.* Diverse psychotomimetics act through a common signaling pathway. *Science*, 2003. **302**(5649):1412–15.

202. Rabiner E. A. Imaging of striatal dopamine release elicited with NMDA antagonists: is there anything there to be seen? *J Psychopharmacol*, 2007. **21**(3):253–8.

203. Davis S. M., Lees K. R., Albers G. W., *et al.* Selfotel in acute ischemic stroke – possible neurotoxic effects of an NMDA antagonist. *Stroke*, 2000. **31**(2):347–54.

204. Moghaddam B., Adams B. W. Reversal of phencyclidine effects by a group II metabotropic glutamate receptor agonist in rats. *Science*, 1998. **281**(5381):1349–52.

205. Hetzler B. E., Wautlet B. S. Ketamine-induced locomotion in rats in an open-field. *Pharmacol Biochem Behav*, 1985. **22**(4): 653–5.

206. Sams-Dodd F. Distinct effects of d-amphetamine and phencyclidine on the social behavior of rats. *Behav Pharmacol*, 1995. **6**(1):55–65.

207. Rung J. P., Carlsson A., Markinhuhta K. R., *et al.* (+)-MK-801 induced social withdrawal in rats: a model for negative symptoms of schizophrenia. *Prog Neuropsychopharmacol Biol Psychiatry*, 2005. **29**(5):827–32.

208. Duncan G. E., Miyamoto S., Leipzig J. N., *et al.* Comparison of brain metabolic activity patterns induced by ketamine, MK-801 and amphetamine in rats: support for NMDA receptor involvement in responses to subanesthetic dose

of ketamine. *Brain Res*, 1999. **843**(1–2):171–83.

209. Duncan G. E., Leipzig J. N., Mailman R. B., *et al.* Differential effects of clozapine and haloperidol on ketamine-induced brain metabolic activation. *Brain Res*, 1998. **812**(1–2):65–75.

210. Duncan G. E., Moy S. S., Knapp D. J., *et al.* Metabolic mapping of the rat brain after subanesthetic doses of ketamine: potential relevance to schizophrenia. *Brain Res*, 1998. **787**(2):181–90.

211. Littlewood C. L., Jones N., O'Neill M. J., *et al.* Mapping the central effects of ketamine in the rat using pharmacological MRI. *Psychopharmacology*, 2006. **186**(1):64–81.

212. Wu J. C., Buchsbaum M. S., Potkin S. G., *et al.* Positron emission tomography study of phencyclidine users. *Schizophr Res*, 1991. **4**(3):415.

213. Cochran S. M., Kennedy M., McKerchar C. E., *et al.* Induction of metabolic hypofunction and neurochemical deficits after chronic intermittent exposure to phencyclidine: differential modulation by antipsychotic drugs. *Neuropsychopharmacology*, 2003. **28**(2):265–75.

214. Wickelgren I. Neurobiology – a new route to treating schizophrenia? *Science*, 1998. **281**(5381):1264–5.

215. Moghaddam B., Adams B., Verma A., *et al.* Activation of glutamatergic neurotransmission by ketamine: a novel step in the pathway from NMDA receptor blockade to dopaminergic and cognitive disruptions associated with the prefrontal cortex. *J Neurosci*, 1997. **17**(8):2921–7.

216. Adams B., Moghaddam B. Corticolimbic dopamine neurotransmission is temporally dissociated from the cognitive and locomotor effects of phencyclidine. *J Neurosci*, 1998. **18**(14):5545–54.

165

217. Liu J., Moghaddam B. Regulation of glutamate efflux by excitatory amino-acid receptors – evidence for tonic inhibitory and phasic excitatory regulation. *J Pharmacol Exp Thera*, 1995. **274**(3):1209–15.

218. Homayoun L., Jackson M. E., Moghaddam B. Activation of metabotropic glutamate 2/3 receptors reverses the effects of NMDA receptor hypofunction on prefrontal cortex unit activity in awake rats. *J Neurophysiol*, 2005. **93**(4):1989–2001.

219. Homayoun H., Moghaddam B. Fine-tuning of awake prefrontal cortex neurons by clozapine: comparison with haloperidol and N-desmethylclozapine. *Biol Psychiatry*, 2007. **61**(5):679–87.

220. Homayoun H., Moghaddam B. NMDA receptor hypofunction produces opposite effects on prefrontal cortex interneurons and pyramidal neurons. *J Neurosci*, 2007. **27**(43): 11496–500.

221. Suzuki Y., Jodo E., Takeuchi S., *et al.* Acute administration of phencyclidine induces tonic activation of medial prefrontal cortex neurons in freely moving rats. *Neuroscience*, 2002. **114**(3):769–79.

222. Jodo E., Suzuki Y., Katayama T., *et al.* Activation of medial prefrontal cortex by phencyclidine is mediated via a hippocampo-prefrontal pathway. *Cereb Cortex*, 2005. **15**(5):663–9.

223. Katayama T., Jodo E., Suzuki Y., *et al.* Activation of medial prefrontal cortex neurons by phencyclidine is mediated via AMPA/kainate glutamate receptors in anesthetized rats. *Neuroscience*, 2007. **150**(2):442–8.

224. Sharp F. R., Tomitaka M., Bernaudin M., *et al.* Psychosis: pathological activation of limbic thalamocortical circuits by psychomimetics and schizophrenia? *Trends Neurosc*, 2001. **24**(6):330–4.

225. Krystal J. H., Abi-Dargham A., Laruelle M., *et al.* (2004). Pharmacological models of psychoses. In *Neurobiology of Mental Illness*. Charney D. S. and Nestler E. J. (Eds.). New York: Oxford University Press, pp. 287–98.

226. Gulyas A. I., Megias M., Emri Z., *et al.* Total number and ratio of excitatory and inhibitory synapses converging onto single interneurons of different types in the CA1 area of the rat hippocampus. *J Neurosci*, 1999. **19**:10082–97.

227. Jones R. S. G., Buhl E. H. Basket-like interneurons in layer II of the entorhinal cortex exhibit a powerful NMDA-mediated synaptic excitation. *Neurosci Lett*, 1993. **149**(1):35–9.

228. Goldberg J. H., Yuste R., Tamas G. Ca2+ imaging of mouse neocortical interneurone dendrites: contribution of Ca2+-permeable AMPA and NMDA receptors to subthreshold Ca2 +dynamics. *J Physiol*, 2003. **551**(1):67–78.

229. Cochran S. M., Fujimura M., Morris B. J., *et al.* Acute and delayed effects of phencyclidine upon mRNA levels of markers of glutamatergic and GABAergic neurotransmitter function in the rat brain. *Synapse*, 2002. **46**(3):206–14.

230. Rujescu D., Bender A., Keck M., *et al.* A pharmacological model for psychosis based on N-methyl-D-aspartate receptor hypofunction: Molecular, cellular, functional and behavioral abnormalities. *Biol Psychiatry*, 2006. **59**(8):721–9.

231. Abdul-Monim Z., Neill J. C., Reynolds G. P. Sub-chronic psychotomimetic phencyclidine induces deficits in reversal learning and alterations in parvalbumin-immuno-reactive expression in the rat. *J Psychopharmacol*, 2007. **21**(2):198–205.

232. Keilhoff G., Becker A., Grecksch G., *et al.* Repeated application of ketamine to rats induces changes in the hippocampal expression of parvalbumin, neuronal nitric oxide synthase and cFOS similar to those found in human schizophrenia. *Neuroscience*, 2004. **126**(3):591–8.

233. Morrow B. A., Elsworth J. D., Roth R. H. Repeated phencyclidine in monkeys results in loss of parvalbumin-containing axo-axonic projections in the prefrontal cortex. *Psychopharmacology*, 2007. **192**(2):283–90.

234. Kinney J. W., Davis C. N., Tabarean I., *et al.* A specific role for NR2A-containing NMDA receptors in the maintenance of parvalbumin and GAD67 immunoreactivity in cultured interneurons. *J Neurosci*, 2006. **26**(5):1604–15.

235. Bartos M., Vida I., Jonas P. Synaptic mechanisms of synchronized gamma oscillations in inhibitory interneuron networks. *Nat Rev Neurosci*, 2007. **8**(1):45–56.

236. Cunningham M. O., Hunt J., Middleton S., *et al.* Region-specific reduction in entorhinal gamma oscillations and parvalbumin-immunoreactive neurons in animal models of psychiatric illness. *J Neurosci*, 2006. **26**(10):2767–76.

237. Lewis D. A., Gonzalez-Burgos G. Pathophysiologically based treatment interventions in schizophrenia. *Nat Med*, 2006. **12**(9):1016–22.

238. Lewis D. A., Hashimoto T. Deciphering the disease process of schizophrenia: the contribution of cortical GABA neurons. *Int Rev Neurobiol*, 2007. **78**:109–31.

239. Lewis D. A., Hashimoto T., Volk D. W. Cortical inhibitory neurons and schizophrenia. *Nat Rev Neurosci*, 2005. **6**(4):312–24.

240. Lewis D. A., Gonzalez-Burgos G. Neuroplasticity of neocortical circuits in schizophrenia. *Neuropsychopharmacology*, 2008. **33**:141–65.

241. Reynolds G. P., Harte M. K. The neuronal pathology of schizophrenia: molecules and mechanisms. *Biochem Soc Trans*, 2007. **35**:433–6.

242. Basar-Eroglu C., Brand A., Hildebrandt H., *et al.* Working memory related gamma oscillations in schizophrenia patients. *Intl J Psychophysiol*, 2007. **64**(1):39–45.

243. Symond M. B., Harris A. W. F., Gordon E., *et al.* "Gamma synchrony" in first-episode schizophrenia: a disorder of temporal connectivity? *Am J Psychiatry*, 2005. **162**(3):459–65.

244. Light G. A., Hsu J. L., Hsieh M. H., *et al.* Gamma band oscillations reveal neural network cortical coherence dysfunction in schizophrenia patients. *Biol Psychiatry*, 2006. **60**(11):1231–40.

245. Spencer K. M. Abnormal neural synchrony in schizophrenia. *Psychophysiology*, 2003. **40**:S17

246. Behrens M. M., Ali S. S., Dao D. N., *et al.* Ketamine-induced loss of phenotype of fast-spiking interneurons is mediated by NADPH-oxidase. *Science*, 2007. **318**(5856):1645–7.

247. Jentsch J. D., Elsworth J. D., Redmond D. E., *et al.* Phencyclidine increases forebrain monoamine metabolism in rats and monkeys: modulation by the isomers of HA966. *J Neurosci*, 1997. **17**(5):1769–75.

248. Jentsch J. D., Tran A., Le D., *et al.* Subchronic phencyclidine administration reduces mesoprefrontal dopamine utilization and impairs prefrontal cortical-dependent cognition in the rat. *Neuropsychopharmacology*, 1997. **17**(2):92–9.

249. Jentsch J. D., Redmond D. E., Elsworth J. D., *et al.* Enduring cognitive deficits and cortical dopamine dysfunction in monkeys after long-term administration of phencyclidine. *Science*, 1997. **277**(5328):953–5.

250. Kristiansen L. V., Huerta I., Beneyto M., *et al.* NMDA receptors and schizophrenia. *Curr Opin Pharmacol*, 2007. **7**(1):48–55.

251. Javitt D. C. Glutamate and schizophrenia: phencyclidine, N-methyl-D-aspartate receptors, and dopamine-glutamate interactions. *Int Rev Neurobiol*, 2007. **78**:69.

252. Catts S. V., Ward P. B., Lloyd A., *et al.* Molecular biological investigations into the role of the NMDA receptor in the pathophysiology of schizophrenia. *Aust NZ J Psychiatry*, 1997. **31**(1):17–26.

253. Carlsson A. The current status of the dopamine hypothesis of schizophrenia. *Neuropsychopharmacology*, 1988. **1**(3):179–86.

254. Carlsson M., Carlsson A. Schizophrenia – a subcortical neurotransmitter imbalance syndrome. *Schizophr Bull*, 1990. **16**(3):425–32.

255. Brody S. A., Geyer M. A., Large C. H. Lamotrigine prevents ketamine but not amphetamine-induced deficits in prepulse inhibition in mice. *Psychopharmacology (Berl)*, 2003. **169**(3–4):240–6.

256. Anand A., Charney D. S., Oren D. A., *et al.* Attenuation of the neuropsychiatric effects of ketamine with lamotrigine – support for hyperglutamatergic effects of N-methyl-D-aspartate receptor antagonists. *Arch Gen Psychiatry*, 2000. **57**(3):270–6.

257. Large C. H., Webster E. L., Goff D. C. The potential role of lamotrigine in schizophrenia. *Psychopharmacology*, 2005. **181**(3):415–36.

258. Kremer I., Vass A., Gorelik I., *et al.* Placebo-controlled trial of lamotrigine added to conventional and atypical antipsychotics in schizophrenia. *Biol Psychiatr*, 2004. **56**(6):441–6.

259. Dursun S. M., Deakin J. F.W. Augmenting antipsychotic treatment with lamotrigine or topiramate in patients with treatment-resistant schizophrenia: a naturalistic case series outcome study. *J Psychopharmacol*, 2001. **15**(4):297–301.

260. Dursun S. M., McIntosh D. Clozapine plus lamotrigine in treatment-resistant schizophrenia. *Arch Gen Psychiatry*, 1999. **56**(10):950.

261. Zoccali R., Muscatello M. R., Bruno A., *et al.* The effect of lamotrigine augmentation of clozapine in a sample of treatment-resistant schizophrenic patients: a double-blind, placebo-controlled study. *Schizophr Res*, 2007. **93**(1–3):109–16.

262. Tiihonen J., Hallikainen T., Ryynanen O. P., *et al.* Lamotrigine in treatment-resistant schizophrenia: a randomized placebo-controlled crossover trial. *Biol Psychiatry*, 2003. **54**(11):1241–8.

263. Ahmad S., Fowler L. J., Whitton P. S. Lamotrigine, carbamazepine and phenytoin differentially alter extracellular levels of 5-hydroxytryptamine, dopamine and amino acids. *Epilepsy Res*, 2005. **63**(2–3):141–9.

264. Harsing L. G., Gacsalyi I., Szabo G., *et al.* The glycine transporter-1 inhibitors NFPS and Org 24461: a pharmacological study. *Pharmacol Biochem Behav*, 2003. **74**(4):811–25.

265. Lane H. Y., Liu Y. C., Huang C. L., *et al.* Sarcosine (N-methylglycine) treatment for acute schizophrenia: a randomized, double-blind study. *Biol Psychiatr*, 2008. **63**(1):9–12.

266. Tsai G. C., Lane H. Y., Yang P. C., *et al.* Glycine transporter I inhibitor, N-methylglycine

(Sarcosine), added to antipsychotics for the treatment of schizophrenia. *Biol Psychiatr*, 2004. **55**(5):452–6.

267. Lane H. Y., Huang C. L., Wu P. L., *et al.* Glycine transporter I inhibitor, N-methylglycine (Sarcosine), added to clozapine for the treatment of schizophrenia. *Biol Psychiatr*, 2006. **60**(6):645–9.

268. Neale J. H., Olszewski R. T., Gehl L. M., *et al.* The neurotransmitter N-acetylaspartylglutamate in models of pain, ALS, diabetic neuropathy, CNS injury and schizophrenia. *Trends Pharmacol Sci*, 2005. **26**(9):477–84.

269. Olszewski R. T., Bukhari N., Zhou J., *et al.* NAAG peptidase inhibition reduces locomotor activity and some stereotypes in the PCP model of schizophrenia via group II mGluR. *J Neuro*, 2004. **89**(4):876–85.

270. Olszewski R. T., Wegorzewska M. M., Monteiro A. C., *et al.* Phencyclidine and dizocilpine induced behaviors reduced by N-acetylaspartylglutamate peptidase inhibition via metabotropic glutamate receptors. *Biol Psychiatr*, 2008. **63**(1):86–91.

271. Schoepp D. D., Johnson B. G., Wright R. A., *et al.* LY354740 is a potent and highly selective group II metabotropic glutamate receptor agonist in cells expressing human glutamate receptors. *Neuropharmacology*, 1997. **36**(1):1–11.

272. Krystal J. H., Abi-Saab W., Perry E., *et al.* Preliminary evidence of attenuation of the disruptive effects of the NMDA glutamate receptor antagonist, ketamine, on working memory by pretreatment with the group II metabotropic glutamate receptor agonist, LY354740, in healthy human subjects. *Psychopharmacology*, 2005. **179**(1):303–9.

273. Patil S. T., Zhang L., Martenyi F., *et al.* Activation of mGlu2/3 receptors as a new approach to treat schizophrenia: a randomized Phase 2 clinical trial. *Nat Med*, 2007. **13**(9):1102–7.

274. Kim J. S., Kornhuber H. H., Schmidburgk W., *et al.* Low cerebrospinal-fluid glutamate in schizophrenic patients and a new hypothesis on schizophrenia. *Neurosci Lett*, 1980. **20**(3):379–82.

275. Wachtel H., Turski L. Glutamate – a new target in schizophrenia. *Trends Pharmacol Sci*, 1990. **11**(6):219–22.

276. Farber N. B., Wozniak D. F., Price M. T., *et al.* Age-specific neurotoxicity in the rat associated with NMDA receptor blockade: potential relevance to schizophrenia? *Biol Psychiatr*, 1995. **38**(12):788–96.

277. Keshavan M. S., Anderson S., Pettegrew J. W. Is schizophrenia due to excessive synaptic pruning in the prefrontal cortex – the Feinberg Hypothesis revisited. *J Psychiatr Res*, 1994. **28**(3):239–65.

278. Glantz L. A., Lewis D. A. Decreased dendritic spine density on prefrontal cortical pyramidal neurons in schizophrenia. *Arch Gen Psychiatr*, 2000. **57**(1):65–73.

279. Halberstadt A. L. The phencyclidine glutamate model of schizophrenia. *Clin Neuropharmacol*, 1995. **18**(3):237–49.

280. Tsai G. C., Coyle J. T. Glutamatergic mechanisms in schizophrenia. *Ann Rev Pharmacol Toxicol*, 2002. **42**:165–79.

281. Hirsch S. R., Das I., Garey L. J., *et al.* A pivotal role for glutamate in the pathogenesis of schizophrenia, and its cognitive dysfunction. *Pharmacol Biochem Behav*, 1997. **56**(4):797–802.

282. Krystal J. H., D'Souza D. C., Mathalon D., *et al.* NMDA receptor antagonist effects, cortical glutamatergic function, and schizophrenia: toward a paradigm shift in medication development. *Psychopharmacology*, 2003. **169**(3–4):215–33.

283. Stone J. M., Morrison P. D., Pilowsky L. S. Glutamate and dopamine dysregulation in schizophrenia – a synthesis and selective review. *J Psychopharmacol*, 2007. **21**(4):440–52.

284. Jarskog L. F., Glantz L. A., Gilmore J. H., *et al.* Apoptotic mechanisms in the pathophysiology of schizophrenia. *Prog Neurosychopharmacol Biol Psychiatry*, 2005. **29**(5):846–58.

285. Catts V. S., Catts S. V., McGrath J. J., *et al.* Apoptosis and schizophrenia: a pilot study based on dermal fibroblast cell lines. *Schizophr Res*, 2006. **84**(1):20–8.

286. Lipska B. K. Using animal models to test a neurodevelopmental hypothesis of schizophrenia. *J Psychiatr Neurosci*, 2004. **29**(4):282–6.

287. Ozawa K., Hashimoto K., Kishimoto T., *et al.* Immune activation during pregnancy in mice leads to dopaminergic hyperfunction and cognitive impairment in the offspring: a neurodevelopmental animal model of schizophrenia. *Biol Psychiat*, 2006. **59**(6):546–54.

288. Paylor R., McIlwain K. L., McAninch R., *et al.* Mice deleted for the DiGeorge/velocardiofacial syndrome region show abnormal sensorimotor gating and learning and memory impairments. *Hum Mol Genet*, 2001. **10**(23):2645–50.

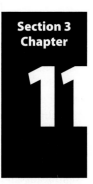

Schizophrenia secondary to cannabis use

Wayne Hall and Louisa Degenhardt

Facts box

- There are good theoretical reasons why cannabis may be a contributor to the development of schizophrenia.

- There is compelling evidence that cannabis use and psychosis are associated, and the debate is on whether cannabis use is a *cause* of psychosis.

- There is strong evidence from longitudinal studies that cannabis use may precipitate schizophrenia in vulnerable individuals.

- The vulnerability to cannabis-induced psychosis may be genetic, but further research is needed to support the preliminary evidence.

- There is also reasonable evidence that cannabis use exacerbates symptoms of psychosis in persons with a psychosis who continue to use cannabis.

- The evidence does not rule out the possibility that persons with psychosis use cannabis to control some of their symptoms or to improve their mood, but the self-medication hypothesis is unlikely to wholly explain the relationship observed between cannabis use and psychosis.

- Cannabis may promote psychosis directly through the cannabinoid system or indirectly through the dopaminergic system. More biological research on these mechanisms is necessary.

Introduction

There are good reasons for suspecting that regular cannabis use may be a contributory cause of schizophrenia. First, tetrahydrocannabinol (THC), the major psychoactive ingredient in cannabis preparations, can produce euphoria, distorted time perception, cognitive and memory impairments [1, 2, 3]. Under controlled laboratory conditions, normal volunteers using THC in high doses have reported visual and auditory hallucinations, delusional ideas, and thought disorder [4, 5]. Second, a putative clinical entity of "cannabis psychosis" has been identified by clinical observers in India, Egypt, and the Caribbean, regions with a long history of heavy cannabis use [1, 6].

A number of possible causal relationships have been suggested between cannabis use and psychosis [3]. The *first* possibility is that cannabis use may produce a specific psychosis de novo. Three variants of this hypothesis can be distinguished: i) that large doses of cannabis may induce a toxic paranoid psychosis that is analogous to that produced by large doses of amphetamine; ii) that heavy cannabis use may produce an acute functional psychosis clinically similar to paranoid schizophrenia; or iii) that chronic cannabis use may produce a psychotic disorder that persists beyond the period of intoxication. A *second* possibility is that cannabis use could precipitate an episode of schizophrenia in a vulnerable or predisposed individual. A *third* possibility is that cannabis use may exacerbate the symptoms of schizophrenia by precipitating more frequent relapses, or the pharmacological effects of THC might impair the effectiveness of the neuroleptic drugs used to treat schizophreniform psychoses.

These possibilities have not always been distinguished, and, until recently, our ability to decide between them has been hampered by a lack of sophistication in research design [3, 7, 8, 9, 10]. Because there is currently compelling evidence that cannabis use and psychosis are associated, the debate now concerns whether cannabis use is or is not a contributory *cause* of psychosis and indeed, what we mean by "cause" [10].

Cannabis use as a precipitant of psychosis

There is consistent evidence that cannabis use occurs at a much higher rate among patients with schizophrenia than among their age peers in the community [11]. There is also good epidemiological evidence for an association between schizophrenia and drug abuse and dependence in the community. The Epidemiological Catchment Area (ECA) study from the USA [12] found that the lifetime prevalence of drug abuse and dependence was 6.2% (7.7% among men and 4.8% among women), with abuse and dependence on cannabis the most common form of drug abuse and dependence, with a lifetime prevalence of 4.4%. The National Survey of Mental Health and Wellbeing (NSMHWB) conducted in Australia in 1997 included a screening questionnaire for psychotic symptoms [13]. A diagnosis of cannabis dependence increased the chances of reporting psychotic symptoms 1.7 times, after adjusting for age, affective and anxiety disorders, smoking status, and alcohol dependence [14]. In the NSMHWB, 11.5% of those who reported that they had been diagnosed with schizophrenia met ICD-10 criteria for a cannabis use disorder in the past 12 months. After adjusting for confounding variables, those who met criteria for cannabis dependence were 2.9 times more likely to report that they had been diagnosed with schizophrenia than those who did not.

Longitudinal studies

The first convincing evidence that cannabis use may precipitate schizophrenia was provided by a study of Swedish conscripts [15]. These investigators conducted a 15-year prospective study of 50,465 Swedish conscripts to investigate the relationship between self-reported cannabis use at age 18 and the risk of receiving a psychiatric diagnosis of schizophrenia in the subsequent period, as indicated by inclusion in the Swedish psychiatric case register. Their results showed that the relative risk of receiving a diagnosis of schizophrenia was 2.4 (95% confidence interval [1.8, 3.3]) for those who had ever tried cannabis compared with those who had not. There was also a dose-response relationship between the risk of a diagnosis of schizophrenia and the number of times that the conscript had tried cannabis by age 18. The relative risk of developing schizophrenia was 1.3 (0.8, 2.3) for those who had used cannabis 1 to 10 times, 3.0 (1.6,

5.5) for those who had used cannabis between 1 and 50 times, and 6.0 (4.0, 8.9) for those who had used cannabis more than 50 times. The size of these risks was reduced by adjustment for confounding variables that were related to the risk of developing schizophrenia (namely, having a psychiatric diagnosis at conscription and having parents who had divorced). Nevertheless, the relationship between cannabis use and schizophrenia remained statistically significant and still showed a dose-response relationship.

Andreasson and colleagues [15] and Allebeck [16] argued from the earlier study that cannabis use precipitated schizophrenia in vulnerable individuals, rejecting as implausible the hypothesis that cannabis use was a consequence of emerging schizophrenia. First, the cannabis users who developed schizophrenia had better premorbid personalities, a more abrupt onset, and more positive symptoms than the nonusers who developed schizophrenia [16]. Second, although more than half of the heavy cannabis users (58%) had a psychiatric diagnosis at the time of conscription, there was still a dose-response relationship between cannabis use and risk of schizophrenia among conscripts who had psychiatric symptoms at baseline.

Critics suggested a number of alternative explanations for the findings by Andreasson and colleagues [15]. First, there was a long delay between self-reported cannabis use – at age 18–20 – and the diagnosis of schizophrenia – over the next 15 years [17, 18], and it was not clear that these individuals continued to use cannabis up until the time that schizophrenia was diagnosed. Andreasson and colleagues showed that self-reported cannabis use at age 18 was strongly related to the risk of attracting a diagnosis of drug abuse, suggesting that cannabis use at age 18 was predictive of continued drug use.

A second explanation was that the excessive rate of "schizophrenia" among the heavy cannabis users was due to cannabis-induced schizophreniform psychoses [17, 18]. Andreasson and colleagues addressed this criticism by a small study of the validity of the schizophrenia diagnoses, which suggested that 80% of those so diagnosed met DSM-III criteria, among which is a requirement of at least 6 months' duration that would exclude transient drug-induced psychoses.

Third, the relationship between cannabis use and schizophrenia may have been confounded by the use of other psychoactive drugs. Frequent cannabis use in late adolescence predicts the later use of amphetamine and cocaine [19, 20] which can produce paranoid psychoses [21, 22, 23, 24, 25]. The major illicit drug of abuse in Sweden during the study period [26, 27, 28], was amphetamine, making it difficult to exclude the hypothesis that amphetamine rather than cannabis explained the association between cannabis use and schizophrenia.

A fourth criticism was that Andreasson and colleagues had not ruled out the possibility that cannabis use at age 18 was a symptom of emerging schizophrenia. Statistical adjustment for a psychiatric diagnosis at conscription did not eliminate the relationship between cannabis use and schizophrenia, but it substantially reduced its size, because more than half of the heavy cannabis users had received a psychiatric diagnosis by age 18.

A number of longitudinal studies have since been reported that have supported the findings of the Andreassen and colleagues study and addressed many of the criticisms made of their study. Zammit and colleagues [29] reported a 27-year follow-up of the Swedish cohort that covered most of the risk period for the onset of psychotic disorders in the cohort. This study improved on the Andreassen and colleagues [15] study in a number of ways. The psychiatric register provided a more complete coverage of all cases diagnosed with schizophrenia; there was better statistical control of more potential confounding variables, including other drug use, IQ, and known risk factors for schizophrenia and social integration; the study distinguished between cases in the first 5 years of the study and those that occurred more than 5 years afterwards in order to look at the possible role of a prodrome; and the study undertook separate analyses in those who only reported using cannabis at the initial assessment.

Zammit and colleagues found that cannabis use at age 18 predicted an increased risk of schizophrenia during the follow-up period, with a dose-response relationship between frequency of cannabis use at age 18 and risk of being diagnosed with schizophrenia during the follow-up. The relationship between cannabis use and schizophrenia persisted after statistically controlling for the effects of other drug use and other potential confounding factors, including psychiatric symptoms at age 18. They estimated that 13% of cases of schizophrenia could be averted if all cannabis use were prevented. The same relationships were observed in the subset of the sample who only reported cannabis use at baseline and among cases diagnosed in the first 5 years after assessment and for the 22 years after-

wards. The relationship was a little stronger in cases observed in the first 5 years, probably reflecting the decline in cannabis use with age.

Zammit's findings have been supported by van Os and colleagues [30] in a 3-year longitudinal study of the relationship between self-reported cannabis use and psychosis in a community sample of 4,848 people in the Netherlands. Subjects were assessed at baseline on cannabis and other drug use and psychotic symptoms were assessed using a computerized diagnostic interview. A diagnosis of psychosis was validated in positive cases by a diagnostic telephone interview with a psychiatrist or psychologist. A consensus clinical judgement was made on the basis of the interview material as to whether individuals had a psychotic disorder for which they were in need of psychiatric care.

Van Os and colleagues substantially replicated the findings of the Swedish cohort and extended them in a number of important ways. First, cannabis use at baseline predicted an increased risk of psychotic symptoms during the follow-up period in individuals who had not reported psychiatric symptoms at baseline. Second, there was a dose-response relationship between frequency of cannabis use at baseline and risk of psychotic symptoms during follow up. Third, the relationship between cannabis use and psychotic symptoms persisted when they statistically controlled for the effects of other drug use. Fourth, the relationship between cannabis use and psychotic symptoms was stronger for persons with more severe psychotic symptoms who were judged to be in need of psychiatric care. Van Os and colleagues estimated the attributable risk of cannabis to psychosis was 13% for psychotic symptoms and 50% for cases with psychotic disorders in need of treatment. Fifth, those who reported any psychotic symptoms at baseline were more likely to develop schizophrenia if they used cannabis than were individuals who were not so vulnerable. They estimated that cannabis use accounted for 80% of the increased risk of developing a psychotic disorder that warranted treatment among vulnerable individuals.

A 1-year follow-up of a cohort of 2,437 adolescents and young adults between 1995 and 1999 in Munich [31] has substantially replicated the Swedish and Dutch studies. Subjects were assessed at baseline on cannabis use and psychotic symptoms using a questionnaire; psychotic symptoms were assessed in early adulthood using the Computerized International Diagnostic Interview. Henquet and colleagues

[31] found a dose-response relationship between self-reported cannabis use at baseline and the likelihood of reporting psychotic symptoms. As in the Dutch cohort, young people who reported psychotic symptoms at baseline were much more likely to experience psychotic symptoms at follow-up if they used cannabis than were peers who did not have such a history.

Arseneault and colleagues [32] reported a prospective study of the relationship between adolescent cannabis use and psychosis in young adults in a New Zealand birth cohort ($N = 759$) whose members had been assessed intensively on risk factors for psychotic symptoms and disorders since birth. Psychotic disorders were assessed according to DSM-IV diagnostic criteria, with corroborative reports from family members or friends on social adjustment. They assessed psychotic symptoms at age 11 *before* the onset of cannabis use and distinguished between early and late onset cannabis use. They also examined the specificity of the association between cannabis use and psychosis by conducting analyses of the effects of: i) other drug use on psychotic symptoms and disorders; and ii) cannabis use on depressive disorders.

Arseneault and colleagues found a relationship between cannabis use by age 15 and an increased risk of psychotic symptoms by age 26. Controlling for other drug use did not affect the relationship. The relationship was no longer statistically significant after adjustment for reporting psychotic symptoms at age 11, which probably reflected the small number of psychotic disorders observed in the sample. The small number of cases also limited the ability of the study to examine predictors of psychotic disorders at age 26. The measurement of cannabis and other drug use was crude (i.e., none, 1, 2, and 3 or more times), although this was more likely to work against finding relationships. There was no relationship between other drug use and psychotic disorders and no relationship between cannabis use and depression. There was also an interaction between psychosis risk and the age of onset of cannabis use, with earlier onset being more strongly related to psychosis. In addition, there was the suggestion of an interaction between cannabis use and vulnerability, with a higher risk of psychosis among cannabis users who reported psychotic symptoms at age 11.

Caspi and colleagues [33] subsequently reported an analysis of data from this cohort on an interaction between risk of psychosis and cannabis use and a functional polymorphism of the COMT gene that codes for dopamine. They found that the 25% of the cohort who were homozygous for a polymorphism and used cannabis were 10.9 times more likely to have developed a schizophreniform disorder than peers with the same polymorphism who did not use cannabis. In the absence of this polymorphism, young adults who used cannabis did not seem to be at any increased risk of a psychosis.

Fergusson, Horwood, and Swain-Campbell [34] have reported a longitudinal study of the relationship between cannabis dependence at age 18 and the number of psychotic symptoms reported at age 21 in the Christchurch birth cohort in New Zealand. They assessed cannabis dependence using DSM-IV criteria and psychotic symptoms were assessed by 10 items from the SCL-90. Because this was a birth cohort that had been assessed throughout childhood and adolescence, Fergusson and colleagues were able to adjust for a large number of potential confounding variables, including self-reported psychotic symptoms at the previous assessment, other drug use, and other psychiatric disorders. They found that cannabis dependence at age 18 predicted an increased risk of psychotic symptoms at age 21 years (*RR* of 2.3). This association was smaller but still significant after adjustment for potential confounders (*RR* of 1.8).

More recently, Fergusson and colleagues examined the association between cannabis and psychotic symptoms until age 25 years with the same cohort of young adults, using a more sophisticated fixed-effects regression analysis and structural equations modeling to account for both observed and nonobserved confounding factors [35]. As with their earlier study, they concluded that the association between cannabis and psychosis did not appear to be explained by measured or unmeasured confounding factors. The structural equations modeling suggested that the direction of the association appeared to be from cannabis use to psychotic symptoms rather than vice versa.

The longitudinal studies have found consistent associations between cannabis use in adolescence and psychotic symptoms in early adult life but all share a weakness: uncertainty about the temporal relationship between cannabis use and the timing of the onset of psychotic symptoms. Subjects in these studies have usually been assessed once a year (or less often) and they have typically reported retrospectively on their cannabis use during the preceding period, often crudely as to the number of times that cannabis was used, or the number of times it was typically used per week or month.

A French study provides greater detail on the temporal relationship between cannabis use and psychotic symptoms using an experience sampling method [36]. These investigators asked 79 college students to report on their drug use and experience of psychotic symptoms at randomly selected time points, several times each day over 7 consecutive days. The ratings were prompted by randomly programmed signals sent to a portable electronic device that the students carried. The students were a stratified sample from a larger group so that high cannabis users ($N = 41$) and students identified as vulnerable to psychosis ($N = 16$) were over-represented in the sample. Vulnerability to psychosis was indicated by reporting one or more psychotic symptoms in the past month during a personal interview.

Verdoux and colleagues [36] found a positive association between self-reported cannabis use and unusual perceptions and a negative association between cannabis use and hostility. That is, in time periods when cannabis was used, users reported more unusual perceptions and less hostility. These relationships depended upon vulnerability to psychosis: in vulnerable individuals cannabis use was more strongly associated with strange impressions and unusual perceptions and its use did not decrease feelings of hostility in the way that it did in individuals who lacked this vulnerability.

The self-medication hypothesis

The reasons that most persons with schizophrenia give for using alcohol, cannabis, and other illicit drugs are similar to those given by persons who do not have schizophrenia, namely, to relieve boredom, to provide stimulation, to feel good, and to socialize with peers [37, 38, 39]. The drugs that are most often used by patients with schizophrenia are also those that are used by their peers, namely, tobacco, alcohol, and cannabis. There is some evidence that some patients with schizophrenia report using cannabis because its euphoric effects help to relieve negative symptoms and depression [37, 40, 41, 42].

Nonetheless, the self-medication hypothesis was not supported by the van Os, Henquet, or Fergusson studies [30, 31, 34]. None of these studies found any relationship between early psychotic symptoms and an increased risk of using cannabis as required by the self-medication hypothesis; the relationship flowed from early cannabis use to psychosis rather than vice versa. Their negative results have been supported by the Verdoux and colleagues study of the temporal relationship between cannabis use and psychotic symptoms using an experience sampling method [43]; and in a recent prospective Australian study of persons with psychosis who used cannabis [37]. This evidence does not rule out the possibility that persons with psychosis use cannabis to control some of their symptoms or to improve their mood but it makes it unlikely that the self-medication hypothesis wholly explains the relationship observed between cannabis use and psychosis.

Intervention studies

If we could reduce cannabis use among patients with schizophrenia, then we could discover if their risk of relapse was reduced. The major challenge in doing so is, knowing how to reduce cannabis use in persons with schizophrenia. There are very few controlled outcome studies of substance abuse treatment in schizophrenia [44] and few of these have produced large enough benefits of treatment or treated a large enough number of patients, to provide an adequate chance of detecting any positive impacts of abstinence from cannabis on the course of the disorder. A recent Cochrane review identified only six relevant studies, four of which were small [45]. The few that have been large enough [46] have not reported results separately by diagnosis. The Cochrane review found no clear evidence that supported any type of substance-abuse treatment in schizophrenia over standard care.

Biological plausibility

Recent evidence from research on the neurobiology of the cannabinoid system provides biological plausibility for a causal relationship between cannabis use and psychotic symptoms. First, the principal psychoactive ingredient of cannabis, THC, acts upon a specific cannabinoid receptor (CB_1) in the brain [47] that appears to interact with the dopaminergic system of neurotransmission. Second, although the dopaminergic system of the brain has been considered to play an important role in psychotic disorders [48], there is increasing evidence that the cannabinoid system may be directly involved in schizophrenia and related psychotic disorders [49, 50, 51]. For example, CB_1 receptor knockout mice show behaviors consistent with some of the symptoms of schizophrenia, such as reduced goal-directed activity and memory for temporal representations [49]. Third, elevated levels of anandamide, an endogenous cannabinoid agonist, have also been found in the cerebrospinal fluid of persons with schizophrenia [52], and a recent case-control study found that persons with schizophrenia had a greater density of CB_1 receptors in the prefrontal cortex than controls [53]. Fourth, D'Souza and colleagues [54] have shown in a double-blind provocation study that intravenous THC provokes positive and negative psychotic symptoms in a dose-dependent way in persons with schizophrenia. Fifth, Caspi and colleagues [33] found a strong interaction between cannabis use and a common polymorphism in the COMT gene that is implicated in dopaminergic neurochemistry. This suggests a biological basis for the relationship that, if replicated, would explain why the risk of developing a psychosis after using cannabis is so modest in the population as a whole.

Cannabis use and the exacerbation of schizophrenia

There have been few controlled studies of relationships between cannabis use and the clinical outcome of schizophrenia. Negrete and colleagues [55] conducted a retrospective study using clinical records of symptoms and treatment seeking among 137 schizophrenic patients with a disorder of at least 6 months' duration, and three visits to their psychiatric service during the previous 6 months. Negrete and colleagues compared the prevalence of hallucinations, delusions, and hospitalizations among the active users ($N = 25$), the past users ($N = 51$), and those who had never used cannabis ($N = 61$). The crude comparison showed higher rates of continuous hallucinations, delusions, and hospitalizations among active users. This pattern of results persisted after statistical control for differences in age and sex between the three user groups. They argued that cannabis use exacerbated schizophrenic symptoms, suggesting three possibilities: i) that cannabis disorganizes psychological functioning; ii) that it causes a toxic psychosis that accentuates schizophrenic symptomatology, or iii) that it interferes with the therapeutic action of antipsychotic medication.

More recently, Cleghorn and colleagues [56], Jablensky and colleagues [57], and Martinez-Arevalo and colleagues [58] have provided supportive evidence. Cleghorn and colleagues [56] compared the

symptom profiles of schizophrenic patients with histories of substance abuse, among whom cannabis was the most heavily used drug. Comparisons revealed that drug abusers had a higher prevalence of hallucinations, delusions, and positive symptoms than those who did not abuse drugs. Jablensky and colleagues [57] reported a 2-year follow-up of 1,202 first-episode schizophrenic patients enrolled in 10 countries as part of a WHO collaborative study. They found that the use of "street drugs," including cannabis and cocaine, during the 2-year follow-up period predicted a poorer outcome, as assessed by psychotic symptoms and periods of hospitalization. Martinez-Arevalo and colleagues [58] also reported that continued use of cannabis during a 1-year follow-up of 62 DSM-diagnosed schizophrenic patients predicted a higher rate of relapse and poorer compliance with antipsychotic drug treatment.

Prospective evidence that cannabis exacerbates schizophrenic symptoms has been provided by Linszen and colleagues [59]. These investigators conducted a prospective study of outcomes in 93 psychotic patients whose symptoms were assessed monthly over a year. Twenty-four of their patients were cannabis abusers (11 were "mild" or less than daily users and 13 were heavy or more than daily cannabis users). They found that the cannabis abusers as a whole relapsed to psychotic symptoms sooner, and had more frequent relapses in the year of follow-up, than the patients who had not used cannabis. There was also a dose-response relationship between cannabis use and the risk of relapse. The heaviest cannabis users relapsed earlier, and more often, than the mild users who, in turn, relapsed sooner, and more often, than the patients who did not use cannabis. These relationships persisted after adjustment for potential confounding variables, including premorbid adjustment, and alcohol and other drug use during the follow-up period.

These results have recently been replicated in a prospective study of 100 patients with schizophrenia in Sydney, Australia [37]. These patients were assessed monthly on medication compliance, cannabis use, symptoms of depression, and symptoms of psychosis over 10 months. Linear regression methods were used to assess relationships between cannabis use and symptoms of psychosis and depression while adjusting for serial dependence, medication compliance, and other demographic and clinical variables. Cannabis use predicted a small but statistically significant increase in symptoms of psychosis but not of depression after controlling for other differences between cannabis users and nonusers. Symptoms of depression and psychosis, by contrast, did not predict cannabis use.

Most but not all (e.g., Zisook and colleagues [60]) of the evidence is consistent with the hypothesis that cannabis use exacerbates psychotic symptoms in patients with schizophrenia. The major cause of uncertainty is assessing the contribution of confounding factors in some of these studies. It is possible, for example, that the difference in the rates of psychotic symptoms between schizophrenia patients who do and do not use cannabis is due to differences in premorbid personality, family history, and other characteristics [61]. This is least likely in the WHO schizophrenia study [57] and the recent study of Linszen and colleagues [59], both of which used multivariate statistical methods to adjust for many of these confounders.

The other difficult issue is separating the contributions that cannabis, alcohol, and other drug use made to exacerbations of schizophrenic symptoms. It is rare for a schizophrenic patient to *only* use cannabis [62]. The concurrent use of alcohol is common, and the heavier their cannabis use, the more likely they are to use psychostimulants and hallucinogens. The Linszen and colleagues [59] and Degenhardt and colleagues [9] studies statistically adjusted for the effects of concurrent alcohol and drug use and found that the relationship persisted. Our confidence that the effect is attributable to cannabis would be increased by replications of these findings.

Future research directions

The following are a number of priorities for research that will assist in sorting out the nature of the relationship between cannabis use and psychosis that has been consistently observed in observational epidemiological studies. First, there needs to be replication of the cannabis-genotype interactions reported by Caspi and colleagues [54] between a COMT allele and cannabis use. If replicated, these findings would provide strong evidence for a causal role of cannabis in the vulnerable. It would also potentially provide a way of identifying young people who are at high risk of developing psychosis if they use cannabis.

Second, replications and extension of studies of the effects of cannabis use on the course of psychosis are needed. These studies might also look at the interaction between the COMT allele and psychosis. It would be useful to conduct these studies as part of intervention studies to reduce cannabis use among persons with schizophrenia.

Third, we need more human studies of the possible mechanism for interactions between cannabinoids and the dopaminergic system. This may include neuroimaging studies of the effects that cannabinoids have on human brain function.

Finally, we need to consider new and innovative ways to reduce cannabis use among persons with psychosis. The effective treatment of drug use is a challenging task and one that is not made easier by comorbid mental health problems such as schizophrenia. Effective pharmacological and psychological interventions, appropriate for this group, are required.

Conclusion

There is strong evidence from longitudinal studies that cannabis use may precipitate schizophrenia in vulnerable individuals. There is also reasonable evidence that cannabis use exacerbates symptoms of psychosis in persons with a psychosis who continue to use cannabis. These are biologically plausible relationships given the known effects of cannabis on dopaminergic and other brain neurotransmitter systems and the results of recent provocation studies of THC in schizophrenia.

Acknowledgments

This chapter is an updated version of two previous reviews of the evidence on cannabis and psychosis published in 2001 and 2004. Thanks to Emma Black and Amanda Roxburgh for assisting with compilation of references and proofreading the paper.

References

1. Brill H., Nahas G. (1984). Cannabis intoxication and mental illness. In *Marijuana in Science and Medicine*, Nahas G. (Ed.). New York: Raven Press.

2. Halikas J. A., Goodwin D. W., Guze S. B. Marihuana effects: a survey of regular users. *JAMA*, 1971. **217**:692–4.

3. Thornicroft G. Cannabis and psychosis: is there epidemiological evidence for association. *Br J Psychiatry*, 1990. **157**:25–33.

4. Georgotas A., Zeidenberg P. Observations on the effects of four weeks of heavy marijuana smoking on group interaction and individual behavior. *Compr Psychiatry*, 1979. **20**:427–32.

5. National Academy of Science (1982). Marijuana and Health. Washington, DC: National Academy Press.

6. Ghodse A. Cannabis psychosis. *Br J Addiction*, 1986. **81**:473–87.

7. Mueser K., *et al.* Prevalence of substance abuse in schizophrenia: demographic and clinical correlates. *Schizophr Bull*, 1990. **16**:31–56.

8. Turner W., Tsuang M. Impact of substance abuse on the course and outcome of schizophrenia. *Schizophr Bull*, 1990. **16**:87–372.

9. Degenhardt L., Hall W. The association between psychosis and problematical drug use among Australian adults: findings from the National Survey of Mental Health and Well-Being. *Psychol Med*, 2001. **31**(4):659–68.

10. Degenhardt L. D., Hall W. Is cannabis a contributory cause of psychosis? *Can J Psychiatry*, 2006. **9**:556–65.

11. Green B., Young R., Kavanagh D. Cannabis use and misuse prevalence among people with psychosis. *Br J Psychiatry*, 2005. **187**:306–13.

12. Anthony J., Helzer J. (1991). Syndromes of drug abuse and dependence. In *Psychiatric Disorders in America*, Robins L. and Regier D. (Eds.). New York: Free Press, Macmillan.

13. Hall W. D., *et al.* (1998). The prevalence in the past year of substance use and ICD-10 substance use disorders in Australian adults: findings from the National Survey of Mental Health and Well-Being. NDARC Technical Report, vol. **63**. Sydney: National Drug and Alcohol Research Centre, University of New South Wales.

14. Degenhardt L., Hall W. D. The association between psychosis and problematical drug use among Australian adults: findings from the National Survey of Mental Health and Well-Being. *Psychol Med*, 2001. **31**(4):659–68.

15. Andreasson S., *et al.* Cannabis and schizophrenia: a longitudinal study of Swedish conscripts. *Lancet*, 1987. **2**:1483–6.

16. Allebeck P. (1991). Cannabis and schizophrenia: is there a causal association?. In *Physiopathology of Illicit Drugs: Cannabis, Cocaine, Opiates*, Nahas G. and Latour C. (Eds.). Oxford: Pergamon Press.

17. Johnson B. A., Smith B. L., Taylor P. Cannabis and schizophrenia. *Lancet*, 1988. **1**:592–3.

18. Negrete J. Cannabis and schizophrenia. *Br Addiction*, 1989. **84**:349–51.

19. Johnson V. (1988). A longitudinal assessment of predominant patterns of drug use among adolescents and young adults. In *Marijuana: An International Research Report*, Chesher G., Consroe P., and Musty R. (Eds.). Canberra: Australian Government Publishing Service.

20. Kandel D., Faust R. Sequence and stages in patterns of adolescent drug use. *Arch Gen Psychiatry*, 1975. **32**:923–32.

21. Angrist B. (1983). Psychoses induced by central nervous system stimulants and related drugs. In *Stimulants: Neurochemical, Behavioral and Clinical Perspectives*, Creese I. (Ed.). New York: Raven Press.

22. Bell D. The experimental reproduction of amphetamine psychosis. *Arch Gen Psychiatry*, 1973. **29**:35–40.

23. Connell P. H. (1958). *Amphetamine Psychosis*. Maudsley Monograph Number **5**. London: Chapman & Hall, Ltd.

24. Gawin F. H., Ellinwood Jr. E. H. Cocaine and other stimulants. Actions, abuse, and treatment. *N Engl J Med*, 1988. **318**(18):1173–82.

25. Grinspoon L., Hedblom P. (1975). *The Speed Culture: Amphetamine Abuse in America*. Cambridge, Massachusetts: Harvard University Press.

26. Inghe G. (1969). The present state of abuse and addiction to stimulant drugs in Sweden. In *Abuse of Central Stimulants*, Sjoqvist F. and Tottie M. (Eds.). New York: Raven Press, pp. 187–214.

27. Goldberg L. Drug abuse in Sweden. Part I. *Bull Narc*, 1968. **20**(1):1–31.

28. Goldberg L. Drug abuse in Sweden. Part II. *Bull Narc*, 1968. **20**(2):9–36.

29. Zammit S., Lewis G. Exploring the relationship between cannabis use and psychosis. *Addiction*, 2004. **99**(10):1353–5.

30. van Os J., *et al.* Cannabis use and psychosis: a longitudinal population-based study. *Am J Epidemiol*, 2002. **156**(4):319–27.

31. Henquet C., *et al.* Prospective cohort study of cannabis use, predisposition for psychosis, and psychotic symptoms in young people. *Br Med J*, 2005. **330**(7481):11–14.

32. Arseneault L., *et al.* Mental disorders and violence in total birth cohort: results from the Dunedin study. *Arch Gen Psychiatry*, 2000. **57**(10): 979–86.

33. Caspi A., *et al.* Moderation of the effect of adolescent-onset cannabis use on adult psychosis by a functional polymorphism in the catechol-O-methyltransferase gene: longitudinal evidence of a gene X environment interaction. *Biol Psychiatry*, 2005. **57**(10): 1117–27.

34. Fergusson D., Horwood J., Swain-Campbell N. Cannabis dependence and psychotic symptoms in young people. *Psychol Med*, 2003. **33**(1): 15–21.

35. Fergusson D. M., Horwood L. J., Ridder E. M. Tests of causal linkages between cannabis use and psychotic symptoms. *Addiction*, 2005. **100**(3): 354–66.

36. Verdoux H., *et al.*, Cannabis use and the expression of psychosis vulnerability in daily life. *Eur Psychiatry*, 2002. **17**: 180S–180S.

37. Degenhardt L., Tennant C., and Gilmour S., *et al.* The temporal dynamics of relationships between cannabis, psychosis and depression among young adults with psychotic disorders: Findings from a ten-month prospective study. *Psychol Med*, 2007. **37**(7):927–34.

38. Mueser K. T., Bellack A. S., Blanchard J. J. Comorbidity of schizophrenia and substance abuse: implications for treatment. *J Consult Clin Psychol*, 1992. **60**(6): 845–56.

39. Noordsy D. L., *et al.* Subjective experiences related to alcohol use among schizophrenics. *J Nerv Ment Dis*, 1991. **179**(7): 410–14.

40. Dixon L., *et al.* Acute effects of drug abuse in schizophrenic patients: clinical observations and patients' self-reports. *Schizophr Bull*, 1990. **16**(1):69–79.

41. Peralta V., Cuesta M. J. Influence of cannabis abuse on schizophrenic psychopathology. *Acta Psychiatr Scand*, 1992. **85**(2): 127–30.

42. Schneier F. R., Siris S. G. A review of psychoactive substance use and abuse in schizophrenia: patterns of drug choice. *J Nerv Ment Dis*, 1987. **175**(11):641–52.

43. Verdoux H., *et al.* Effects of cannabis and psychosis vulnerability in daily life: an experience sampling test study. *Psychol Med*, 2003. **33**(1):23–32.

44. Lehman A. F., *et al.* Rehabilitation for adults with severe mental illness and substance use disorders: a clinical trial. *J Nerv Ment Dis*, 1993. **181**(2):86–90.

45. Epstein J. N., *et al.* The effects of anxiety on continuous performance test functioning in an ADHD clinic sample. *J Atten Disord*, 1997. **2**(1):45–52.

46. Jerrell J. M., Ridgely M. S. Comparative effectiveness of three approaches to serving people with severe mental illness and substance abuse disorders. *J Nerv Ment Dis*, 1995. **183**(9): 566–76.

47. Hall W., Degenhardt L., Lynskey M. (2001). *The Health and Psychological Consequences of Cannabis Use*. Canberra: Australian Publishing Service.

48. Julien R. (2001). *A Primer of Drug Action. A Concise, Nontechnical Guide to the Actions, Uses, and Side Effects of Psychoactive Drugs*. 9th ed. New York: Worth Publishers.

49. Fritzsche M. Are cannabinoid receptor knockout mice animal models for schizophrenia? *Med Hypotheses*, 2001. **56**(6): 638–43.

50. Glass M. The role of cannabinoids in neurodegenerative diseases. *Prog Neuropsychopharmacol Biol Psychiatry*, 2001. **25**(4): 743–65.

51. Skosnik P. D., Spatz-Glenn L., Park S. Cannabis use is associated with schizotypy and attentional dysinhibition. *Schizophr Res*, 2001. **48**:83–92.

52. Leweke F. M., *et al.* Elevated endogenous cannabinoids in schizophrenia. *Neuroreport*, 1999. **10**(8):1665–9.

53. Dean B., *et al.* Studies on [3H]CP-55940 binding in the human central nervous system: regional specific changes in density of cannabinoid-1 receptors associated with schizophrenia and cannabis use. *Neuroscience*, 2001. **103**(1): 9–15.

54. D'Souza D. C., *et al.* The psychotomimetic effects of intravenous delta-9-tetrahydrocannabinol in healthy individuals: implications for psychosis. *Neuropsychopharmacology*, 2004. **29**(8):1558–72.

55. Negrete J. C., *et al.* Cannabis affects the severity of schizophrenic symptoms: results of a clinical survey. *Psychol Med*, 1986. **16**:515–20.

56. Cleghorn J. M., *et al.* Substance abuse and schizophrenia: effect on symptoms but not on neurocognitive function. *J Clin Psychiatr*, 1991. **52**:26–30.

57. Jablensky A., Sartorius N., Ernberg G. Schizophrenia: manifestations, incidence and course in different cultures. A World Health Organization Ten-Country Study. *Psychol Med*, 20(Suppl), 1991.

58. Martinez-Arevalo M. J., Calcedo-Ordonez A., Varo-Prieto J. R. Cannabis consumption as a prognostic factor in schizophrenia. *Br J Psychiatry*, 1994. **164**:679–81.

59. Linszen, D. H., Dingemans P. M., Lenior M. E., Cannabis abuse and the course of recent-onset

schizophrenic disorders. *Arch Gen Psychiatry*, 1994. **51**: 273–9.

60. Zisook S., *et al.* Past substance abuse clinical course of

schizophrenia. *Am J Psychiatry*, 1992. **149**:552–3.

61. Kavanagh D. An intervention for substance abuse in schizophrenia. *Behav Change*, 1995. **12**:20–30.

62. Mueser K., Bellack A., Blanchard J. Comorbidity of schizophrenia and substance abuse: implications for treatment. *J Consult Clin Psychol*, 1992. **60**(6):845–56.

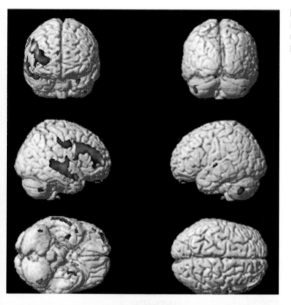

Figure 1.1 Brain MRI images showing grey-matter volume reductions in first-episode schizophrenia subjects compared to healthy controls using Voxel Based Morphometry (VBM). [From the University of Pittsburgh.]

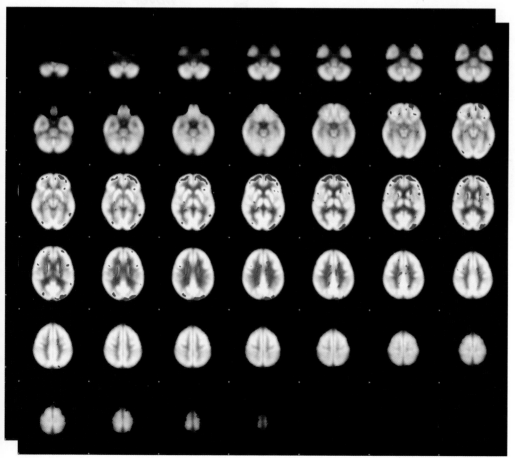

Figure 5.3 Significance probability mapping [184] test areas of decrease in FDG relative metabolic rate and D2 receptor binding.

(A)

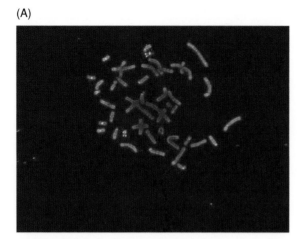

(B)

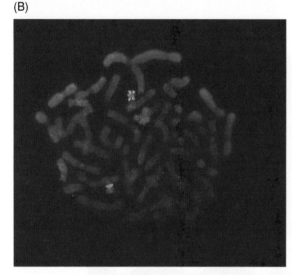

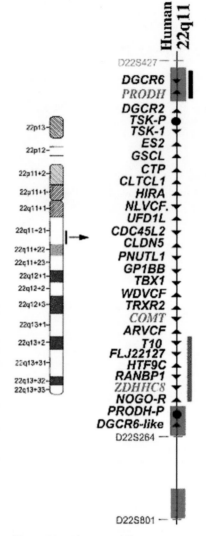

Figure 24.3 Fluorescence *in-situ* hybridization showing the presence of both 22q11.2 regions (a) and the deletion (b) with the commercially available probe (Vysis, Gaithersburg, MD. Courtesy: Mark Pettenati, PhD, Department of Pediatrics, Wake Forest University School of Medicine.)

Figure 24.5 Ideogram of Chromosome 22, with a listing of all the genes in the 1.5 Mb interval in the q11.2 region, thought to be critical for schizophrenia. The genes denoted in red are thought to be most likely related to psychosis.

Toxic psychosis

Rajeev Kumar and Jeffrey C. L. Looi

Facts box

- Toxic psychosis is characterized by the presence of psychotic symptoms usually associated with acutely impaired cognitive functions.
- A number of centrally active prescription drugs taken in excessive amount can cause neurotoxicity.
- Clinical manifestations include delirium with features of altered consciousness, impairment of general cognitive functions, acute onset, fluctuating course, nocturnal worsening, and presence of delusions, hallucinations, and thought disorder.
- It is sometimes difficult to differentiate between toxic psychosis and primary psychiatric conditions.
- General risk factors include older age, underlying dementia, and severe physical illness.
- Several classes of drugs have been implicated.
- Pathogenesis of toxic psychosis is poorly understood. However, current knowledge is that there is dysfunction of a number of neurotransmitters such as acetylcholine, dopamine, GABA, and glutamate.
- Management includes the identification and treatment of the underlying cause, which is often multifactorial.
- Common clinical situation: clinicians should be able to correctly identify this state to reduce mortality.
- Current research is flawed by methodological issues. Future research should include a large number of patients, use standardized measurements, study individual drugs, and control confounders.

Introduction

A number of terms have been used in literature to describe psychosis associated with acutely impaired cognitive functions [1]. These include toxic psychosis, acute brain syndrome, acute organic psychosis, acute confusional state, ICU psychosis, metabolic encephalopathy, toxic confusional state, and delirium. The multiple terms used to denote this state lead to confusion both in clinical and research practice. Therefore, the more recent psychiatric diagnostic and classification systems (DSM-IV and ICD-10) opted to use the term "delirium." This chapter reviews the current evidence related to the occurrence of toxic psychosis (delirium) caused by commonly prescribed drugs consumed in excessive amounts. The most common presentation is clearly that of delirium. Therefore, the clinical features of this are discussed briefly, followed by a discussion of the literature relevant to the association between commonly prescribed drugs and delirium.

Clinical features of delirium

Without careful assessment, delirium can easily be mistaken for a number of primary psychiatric disorders such as dementia, depression, and psychosis. The key characteristics of delirium are a disturbance in the level of consciousness, an impairment of cognition and perception, acute onset and fluctuating course, a medical history of illnesses or toxic exposure to drugs, and presence of other features such as a reversal of the sleep-wake cycle [2]. Table 12.1 shows the DSM-IV criteria for the diagnosis of delirium.

An important challenge for the clinician is to differentiate delirium from other conditions such as depression, dementia, and functional psychoses. However, certain signs and symptoms can assist clinicians to distinguish between delirium and other conditions [3]. Table 12.2 provides the salient features of delirium, dementia, and psychosis. Electroencephalography can

Table 12.1 DSM-IV diagnostic criteria of delirium

a) Disturbance of consciousness (that is, reduced clarity of awareness of the environment, with reduced ability to focus, or shift orientation)

b) A change in cognition (such as memory deficit, disorientation, language disturbance) or the development of a perceptual disturbance that is not better accounted for by a pre-existing established or evolving dementia.

c) The disturbance developed over a short period of time (usually hours to days) and tends to fluctuate during the course of the day.

d) Where the delirium is due to a general medical condition-there is evidence from the history, physical examination, or laboratory findings that the disturbance is caused by the direct physiological consequences of a general medical condition. Where the delirium is due to substance intoxication-there is evidence from the history, physical examination, or laboratory findings of either 1 or 2:

    1) The symptoms in criteria (a) and (b) developed during substance intoxication

    2) Medication use – etiologically related to the disturbance

    Where the delirium is due to substance withdrawal- there is evidence from the history, physical examination, or laboratory findings that the symptoms in criteria (a) and (b) developed during or shortly after the withdrawal syndrome. Where delirium is due to multiple etiologies- there is evidence from the history, physical examination, or laboratory findings that the delirium has more than one aetiology (for example: more than one etiological general medical condition, a general medical condition plus substance intoxication, or medication side effects).

(e) Delirium not otherwise specified: this category should be used to diagnose a delirium that does not meet criteria for any of the specific types of delirium described. Examples include a clinical presentation of delirium that is suspected to be due to a general medical condition or substance use but for which there is insufficient evidence to establish a specific aetiology, or where delirium is due to causes not listed (for example, sensory deprivation)

Reprinted with permission from the Diagnostic and Statistical Manual of Mental Disorders, Text Revision, Fourth Edition (Copyright 2000). American Psychiatric Association.

be useful in differentiating delirium from other conditions, particularly primary psychiatric states such as schizophrenia.

Epidemiology

A number of methodological shortcomings are reported to be associated with the studies on the prevalence of delirium. These include under-reporting due to short duration in some cases, lack of consensus in the definition, use of different screening tools, sample bias, and study settings. As a result, the reported prevalence and incidence rates of delirium varied significantly in different studies.

In general hospital patients, Hodkinson [4] has reported a prevalence of 35% in patients older than 65 years of age. O'Keefe and Lavan [5] reported a prevalence of 18% at admission and an additional 24% during hospital stays in an acute geriatric setting. Chisholm and colleagues [6] reported a rate of more than 50% in a mixed group of medical and surgical patients over the age of 60 years. Most studies found a higher prevalence in surgical patients [7, 8]. A higher prevalence has also been found in oncology settings [9]. Most published data on prevalence and incidence are restricted to hospitalized, medically ill elderly. In general, 10%–15% of medical and surgical general hospital patients suffer from delirium at any time and the rate increases with age.

General risk factors

Burns and colleagues [10] suggested that the risk factors could be categorized into predisposing factors, such as older age, underlying cognitive impairment, or physical illnesses; precipitating factors, such as an infection, or even a combination of these two factors. Even though physical frailty is a major confounding factor in ageing, Schor and colleagues reported that age more than 80 years was an independent risk factor for the occurrence of delirium [11]. It has been noted that alterations in the metabolism of drugs with age may cause increased vulnerability to side effects. Other reported risk factors include dementia [12], poor physical health [13], and depression [12]. One of the most common biochemical abnormalities associated with delirium is hypoalbuminemia. This is a very important risk factor for drug-induced delirium, because low albumin level can enhance brain toxicity by making the blood concentration of the unbound, centrally acting drug higher [14].

General etiological factor

Delirium is viewed as a potential medical emergency. Several causes of delirium have been identified, but

Table 12.2 Differentiating characteristics of delirium, dementia, and psychosis

Salient features	Delirium	Dementia	Psychosis
Onset	Acute	Gradual	Acute
Course	Fluctuates, worse at night	No change	No change
Level of consciousness	Altered	Clear sensorium	Clear sensorium
Attention and concentration	Reduced	Generally intact, but may be impaired	Generally intact, but may be impaired
Orientation	Usually disorientated in time	Often impaired	May be impaired
Delusions	Usually paranoid in nature, fleeting and poorly systematized	May occur in some cases	Multiple systematized delusions or singe well formed
Hallucinations	Usually visual	Often absent, but may be present in Lewy body Dementia	Usually auditory, but can occur in any modalities
Psychomotor activity	Increased, reduced, or shifting	Often normal	Sometimes varies
Speech	Often incoherent (formal thought disorder)	Nominal dysphasia and sometimes perseveration	Normal, or formal thought disorder in disorganized patients
Physical findings	Present in some conditions such as metabolic encephalopathy	Often absent	Often absent
Medical conditions or drug toxicity	Usually present	Often absent	Usually absent

the links between this condition and the underlying mechanisms are poorly understood. The list of conditions associated with delirium include intracerebral infections, drug and alcohol withdrawal, acute metabolic encephalopathy from renal or hepatic failure, head injury, brain tumors, epilepsy, brain hypoxia, thiamine, vitamin B12 and folate deficiencies, various endocrine disorders, acute cerebrovascular episodes, toxins or drugs, and heavy metal poisoning [15].

Delirium (toxic psychosis) due to commonly used drugs

Several classes of drugs have been reported to cause delirium and toxic delirium, especially in elderly patients. Table 12.3 shows the common classes of drugs that cause delirium. Review of every single agent is beyond the scope of this chapter, because nearly every class of drug has been associated with neurotoxicity in susceptible individuals. Interested readers should read the *Medical Letter* [16, 17], which publishes an updated list biannually. Additional lists can also be found in other sources [18, 19, 20]. Literature on drug-induced delirium is mainly based on case reports and uncontrolled case series. Delirium is usually multifactorial in etiology and there is often an interplay of several factors such as the effect of a particular drug or drugs in an elderly patient with multiple medical problems such as

Table 12.3 Classes of drugs reported to cause delirium

1. Anticholinergics
2. Anticonvulsants
3. Antidepressants
4. Antiemetics
5. Antipsychotics
6. Antiparkinsonians
7. Benzodiazepines
8. Corticosteroids
9. Histamine H2 receptor antagonists
10. Opioids and Nonsteroidal antiinflammatory drugs
11. Antibiotics

dementia, infection, and metabolic abnormalities. Psychotropic medications are reported to cause delirium often, as they were involved in 15%–75% of delirium–cases [9, 21, 22, 23, 24, 25, 26, 27]. However, only 2%–14% of cases were accounted for delirium exclusively due to drugs [21, 22, 23, 24, 25, 26, 27].

Anticholinergics

Pure anticholinergics or drugs with anticholinergic properties are well known to cause toxic psychosis, especially in older patients [28, 29]. However, this effect has not been confirmed in several other clinical studies [11, 21, 30, 31, 32, 33, 34]. Nonetheless, serum anticholinergic activity measured using a radioactive assay gives a more accurate estimate of anticholinergic activity, and did show a robust relationship to toxic psychosis [35, 36].

Anticonvulsants

Anticonvulsants can cause toxic psychosis when it reaches toxic blood levels [37]. Inouye and colleagues examined the risk associated with anticonvulsant medications and found an increased risk [34].

Antidepressants

Antidepressants are known to increase the risk of toxic psychosis, especially in elderly subjects [32]. It is clearly known that tricyclic antidepressants have anticholinergic properties, amitriptyline being the strongest and nortriptyline the weakest. These groups of drugs are particularly at high risk [38]. Among SSRI antidepressants, fluoxamine [39] and paroxetine [40] can cause toxic psychosis in high-risk patients.

Antiemetics

One study that examined the risk associated with antiemetics found a positive result [34].

Antipsychotics

Antipsychotics with anticholinergic properties, alpha-receptor blocking abilities, and with prominent dopamine D2 receptor binding are particularly at an increased risk of causing neurotoxicity [41]. Two studies that examined the risk reported positive results with antipsychotics [11, 32]. Some of the newer drugs with minimal anticholinergic effects are probably safer compared to the older generation drugs.

Antiparkinsonians

All antiparkinsonian drugs by their dopamine activating property can induce delirium [42, 43, 44]. However, one study that examined the risk reported negative results [32]. Delirium is a dose-related side effect. Therefore, reduction of appropriate antiparkinsonian drugs is necessary to manage parkinsonian symptoms.

Benzodiazepines

Benzodiazepines are commonly prescribed drugs and they are associated with toxic psychosis. Several studies have examined the associated risk and reported mixed results; with some reporting positive results [11, 30, 45, 46], and some negative [31, 32, 33, 34, 47, 48, 49]. Drugs with a prolonged half-life when used in the elderly can lead to high blood levels causing toxicity.

Corticosteroids

Following a review of the literature on this topic, Sirios and colleagues [50] suggested that two clinical profiles have been reported: an affective profile and a toxic-organic profile. Toxic psychosis was reported in 13% of cases and pure psychosis in 11% [51, 52]. An affective psychosis with normal cognition can occur that may be very similar to a primary psychiatry condition. The toxic-organic profile comprises delusions, hallucinations, thought disorder, confusion, agitation, and perplexity. It has been shown that prednisone is better than high-dose cortisone or adrenocorticotropic hormone in causing toxic psychosis. However, high-dose steroids and female gender have been associated with increased risk of toxicity [53, 54].

Histamine H2 receptor antagonists

Histamine H2 receptor antagonists are linked to toxic psychosis [33, 55]. Others also reported that the drugs cimetidine [56], ranitidine [56], and famotidine [57] can induce a toxic psychosis.

Opioids and nonsteroidal anti-inflammatory drugs

Opioid and nonopioid medications have been reported to cause toxic psychosis. Several studies have examined opioid analgesics and found a correlation with toxic psychosis [11, 45, 46, 58]. Among opioids, pethidine is found to be more problematic because of its metabolite norpethidine, which has anticholinergic and central nervous system excitatory properties [30]. Nonsteroidal anti-inflammatory drugs (NSAIDs) have also been associated with toxic psychosis [59, 60].

Antibiotics

Antibiotics in toxic concentration in the blood have been reported to be associated with toxic psychosis

[61]. It may be difficult at times to distinguish between psychosis induced by an infectious disease and that induced by the prescribed antibiotic.

Pathogenesis of drug-induced toxic psychosis

Centrally acting drugs may be present in toxic concentrations due to excessive intake or impaired clearance. Elderly patients and patients with multiple medical problems and organ damage are particularly vulnerable because of pharmacokinetic changes. A number of mechanisms involving various neurotransmitters have been reported. Cholinergic hypoactivity, dopaminergic hyperactivity [62] and involvement of γ-amino-butyric acid (GABA) and glutamatergic diffuse modulatory pathways [63] have been the foci of research in this area. Gaudreau and colleagues [64] proposed a model that suggested the central role of thalamus in the causation of toxic psychosis. According to this model, psychotic symptoms could originate from a transitory dysfunction of thalamus leading to sensory overload and hyperarousal. Psychoactive medications such as benzodiazepines and opioids could exert this effect by compromising the thalamic gating functions by interfering with central glutamatergic, GABAergic, dopaminergic, and cholinergic pathways.

Management

Management, including the identification and treatment of acute precipitants and implementation of supportive and restorative care, is most important. A thorough review of medications taken is crucial as this is often the most common reversible cause of toxic psychosis. The review should include exploring the temporal association between the drug and the onset of psychosis, a recent change in prescription or dose increase, and a history of over-the-counter medications. Once a medication was found to cause the psychosis, it should be stopped as soon as possible. Most importantly, drugs that are well known to cause toxic psychosis in high-risk patients should be avoided.

Implications for clinical practice

A number of centrally acting drugs are associated with brain toxicity that leads to a psychotic state with acute cognitive impairment. This is often seen in clinical practice and is sometimes difficult to differentiate from primary psychiatric conditions such as an affective psychosis or schizophreniform psychosis. In an acute setting, it may not always be possible to test the cognition of an acutely agitated patient. Recognition and management of toxic psychosis are vital for saving the lives of such patients.

Summary and conclusions

Toxic psychosis is a medical emergency and a manifestation of an underlying serious insult to the brain, due to an excessive amount of commonly prescribed drugs in the blood. Often the causes are multifactorial with several risk factors operating at the same time. Almost all classes of prescription drugs can cause toxicity when consumed in large amounts. Therefore, clinicians should be aware of this condition when prescribing to patients, particularly high-risk groups such as the elderly and the medically compromised.

Future research directions

Good-quality, well-controlled studies are lacking in this area and the studies examining the risk of drugs causing toxic psychosis often reported mixed results. Therefore, more studies are needed in this area. Future studies should be large enough to find meaningful associations and individual drugs should be studied separately. Instruments that are used to diagnose and monitor the progress of toxic psychosis (delirium) should be standardized to make comparisons easy across different settings. Additionally, researchers should study all the potential confounders and should control for these in their analyses.

References

1. Brown T. M., Boyle M. F. Delirium. *Br Med J*, 2002. **325**:644–7.

2. Francis J. Drug-induced delirium. *CNS Drugs*, 1996. **5**:103–14.

3. Lipowski Z. J. Delirium in the elderly patient. *New Engl J Med*, 1989. **320**:578–82.

4. Hodkinson H. M. Mental impairment in the elderly. *J R Coll Physicians Lond*, 1973. **7**:305–17.

5. O'Keefe S., Lavan J. The prognostic significance of delirium in older hospital patients. *J Am Geriatr Soc*, 1997. **45**:174–8.

6. Chisholm S. E., Deniston O. L., Igrisan R. M., *et al.* Prevalence of confusion in elderly hospital patients. *J Gerontol Nurs*, 1982. **8**:87–96.

7. Marcantonio E. R., Flacker J. M., Michaels M., *et al.* Delirium is independently associated with poor functional recovery after hip fracture. *J Am Geriatr Soc*, 2000. **48**:618–24.

8. Milstein A., Barak Y., Kleinman G., *et al.* The incidence of delirium immediately following cataract surgery: a prospective study in the elderly. *Aging Mental Health*, 2000. **4**:178–81.

9. Lawlor P. G., Gagnon B., Mancini I. L., *et al.* Occurrence, causes and outcome of delirium in patients with advanced cancer: a prospective study. *Arch Intern Med*, 2000. **160**:786–94.

10. Burns A., Gallagley A., Byrne J. Delirium. *J Neurol Neurosurg Psychiatry*, 2004. **75**:362–7.

11. Schor J. D., Levkoff S. E., Lipsitz L. A., *et al.* Risk factors for delirium in hospitalised elderly. *JAMA*, 1992. **267**:827–31.

12. Elie M., Cole M. G., Primeau F. J., *et al.* Delirium risk factors in elderly hospitalised patients. *J Gen Intern Med*, 1998. **13**:204–12.

13. Marcantonio E. R., Goldman L., Mangione C. M. A clinical prediction rule for delirium after elective noncardiac surgery. *JAMA*, 1994. **247**:134–9.

14. Trzepacz P. T., Francis J. Low serum albumin and risk of delirium. *Am J Psychiatry*, 1990. **147**:675.

15. Wise M. G., Hilty D. M., Cerda G. M., *et al.* (2005). Delirium (confusional states). In *The American Psychiatric Publishing Textbook of Consultation-Liaison Psychiatry*, Wise M. G., Rundell J. R. (Eds.). 2nd ed. Washington, DC: American Psychiatric Press, pp. 257–72.

16. Drugs that cause psychiatric symptoms. *Med Lett Drugs Ther*, 1993. **35**:65–70.

17. Drugs that may cause psychiatric symptoms. *Med Lett Drugs Ther*, 2002. **44**:59–62.

18. Lipowski Z. J. (1990). *Delirium: Acute Confusional States*. New York: Oxford University Press.

19. American Hospital Formulary Service. *Drug Information*. Bethesda, Maryland: American Society of Hospital Pharmacists. 1995.

20. Cassem E. H., Lake C. R., Boyer W. F. (1994). Psychopharmacology in the ICU. In *The Pharmacologic Approach to the Critically Ill Patient*, Chernow B. (Ed.). 3rd ed. Baltimore, Maryland: Williams and Wilkins, pp. 651–65.

21. Francis J., Martin D., Kapoor W. N. A prospective study of delirium in hospitalised elderly. *JAMA*, 1990. **263**:1097–101.

22. Brauer C., Morrison R. S., Silberzweig S. B., *et al.* The cause of delirium in patients with hip fracture. *Arch Intern Med*, 2000. **160**:1856–60.

23. Breitbart W., Gibson C., Tremblay A. The delirium experience: delirium recall and delirium-related distress in hospitalised patients with cancer, their spouse/care givers, and their nurses. *Psychosomatics*, 2002. **43**:183–94.

24. Olofson S. M., Weitzner M. A., Valentine A. D., *et al.* A retrospective study of the psychiatric management and outcome of delirium in the cancer patient. *Support Care Cancer*, 1996. **4**:351–7.

25. O'Keefe S. T., Lavan J. N. Clinical significance of delirium subtypes in older people. *Age Ageing*, 1999. **28**:115–19.

26. Morita T., Tei Y., Tsunoda J., *et al.* Underlying pathologies and their associations with clinical features in terminal delirium of cancer patients. *J Pain Sympt Manage*, 2001. **22**:997–1006.

27. Tuma R., DeAngelis L. M. Altered mental status in patients with cancer. *Arch Neurol*, 2000. **57**:1727–31.

28. Feinberg F. The problems of anticholinergic effects in older patients. *Drugs Ageing*, 1993. **3**:335–48.

29. Peters N. L. Snipping the thread of life: antimuscarinic side effect of medications in the elderly. *Arch Intern Med*, 1989. **149**:2414–20.

30. Macantonio E. R., Juarez G., Goldman L., *et al.* The relationship of postoperative delirium with psychoactive medications. *JAMA*, 1994. **272**:1518–22.

31. Inouye S. K., Viscoli C. M., Horwitz R. I., *et al.* A predictive model for delirium in hospitalised elderly medical patients based on admission characteristics. *Ann Intern Med*, 1993. **119**:474–81.

32. Gustafson Y., Berggren D., Brannstrom B., *et al.* Acute confusional states in elderly patients treated for femoral neck fracture. *J Am Geriatr Soc*, 1988. **36**:525–30.

33. Martin N. J., Stones M. J., Young J. E., *et al.* Development of delirium:

a prospective cohort study in a community hospital. *Int Psychogeriatr*, 2000. **12**:117–27.

34. Inouye S. K., Charpentier P. A. Precipitating factors for delirium in hospitalised elderly persons. Predictive model and interrelationship with baseline vulnerability. *JAMA*, 1996. **275**:852–7.

35. Tune L. E., Blysma F. W. Benzodiazepine-induced and anticholinergic-induced delirium in the elderly. *Int Psychogeriatr*, 1991. **3**:397–408.

36. Mach J. R., Dysken M. W., Kuskowski M., et al. Serum anticholinergic activity in hospitalised older persons with delirium: a preliminary study. *J Am Geriatr Soc*, 1995. **43**:491–5.

37. Meador K. J. Cognitive side effects of antiepileptic drugs. *Can J Neurol*, 1994. **21**:512–16.

38. Preskorn S. H., Jerkovich G. S. Central nervous system toxicity of tricyclic antidepressants: phenomenology, course, risk factors and role of therapeutic drug monitoring. *J Clin Psychopharmacol*, 1990. **10**:88–95.

39. Jefferson J. W., Griest J. H., Perse T. L., et al. Fluoxetine-associated mania/hypomania in patients with obsessive compulsive disorders. *J Clin Psychopharmacol*, 1991. **11**:391–2.

40. Richelson E. Treatment of acute depression. *Psychopharmacology*, 1993. **16**:461–478.

41. Rosen J., Bohon S., Gershon S. Antipsychotics in the elderly. *Acta Psychiatr Scand*, 1990. **82**:170–5.

42. Bowen J. D., Larson E. B. Drug-induced cognitive impairment. Defining the problem and finding the solutions. *Drugs Ageing*, 1993. **3**:349–57.

43. Friedman A., Sienkiewicz Z. Psychotic complications of long-term levodopa treatment of Parkinson's disease. *Acta Neurol Scand*, 1991. **84**:111–3.

44. Vezina P., Mohr E., Grimes D. Deprenyl in Parkinson's disease: mechanisms, neuroprotective effect, indications and adverse effects. *Can J Neurol Sci*, 1992. **19**:142–6.

45. Dubois M. J., Bergeron N., Dumont M., et al. Delirium in an intensive care unit: a study of risk factors. *Intensive Care Med*, 2001. **27**:1297–1304.

46. Litaker D., Locala J., Franco K., et al. Preoperative risk factors for postoperative delirium. *Gen Hosp Psychiatry*, 2001. **23**:84–9.

47. Fann J. R., Roth-Roemer S., Burington B. E., et al. Delirium in patients undergoing haematopoietic stem cell transplantation. *Cancer*, 2002. **95**:1971–81.

48. Ljubisavljevic V., Kelly B. Risk factors for development of delirium among oncology patients. *Gen Hosp Psychiatry*, 2003. **25**:345–52.

49. Foy A., O'Connell D., Henry D., et al. Benzodiazepine use as a cause of cognitive impairment in elderly hospital inpatients. *J Gerontol A Biol Sci Med Sci*, 1995. **50**:M99–M106.

50. Sirios F. Steroid psychosis: a review. *Gen Hosp Psychiatry*, 2003. **25**:27–33.

51. Lewis D. A., Smith R. E. Steroid-induced psychiatric syndromes: a report of 14 cases, and a review of the literature. *J Affect Disord*, 1983. **5**:319–32.

52. Stoudemire A., Anfinson T., Edwards J. Corticosteroid-induced delirium, and dependency. *Gen Hosp Psychiatry*, 1996. **18**:196–202.

53. Ling M. H. M., Perry P. J., Tsuang M. T. Side effects of corticosteroid therapy: psychiatric aspects. *Arch Gen Psychiatry*, 1981. **38**:471–7.

54. Lacomis D., Samuels M. A. Adverse neurological effects of glucocorticosteroids. *J Gen Intern Med*, 1991. **6**:367–76.

55. Cantu T. G., Korek J. S. Central nervous system reactions to histamine-2 receptor blockers. *Ann Intern Med*, 1991. **114**:1027–34.

56. Morrison R. L., Katz I. R. Drug-related cognitive impairment: current progress and recurrent problems. *Am Rev Gerontol Geriatr*, 1989. **9**:233–79.

57. Henmann N. E., Carpenter D. U., Janda S. M. Famotidine-associated mental confusion in elderly patients. *Drug Intell Clin Pharm*, 1988. **22**:976–8.

58. Morrison R. S., Magaziner J., Gilbert M., et al. Relationship between pain and opioid analgesics on the development of delirium following hip fracture. *J Gerontol A Biol Sci Med*, 2003. **58**:76–81.

59. Jobst W. F., Bridges C. R., Regan-Smith M. G. Antirheumatic agents: CNS toxicity and its avoidance. *Geriatrics*, 1989. **44**:95–102.

60. Goodwin J. S., Regan M. Cognitive dysfunction associated with naproxen and ibuprofen in the elderly. *Arthritis Rheum*, 1982. **25**:1013–5.

61. Sharon R. S., Glenn R. H. The neurotoxicity of antibacterial agents. *Ann Intern Med*, 1984. **101**:92–104.

62. Trezpacz P. T. Is there a final common neural pathway in delirium? Focus on acetylcholine and dopamine. *Semin Clin Neuropsychiatry*, 2005. **5**:132–48.

63. Flacker J. M., Lipsitz L. A. Neural mechanisms of delirium: current hypotheses are evolving concepts. *J Gerontol A Biol Sci Med*, 1999. **54**:B239–46.

64. Gaudreau J-D., Gagnon P. Psychotogenic drugs and delirium pathogenesis: the central role of thalamus. *Med Hypotheses*, 2005. **64**:471–5.

13 Schizophrenia-like psychosis and traumatic brain injury

Perminder S. Sachdev

Facts box

- The many anecdotal reports of schizophrenia-like psychosis (SLP) following traumatic brain injury (TBI) do not provide strong evidence for a link between the two because of the likelihood of chance association and the subjective nature of the determination.

- One large cross-sectional study did not provide strong evidence for an association between head injury and schizophrenia.

- The case control studies provide strong evidence that TBI does not substantially increase the risk of schizophrenia in the general population, although a small increase cannot be ruled out.

- The association may be stronger in those with a genetic vulnerability to schizophrenia or the presence of preinjury psychopathology.

- Psychosis following TBI has considerable overlap with primary schizophrenic disorder, with a prominence of persecutory and other delusions, auditory hallucinations, and a dearth of negative symptoms.

- More severe and diffuse brain injuries, especially those involving the temporal and frontal lobes, are the most prominent risk factor, and EEG and neuroimaging abnormalities are often present.

Traumatic brain injury (TBI) is a common problem with major public health implications. A conservative estimate of the annual incidence of TBI in the United States is 200 per 100,000 per year [1], and estimates of its prevalence range from 2.5 to 6.5 million individuals [2]. Disorders arising from traumatic injuries to the brain are more common than any other neurological disease, with the exception of headache [3]. The impact of severe TBI on the victim is almost always devastating, but even mild TBI can result in serious and disabling neuropsychiatric disorders, ranging from cognitive deficits and personality change to severe and chronic psychosis.

The association between TBI and schizophrenia-like psychosis (SLP) has generated research interest for more than a century [4], but systematic studies have been relatively few. The most important question is whether TBI predisposes an individual to schizophrenia or SLP. If this can be unequivocally established, a number of other questions become relevant: What is the prevalence of SLP following TBI? Are the clinical features of SLP related to TBI different from schizophrenia? What is its prognosis? What factors, related to the injury as well as to the individual, predispose the person with TBI to develop SLP? Is the development of SLP particularly related to injury to specific brain regions? Does the study of SLP advance our understanding of the etiopathogenesis of schizophrenia? We first examine the epidemiological evidence and then attempt to answer some of these questions.

Epidemiology

The evidence for an association between SLP and TBI has come from a number of sources, and the various studies can be grouped according to their design. The most definitive study would be a longitudinal cohort design, in which a large number of head-injured individuals across a wide age range, and a matched not head-injured control group, would be followed up prospectively using standard instruments and well-defined diagnostic criteria. Because this ideal study does not exist, the evidence must be pooled from a variety of sources.

Case reports

Observations by clinicians have been a major factor in focusing the attention on this association. A systematic review of published case reports was performed recently [5], which included 69 cases from 39 reports in the period 1971 to 1994. The authors applied DSM-IV criteria of "psychotic disorder due to traumatic brain injury (PDTBI)" with hallucinations or delusions being present, the psychosis being considered a direct consequence of the injury, and not being accounted for by another mental disorder or delirium. The crucial decision in such cases is meeting the "direct consequence" criterion. The usual approach taken by clinicians is that there is a temporal association (TBI preceding SLP, generally by a short interval but with no upper time limit), the individual was free of psychopathology, in particular, prepsychotic symptoms prior to the TBI, and there was no apparent genetic vulnerability to the development of schizophrenia (i.e. no family history of psychosis). They might also take the type of injury into consideration. A closed-head injury with concussion and presumed fronto-temporal injury, and an open injury with trauma to the frontal or temporal lobes may be considered as "sufficient evidence."

On the other hand, an injury exclusively to the parietal or occipital lobe is considered as insufficient evidence for such an association, based on the functional neuroanatomy of schizophrenia. Neuropsychological deficits may also be considered in the determination, with fronto-subcortical or temporal lobe deficits suggesting plausibility. Unfortunately, because the anatomical and neuropsychological deficits in schizophrenia are not specific, they do not offer clear guidelines for meeting the "direct consequence" criterion, and clinical judgment is generally relied upon.

In conclusion, anecdotal reports of SLP following TBI do not and cannot provide strong evidence for the association because of the likelihood of chance association and the subjective nature of the determination. However, they have prompted more systematic studies.

Cross-sectional surveys

The noteworthy cross-sectional study was conducted as part of the U.S. National Epidemiological Catchment Area study based in New Haven, Connecticut [6], with any heads injury leading to loss of consciousness or confusion being included. Of the 361 (7.2%) head-injured individuals in the sample, 3.4% were diagnosed with schizophrenia (cf. 1.9% of controls without head injury), a statistically nonsignificant result (chi^2 = 2.8, p = 0.093). Although this was a large population-

based study and the ascertainment of schizophrenia used a standard instrument (albeit one that has been questioned in its validity), the ascertainment of head injury was crude and relied on self-report alone. The cross-sectional nature of the study means that both schizophrenia and TBI are measured at the same time, and the nature of causality can be difficult to determine. It could be argued, for example, that individuals predisposed to schizophrenia are behaviorally more predisposed to a head injury, an instance of *reverse causality*, which this design cannot clarify.

Case control studies

These studies have been used to both examine the strength of the association and identify risk factors for the development of SLP following TBI.

Studies examining the strength of the association

Evidence has been presented [7, 8] to implicate pregnancy and delivery complications, some of which result in TBI, as an increased risk for the development of schizophrenia. In a large case-control study, Wilcox and Nasrallah [9] used medical records of patients admitted to a university hospital between 1934 and 1944 with schizophrenia (n = 200), depression (n = 203), mania (n = 122) and "surgical" controls (n = 134) to examine the prevalence of head injury before age 10 years. The odds ratio (OR) for schizophrenia for those with childhood head injury was 16.6 (CI 2.6 to 689), a highly significant result. The odds for bipolar disorder (OR 6.9, CI 0.8 to 321) and depression (OR 2.0, CI 0.2 to 10.5) were nonsignificantly elevated. These authors did not find any significant relationship with a particular location of the injury. Gureje and colleagues [10], in a case-control study in a Nigerian sample, also found an association between childhood brain trauma and schizophrenia. These patients also had mixed laterality in adulthood, possibly attributable to left hemispheric damage.

The major limitation of studies that rely on historical information is recall bias, with the suspicion that subjects with schizophrenia and their family members are more likely to report past TBI than matched controls. There is also a likelihood of observer bias, with a clinician more likely to inquire and record an episode of head injury in a neuropsychiatric patient than a control patient. The issue of a suitable control population is another consideration. These limitations have been overcome by two case register linkage studies from countries in which population-based case registers are maintained and most of medical encounters occur in the public sector.

The study by Nielsen and colleagues [11], a nested case-control study, identified 8,288 individuals with ICD-8 schizophrenia who had been admitted to a Danish psychiatric hospital between 1978 and 1993, and matched each case to 10 controls from the general population, based on the Central Persons Register. The subjects were linked to the National Patient Register to identify any admission secondary to TBI between 1978 and the date of the index psychiatric admission. The authors also noted the occurrence of fractures affecting other parts of the body in this period, as an index of proneness to accidents and injury. Overall, there was no excess of concussion or severe head injury in the schizophrenia patients (OR 0.94 and 0.89, respectively; not a significant result). Individuals with schizophrenia were less likely to have had another fracture (ORT = 0.71, p < 0.01), and if this was corrected for, head injury was slightly but significantly more likely to be associated with schizophrenia (OR 1.37 and 1.29, respectively, p < 0.01). The interpretation of fewer fractures in schizophrenic patients is problematic, appearing to suggest that in the prodromal phase of schizophrenia, their behavior such as social withdrawal, made them less likely to suffer fractures (a case of reverse causality). This was complicated by the fact the rates of fractures differed depending upon the lag periods between injury and psychosis. The authors also examined the risk in relation to the interval between TBI and schizophrenia, and reported that head injury was more likely in the schizophrenia group in the 12 months preceding the index admission (OR 2.0 and 1.84, respectively, p < 0.01) and less likely beyond the 1-year interval.

Although this study should be considered to be largely negative, it does not rule out a small but significant increase in the risk of schizophrenia in the year following TBI. The study, through the linkage of registers, overcame recall bias. However, observer bias is not ruled out, as it is possible that the history of head injury prompted clinicians to make a diagnosis of an "organic" psychosis rather than schizophrenia, leading to an underestimate of the association; the retrospective design does not pick up this detail.

The recent nested case-control study by Harrison and colleagues [12] has the added advantage of having identified a large birth cohort (n = 785,051), in whom 748 cases of schizophrenia and 14,960 matched controls were identified and a documented history of head injury obtained through linkage with the various health registers in Sweden, which is recognized for the comprehensive nature of such documentation. This study found no increase in schizophrenia after head injury (OR 1.10, CI 0.82 to 1.47), and a small increase of nonschizophrenic, nonaffective psychosis (OR 1.37, CI 1.14 to 1.66), which occurred only in head injuries during adolescence or later. The association was not appreciably influenced by the inclusion of various confounding factors (year of birth, highest parental income, highest parental education, highest parental occupation, area of birth, family history of psychosis, Apgar score at 5 min, gestational age, paternal age, birth weight, birth length) in the model.

This is the largest case-control study in this field and its reliance on record linkage and a birth cohort gives it much strength, although it suffers from the same limitation as the Danish study in terms of the diagnoses being made in different centers with lack of standardization, because organic psychoses were not included. Overall, this excellent study, in combination with the previous literature, makes it very unlikely that there is a strong link between head injury and schizophrenia, but a weak association is not ruled out.

Two other studies used the case-control method to ask the question whether TBI increased the risk of schizophrenia in individuals at genetically increased risk of the disorder. Corcoran and Malaspina [13] used the diagnostic interview for genetic studies to inquire about a history of significant head injury in individuals from multiplex schizophrenia pedigrees (n = 561) and multiplex bipolar disorder pedigrees (n = 1,271) participating in a genetics study. Overall, the individuals with schizophrenia were > 3 times more likely to report a previous TBI than unaffected individuals. This risk increased with the genetic risk of schizophrenia. In the bipolar pedigree, there was no increased risk, and it was four-fold in those with a high genetic risk for schizophrenia (OR 4.27, CI 1.40 to 13.0). The authors did not test for an interaction effect, and we therefore are not certain whether the increased risk is specific to the high genetic risk group.

A Canadian study [14] also used the case-control design in 23 multiply-affected families with schizophrenia and reported that schizophrenia patients had an excess of TBI sustained before 10 years (OR 2.34, CI 1.03 to 5.03) or before 17 years (OR 1.90, CI 0.95 to 3.79), the former being statistically significant.

In summary, the case-control studies provide strong evidence that TBI does not substantially increase the risk of schizophrenia in the general population, although a small increase cannot be ruled out. In individuals with a genetic risk for schizophrenia, this increase in risk may be greater, although the retrospective nature of the studies make the data prone to bias.

Studies that examined risk factors for schizophrenia following TBI

The study by Sachdev and colleagues [15] included 45 patients with SLP following TBI who had been referred for a medicolegal opinion and were so determined by the authors, and matched them with 45 head-injured patients without SLP or other psychiatric disorder. The authors found that a family history of schizophrenia was a risk factor for SLP, but the nature and degree of head injury did not produce a significant effect, although the study was not powered for subtle effects.

A similar case-control study by Fujii and Ahmed [16] included 25 cases of PDTBI and 25 controls, and reported that those with psychosis had history of prior head injury or evidence of neurological disorder, suggesting brain damage as a source of vulnerability. The small size of the study and the broad and heterogeneous nature of brain damage make the results inconclusive. Moreover, the authors excluded patients who had a family history of psychosis, thereby making it impossible to examine an interaction with genetic vulnerability.

Some of the findings of these studies in relation to the nature of the psychosis will be discussed later.

Cohort studies

The earliest attempt to review the cohort studies was by Davison and Bagley [17] who examined 8 studies published between 1917 and 1964, 7 of which were in war veterans, with follow-up periods of 10 to 20 years (except for 2 studies with 2 years or less). The cumulative incidence of schizophrenia in the TBI subjects ranged from 0.07% to 9.8%, with the median figure of 1.35%. Using a comparison figure of 0.8% incidence over 25 years in the general population, the

authors concluded that the risk in the brain-injured group was two- to threefold. The limitations of heterogeneity of diagnostic criteria applied, and the use of a population based incidence figure derived by different methodology, are obvious.

The most well-known cohort study was published from Finland [18] and was a 22–26 year follow-up of 3,552 Finnish veterans of World War II. Almost all (98.8%) suffered injuries from bullets or shrapnel and 42% of injuries were open, making them atypical of peacetime injuries. Medical care for the veterans was provided by one hospital, and the records of this hospital were examined for history of psychosis. Defined broadly, 317 (8.9%) individuals had the onset of psychosis following brain injury; of these, 2.1% had schizophrenic psychoses and another 2.0% paranoid psychoses, giving an incidence of SLP of about 4.1% (CI 3.5 to 4.7%). A significant proportion (42%) had the onset of psychosis more than 10 years after the injury. Although the study strongly supported an increased incidence of SLP, it suffers from the limitations of observer bias, lack of standardized diagnostic assessments, the atypical nature of brain injury, the possibility of psychological factors such as combat stress being contributory, and the lack of generalizability from a special population.

A study from Belgium [19] retrospectively studied 530 brain-injured patients who had been assessed at a neuropsychological center and followed up for 1–10 years. Eighteen were diagnosed with a major psychiatric disorder, mostly (83%) within 6 months of the injury, of which 12 (2.3%) had DSM-III schizophrenia or schizophreniform disorder. The authors reported high rates of premorbid psychopathology and suggested that the injury aggravated or precipitated a pre-existing condition rather than caused it.

Roberts [20] attempted to follow up 479 patients with severe head injury (post-traumatic amnesia > 1 week) admitted to the Radcliffe Infirmary, Oxford, after 10–24 years. Of the 291 survivors with sufficient clinical data, 7 had a diagnosis of "paranoid dementia" and 2 of SLP (9/291 = 3.09%). In the 2 with SLP, the onset was 9 and 17 years postinjury, and affective symptoms were prominent.

There have been some other noteworthy studies. Ota [21] studied 1,168 adults who were admitted to hospital following TBI and reported psychosis, which could be either "functional" or "organic", in 2.7%. Miller and Stern [22], in a long-term follow-up of 100 TBI subjects, found 10 with psychosis, all of whom

Table 13.1 Association between traumatic brain injury (TBI) and schizophrenia-like psychosis (SLP): epidemiological evidence

Authors	N	Duration of follow-up	Risk	Comment
Case Reports				
Fujii & Ahmed, 2002 [5]	69	–	–	Anecdotal reports
Cross-sectional Studies				
Silver *et al.*, 2001 [6]	361	–	1.8	3.4% vs. 1.9%
Case control studies				
Wilcox & Nasrallah, 1987 [9]	200 (controls = 137)	–	OR 16.6** (95% CI 2.6–689)	TBI < 10 years
Nielsen *et al.*, 2002 [11]	8,288	–	OR 0.94/0.89 (0.71*, corrected)	N.S. (corrected for fractures)
Harrison *et al.*, 2006 [12]	748 (204 controls)	–	OR1.10 (CI 0.82–1.47) [OR1.37 (CI1.14–1.66)]	Nonschizophrenic, nonaffective psychosis
Corcoran & Malaospina, 2001 [13]	581	–	OR 4.27 (CI 1.4–3.0)	
Malik *et al.*, 2003 [14]	23 families	–	OR 2.34 (CI 1.03–5.03)	TBI < 10 years

suffered from dementia. A study by Lishman [23], using contemporary diagnostic criteria, identified only 5 patients with schizophrenia-like illness in 670 patients with penetrating head injury.

A recent historical cohort study is of interest [24]. It included 939 adults diagnosed with TBI in a emergency department during 1993 and searched their medical records for the period of 1 year before and 3 years following the injury for psychiatric diagnoses or treatment. An unexpected finding of the study was that patients with TBI had a higher rate of pre-existing psychosis (OR 10.0 for moderate to severe TBI, and 1.7 for mild TBI). In those with no pre-existing psychiatric disorder (n = 85), the risk of psychosis was significantly elevated by moderate to severe head injury in the second year (OR 5.9, CI 1.6 to 22.1) and third year (OR 3.6, CI 1.0 to 1.3) of follow-up. The limitations of this study include the reliance on case notes for diagnosis, the short preinjury period covered, and the relatively small sample size.

The diversity of the evidence discussed earlier makes for a difficult synthesis, but the conservative conclusion is that population-based studies suggest that civilian TBI leads to only a small increase in the risk of SLP if at all, and the evidence for this is not consistent. The association may be stronger in those with a genetic vulnerability to schizophrenia or the presence of preinjury psychopathology. War-related brain injury may be a special case that cannot be generalized to civilian populations, and the reported increase of risk may well be due to psychological rather than neurological factors. Because the increase in risk, albeit small, cannot be dismissed, the clinical characteristics of putative post-traumatic SLP to determine if it is distinct from schizophrenia in its phenomenology, clinical associations, and prognosis will now be examined.

Clinical presentation

This description is based primarily on the review by Davison and Bagley [17] and 2 recent reports of SLP-TBI [5, 25], 1 of which [5] is an analysis of 69 published cases.

The majority of the subjects are young, with a male preponderance in the case reports. The mean age of onset of psychosis was 26.3 (SD 10.2) years and 33.4 (SD 15.4) years in the 2 studies, with 80% and 90% being men. Because TBI is more common in young men, it is uncertain whether the SLP rates merely reflect this. It has been suggested [5] that men may be over-represented after accounting for the base rates for TBI, but this is far from established. In the large Danish study, the authors examined the effect of sex and found that the mean interval between the TBI and the development of psychosis was 4.6 [15] and 4.1 [5] years in the 2 reports, with a wide range (0–34 years). Although most civilian TBI is due to motor vehicle accidents; assaults, gunshot injuries, and falls are all represented.

Characteristics of head injury

The TBI is more likely to be closed, but an open injury is not necessarily protective against future SLP, as has sometimes been suggested [18]. The severity of the injury is usually moderate to severe intensity. The severity of the head injury, by neuroimaging and neuropsychological criteria, was greater in the SLP-TBI group than the TBI group without psychosis [15]. Although many SLP-TBI occur after head injury in childhood, early head injury was not over-represented in one large study [15]. In about 40% cases in this study [15], the head injury was followed by personality or behavioral change, the main characteristics of which were impulsivity, aggressiveness, loss of social graces, moodiness, and, less commonly, apathy. There was evidence for brain damage in the temporal, parietal, and frontal lobes, more often unilateral than bilateral, on the basis of neuroimaging, clinical, and neuropsychological data. The SLP-TBI subjects had more widespread neuropsychological deficits than the control group [15].

Psychopathology

Prodromal symptoms are common and include bizarre or antisocial behavior, social withdrawal, affective instability, and deterioration in work, often lasting for months. Depressive symptoms are often present at the time of presentation but confusional symptoms at onset are unusual.

The psychosis is delusional-hallucinatory in nature. A range of delusional symptoms, similar to that seen in schizophrenia, is present and includes first rank Schneiderian symptoms. In the study by Sachdev and colleagues [15], one or more delusions were present in all subjects, with persecutory (55.5%), referential (22.2%), control (22.2%), grandiose (20%), and religious (15.4%) delusion being the most common types. Delusions of thought alienation, thought insertion, withdrawal, or broadcast were present in six (13.3%) and somatic passivity in three (6.7%). The review by Fujii and Ahmed [5] emphasized the presence of persecutory delusions. Organic themes, described by Cutting [26], were absent in the Sachdev and colleagues [15] study. However, the review of published cases [5] did find 5 cases with the Capgras delusion and 3 cases each with reduplicative amnesia, erotomania, and stealing. Delusions relating to misidentification, stealing, or hiding that are prone to occur in dementia patients with psychosis, are not generally seen in SLP-TBI. Hallucinations were predominantly auditory or visual, with the former being more likely. Formal thought disorder and catatonic features are usually absent. The psychosis is therefore predominantly a positive syndrome, with only 22% and 15% of patients in the two studies demonstrating negative symptoms such as flattening of affect, avolition, or asociality. Agitated and aggressive behavior are common.

Diagnostic criteria

As is apparent from the earlier description, the clinical picture resembles schizophrenia, with the difference being that like other secondary schizophrenias, the emphasis is on a paranoid-hallucinatory psychosis with few negative symptoms. To meet the DSM-IV criteria for a Psychotic Disorder due to Traumatic Brain Injury, it is crucial to establish that i) the psychosis is a direct physiological consequence of a brain disorder, and ii) the psychosis is not better accounted for by a primary psychiatric disorder such as schizophrenia. The pathophysiology of SLP is discussed later, but the association between TBI and SLP cannot be considered proof of causality even though it is a recognized association, psychosis as a consequence of brain injury is plausible, and many of the patients are not otherwise vulnerable to schizophrenia.

Course

The long-term course of SLP-TBI is poorly studied. Fujii and Ahmed [5] found some follow-up information on 39 out of the 69 cases reviewed: of these, 25 patients were reported to have improved, 11 did not improve, and 3 worsened. Sachdev and colleagues [15] did not follow patients systematically; but it is not unusual for clinicians to encounter TBI related psychosis that, despite its prominence of positive symptoms, responds poorly to neuroleptic medication.

Risk factors and pathophysiology

Are there specific neuroanatomical substrates of SLP-TBI?

Psychosis following focal brain injury is a relatively rare event, but several consistent observations relating right brain dysfunction to delusional disorders have emerged. Anatomically, lesions of the temporo-parietal region are associated with the highest frequency of lesion-related psychosis [26, 27]. The data on anatomical localization in relation to TBI have not been consistent, and no convincing theoretical framework has emerged. In the study by Sachdev and colleagues [15], the comparison of the two groups on neuroimaging data suggested greater damage in the SLP group in the left temporal and right parietal regions, but the differences were not significant after Bonferroni correction. The Fujii and Ahmed [5] review suggested a trend toward focal lesions affecting, in particular, the frontal and temporal lobes. Although 65% cases reported positive findings on CT/MRI, no brain region emerged as being necessarily affected in patients with SLP, however, in closed, head injury, the lack of involvement of specific brain regions becomes difficult to prove. Similarly, laterality has not emerged as a significant factor in the development of psychosis, although a suggestion has been made that left temporal lesions may be more common in those who develop SLP [15].

Is there a specific cognitive syndrome underlying the development of SLP following TBI?

Cognitive deficits have the potential of providing continuity between the brain damage of TBI and the development of psychosis. If the cognitive deficits of SLP-TBI patients resemble those seen in schizophrenia and differ from the deficits seen in TBI patients who do not develop psychosis, an argument relating to their specificity can be supported. The difficulty is that what constitutes core deficits in schizophrenia is still in dispute, although attention, memory, and executive deficits are broadly recognized as being characteristic. In the study by Sachdev and colleagues [15], SLP-TBI subjects were more likely to have abnormalities on measures of verbal and nonverbal memory and frontal-executive functioning, when compared to TBI subjects without psychosis. However, they also tended to have more of a disturbance in language and parietal lobe functioning, suggesting a diffuse impairment in neuropsychological functioning in comparison with the non-SLP group. In the other review [5] mentioned earlier, 88% of cases reported impairments on neuropsychological testing. The most common impaired function was memory, followed by executive and visuospatial functions. Clearly, more work is necessary to establish the salience and specificity of some neurocognitive deficits in the development of SLP.

Are TBI patients who develop SLP predisposed to psychosis due to some pre-existing vulnerability?

The cohort studies mentioned earlier are informative on this question. In the study by Corcoran and Malaspina [13], there was no increase in risk for schizophrenia after TBI in the members of bipolar pedigrees (OR 0.75, CI 0.10 to 5.93), but a fourfold increase in families with two or more first-degree relatives affected with schizophrenia (OR 4.27, CI 1.40 to 13.0). The authors did not, however, test for interaction effects to confirm that this difference was greater than a chance effect. In the Sachdev and colleagues [15] study, it emerged that the most significant risk factor for SLP-TBI was a genetic vulnerability to psychosis as reflected in the family history, even though this was present in only a fraction of patients. Family history has been used as a marker of genetic predisposition for schizophrenia and other psychiatric disorders. For schizophrenia, the lifetime risks of psychosis reported for first-degree relatives have varied from 3.1 to 16.9% [28]. The Sachdev and colleagues [15] finding of 24% risk in first-degree relatives, compared to 3% for controls, is therefore high, even if an upward reporting bias in the SLP group is considered as a factor. In a study of schizophrenia secondary to a variety of neurological disorders, Feinstein and Ron [29] found a positive family history in only 3.8%. In epilepsy patients with chronic SLP, the risk of schizophrenia in first degrees was reported by Slater and Glithero [30] to be no higher than the general population. It is possible that head injury brings out a vulnerability to schizophrenia due to genetic or other factors in at least some patients. Further, Malik and colleagues [14] reported that in those with a family history of schizophrenia, TBI before 10 years was related with an earlier age of onset of schizophrenia.

Relationship with epilepsy?

A varying percentage of patients, depending on the location and severity of injury, will have seizures during the acute period after the trauma. Post-traumatic epilepsy, with repeated seizures and the requirement for anticonvulsant medication, occurs in approximately 12%, 2%, and 0.8% of patients with severe, moderate, and mild head injuries, respectively, within 5 years of the injury [31]. The rate of epilepsy reported by Fujii and Ahmed in their review of SLP-TBI was 34%, which is an over-representation [32]. On the other hand, in the case-control study presented by Sachdev and colleagues [15], the SLP subjects had a nonsignificantly lower epilepsy rate, and epilepsy in these patients was well-controlled, unlike those TBI patients who were not psychotic who had medication-resistant epilepsy. These authors speculated that epileptic seizures might in some way be protective against the development of psychosis. An interesting observation from the Fujii and Ahmed [5] review was that SLP patients with epilepsy were less likely to have delusions than those without epilepsy.

Is age of TBI important?

The schizophrenia literature suggests that brain injury early in childhood may be more important in relation to the risk for schizophrenia [7, 8] because it is likely to disrupt normal neurodevelopment. The SLP-TBI literature does not consistently support this conclusion, however, and head injury in these individuals occurred across a wide age span, including childhood, adolescence, and adulthood. The Wilcox and Nasrallah [9] and Gureje and colleagues [10] studies, designed specifically to examine the effect of head injury in childhood, reported a strong association with SLP. In the Canadian study of multiply affected families, injury <10 years was over-represented in the schizophrenia cases (OR 2.34, CI 1.03 to 5.36). However, in the large Swedish case control study [12], the small increase in incidence of nonschizophrenic, nonaffective psychosis occurred only in those with injury during adolescence or later. In the Sachdev and colleagues [15] study, childhood injury was not over-represented.

Birth trauma and schizophrenia

The proposal that pregnancy and birth complications are associated with an increased risk of schizophrenia has been extensively studied and is generally accepted despite some controversy [7]. In a cohort study mentioned earlier, Wilcox and Nasrallah [9] concluded that childhood head trauma at less than 5 years of age was more likely to have occurred in schizophrenic patients. Gureje and colleagues [10], in another retrospective study, also found an association between childhood brain trauma and schizophrenia. The markers used to indicate these perinatal insults include low birth weight, prematurity, preeclampsia, prolonged labor, hypoxia, and fetal distress [33]. The overall effect of perinatal accidents when calculated is small, increasing risk of disease by only 1%. The evidence only points to an association and not causality.

Conclusion and future directions

SLP is a relatively uncommon psychiatric consequence after brain injury. The epidemiological literature on the association between SLP and TBI is considerable, but a definitive longitudinal study has never been conducted. The two Scandinavian studies [11, 12] present the best current evidence for the association and support only a marginally increased risk, if at all. The risk may be significantly greater, however, in those with a genetic vulnerability to schizophrenia. It is also possible that TBI may exacerbate pre-existing psychosis. Whether an individual in the prodrome of a schizophrenic illness has an altered risk of having a TBI is not certain from the data.

When it does develop, the clinical presentation of the psychosis following TBI has considerable overlap with primary schizophrenic disorder, with a prominence of persecutory and other delusions, auditory hallucinations, and a dearth of negative symptoms. The interval between TBI and the onset of SLP is very variable. The onset is often gradual, with a subacute or chronic course. More severe and diffuse brain injury, especially one that involves the temporal and frontal lobes, is the most prominent risk factor, and EEG and neuroimaging abnormalities are often present. The presence of epilepsy does not appear to increase the risk of SLP and could possibly be protective.

The interaction of TBI with genetic risk factors for schizophrenia is worthy of further examination, and this should include the study of candidate genes implicated in schizophrenia. Detailed studies of SLP-TBI patients with newer imaging techniques, combined with electrophysiology, should enable us to better understand the nature of brain injury that is associated with the development of psychosis. These patients must also be examined for neurobiological and neuropsychological abnormalities commonly associated with schizophrenia to determine the relative contributions of a diathesis and brain injury toward the genesis of SLP.

What are the implications of the conclusion for medicolegal practice? Although the evidence for the association is not overwhelming, as noted earlier, the possibility that TBI might make a contribution toward the development of schizophrenia, especially in vulnerable individuals cannot be dismissed. Medicolegal determination must therefore occur on an individual basis, after considering the premorbid status of the individual, the nature of the TBI, the psychological trauma and social factors related to the injury, neuropsychological and anatomical deficits from the injury, and the nature of the psychosis that follows.

The level of evidence needed for medicolegal purposes is different from that required for scientific inquiry, and it may be possible that some injuries could be compensable, at least partially, due to the subsequent development of SLP.

References

1. Kraus J. F., Sorenson, S. B. (1994). Epidemiology. In *Neuropsychiatry of Traumatic Injury*, Silver J. M., Yudofsky S. C., Hales R. E. (Eds.). Washington, DC: APPI, pp. 3–41.

2. NIH Consensus Development Panel on rehabilitation of persons with traumatic brain injury: rehabilitation of persons with traumatic brain injury. *JAMA*, 1999. **282**:974–83.

3. Kurtzke, J.F. Neuroepidemiology. *Ann Neurol*, 1984. **16**:265–77.

4. Von Krafft-Ebing, R. (1868). Ueber die durch Gehirnerschutterung und kopfverletzung hervogerufenen psychischen krankheiten. Eine klinisch-forensische studie. Verlag von Ferdinand enke: Erlngen.

5. Fujii D. E., Ahmed I. Characteristics of psychotic disorder due to traumatic brain injury: an analysis of case studies in the literature. *J Neuropsychiatry Clin Neurosci*, 2002. **14**:130–140.

6. Silver J. M., Kramer R., Greenwald S., *et al.* The association between head injuries and psychiatric disorders: findings from the New York NIMH epidemiologic catchment area study. *Brain Inj*, 2001. **15**:935–45.

7. Lewis S. W., Murray R. M. Obstetrical complications, neurodevelopmental deviance, and risk of schizophrenia. *J Psychiatr Res*, 1987. **21**:413–21.

8. Dalman C., Allebeck P., Cullberg J., *et al.* Obstetric complications and the risk of schizophrenia. *Arch Gen Psychiatry*, 1999. **56**:234–40.

9. Wilcox J. A., Nasrallah H. Childhood head trauma and psychosis. *Psychiatr Res*, 1987. **21**:303–6.

10. Gureje O., Bamidele R. Raji O. Early brain trauma and schizophrenia in Nigerian patients. *Am J Psychiatry*, 1994. **151**:368–71.

11. Nielsen A. S., Mortensen P. B., O'Callagahn E., *et al.* Is head injury a risk factor for schizophrenia? *Schizophr Res*, 2002. **55**:93–8.

12. Harrison G., Whitley E., Rasmussen F., *et al.* Risk of schizophrenia and other nonaffective psychosis among individuals exposed to head injury: case control study. *Schizophr Res*, 2006. **88**: 119–26.

13. Corcoran C., Malaspina D. Traumatic brain injury and risk for schizophrenia. *Int J Ment Health*, 2001. **30**:17–32.

14. Malik P. A., Husted J., Chow E. W. C., *et al.* Childhood head injury and expression of schizophrenia in multiply affected families. *Arch Gen Psychiatry*, 2003. **60**: 231–6.

15. Sachdev P., Smith J. S., Cathcart S. Schizophrenia-like psychosis following traumatic brain injury: a chart-based descriptive and case-control study. *Psychol Med*, 2001. **31**:231–9.

16. Fujii D. E., Ahmed I. Risk factors in psychosis secondary to traumatic brain injury. *J Neuropsychiatry Clin Neurosci*, 2001. **13**:61–9.

17. Davison K., Bagley C. R. (1969). Schizophrenia-like psychosis associated with organic disorders of the central nervous system: a review of the literature. In *Current Problems in Neuropsychiatry: Schizophrenia, Epilepsy, the Temporal Lobe*. Special Publication No. 4, Herrington, R. (Ed.). London: British Psychiatric Association, pp. 1–89.

18. Achte K., Hillbom E., Aalberg V. Psychoses following war injury. *Acta Psychiatr Scand*, 1969. **45**:1–18.

19. De Mol J., Violon A., Brihaye J. Post-traumatic psychoses: a retrospective study of 18 cases. *J Arch Psychol Neurol*, 1987. **48**:336–50.

20. Roberts A. H. (1979). *Severe Accidental Head Injury: an Assessment of Long-Term Prognosis*. London: MacMillan Press.

21. Ota Y. (1969). Psychiatric studies on civilian head injuries. In *The Late Effects of Head Injury*, Walker A. E., Caveness W. F., and Critchley M. (Eds.). Springfield, Illinois: C C Thomas, pp. 110–19.

22. Miller H., Stern G. The long-term prognosis of severe head injury. *Lancet*, 1965. **1**:225–9.

23. Lishman A. Brain damage in relation to psychiatric disability after head injury. *Br J Psychiatry*, 1968. **114**:373–410.

24. Fann J. R., Burington B., Leonetti A., *et al.* Psychiatric illness following traumatic brain injury in a adult health maintenance organization population. *Arch Gen Psychiatry*, 2004. **61**: 53–61.

25. Buckley P., Stack J. P., Madigan C., *et al.* Magnetic resonance imaging of schizophrenia-like psychosis associated with cerebral trauma: clinicopathological correlates. *Am J Psychiatry*, 1993. **150**:146–8.

26. Cutting J. The phenomenology of acute organic psychosis: comparison with acute schizophrenia. *Br J Psychiatry*, 1987. **151**:324–32.

27. Miller B. L., Benson D. F., Cummings J. L., *et al.* Late -life paraphrenia: an organic delusional syndrome. *J Clin Psychiatry*, 1986. **47**:204–7.

28. Gershon E. S., Delisi L. E., Hamovit J., *et al.* A controlled study of chronic psychoses. Schizophrenia and schizoaffective disorder. *Arch Gen Psychiatry*, 1988. **45**:328–36.

29. Feinstein A., Ron M. A. Psychosis associated with demonstrable brain disease. *Psychol Med*, 1990. **20**:793–803.

30. Slater E., Glithero E. The
    schizophrenia-like psychoses of
    epilepsy 3. Genetic aspects. *Br J
    Psychiatry*, 1963. **109**:130–3.

31. Annegers J. F., Grabow J. D.,
    Groover R. V., *et al.* Seizures
    after head trauma: a population

    study. *Neurology*, 1908. **30**:
    683–9.

32. Fujii D. E., Ahmed I. Psychosis
    secondary to traumatic brain
    injury. *Neuropsychiatr
    Neuropsychol Behav Neurol*, 1996.
    9:133–8.

33. McGrath J., Murray R. M. (1995).
    Risk factors for schizophrenia:
    from conception to birth. In
    Schizophrenia, Hirsch S. R. and
    Weinberger D. R. (Eds). Oxford,
    England: Blackwell Scientific,
    pp. 187–205.

Cerebrovascular disease and psychosis

Osvaldo P. Almeida and Sergio E. Starkstein

Facts box

- Poststroke psychosis is uncommon, and the vast majority of stroke patients will never develop psychotic symptoms.
- Psychosis can occur in association with cerebrovascular disease, but poststroke schizophrenia is rare.
- Temporo-parietal-occipital lesions are more likely to be found in association with psychosis, although strokes in almost all other brain areas have been reported in association with psychotic symptoms.
- The prevalence of psychosis in vascular dementia and Alzheimer's Disease is similar, which suggests that it is not so much vascular pathology but the disruption of neuronal networks associated with dementia that contributes to the development of delusions and hallucinations.
- Currently available evidence suggests that, in isolation, cerebrovascular disease plays a limited role in the development of schizophrenia-like symptoms in later life.

Introduction

The neurobiological mechanisms that ultimately lead to the development of psychotic symptoms are poorly understood, but tentative evidence suggests that cerebrovascular disease might contribute to the onset of delusions and hallucinations, particularly in later life. This chapter aims to critically review the available literature on this topic. It is divided into two major subsections: the first examines studies investigating the emergence of psychotic symptoms in association with established cerebrovascular accidents; the second evaluates the presence of cerebrovascular disease in association with schizophrenia and delusional disorder.

Psychotic symptoms arising after stroke

A case report

JB was a 63-year-old engineer who presented with left-sided weakness, left homonymous hemianopia, spatio-temporal disorientation and visual hallucinations. There was no past history of psychiatric disorders. He was alert and cooperative and showed no agitation. JB had impaired memory for recent events, confabulated spontaneously and often mistook one physician for another. His visual hallucinations were orientated to the right visual space only. He reported seeing three young girls dressed in colorful clothes who were mocking him because of his poor performance on the neurological examination. During the following days, he reported seeing a soldier through the ceiling and a clergyman beside his bed. These complex hallucinations rarely occurred in the evening, and only once did he report tactile (a dog's cold nose touching him) and auditory hallucinations (e.g., hearing a Spanish song). Additional findings on neuropsychological evaluation were a severe hemispatial neglect, motor impersistence, constructional apraxia, and spatial dysgraphia. Two weeks after the stroke, the patient became euphoric and jocular. He reduplicated body parts (e.g., he reported having three arms) and also showed anosognosia, personification of his weak left arm and misoplegia (morbid dislike or hatred of paralyzed limb). He obtained a score of 97 on the verbal scale of the WAIS-R, a score of 77 on WAIS-R performance scale and a score of 91 on the Wechsler Memory Scale. A CT scan showed an extensive right fronto-temporo-parietal infarction. JB was re-examined 6 months after his acute admission. There were no visual hallucinations, and he attributed his past hallucinations to "mistaken impressions" [1].

Phenomenology of post-stroke psychosis

Different terms have been used to refer to post-stroke psychosis, namely, atypical psychosis, peduncular hallucinosis, release hallucinations, organic psychosis, and agitated delirium. The term "peduncular hallucinosis" was coined by L'Hermitte [2] to describe the clinical presentation of a patient with visual hallucinations after a brainstem lesion and preserved insight into the lack of reality of the perception.

Post-stroke psychosis should be diagnosed using the DSM-IV criteria for "Psychotic Disorder Due to a General Medical Condition." The essential features of this diagnosis are "prominent hallucinations or delusions that are judged to be due to the direct physiological effects of a general medical condition." However, this is difficult to ascertain in the case of strokes, given the relatively low incidence of psychotic symptoms after stroke. The DSM-IV acknowledges that "there are no infallible guidelines for determining whether the relationship between the psychotic disturbance and the general medical condition is etiological" and suggests that the temporal association between psychosis and the medical condition, as well as the presence of features that are atypical for a primary psychotic disorder, are helpful diagnostic considerations. The DSM-III revision (DSM-111-R) had specific criteria for atypical psychosis, which was considered "a residual category for cases in which there are psychotic symptoms (delusions, hallucinations, incoherence, loosening of associations, markedly illogical thinking or behavior that is grossly disorganized or catatonic) that do not meet criteria for any mental disorder." This category is now subsumed under the DSM-IV category of "Psychotic Disorder Not Otherwise Specified." The ICD-10 includes specific criteria for "Organic Hallucinosis" and for "Organic Delusional [schizophrenia-like] Disorder." For both diagnoses there has to be objective evidence of cerebral damage and clear consciousness, as well as persistent or recurrent hallucinations for the former and delusions with a varying degree of systematization for the latter. Finally, the DSM-III-R listed the following as specific criteria for "organic hallucinosis": i) prominent persistent or recurrent hallucinations, ii) evidence of a specific organic factor judged to be etio-

logically related to the disturbance, and iii) not occurring exclusively during the course of delirium. However, this category has been deleted from the DSM-IV revision.

Starkstein and colleagues [3] described two types of hallucinatory phenomena in stroke patients. *Hallucination* refers to a perception in the absence of a stimulus, with the qualification that the patient believes that the perception is real. When these hallucinations occur after a stroke, they should be considered *secondary hallucinations*. *Hallucinosis* also involves a perception without a stimulus, but the patient does not believe the perception is real. They listed the following as characteristic of hallucinosis: i) vivid imagery, ii) anomalous presentation of the images, iii) ego-dystonia (the false perceptions are not integrated to the patient's perception of reality), and iv) preserved awareness on the nonreality of the perception. Based on this diagnostic scheme, hallucinosis occurring after a stroke should be labeled *secondary hallucinosis*.

Prevalence of post-stroke psychosis

Few studies have systematically looked into the association between stroke and psychosis (i.e. delusions and hallucinations) [4, 5]. Not surprisingly, the prevalence of psychotic symptoms after stroke remains largely unknown. The results from the Study of Assets and Health Dynamics in the USA showed that stroke is associated with increased odds of delusions (odds ratio (OR): 16.1, 95% confidence interval (CI): 8.87, 29.5) and hallucinations (OR: 7.4, 95% CI: 4.1, 13.2)[35]. More recently, Kumral and Öztürk [6] reported that 15 out of 360 consecutive patients admitted to hospitals after a stroke developed delusions within 3 months (4.2%). In most cases, symptoms became apparent during the first week after the stroke. In a record-linkage study of 1,008 incident cases of stroke admitted to hospitals in Western Australia, Almeida and Xiao [7] found that 35 people developed a delusional or schizophreniform disorder during the subsequent 2 years (3.5%), with an estimated cumulative incidence of psychosis of 1.1 per 1,000 persons over 12 years. As these estimates are based on stroke patients who are in contact with hospital services, it seems likely that the true incidence of post-stroke psychosis in the community will be lower than 1 per 1000 person-years.

Table 14.1 Selected case reports and case series of psychotic symptoms associated with cerebrovascular lesions

Author	Psychotic symptoms	Lesion location
Berthier and Starkstein, 1987 [1]	Complex visual hallucinations associated with sporadic auditory and tactile hallucinations. Reduplicative paramnesia	Extensive right fronto-temporo-parietal ischemic infarct
Kumral and Öztürk, 2004 [6]	Paranoid (jealousy or persecutory) or somatic delusions in a selected series of 15 patients	Lesions involving most frequently the right posterior temporo-parietal cortex, although lenticular, thalamic, and medullar lesions were also observed
Rabins et al., 1991 [8]	Unspecified delusions and hallucinations in a select series of 5 patients. Subjects met DSM-III criteria for the diagnosis of schizophrenia or schizophreniform disorder	Right hemisphere lesions involving one or more of the following structures: frontal, temporal, parietal, and occipital cortices or caudate, putamen, and internal capsule
Filley et al., 1999 [27]	Delusion of jealousy	Extensive diffuse and symmetric confluent white-matter changes on MRI associated with small infarcts in the centrum semiovale and left thalamus (CADASIL)
Nagaratnam and O'Neile, 2000 [28]	Tactile hallucinations and delusions of parasitic infestation	Left temporo-occipital ischemic stroke
Cerrato et al., 2001 [29]	Musical hallucinations	Hemorrhagic lesion involving the left putamen and internal capsule
Beniczky et al., 2002 [30]	Complex visual and tactile hallucinations	Right medial occipital ischemic infarct
Suzuki et al., 2003 [31]	Auditory hallucinations (commanding and derogatory voices)	Bilateral hippocampi lesions (more prominent on the left)
ffytche DH et al., 2004 [32]	Complex visual hallucinations (written sentences and people)	Bilateral temporo-occipital ischemic lesion (more extensive in the right hemisphere)
Predescu et al., 2004 [33]	Auditory hallucinations and paranoid delusions	Bilateral mesencephalo-thalamic ischemic lesion (more extensive in the left hemisphere)
Narumoto et al., 2005 [34]	Delusion of persecution	Bilateral caudate ischemic infarct (head of caudate)
Nye and Arendts, 2002 [35]	Episodic olfactory hallucinations	Hemorrhagic lesion to the left uncus

Mechanisms leading to post-stroke psychosis

Kumral and Öztürk [6] found that delusional ideation was predominantly associated with right posterior temporo-parietal lesions in a selected series of 15 stroke patients. However, as outlined in Table 14.1, delusions and hallucinations may also arise in association with lesions to the left cerebral cortex and subcortical structures. Rabins and colleagues [8] described a series of 5 patients who developed psychotic symptoms shortly after a stroke (a few hours after the stroke in 2 cases, within several days in another 2 cases, and 2 months post-stroke in the remaining patient). All patients had right hemisphere lesions involving the frontal operculum and parietal cortex (1 case), basotemporal and occipital cortex (1 case), fronto-temporo-parietal cortex (1 case), occipital cortex (1 case), and head of the caudate, putamen, and internal

capsule (1 case). These 5 patients with post-stroke psychosis were compared with 5 stroke patients who were within 2 years of the patient's age and whose strokes were in a similar brain region. Neurological findings were similar for both groups, except that seizures were more frequent in those with psychosis (3/5 vs. 0/5). However, there was no significant association between the onset of seizures and of hallucinations. Robinson [9] compared these 5 psychotic subjects with a consecutive series of 301 people with acute stroke lesions assessed for other psychiatric disorders. Patients with psychotic symptoms were significantly older and had higher frequency of family history of psychiatric disorders than stroke patients without psychosis. Finally, 4/5 patients with post-stroke psychosis had cortical lesions, as compared to 42% of the unselected stroke group. On the other hand, there were no differences in lesion volume between the post-stroke psychotic patients, the lesion-matched controls, or the overall stroke population. There were no significant between-group differences in measures of cortical atrophy, but patients with post-stroke psychosis had significantly more severe subcortical atrophy (as determined by frontal horn and third ventricle-to-brain size ratios) than stroke patients without psychosis. Starkstein and colleagues [3] suggested that the reason post-stroke psychosis is uncommon is that several factors may be required to produce psychotic symptoms: right hemisphere lesion involving the temporo-parieto-occipital junction in combination with seizures, genetic vulnerability, and subcortical atrophy probably preceding the brain lesion.

The mechanism of secondary hallucinosis after peduncular lesions is even less well known. L'Hermitte [2] suggested that disturbance of the wake/sleep cycle in association with attentional deficits and a tendency to confabulate may play an important role. Starkstein and colleagues [3] considered that secondary hallucinosis could be a "release phenomenon" secondary to damage to reticular activating brainstem pathways and that the presence of primary sensory deficits could be an important predisposing factor. Levine and Finklestein [10] reported that prominent hallucinations, delusions, and agitation might be associated with right temporo-parietal strokes or trauma.

There are no systematic studies comparing patients with secondary hallucinations and patients with secondary hallucinosis, and it is unclear whether these entities are independent phenomena or are symptoms of the same syndrome. Starkstein and colleagues [3] compared patients with secondary hallucinations reported in the literature with patients with secondary hallucinosis. They found that patients with secondary hallucinations had a higher frequency of visual and auditory phenomena, delusions, and depression when compared to those with hallucinosis. On the other hand, sensory deficits (mainly hemianopia) were significantly more frequent in patients with secondary hallucinosis. Finally, there were no significant between-group differences in the frequency of confusional states.

Vascular dementia and psychosis

Compared to Alzheimer's Disease (AD) and dementia with Lewy bodies (DLB), few clinical and epidemiological investigations have explored the association between psychotic symptoms and vascular dementia (VaD). As a consequence, little is known about the prevalence and characteristics of psychotic symptoms among these patients. Ballard and O'Brien [11], in their review of the available literature, identified eleven cross-sectional studies (mostly of clinical samples). They described a wide variation in the reported prevalence of delusions and hallucinations: 9–70% (total number of patients included in these studies=288). For example, a retrospective analysis of data collected as part of the assessment of 92 patients with VaD and 92 with AD in the Tyneside Hospital, UK, found psychotic symptoms in 42 patients (45.6%) with VaD. Visual and auditory hallucinations were observed in 20 (21.7%) and 7 (7.6%) people with VaD, whereas delusions and misidentification syndromes were recorded for 33 (35.9%) and 21 (22.8%) patients. The frequency distribution of psychotic symptoms in people with AD was similar to VaD.

In the largest community-based study available to date, Lyketsos and colleagues [12] observed delusions and hallucinations in 5 (8.1%) and 8 (12.9%) of their 62 patients with VaD. All subjects were assessed with the Neuropsychiatric Inventory and were part of a large community-based study (Cache County Study) [12]. There was no obvious association between the presence of psychotic symptoms and the severity of the dementia, as measured by the Clinical Dementia Rating. In a later publication [13], this same group described the types of psychotic symptoms present among these patients. They included the belief that others were stealing (4/59) or planning to abandon them (2/59), that intruders were living in their house (3/59), that people were not who they claimed to be (3/59), that their house was not their real home (2/59), or that media figures were in the home (1/59). The frequency distribution of these beliefs was similar to that observed among patients with AD. Hallucinations in the form of audible voices (4/58), talking to people who were not there (5/58) and seeing things others could not see (5/59) were also reported. Again, subjects with VaD and AD had a similar frequency distribution of hallucinations.

There is debate as to whether the psychotic symptoms associated with dementia correlate with the severity of the cognitive impairment. Tentative evidence suggests that delusional ideation is more likely to arise in people with moderate dementia, whereas hallucinations may be more prevalent amongst those with severe cognitive impairment [14, 15]. However, it remains unclear whether psychosis in VaD is associated with the disruption of particular neuronal networks or simply represents a nonspecific response associated with dementia.

Cerebrovascular disease in delusional disorder and schizophrenia

Schizophrenia and delusional disorder with late onset have been associated with a variety of structural brain abnormalities compared to healthy controls, including increased ventricular-to-brain ratio, third ventricular enlargement, generalized cerebral cortical atrophy, smaller superior temporal gyrus, and greater white-matter disease burden [16]. The purported changes in white-matter tracts have attracted a great deal of attention and led to the suggestion that the onset of psychotic symptoms in later life might be partly mediated by cerebrovascular pathology [17]. However, findings from studies using MRI are far from conclusive. To date, four studies reported greater burden of white-matter disease among patients than controls [18, 19, 20, 21], with another four studies observing no obvious difference between these groups [22, 23, 24, 25].

More recently, Jones and colleagues [26] reported the results of the first diffuse tensor imaging study investigating the integrity of white-matter tracts in a sample of 12 patients with late-onset schizophrenia and 12 controls. There was no difference between the groups regarding fractional anisotropy or mean diffusivity, which argues against the presence of specific structural abnormalities within the white-matter tracts of patients.

Existing data does not support the hypothesis that schizophrenia and delusional disorder with onset in later life are strongly associated with cerebrovascular disease.

Conclusion

Cerebrovascular disease has been associated with behavioral changes, including psychosis, for decades, if not centuries. Surprisingly, however, systematic information on this topic remains sparse and, on the whole, inconclusive. After stroke, the onset of psychotic symptoms is uncommon and the development of typical schizophrenic symptoms rare. Preliminary evidence suggests that lesions to the right temporo-parietal-occipital cortex are more likely to be found in association with psychosis, although strokes in almost all other areas of the brain have been observed in association with psychotic symptoms. It is also important to note that most stroke patients never experience delusions or hallucinations, even when the stroke affects the right temporo-parietal-occipital cortex.

There is also limited evidence about the association between psychosis and vascular dementia. The reported prevalence of psychotic symptoms in people with vascular dementia and Alzheimer's Disease is similar [13, 14], and it might be argued that it is not so much the vascular pathology but the disruption of neuronal networks associated with dementia that leads to the expression of delusional ideation and hallucinations.

Cerebrovascular disease has also been associated with late-onset schizophrenia and delusional disorder, particularly in the form of subcortical infarcts or white-matter hyperintensities. However, the results from MRI studies have been inconsistent and the only investigation using diffuse tensor imaging techniques did not find any difference between patients with late-onset schizophrenia and age-gender-education matched controls [26].

Currently available evidence suggests that cerebrovascular disease per se plays a limited role in the development of schizophrenia-like symptoms in later life.

References

1. Berthier M., Starkstein S. Acute atypical psychosis following a right hemisphere stroke. *Acta Neurol Belg*, 1987. **87**:125–31.

2. L'Hermitte J. Syndrome de la callotte du pedoncle cerebral. Les troubles psychosensorieles dans les lesions du mesencephale. *Rev Neurologique*, 1922. **38**:1359–65.

3. Starkstein S. E., Berthier M., Robinson R. G. Post-stroke hallucinatory delusional syndromes. *Neuropsychiatr Neuropsychol Behav Neurol*, 1992. **5**:114–18.

4. Carota A., Staub F., Bogousslavsky J. Emotions, behaviours and mood changes in stroke. *Curr Opin Neurol*, 2002. **15**:57–69.

5. Turkey C. L., Schultz S. K., Arndt S., *et al.* Caregiver report of hallucinations and paranoid delusions in elders aged 70 or older. *Int Psychogeriatr*, 2001. **13**:241–9.

6. Kumral E., Öztürk Ö. Delusional state following acute stroke. *Neurology*, 2004. **62**:110–13.

7. Almeida O. P., Xiao J. Morbidity and mortality associated with incident mental health disorders after stroke: results from a population-based record linkage study. *Aust N Z J Psychiatry*, 2007. **41**:274–81.

8. Rabins P. V., Starkstein S. E., Robinson R. G. Risk factors for developing atypical (schizophreniform) psychosis following stroke. *J Neuropsychiatr Clin Neurosci*, 1991. **3**:6–9.

9. Robinson R. G. (1998). *The clinical neuropsychiatry of stroke.* Cambridge: Cambridge University Press.

10. Levine D. N., Finklestein S. Delayed psychosis after right temporoparietal stroke or trauma: relation to epilepsy. *Neurology*, 1982. **32**:267–73.

11. Ballard C., O'Brien J. T. (2002). Behavioural and psychological symptoms. In: *Vascular Cognitive Impairment.* Erkinjuntti T. and Gautheir S. (Eds.). London: Martin Dunitz, pp. 237–51.

12. Lyketsos C. G., Steinberg M., Tschanz J., *et al.* Mental and behavioral disturbances in dementia: findings from the Cache County Study on memory and aging. *Am J Psychiatry*, 2000. **157**:708–14.

13. Leroi I., Voulgari A., Breitner J. C. S., *et al.* The epidemiology of psychosis in dementia. *Am J Geriatr Psychiatry*, 2003. **11**:83–91.

14. Ballard C., Neill D., O'Brien J., *et al.* Anxiety, depression and psychosis in vascular dementia: prevalence and associations. *J Affect Disord*, 2000. **59**:97–106.

15. Hope T., Keene J., Gedling K., *et al.* Behaviour changes in dementia 1: point of entry data of a prospective study. *Int J Geriatr Psychiatry*, 1997. **12**:1062–73.

16. Howard R., Rabins P. V., Seeman M. V., *et al.* Late-onset schizophrenia and very-late-onset schizophrenia-like psychosis: an international consensus. The International Late-Onset Schizophrenia Group. *Am J Psychiatry*, 2000. **157**:172–8.

17. Miller B. L., Lesser I. M., Boone K. B., *et al.* Brain lesions and cognitive function in late-life psychosis. *Br J Psychiatry*, 1991. **158**:76–82.

18. Breitner J. C., Husain M. M., Figiel G. S., *et al.* Cerebral white matter disease in late-onset paranoid psychosis. *Biol Psychiatry*, 1990. **28**:266–74.

19. Keshavan M. S., Mulsant B. H., Sweet R. A., *et al.* MRI changes in schizophrenia in late life: a preliminary controlled study. *Psychiatry Res*, 1996. **60**:117–23.

20. Lesser I. M., Jeste D. V., Boone K. B., *et al.* Late-onset psychotic disorder, not otherwise specified: clinical and neuroimaging findings. *Biol Psychiatry*, 1992. **31**:419–23.

21. Sachdev P., Brodaty H., Rose N., *et al.* Schizophrenia with onset after age 50 years. 2: Neurological, neuropsychological and MRI investigation. *Br J Psychiatry*, 1999. **175**:416–21.

22. Corey-Bloom J., Jernigan T., Archibald S., *et al.* Quantitative magnetic resonance imaging of the brain in late-life schizophrenia. *Am J Psychiatry*, 1995. **152**:447–9.

23. Howard R., Cox T., Almeida O., *et al.* White matter signal hyperintensities in the brains of patients with late paraphrenia and the normal, community-living elderly. *Biol Psychiatry*, 1995. **38**:86–91.

24. Rivkin P., Kraut M., Barta P., *et al.* White matter hyperintensity volume in late-onset and early-onset schizophrenia. *Int J Geriatr Psychiatry*, 2000. **15**:1085–9.

25. Symonds L. L., Olichney J. M., Jernigan T. L., *et al.* Lack of clinically significant gross structural abnormalities in MRIs of older patients with schizophrenia and related psychoses. *J Neuropsychiatr Clin Neurosci*, 1997. **9**:251–8.

26. Jones D. K., Catani M., Pierpaoli C., *et al.* A diffusion tensor magnetic resonance imaging study of frontal cortex connections in very-late-onset schizophrenia-like psychosis. *Am J Geriatr Psychiatry*, 2005. **13**:1092–9.

27. Filley C. M., Thompson L. L., Sze C. I., *et al.* White matter dementia in CADASIL. *J Neurol Sci*, 1999. **163**:163–7.

28. Nagaratnam N., O'Neile L. Delusional parasitosis following occipito-temporal cerebral infarction. *Gen Hosp Psychiatry*, 2000. **22**:129–32.

29. Cerrato P., Imperiale D., Giraudo M., *et al.* Complex musical

hallucinosis in a professional musician with left subcortical haemorrhage. *J Neurol Neurosurg Psychiatry*, 2001. **71**:280–1.

30. Beniczky S., Kéri S., Vörös E., *et al*. Complex hallucinations following occipital lobe damage. *Eur J Neurol*, 2002. **9**:175–6.

31. Suzuki K., Takei N., Toyoda T., *et al*. Auditory hallucinations and cognitive impairment in a patient with a lesions restricted to the hippocampus. *Schizophr Res*, 2003. **64**:87–9.

32. ffytche D. H., Lappin J. M., Philpot M. Visual command hallucinations in a patient with pure alexia. *J Neurol Neurosurg Psychiatry*, 2004. **75**:80–6.

33. Predescu A., Damsa C., Riegert M., *et al*. Persistent psychotic disorder following bilateral mesencephalo-thalamic ischaemia: case report [French]. *Encephale*, 2004. **30**:404–7.

34. Narumoto J., Matsushima N., Oka S., *et al. Psychiatr Clin Neurosci*, 2005. **59**:109–10.

35. Nye E., Arendts G. Intracerebral haemorrhage presenting as olfactory hallucinations. *Emerg Med (Fremantle)*, 2002. **14**:447–9.

15

Neurodegenerative disorders (Alzheimer's Disease, fronto-temporal dementia) and schizophrenia-like psychosis

Nicola T. Lautenschlager and Alexander F. Kurz

Facts box

- Delusions, misidentifications, and hallucinations are common neuropsychiatric symptoms in Alzheimer's Disease.
- Psychotic symptoms in Alzheimer's Disease can significantly affect the well-being of patients and caregivers.
- Psychotic symptoms in Alzheimer's Disease differ from psychotic symptoms in schizophrenia.
- Clinical criteria for diagnosis of psychosis in Alzheimer's Disease have been proposed.
- Several biological markers as risk factors for psychosis in Alzheimer's Disease have been suggested.
- There is ongoing discussion whether Alzheimer's Disease with psychotic symptoms is a specific subtype of Alzheimer's Disease or whether genetic factors determine a person's underlying vulnerability to psychotic symptoms, independent of the primary mental illness.
- Psychotic symptoms in fronto-temporal dementias are less common than in Alzheimer's Disease.

Introduction

Although descriptions of psychotic symptoms in senile dementia existed in earlier reports, Emil Kraepelin documented delusions, illusionary misidentifications, and hallucinations as part of the clinical picture in some detail [1]. He characterized psychotic symptoms of dementia patients as simple, unelaborated, fluctuating, inconsistent, and often contradictory. The most frequent delusional contents were described as being hypochondriac concerns, unwarranted mistrust

and suspiciousness, and fear of theft. Kraepelin also discussed the pathogenesis of delusions in dementia. In the eighth edition of his textbook, in which he introduced the term "Alzheimer's Disease (AD)," he postulated that reduced mental equipment (*geistiges Rüstzeug*) and poor judgment resulted in credulity and prepared the ground for delusional interpretations [2]. Hallucinations were described as being auditory or visual, but never bizarre.

In relation to presenile dementia, neither Arnold Pick's original descriptions of the lobar atrophies [3, 4, 5] nor subsequent reviews [6] mentioned delusions or hallucinations. In his famous case report from 1907 on Auguste D ("*Über eine eigenartige Erkrankung der Hirnrinde*"), Alois Alzheimer mentioned that jealousy was the initial symptom in the 51-year-old patient, followed by progressive memory loss that was accompanied by paranoid ideas, manifest in her behavior of hiding objects and the fear that she would be sexually abused or even killed by the doctor [7]. She also appeared to experience auditory hallucinations.

Little was added to Kraepelin's description of psychotic symptoms in senile dementia in subsequent years. Walther Spielmeyer characterized, in 1912, paranoid symptoms in senile dementia patients as being poor, unstable, and lacking in judgment [8]. In 1930, W. Runge contributed the observation that paranoid symptoms in patients with senile dementia were facilitated by hearing loss [9].

The association between impaired cognitive ability and delusional thinking in dementia was further emphasized by Gertrud Jacob in 1928 [10]. She argued that the apperception of reality becomes increasingly vague and fragmented, allowing emotionally charged imaginations to occupy the foreground of consciousness. Hans Lauter also maintained in 1968 that, in contrast to schizophrenia, delusions in dementia retain a close connection with reality, lack systematization, and are related to the loss of intellectual ability [11].

Table 15.1 Comparison of psychosis in AD and schizophrenia in older adults

Presentation	Psychosis in AD	Schizophrenia in old age
Complex delusions	Rare	Common
Type of hallucination	Visual > auditory	Auditory > visual
Misidentifications	Common	Rare
Schneiderian first-rank symptoms	Rare	Common
Suicidal ideation	Rare	Common
History of psychotic symptoms	Rare	Common

Adapted from Jeste and Finkel, 2000 [13].

Definition and clinical features

Psychotic symptoms in Alzheimer's Disease

Psychotic symptoms in AD differ from those typically seen in schizophrenia. The most common psychotic symptoms observed in patients with AD are delusions, delusional misidentifications, and hallucinations. Delusions tend to be simple and of the paranoid type. Burns and colleagues identified delusions of theft as the most common form, followed by delusions of suspicion [12]. Around 20% of AD patients in their study had experienced persecutory ideas. Misidentifications are common in AD. In reduplicative phenomena, which may be temporal, personal, or environmental, patients believe that a place, person, or time exists more than once or has been replaced by something else. These include syndromes such as the *Capgras syndrome*, in which the patient is convinced that a familiar person has been replaced by an impostor, and the *Frégoli syndrome*, in which an unknown person is believed to be someone familiar. Misidentifications of television and mirror images are also common. Hallucinations are less common than delusions.

Unlike schizophrenia, hallucinations are more often visual than auditory, and when auditory they usually lack the complexity described in the Schneiderian first-rank symptoms. In contrast to schizophrenia, suicidal ideation or suicide attempts due to psychotic symptoms are uncommon in AD, as is a history of psychotic symptoms prior to the onset of AD [13].

Table 15.1 describes typical differences between psychotic features in AD and older adults with schizophrenia.

Table 15.2 Proposed diagnostic criteria for "psychosis of Alzheimer's Disease" [13]

Characteristic symptoms

Presence of visual or auditory hallucinations and/or delusions.

Primary diagnosis

Clinical criteria for AD are met.

Chronology of onset of symptoms of psychosis

Psychotic symptoms have not been present continuously prior to the onset of dementia.

Duration

Psychotic symptoms have been present (even if intermittently) for at least 1 month.

Severity

Psychotic symptoms are severe enough to affect patients' or others' level of functioning.

Exclusion of other psychotic disorders

Criteria for schizophrenia or other functional psychiatric disorders with psychotic symptoms have never been met. Psychotic symptoms are also not better explained for by other medical conditions.

Relationship to delirium

The psychotic symptoms do not occur exclusively in the context of a delirium.

Adapted from Jeste and Finkel, 2000 [13].

Evidence of associations of psychotic symptoms with specific stages of the illness is inconsistent [14], although more complex delusions have been described in patients with better preserved intellectual functions [15]. Visual hallucinations have been associated with severe AD [16].

There has been a recent attempt to establish specific diagnostic criteria for the psychosis of AD, to help improve diagnostic consistency for communication in the areas of epidemiology, diagnosis, management, and research. Table 15.2 list the criteria suggested by Jeste and Finkel [13]. The authors point out that the psychosis can be associated with agitation, depressive symptoms, or negative symptoms. They also stress that the clinical usefulness of these criteria relies on the experience and judgment of the clinician applying them, for example, confabulations may be confused with delusions by some. The criteria were proposed as guidelines to help clinicians to distinguish psychosis in AD from other primary psychotic disorders and delirium.

Lyketsos and colleagues proposed a different approach. Based on data from the Cache County Study using a latent class analysis, several subgroups

Table 15.3 Diagnostic criteria for "Alzheimer-associated psychotic disorder"

A. Alzheimer's Disease according to NINDS/ADRDA criteria

B. Delusions or hallucinations that have an impact on the patient's behavior and his care.

C. One or more associated symptoms must be present: depression, irritability, anxiety, euphoria, aggression, and/or psychomotor agitation.

D. Duration must be 2 weeks or longer.

E. Should occur in a temporal relationship with the cognitive symptoms.

F. Can not be explained by other causes.

Adapted from Lyketsos *et al.* (2001) [17].

of patients with AD were identified according to their neuropsychiatric symptoms measured with the Neuropsychiatry Inventory (NPI) [17]. Table 15.3 lists the criteria for the psychotic subgroup. The authors favor this empirical approach because their proposed method to identify clusters of symptoms allows for co-occurrence of neuropsychiatric symptoms.

It also has been suggested that a further subclassification of the psychotic syndrome might be clinically relevant. Investigators from Pittsburgh identified two psychotic subtypes: a "misidentification subtype" and a "persecutory delusions subtype," which showed different profiles of cognitive impairment [18, 19].

Psychotic symptoms in fronto-temporal dementias

Descriptions of specific psychotic symptomatology in patients with fronto-temporal dementias (FTD) are sparse in the recent literature, and it has been suggested that hallucinations are an uncommon clinical presentation for tauopathies [20]. However, Gustafson and colleagues reported psychotic symptoms in up to 20% of all patients with FTD [21], and delusions have also been reported in FTD, usually in association with a more prominent atrophy of the right anterior temporal lobe [22].

Psychotic symptoms have been reported in some of the more rare, familial FTDs. One such group is "frontotemporal dementia with parkinsonism linked to chromosome 17" (FTDP-17) [23, 24], which accounts for 6%–18% of all FTDs [25, 26, 27], and for which more than 30 tau mutations in more than 80 families have been reported [28]. Chromosome 17 mutations can lead to a broad variety of phenotypes [29]

between different mutations, but also within a single family [30]. Bird and colleagues described a family with an autosomal-dominant pattern of inheritance of a dementia syndrome in which affected family members developed schizophrenia-like symptoms in the fifth or sixth decade [31], often leading to an initial diagnosis of schizophrenia. The psychotic symptoms were described as "suspiciousness, paranoid ideas, auditory hallucinations, loose associations, and intrusive thoughts" associated with social withdrawal, compulsions, and aggressive behavior. The clinical presentation of affected family members of the same family has been described elsewhere in more detail [32, 33]. Autopsy revealed the presence of neurofibrillary tangles (NFT) in several regions such as the neocortex, amygdala, and parahippocampal gyrus.

This family showed a strong linkage to the marker D17S934 and the V337M mutation was identified as the causative mutation.

Prevalence and incidence

Prevalence and incidence rates for psychotic symptoms in AD differ depending on whether the data are based on population based or clinical samples, partly explaining the wide ranges in published reports. Delusions have been reported to occur in 10%–73% and hallucinations in 3%–49% of patients with AD [34]. In a recent review of 55 studies by Ropacki and Jeste, the overall prevalence for psychotic symptoms in AD was estimated as 41%, with 36% of patients experiencing delusions and 18% hallucinations [35]. Delusional misidentifications have been reported to be present in up to 30% of patients with AD [12, 36, 37].

Psychotic symptoms have been shown to co-occur with other neuropsychiatric symptoms, such as aggression, agitation, apathy, and depression [38]. Bassiony and colleagues, for example, found that the presence of depression significantly increased the risk for delusions in their 303 patients with AD living in the community ($OR = 6.8$, 95% $CI = 2.1$–21.6) [39]. Incidence rates for psychotic symptoms in AD are lower in population-based studies as compared to clinical studies.

Lyketsos and colleagues reported for the community-based Cache County Study an annual incidence rate of 18% for delusions and 11% for hallucinations [17], whereas Paulsen and colleagues found, in a longitudinal study of clinic patients with AD who did not show psychotic symptoms at study entry, an increasing overall incidence rate for psychotic symptoms (20% at year 1, 36% at year 2, and 50% at year 3) [40].

Risk factors and outcomes

Many risk factors for psychotic symptoms have been discussed in the literature, but the results frequently differ depending on characterization of risk factors, nature of patient cohort, methods of analysis, and the interpretation of the results [41]. The finding that psychotic symptoms are less common in advanced AD might be due to the fact that psychotic symptoms are harder to detect in patients with severe AD due to their reduced abilities to communicate. On the other hand, it is also possible that the severely reduced mental abilities of these patients no longer allow them to generate these symptoms. Risk factors may differ between delusions and hallucinations. Bassiony and colleagues, for example, found in a cross-sectional study of 342 community-dwelling patients with AD that delusions were associated with poor general health, older age, aggression, and depression, whereas hallucinations were associated with more severe cognitive impairment and longer disease course, falls, lower education, and African-American race [42, 43].

Neurobiological factors

A variety of hypotheses have been discussed on how neurobiological factors contribute to the development of psychotic symptoms in AD. An overview on reported associations is presented in Table 15.4.

Neuropsychological profile

The published literature suggests that AD patients with psychotic symptoms experience more significant impairment in neuropsychological functions compared to AD patients free from psychotic symptoms [41, 60, 61, 62], with some exceptions [59]. Paulsen and colleagues suggested that AD patients with psychotic symptoms had more neurobehavioral dysfunction such as disinhibition, which is connected to frontal lobe impairment [40]. When Hopkins and Libon compared 24 outpatients with AD or vascular dementia with psychosis with 24 outpatients without psychosis, they found that patients with psychosis performed less well in executive control measured with the mental control subtest of the Wechsler Memory Scale ($F[3, 43] = 4.17, p < .001$) [63]. Interestingly, they performed better than nonpsychotic patients on a language task

Table 15.4 Neurobiological factors discussed for psychosis in AD

Delusions and misidentifications

- Basal ganglia calcification [12].
- Lower neuronal counts in the hippocampus (CA1) [44].
- Elevated muscarinic M2 receptor binding in the cortex [45].
- Temporal lobe asymmetry [46].
- Metabolic and perfusion abnormalities in frontal, temporal, and parietal cortex [47, 48, 49].
- Serotonin receptor 5-HT2A polymorphism 102T [50].

Delusions and hallucinations

- Higher neuronal counts the parahippocampal gyrus and lower counts in the dorsal raphe nucleus [44].
- Higher neurofibrillary burden [51].
- Genetic variations of 5-hydroxytryptamine (5-HT) receptors [52].
- Genetic variations of dopaminergic receptors [53].
- Elevation of glycerophosphoethanolamine and reduction of N-acetyl-L-aspartate [54].
- Metabolic and perfusion abnormalities in frontal, temporal, and parietal cortex [34, 55, 56, 57].
- Left- and right-brain hemisphere differences in size, blood flow, and glucose metabolism [58].
- Cholinergic-serotonergic imbalance [59].

(Boston naming test) and a memory task (CVLT delayed recognition). The authors hypothesized that the reduced capability to perform frontal lobe functions prevented successful self-monitoring and reality testing, which impaired the individual's abilities to interpret and integrate experiences [63, 64, 65]. It has been suggested that relatively preserved language and memory functions might be necessary "to rehearse and store incorrect hypotheses or judgements as 'long-term memory traces' to produce delusions" [64].

Genetic factors

It has been suggested that genetic factors might increase the susceptibility for AD with psychotic symptoms as a specific phenotype [14, 54, 66, 67, 68, 69]. Sweet and colleagues reported in a case-control study, with 371 patients with AD and psychotic symptoms and their 461 siblings, that the risk for AD with psychosis for the siblings was significantly increased with $OR = 2.41$ (95% $CI = 1.46$–4.0, $p = .0006$) [54].

Bacanu and colleagues estimated, with data from the National Institute of Mental Health AD Genetics Initiative on 826 patients with AD, that heritability for siblings for AD patients who displayed at least one symptom of psychosis during their illness was 30%, and for siblings of AD patients with multiple psychotic symptoms was 61% [68]. Two popular hypotheses to explain findings of increased heritability of psychosis in AD are: (i) AD with psychotic symptoms represents a "purer" or "less heterogeneous form of AD" or (ii) susceptibility for psychosis is a "quantitative trait in the population" that can emerge either because of environmental factors or an increased vulnerability of the brain because of neurodegeneration [69]. Interestingly, Bacanu and colleagues reported, in studies with families of AD patients with psychosis, linkages to loci on chromosome 2p and 6p that have also been identified for schizophrenia [67]. Rare types of autosomal-dominant inherited forms of familial AD can present early in the disease course with psychotic symptoms. Rippon and colleagues reported an African-American family with a presenilin 1 point mutation (M139V) in which affected family members developed a rapidly progressive dementia with personality change, delusions, and auditory and visual hallucinations [70]. There have been conflicting results for the association of the apolipoprotein E genotype and psychotic symptoms in AD [58, 71].

Personality

More recently, it has been suggested that symptoms of psychosis may be present before a diagnosis of dementia has been established as part of a prodromal syndrome or on a subsyndromal level as part of a personality structure. Östling and colleagues conducted a prospective population-based study in Göteborg, Sweden, and observed 305 nondemented older adults for psychotic symptoms.

Participants received neuropsychiatric and medical assessments at ages 85 and 88 years, which included an interview with a next of kin [72]. Sixty-three participants developed a dementia syndrome on follow-up. Delusions ($OR = 2.7$; 95% $CI = 1.2$–6.2), hallucinations ($OR = 3.1$; 95% $CI = 1.24$–6.8), and paranoid ideations ($OR = 2.7$; 95% $CI = 1.2$–6.2) were all associated with an increased incidence of dementia from the first to the second assessment. Eror and colleagues investigated prodromal psychotic symptoms in a retrospective study with 61 patients with probable and possible AD [73]. Fifty-one percent were classified as "ever psychotic," whereas 26% had displayed "multiple psychotic symptoms" during their illness so far. Primary care givers were asked in a standardized way whether the patient had shown psychotic

symptoms or subsyndromal psychotic symptoms prior to diagnosis of AD. The authors identified "elevated schizotypal personality scores" in those participants who later displayed psychotic symptoms in the course of their illness at "trend level" ($p = .06$) and a significant association between "severity of schizotypal symptoms and multiple psychotic symptoms during AD" ($p = .008$). They suggested that schizotypal personality symptoms during life change into clinical significant psychotic symptoms in the context of a neurodegenerative process [73]. The retrospective nature of the study, however, raises concerns regarding recall bias for the caregiver who frequently gave the information after having observed psychotic symptoms in their demented next of kin.

Environment

In addition to sensory deficits [74, 75], the environment the patient is exposed to might contribute to the development and persistence of psychotic symptoms.

Insufficient illumination indoors was identified as an important risk factor [76], and bright light therapy has been reported as being effective in reducing psychotic symptoms in AD [77]. The behavior and coping skills of the caregiver represent additional environmental factors that have been shown to have an effect on psychotic symptoms [78].

Cognitive and functional decline, institutionalization, and mortality

Numerous authors have described a more rapid cognitive [61, 79, 80, 81, 82, 83, 84, 85, 86] or functional decline [61, 86, 87, 88] in psychotic patients with AD compared to those without psychotic symptoms, although this is not a consistent finding for either rapid cognitive [12, 61, 88, 89, 90, 91] or functional decline [90, 92]. The discrepancy may be accounted for by differences in ascertainment, criteria for diagnosing psychotic symptoms, infrequency of assessments, dementia severity, and variations in treatment. Jeste and colleagues reported that patients with psychotic symptoms in their study [41] tended to have a more severe dementia with especially poorer performance on fronto temporal cognitive tests, despite a similar duration of illness compared to those without psychotic symptoms. The authors interpreted this as indicating that patients with psychotic symptoms might experience a more rapid decline. Stern and colleagues observed in a prospective study with

266 participants that patients with AD and psychosis had a more rapid cognitive decline (declined 1.15 points more on the mMMS per 6-month interval; 95% $CI = 0.52–1.77$) compared to patients with AD without psychosis [60].

Psychotic symptoms are frequently associated with agitated and aggressive behavior [38, 85, 93] and therefore often contribute to increased caregiver burden [94, 95] and early institutionalization [87, 96, 97]. Stern and colleagues followed 236 patients with AD at 3 research centers in the United States for up to 7 years to determine predictive factors for nursing home admission and death [97]. Delusions and hallucinations were assessed with a semistructured interview (the Columbia University Scale for Psychopathology in Alzheimer's Disease, CUSPAD) during the month prior to the assessment. The CUSPAD asked for paranoid delusions, delusions of abandonment, somatic delusions, and misidentifications. One hundred and three patients had one or more psychotic symptoms at baseline. Cox proportional hazard models showed that the presence of psychotic symptoms at baseline was associated with a significantly increased risk for requiring nursing home care in the future ($RR = 1.50$; 95% $CI = 1.04–2.15$).

Interestingly, patients with psychotic symptoms did not have a significant higher mortality. One of the most recent studies on the association of presence of psychotic symptoms and disease course in AD is a large multicenter study by Scarmeas and colleagues [98]. The authors described psychotic symptoms in 456 patients with mild AD who were followed from 0.11 to 14 years. Patients were assessed on average seven times, usually at 6-month intervals. At study entry, 34% of the patients experienced delusions and 7% hallucinations. Seventy percent developed delusions and 33% hallucinations at any time during follow-up. The authors interpreted this finding as an indication of fluctuation of symptoms, but also as an increase in the prevalence of psychotic symptoms during the course of the illness.

Delusions, and even more so hallucinations, were associated with an increased risk of cognitive and functional decline. Hallucinations were associated with an increased risk of institutionalization ($RR = 1.94$; 95% $CI = 140–2.70$) and death ($RR = 1.52$; 95% $CI = 1.08–2.15$) during follow-up, whereas delusions were not. The authors highlight the new finding of increased cognitive deterioration and mortality in AD patients with hallucinations compared to previous studies.

They give as possible explanations the possibility of a higher neuropathological burden, higher risk-taking behavior, and lower level of attention to medical problems in patients who hallucinate.

Implications for clinical practice

The medical care of patients with AD should include a regular screening for psychotic symptoms with the help of structured interview questionnaires such as the NPI. It has been suggested that roughly a third of patients with AD are significantly distressed by their psychotic symptoms [99]. In these cases, early identification and management are crucial to improve quality of life and nonpharmacologic management is considered the first line of treatment [100]. On the other hand, if patients are not distressed by psychotic symptoms and are not acting on them in a way that would increase health risks for themselves or others, management of these symptoms is not necessarily warranted. If psychotic symptoms are identified, a more thorough medical check-up may be indicated to avoid overlooking a superimposed delirium.

Suggestions for future research

An important goal within the vast research field of AD will be to refine diagnostic criteria for specific neuropsychiatric symptoms, such as psychosis in AD [101]. With growing knowledge, especially from longitudinal studies, it is likely that more subtypes will be identified with a clearer understanding of the relationship of the presentation of psychotic symptoms and disease course. Already there seems to be some evidence that delusions, misidentifications, and hallucinations in AD may have a different underlying pattern of risk factors and clinical outcomes. Psychosis in AD has been the topic of a meeting of the Federal Drug Administration in the United States as a possible future target for drug development [102]. Larger nonpharmacological intervention studies targeting specific psychotic symptoms are also needed [100].

A future scenario in which subtypes of AD would be identifiable with the help of genetic and neurobiological markers, and specific psychotic symptoms might be treatable with genetically engineered drugs, is still outside our immediate reach. However, research already has started on this path in trying to better identify and describe phenotypes and corresponding genotypes of subtypes of AD.

References

1. Kraepelin E. 1899. Psychiatrie. Ein Lehrbuch für Studirende und Ärzte. 6th Ed., Vol. II. Nijmegen: Reprint, Arts & Boeve.

2. Kraepelin E. 1910. Psychiatrie. Ein Lehrbuch für Studierende und Ärzte. 8th Ed., Vol. II. Leipzig: Johann Ambrosius Barth.

3. Pick A. Senile Hirnatrophie als Grundlage von Herderscheinungen. *Wiener klin Wschr*, 1901. **14**:1–2.

4. Pick A. Zur Symptomatologie der linksseitigen Schläfenlappenatrophie. *Mschr Psychiat Neurol*, 1904. **16**: 378–88.

5. Pick A. Über einen weiteren Symptomenkomplex im Rahmen der Dementia senilis, bedingt durch umschriebene stärkere Hirnatrophie (gemischte Apraxie). *Monatsschr Psychiatr*, 1906. **19**:97–108.

6. Stertz G. Über die Picksche Atrophie. *Z Gesaimte Neurol Psychiatr*, 1926. **101**: 729–47.

7. Alzheimer A. Über eine eigenartige Erkrankung der Hirnrinde. *Allg Z Psychiatr*, 1907. **64**:146–8.

8. Spielmeyer W. (1912). Die Psychosen des Rückbildungs- und Greisenalters. In *Handbuch der Psychiatrie*, Aschaffenburg, G. (Ed.). Leipzig, Wien: Deuticke.

9. Runge W. (1930). Psychotisch ausgebaute Sonderformen der senilen Demenz. In *Handbuch der Geisteskrankheiten*, vol 8. Bumke, O. (Ed.). Berlin: Julius Springer.

10. Jacob G. Analyse eines Falles von seniler Demenz. (Störungen der Orientierung, des Denkens, der Realitätserfassung.) *Z ges Neurol.*, 1928; **116**:25–43.

11. Lauter H. Zur Klinik und Psychopathologie der Alzheimerschen Krankheit. *Psychiat Clin*, 1968. **1**:85–108.

12. Burns A., Jacoby R., Levy R. Psychiatric phenomena in Alzheimer's disease, II: disorders of perception. *Br J Psychiatry*, 1990. **157**:78–81, 92–4.

13. Jeste D. V., Finkel S. I. Psychosis of Alzheimer's disease and related dementias. *Am J Geriatr Psychiatry*, 2000. **8**(1):29–34.

14. Sweet R. A., Nimogaonkar V. L., Devlin B., *et al.* Psychotic symptoms in Alzheimer disease: evidence for a distinct phenotype. *Mol Psychiatry*, 2003; **8**:383–92.

15. Cummings J. L. Organic delusions: phenomenology, anatomical correlations, and review. *Br J Psychiatry*, 1985; **146**:184–97.

16. Ballard C., Holmes C., McKeith I., *et al.* Psychiatric morbidity in dementia with -Lewy bodies: a prospective clinical and neuropathological comparison study with Alzheimer's disease. *Am J Psychiatry*, 1999. **156**:1039–45.

17. Lyketsos C. G., Breitner J. C. S., Rabins P. An evidence-based proposal for the classification of neuropsychiatric disturbance in Alzheimer's disease. *Int J Geriatr Psychiatry*, 2001. **16**:1037–42.

18. Cook S. E., Miyahara S., Bacanu S-A., *et al.* Psychotic symptoms in Alzheimer disease. *Am J Geriatr Psychiatry*, 2003. **11**: 406–13.

19. Perez-Madrinan G., Cook S. E., Saxton J. A., *et al.* Alzheimer disease with psychosis. Excess cognitive impairment is restricted to the misidentification subtype. *Am J Geriatr Psychiatry*, 2004. **12**:449–56.

20. Cummings J. L. Toward a molecular neuropsychiatry of neurodegenerative diseases. *Ann Neurol*, 2003. **54**:147–54.

21. Gustafson L., Brun A., Passant U. Frontal lobe degeneration of non-Alzheimer type. *Baillieres Clin Neurol*, 1992. **1**:559–82.

22. Edwards-Lee T., Miller B. L., Benson D. F., *et al.* The temporal variant of frontotemporal dementia. *Brain*, 1997. **120**:1027–40.

23. Wilhelmsen K. C., Lynch T., Pavlou E., *et al.* Localization of disinhibition-dementia-Parkinsonism-amyotrophy complex to 17q21–22. *Am J Hum Genet*, 1994. **55**:1159–65.

24. Foster N. L., Wilhelemsen K., Sima A. A., *et al.* Frontotemporal dementia and parkinsonism linked to chromosome 17: a consensus conference. *Ann Neurol*, 1997. **41**(6):706–15.

25. Houlden H., Baker M., Adamson J., *et al.* Frequency of tau mutations in three series of Non-Alzheimer's degenerative dementia. *Ann Neurol*, 1999. **46**:243–8.

26. Poorkaj P., Grossman M., Steinbart E., *et al.* Frequency of tau gene mutations in familial and sporadic cases of non-Alzheimer dementia. *Arch Neurol*, 2001. **8**(3):383–7.

27. Rosso S. M., Kaar L. D., Baks T., *et al.* Frontotemporal dementia in The Netherlands: patient characteristics and prevalence estimates from a population-based study. *Brain*, 2003. **126**:2016–22.

28. van Swieten J., Spillantini M. G. Hereditary frontotemporal dementia caused by *tau* gene mutations. *Brain Pathol*, 2007. **17**:63–73.

29. Forman M. S. Genotype-phenotype correlations in FTDP-17: does form follow function? *Exp Neurol*, 2004. **187**:229–34.

30. Ingram E. M., Spillantini M. G. Tau gene mutations: dissecting the pathogenesis of FRTD-17. *Trends Mol Med*, 2002. **8**(12):555–62.

31. Bird T. D., Wijsman E. M., Nochlin D., *et al.* Chromosome 17 and hereditary dementia: linkage studies in three non-Alzheimer

families and kindreds with late-onset FAD. *Neurology*, 1997. **48**:949–54.

32. Sumi S. M., Bird T. D., Nochlin D., *et al.* Familial presenile dementia with psychosis associated with cortical neurofibrillary tangles and degeneration of the amygdala. *Neurology*, 1992. **42**(1):120–7.

33. Reed L. A., Grabowski T. J., Schmidt M. L., *et al.* Autosomal dominant dementia with widespread neurofibrillary tangles. *Ann Neurol*, 1997. **42**:564–72.

34. Mega M. S., Lee L., Dinov I. D., *et al.* Cerebral correlates of psychotic symptoms in Alzheimer's' disease. *J Neurol Neurosurg Psychiatry*, 2000. **69**:167–71.

35. Ropacki S. A., Jeste D. V. Epidemiology of and risk factors for psychosis of Alzheimer's disease: a review of 55 studies published from 1990 to 2003. *Am J Psychiatry*, 2001. **162**:2022–30.

36. Mendez M. F., Martin R. J., Smyth K. A., *et al.* Psychiatric symptoms associated with Alzheimer's disease. *J Neuropsychiatry Clin Neurosci*, 1990. **2**:28–33.

37. Förstl H., Almeida O. P., Owen A. M., *et al.* Psychiatric, neurological and medical aspects of misidentification syndromes: a review of 260 cases. *Psychol Med*, 1991. **21**:905–10.

38. Rapoport M. J., van Reekum R., Freedman M., *et al.* Relationship of psychosis to aggression, apathy and function in dementia. *Int J Geriatr Psychiatry*, 2001. **16**:123–30.

39. Bassiony M. M., Warren A., Rosenblatt A., *et al.* The relationship between delusions and depression in Alzheimer's disease. *Int J Geriatr Psychiatry*, 2002a. **17**:549–56.

40. Paulsen J. S., Ready R. E., Stout J. C., *et al.* Neurobehaviours and psychotic symptoms in Alzheimer's disease. *J Int Neuropsychol Soc*, 2000. **6**(7):815–20.

41. Jeste D. V., Wragg R. E., Salmon D. P., *et al.* Cognitive deficits of patients with Alzheimer's disease with and without delusions. *Am J Psychiatry*, 1992. **149**(2):148–9.

42. Bassiony M. M., Steinberg M. S., Warren A., *et al.* Delusions and hallucinations in Alzheimer's disease: prevalence and clinical correlates. *Int J Geriatr Psychiatry*, 2000. **15**:99–107.

43. Bassiony M. M., Warren A., Rosenblatt A., *et al.* Isolated hallucinosis in Alzheimer's disease is associated with African-American race. *Int J Geriatr Psychiatry*, 2002b. **17**:205–10.

44. Förstl H., Burns A., Levy R., *et al.* Neuropathological correlates of psychotic phenomena in confirmed Alzheimer's Disease. *Br J Psychiatry*, 1994. **165**:53–9.

45. Lai M. K. P., Lai O-F., Keene J., *et al.* Psychosis of Alzheimer's disease is associated with elevated muscarinic M2 binding in the cortex. *Neurology*, 2001. **57**:805–11.

46. Geroldi C., Akkawi N. M., Galluzzi S., *et al.* Temporal lobe asymmetry in patients with Alzheimer's disease with delusions. *J Neurol Neurosurg Psychiatry*, 2000. **69**:187–91.

47. Mentis M. J., Weinstein E. A., Horwitz B., *et al.* Abnormal brain glucose metabolism in the delusional misidentification syndromes: a positron emission tomography study in Alzheimer disease. *Biol Psychiatry*, 1995. **38**:438–49.

48. Fukuhara R., Ikeda M., Nebu A., *et al.* Alteration of rCBF in Alzheimer's disease patients with delusions of theft. *Neuro report*, 2001. **12**(11):2473–6.

49. Lopez O. L., Smith G., Becker J. T., *et al.* The psychotic phenomenon in probable Alzheimer's disease: a positron emission tomography study. *J Neuropsychiatry Clin Neurosci*, 2001. **13**(1):50–5.

50. Assal F., Alacon M., Solomon E. C., *et al.* Association of the serotonin transporter and receptor gene polymorphisms in neuropsychiatric symptoms in Alzheimer disease. *Arch Neurol*, 2004. **61**(8):1249–53.

51. Faber N. B., Rubin E. H., Newcomer J. W., *et al.* Increased neocortical neurofibrillary tangle density in subjects with Alzheimer disease and psychosis. *Arch Gen Psychiatry*, 2000. **57**:1165–73.

52. Nacmias B., Tedde A., Forleo P., *et al.* Association between 5-HT2A receptor polymorphism and psychotic symptoms in Alzheimer disease. *Biol Psychiatry*, 2001. **50**:472–5.

53. Holmes C., Smith H., Ganderton R., *et al.* Psychosis and aggression in Alzheimer's disease: the effect of dopamine receptor gene variation. *J Neurol Neurosurg Psychiatry*, 2001. **71**:777–9.

54. Sweet R. A., Nimgaonkar V. L., Devlin B., *et al.* Increased familial risk of the psychotic phenotype of Alzheimer disease. *Neurology*, 2002. **58**:907–11.

55. Starkstein S. E., Vazquez S., Petracca G., *et al.* A SPECT study of delusions in Alzheimer's disease. *Neurology*, 1994. **44**:2055–9.

56. Kotrla K. J., Chacko R. C., Harper R. G., *et al.* Clinical variables associated with psychosis in Alzheimer's disease. *Am J Psychiatry*, 1995. **152**:1377–9.

57. Sultzer D. L., Mahler M. E., Mandelkern M. A., *et al.* The relationship between psychiatric symptoms and regional cortical metabolism in Alzheimer's disease. *J Neuropsychiatr Clin Neurosci*, 1995: 7(4):476–84.

58. Karim S., Burns A. The biology of psychosis in older people. *J Geriatr Psychiatr Neurol*, 2003. **16**(4):207–12.

59. Garcia-Alloza M., Gil-Bea F. J., Diez-Ariza M., *et al.* Cholinergic-serotonergic imbalance contributes to cognitive and behavioural symptoms in Alzheimer's disease. *Neuropsychologia*, 2005. **43**: 442–9.

60. Stern Y., Albert M., Brandt J., *et al.* Utility of extrapyramidal signs and psychosis as predictors of cognitive and functional decline, nursing home admission, and death in Alzheimer's disease: prospective analyses from the Predictors Study. *Neurology*, 1994. **44**(12):2300–7.

61. Lopez O. L., Wisneiwski S. R., Becker J. T., *et al.* Psychiatric medication and abnormal behavior as predictors of progression in probable Alzheimer disease. *Arch Neurol*, 1999. **56**:1266–72.

62. Swanberg M. M., Tractenberg R. E., Mohs R., *et al.* Executive dysfunction in Alzheimer disease. *Arch Neurol*, 2004. **61**(4):556–60.

63. Hopkins M. W., Libon D. J. Neuropsychological functioning of dementia patients with psychosis. *Arch Clin Neuropsychol*, 2005. **20**:771–83.

64. Cloud B., Carew T. G., Rothenberg H., *et al.* A case of paraphrenia: integrating neuropsychological and SPECT data. *J Geriatr Psychiatry Neurol*, 1996. **9**:146–53.

65. Fleminger S. Delusional misidentification: an exemplary symptom illustrating an interaction between organic brain disease and psychological processes. *Psychopathology*, 1994. **27**:161–7.

66. Tunstall N., Owen M. J., Williams J., *et al.* Familial influence on variation in age at onset and behavioural phenotype in Alzheimer's disease. *Br J Psychiatry*, 2000. **174**:156–9.

67. Bacanu S-A., Devlin B., Chowdari K. V., *et al.* Linkage analysis of Alzheimer disease with psychosis. *Neurology*, 2002. **59**(1): 118–20.

68. Bacanu S-A., Devlin B., Chowdari K. V., *et al.* Heritability of psychosis in Alzheimer disease. *Am J Geriatr Psychiatry*, 2005. **13**:624–7.

69. Lovestone S., Hardy J. Psychotic genes or forgetful ones? *Neurology*, 2002. **59**(1):11–12.

70. Rippon G. A., Crrok R., Baker M., *et al.* Presenilin 1 mutation in an African American family presenting with atypical Alzheimer dementia. *Arch Neurol*, 2003. **60**(6):884–8.

71. Levy M. L., Cummings J. L., Fairbanks L. A., *et al.* Apolipoprotein E genotype and non-cognitive symptoms in Alzheimer's disease. *Biol Psychiatry*, 1999. **45**:422–5.

72. Östling S., Skoog I. Psychotic symptoms and paranoid ideation in a non-demented population-based sample in the very old. *Arch Gen Psychiatry*, 2002. **59**:53–9.

73. Eror E. A., Lopez O. L., Dekosky S. T., *et al.* Alzheimer Disease subjects with psychosis have increased schizotypal symptoms before dementia onset. *Biol Psychiatry*, 2005. **58**: 325–30.

74. Ballard C., Bennister C., Graham C., *et al.* Associations of psychotic symptoms in dementia sufferers. *Br J Psychiatry*, 1995a. **167**:537–40.

75. McShane R., Gelding K., Reading M., *et al.* Prospective study of relations between cortical Lewy bodies, poor eyesight, and hallucinations in Alzheimer's disease. *J Neurol Neurosurg Psychiatry*, 1995. **59**: 185–8.

76. Murgatroyd C., Prettyman R. An investigation of visual hallucinosis and visual sensory status in dementia. *Int J Geriatr Psychiatry*, 2001. **16**:709–13.

77. Schindler S. D., Graf A., Fischer P., *et al.* Paranoid delusions and hallucinations and bright light therapy in Alzheimer's disease. *Int J Geriatr Psychiatry*, 2002. **17**:1071–2.

78. Riello R., Geroldi C., Parrinello G., *et al.* The relationship between biological and environmental determinants of delusions in mild Alzheimer's disease patients. *Int J Geriatr Psychiatry*, 2002. **17**:683–8.

79. Mayeux R., Stern Y., Spanton S. Heterogeneity in dementia of the Alzheimer type: evidence of subgroups. *Neurology*, 1985. **35**:453–61.

80. Stern Y., Mayeux R., Sano M., *et al.* Predictors of disease course in patients with probable Alzheimer's disease. *Neurology*, 1987. **37**:1649–53.

81. Drevets W. Rubin E. H. Psychotic symptoms and the longitudinal course of senile dementia of the Alzheimer type. *Biol Psychiatry*, 1989. **25**:39–48.

82. Rosen J., Zubenko G. S. Emergence of psychosis and depression in the longitudinal evaluation of Alzheimer's disease. *Biol Psychiatry*, 1991. **29**:224–32.

83. Chui H. C., Lyness S. A., Sobel E., *et al.* Extrapyramidal signs and psychiatric symptoms predict faster cognitive decline in Alzheimer's disease. *Arch Neurol*, 1994. **51**:676–81.

84. Levy M. L., Cummings J. L., Fairbanks L. A., *et al.* Longitudinal assessment of symptoms of depression, agitation, and psychosis in 181 patients with Alzheimer's disease. *Am J Psychiatry*, 1996. **153**:1438–43.

85. Lopez O. L., Becker J. T., Brenner R. P., *et al.* Alzheimer's disease with delusions and hallucinations: neuropsychological and electroencephalographic correlates. *Neurology*, 1991. **41**:906–12.

86. Lopez O. L., Brenner R. P., Becker J. T., *et al.* EEG spectral abnormalities and psychosis as predictors of cognitive and functional decline in probable Alzheimer's disease. *Neurology*, 1997. **48**:1521–5.

87. Steele C., Rovner B., Chase G. A., *et al.* Psychiatric symptoms and nursing home placement of patients with Alzheimer's disease. *Am J Psychiatry*, 1990. **147**(8): 1049–51.

88. Mortimer J. A., Ebbitt B., Finch M. D. Predictors of cognitive and functional progression in patients with probable Alzheimer's disease. *Neurology*, 1992. **42**:1689–96.

89. Teri L., Hughes J. P., Larson E. B. Cognitive deterioration in Alzheimer's disease: behavioural and health factors. *J Gerontol*, 1990. **45**:58–63.

90. Corey-Bloom J., Galasko D., Hofstetter C. R., *et al.* Clinical features distinguishing large cohorts with possible AD, probable AD, and mixed dementia. *J Am Geriatr Soc*, 1993. **41**:31–7.

91. Miller T. P., Tinklenberg J. R., Brooks J. O., *et al.* Selected psychiatric symptoms associated with rate of cognitive decline in patients with Alzheimer's disease. *J Geriatr Psychiatry Neurol*, 1993. **6**:235–8.

92. Drachman D. A., O'Donnell B. F., Swearer J. M. The prognosis in Alzheimer's disease: how far rather than how fast best predicts the course. *Arch Neurol*, 1990. **47**:851–6.

93. Gilley D. W., Wilson R. S., Beckett L. A., *et al.* Psychotic symptoms and physically aggressive behaviour in Alzheimer's disease. *J Am Geriatr Soc*, 1997. **45**(9): 1974–9.

94. Rabins P. V., Mace N. L., Lucas M. J. The impact of dementia on the family. *JAMA*, 1982. **248**:333–5.

95. Haupt M., Romero B., Kurz A. Delusions and hallucinations in Alzheimer's disease: results from a two year long longitudinal study. *Int J Geriatr Psychiatry*, 1996. **11**:965–72.

96. Haupt M., Kurz A. Predictors of nursing home placment in patients with Alzheimer's disease. *Int J Geriatr Psychiatry*, 1993. **8**:741–6.

97. Stern Y., Tang M-T., Albert M. S., *et al.* Predicting time to nursing home care and death in individuals with Alzheimer's disease. *JAMA*, 1997. **277**: 806–12.

98. Scarmeas N., Brandt J., Albert M., *et al.* Delusions and hallucinations are associated with worse outcome in Alzheimer disease. *Arch Neurol*, 2005. **62**: 1601–08.

99. Ballard C., Saad K., Patel A., *et al.* The prevalence and phenomenology of psychotic symptoms in dementia sufferers. *Int J Geriatr Psychiatry*, 1995b. **10**:477–85.

100. Cohen-Mansfield J. Nonpharacologic interventions for inappropriate behaviours in dementia: a review, summary, and critique. *Am J Geriatr Psychiatry*, 2001. **9**:361–81.

101. McKeith I., Cummings J. Behavioural changes and psychological symptoms in dementia disorders. *Lancet Neurol*, 2005. **4**:735–42.

102. Schneider L. S., Katz I. R., Park S., *et al.* Psychosis in Alzheimer disease. Validity of the construct and response to Risperidone. *Am J Geriatr Psychiatry*, 2003. **11**:414–25.

16

Storage disorders and psychosis

Mark Walterfang and Dennis Velakoulis

Facts box

- Storage disorders including GM2 gangliosidosis, Niemann-Pick Disease type C, cerebrotendinous xanthomatosis, alpha mannosidosis, and adult neuronal ceroid lipofuscinosis all have adult-onset forms.

- Adult-onset storage disorders present with a higher than expected rate of psychosis due to the presumed interaction between neuropathology and late neurodevelopment.

- Storage disorders should be suspected in the presence of psychosis in individuals with movement or other neurological disorders, an atypical course of illness, or a suggestive family history.

- Investigations for storage disorders in the setting of psychosis are guided by clinical features of the illness, and most disorders can be diagnosed using serum and/or skin biopsy testing.

- Substrate reduction therapy is likely to be an illness-modifying treatment in the future, although for most disorders antipsychotic medication is the mainstay of treatment with electroconvulsive therapy having anecdotal support.

Introduction

As already described in previous chapters, neuronal assemblies in key circuits can be disrupted to produce the characteristic symptoms and signs of a schizophrenia-like psychosis. This disruption can occur due to a range of perturbations of neuronal function, one of which is the accumulation of metabolic or other products that may impair key neuronal processes or result in neuronal death. The pathological accumulation of cellular products occurs in a range of disorders, particularly the dementias in which accumulation of β–amyloid, tau, and other proteins can result in neurodegeneration. This chapter restricts its discussion to specific storage disorders that predispose to psychosis and are due to the disruption to a metabolic pathway that results in the abnormal accumulation of one of the key substrates or byproducts of that pathway.

Neuronal storage disorders are a diverse group of metabolic disorders in which alterations in key pathways in neuronal metabolism result in the accumulation of a substance, usually a lipid or related molecule, which interferes with normal cellular function and may ultimately cause neuronal loss. Lysosomes are intracellular organelles containing enzymes necessary for the processing or degradation of proteins, nucleic acids, carbohydrates, and lipids. Many neuronal storage disorders involve the deficiency of a lysosomal enzyme, usually a hydrolase, which results in an abnormal accumulation of sphingolipids. Some of these disorders, such as the leukodystrophies, are covered in Chapter 18.

Lysosomal storage disorders

A multiplicity of cellular processes occur within lysosomes, where most cellular macromolecules (proteins, glycoproteins, lipids, and phospholipids) are degraded by enzymatic "factories," which then pass out their monomeric components for reutilization. Impairment in function of a lysosomal enzyme occurs if it is structurally altered, if alteration occurs to a cofactor protein, or if enzyme transport is affected. Each enzyme is specific for breaking a particular chemical bond, as opposed to a particular substrate macromolecule. More than 70 lysosomal enzymes are known, and more than 40 disease syndromes involving defective enzyme function have been characterized.

Neuronal storage disorders can be broadly broken up into the *mucopolysaccharidoses, glycoproteinoses, sphingolipidoses, other lipid storage disorders, multiple*

Table 16.1 Lysosomal storage disorders affecting the central nervous system

Mucopolysaccharidoses	Glycoproteinoses	Sphingolipidoses	Lipid storage disorders	Multiple enzyme defects	Transport disorders
Mucopolysaccharidosis II Mucopolysaccharidosis III Mucopolysaccharidosis V Mucopolysaccharidosis VII	Aspartylglycosaminuria Fucosidosis Mannosidosis Sialidosis Neuroaxonal dystrophy	Niemann-Pick Disease type A Glucocerebrosidase type II GM2 gangliosidosis Metachromatic leukodystrophy Globoid cell leukodystrophy	Niemann-Pick Disease type C GM2 gangliosidosis	Mucolipidosis type II Mucolipidosis type III	Cystinosis Sialic acid storage disease

Table 16.2 Neuronal storage disorders that present with psychosis in adulthood

Disorder	Eponym	Altered enzyme or protein	Accumulated product	Inheritance	Chromosomal location	Rate of psychosis
GM2 gangliosidosis type I	Tay Sach's Disease	α subunit of β-hexosaminidase A	GM2 gangliosides	Autosomal recessive	15q23–24	30–50%
Niemann-Pick Disease type C	Niemann-Pick Disease type C	NPC1 or NPC2	Unesterified cholesterol	Autosomal receissive	18q11–12 or 14q24.3	Up to 40%
Neuronal ceroid lipofuscinosis	Kuf's Disease	CLN4	Unknown	Autosomal recessive, autosomal dominant	Unknown	Up to 20%
Mannosidosis	–	Lysosomal α-mannosidase	Undegraded N-linked oligosaccharides	Autosomal recessive	19p13.2-q12	25%
Cerebrotendinous xanthomatosis	–	Serol-27-hydrolase	Cholestanol	Autosomal recessive	2q35	5–10%, higher rates reported

enzyme deficiencies, and *transport defects* (Table 16.1). Most of these disorders result in significant impairment of early neurodevelopment, producing severe developmental delay or loss of learned skills, and often death in infancy or childhood. Because of the early age of onset and significant neurological impact, most patients do not progress to psychosis. This is primarily because schizophrenia-like psychosis is a disorder of adolescence and early adulthood, and many of these disorders confer a limited lifespan. Additionally, for many affected individuals who enter adulthood, the degree of neuropathology already present in the central nervous system (CNS) may greatly modify the pathoplastic effects of a process that would otherwise predispose to psychosis when impacting upon an intact brain. A small number of these disorders, however, are associated with mutation-driven variations in enzyme levels and may present at any stage of the human neurodevelopmental lifecycle including adulthood (Table 16.2). Whereas patients with little or no

enzyme levels will present in infancy, those with low levels may not present until childhood and those with moderate enzyme levels may not present until adolescence or early adulthood [1]. Secondary schizophrenia has been associated with the latter group, that is, those patients with moderate enzyme levels who do not present until adolescence. This pattern of presentation is well characterized in metachromatic leukodystrophy, where psychosis is very common in its adult-onset form (Chapter 18) [2]. It is presumed that the neuropathological process interacts with the developmental maturity of the CNS during adolescence and adulthood to produce the key symptoms and signs of schizophrenia [2, 3]. This appears to be the result of disruptions to, or interactions with, a number of key developmental processes, such as synaptic pruning [4, 5], myelination of frontotemporal tracts [6], the development of dopaminergic projections into frontal GABA-ergic neurons [7] and a massive growth in fronto-limbic connections, particularly from the amygdala to the cingulate cortex [8]. Disruptions to any of these processes, either through alterations to the nature and timing of the processes themselves or the integrity of the substrate they affect, may provide a neurodevelopmental model for at least some of the symptoms of schizophrenia [3].

GM2 gangliosidosis type I: Tay-Sachs Disease

Tay-Sachs Disease (TSD) was first described by Sachs in 1887 [9, 10] and is an autosomal recessive lipid storage disorder caused by the accumulation of GM2-gangliosides within neurons due to a deficiency in β–hexosaminidase A (HEX-A)[11]. In its classic, or infantile, form, TSD is a rapidly progressive illness characterized by developmental retardation, paralysis, and blindness and usually results in death by the third year of life [10]. The characteristic "cherry red spot" on the fundus of an affected infant was first described by Tay, who shares the eponym of this disease [12]. The juvenile form generally presents by the fifth year, with weakness, seizures dysarthria, dysmetria, and death by the mid-teens [13]. More recently, a late-onset form of TSD has been described where psychiatric symptoms may co-present with or predate the development of neurological disturbances in early adulthood [14].

HEX-A is composed of α and β subunits, and the related enzyme HEX-B is composed of β-subunits alone. The α–subunit gene is located on chromosome 15q [15], mutations of which cause absent or low levels of HEX-A [16] and produce a predominantly neurological syndrome. Mutations of the β–subunit gene on chromosome 5 cause low levels of both HEX-A and HEX-B [17] and cause GM2-gangliosidosis type II (Sandhoff Disease), where the viscera as well as the CNS is affected [18]. Mutations to different regions of the α–subunit gene result in variably stable transcripts and thus variable resultant enzyme levels, which may correspond to the variable onset of the disease [14, 19]. In most adult-onset patients the mutations G269S or W474C are present [19]. HEX-A deficiency in lysosomes impairs the catabolism of gangliosides from the neuronal cell membrane, resulting in accumulation of lysosomal gangliosides. This leads to secondary neuronal changes, particularly axon hillock outgrowth to form "meganeurites" with ectopic dendritogenesis [20] and focal axonal enlargements known as "axonal spheroids" [21], both

of which may alter neuron-to-neuron microconnectivity. The relationship of ganglioside accumulation with alterations to neuronal structure, and how it results in neuropathology, remains unclear, although this may occur through direct neurotoxicity [22], altered neuronal electrical properties [23], inappropriate apoptosis [23, 24], or a CNS inflammatory response [25].

The neurological presentation of late-onset TSD is quite variable, and no distinct phenotype–genotype correlations exist [26]. Speech disorder, gait disturbance, and tremor are the most common presentations [27]. Many patients have normal or near-normal cognitive function [27], although subtle deficits in executive function, information processing speed, and memory may be present in up to half of patients [28, 29]. In a number of patients, these deficits progress in concert with their neurological symptoms [29]. Neuroimaging findings in TSD describe cerebellar atrophy in most patients [19, 29, 30], although cerebral atrophy may be present in up to a quarter of patients [29]. Diagnosis generally rests on demonstration of deficient hexosaminidase activity. Treatment options are limited to bone marrow transplantation [31], although substrate reduction therapy – potentially a promising short-term treatment for all lipid storage disorders – with miglustat, has shown promise in animal models [25].

Neuropsychiatric presentations occur in up to half of late-onset TSD patients described in unselected series, and the predominant neuropsychiatric presentation appears to be psychosis [19, 29, 32, 33, 34]. Rates of psychosis in late-onset TSD patients range from 30% [33] to 50% [32]. In a review of all published cases before 1998, MacQueen [27] estimated the conservative prevalence at 33% of late-onset patients. The form of this psychosis has been described as "hebephrenic" with disorganization, auditory and visual hallucinations, but also clouding of consciousness and cognitive impairment. Cases have been described where the presenting feature was catatonia [30, 35, 36].

Treatment of psychosis in TSD appears problematic, with often only partial response to neuroleptics and mood stabilizers such as lithium [27, 30, 36, 37]. Importantly, patients with late-onset TSD are exquisitely sensitive to the motor side effects of many neuroleptic medications [30, 36]. For severe psychotic or affective illness, electroconvulsive therapy (ECT) appears to be a safe and effective treatment to offer this patient group [35, 37].

Niemann-Pick Disease type C

Niemann-Pick Disease type C (NPC) is an autosomal recessive neurovisceral disorder of lipid storage, with a frequency of 1 in 100,000 live births [38]. It is characterized by variable degrees of cognitive decline, behavioral disturbance, and neurological impairment, predominantly ataxia, and vertical supranuclear opthalmoplegia [39]. It is biochemically and phenotypically distinct from Niemann-Pick Disease types A and B, which result from a deficiency of lysosomal sphingomyelinase [40, 41]. Genetic analysis reveals two distinct genetic foci, with 95% of the disease caused by aberrations in the NPC1 gene on 18q11–12 [42], coding for the lysosomal NPC1 protein [43]. The less common NPC2 variant is caused by mutations in the NPC2 gene, mapping to chromosome 14q24.3 [44] and whose product resides in the Golgi apparatus and late endosomes. These proteins are involved in cyclical movement of sterols within cells [45, 46, 47], performing cholesterol trafficking and homeostatic functions [48, 49].

Mutation and dysfunction of NPC1 and NPC2 appear to result in late endosomal accumulation of cholesterol, some glycolipids, and selected gangliosides [50, 51] leading to Alzheimer-like neurofibrillary tangles (NFTs), neuronal degeneration, neuroaxonal dystrophy, and demyelination [47, 52, 53, 54]. This intracellular cholesterol "traffic jam" impairs the transport of endogenously synthesized cholesterol to distal axons, where it is required for membrane maintenance [55] and response to axonal injury [56]. Axonal structures are therefore particularly vulnerable and are affected early with axonal spheroid formation, hypomyelination, and eventual demyelination [57]. As a result, white-matter tracts are severely affected [51, 58, 59], with the corpus callosum showing the most striking axonal loss [60].

The neuronal cells most vulnerable to NFT accumulation are the Purkinje cells of the cerebellum, basal ganglia, and thalamus followed by neurons in hippocampal and cortical regions [59, 61, 62, 63]. Affected neurons often show ectopic dendritogenesis with stunted dendrites and greatly reduced dendritic arborization [64]. Altered phosphorylation of the microtubule-associated protein MAP2 results in dendritic microtubule depolymerization [65], and a reduced availability of arborization-promoting neurosteroids secondary to cholesterol unavailability [66].

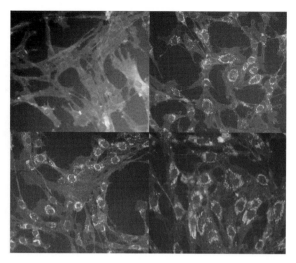

Figure 16.1 Filipin staining of cultured fibroblasts in Niemann-Pick Disease type C. Top left shows normal cells with minimal staining; top right and bottom left and right show staining of perinuclear cholesterol in three NPC-sufferers who presented with psychosis in adulthood and are described in Walterfang *et al.*, 2006 [86].

The diagnosis of NPC can be confirmed by demonstrating a low esterification rate of exogenous cholesterol in cultured skin fibroblasts (Figure 16.1), or by testing for lysosomal accumulation of free cholesterol by filipin staining [67]. The "classical" biochemical phenotype shows markedly reduced esterification and greater than 70% to 80% of cells staining positive for filipin, whereas the "variant" phenotype shows near-normal esterification rates and lower filipin-positive cell counts while still demonstrating clinical symptoms [67].

NPC may present in infancy, adolescence, or adulthood [68] with a clinically variable picture, although its core features include dementia, dysarthria, ataxia, vertical supranuclear opthalmoplegia, and hepatosplenomegaly. It may also commonly present with dystonia and choreoathetosis [68, 69]. Seizures, dysphagia, and pyramidal signs may appear with disease progression. The range of NPC1 and NPC2 mutations results in marked heterogeneity of clinical presentations [70].

Structural imaging in NPC commonly shows diffuse cerebral and/or cerebellar atrophy [68, 71, 72, 73, 74] or callosal pathology [58, 75] (Figure 16.2). Occasionally, white matter hyperintensities may present [68, 74, 75, 76, 77], which may radiologically mimic multiple sclerosis [75]. Single photon emission computed tomography (SPECT) and positron

(B)

(A)

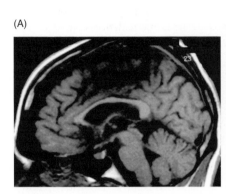
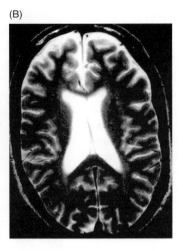

Figure 16.2 Magnetic resonance imaging scan in Niemann-Pick Disease type C in a 23-year-old patient with adult-onset disease and a 10-year history of schizophrenia-like psychosis. Left, a sagittal T1-weighted image showing callosal thinning; right, a T2-weighted axial section showing frontal atrophy.

emission tomography (PET) [78] imaging may show hypoperfusion in frontal regions [77, 79, 80], whereas magnetic resonance spectroscopy (MRS) in psychotic and nonpsychotic patients shows reductions in N-acetyl-aspartate:creatine ratios suggestive of pathology in the frontal and parietal cortices and basal ganglia [72, 74], where changes appear to correlate with clinical dysfunction [74]. Some of these features overlap with those found in schizophrenia, including hypofrontality [81], striatal pathology [82], and white-matter changes [83]. Electro-encephalography (EEG) may demonstrate diffuse slowing [68, 73, 80, 84]. Neuropsychological testing in adolescent/adult-onset cases often reveals a steady decline in function throughout adulthood with significant deficits in executive function and memory [71, 72, 80, 84].

Psychosis is not an uncommon sign later in the presentation of adolescent or adult-onset NPC, but in 25%–40% of adult-onset cases it may present alongside motor symptoms and cognitive impairment as an initial manifestation [85, 86]. When psychosis has been reported, features have included persecutory delusions, auditory hallucinations, and ideas of reference, as well as behavioral disorganization [71, 80, 84, 85, 87]. A small number of cases have been reported where psychosis was the sole initial manifestation [71, 84, 86, 88, 89]. There have been a limited number of cases described where a diagnosis of schizophrenia was made, and the patient treated with neuroleptics alone for a number of years, before gait impairment and steep cognitive decline resulted in a diagnostic revision [71, 85, 86]. Additionally, we have also described a presentation in adulthood with rapid-cycling bipolar disorder that responded to anticonvulsant medication [90].

Cerebrotendinous xanthomatosis

Cerebrotendinous xanthomatosis (CTX) is a rare autosomal recessive disorder caused by mutations of the serol-27-hydroxylase gene on 2q35 [91], which results in increased tissue cholestanol and defective bile acid synthesis [92]. Accumulation of cholestanol in white and grey matter leads to neuroaxonal dystrophy and possibly accelerated apoptosis [93]. Individuals with CTX develop xanthomas, cataracts, mental retardation, or dementia, and varying movement disorders. Global reduction in grey- and white- matter volume, reduced white-matter intensity, and callosal atrophy are noted on structural imaging [94, 95], which may – like NPC – mimic the demyelination of multiple sclerosis [96]. MRS findings suggest that axonal metabolic dysfunction rather than demyelination is responsible for the diffuse white-matter findings [97].

Two case series of CTX patients with psychiatric disturbance have been reported; in one, 4 of 35 cases suffered psychiatric disturbance, 3 of these being neuroleptic-responsive psychotic disorders [98]. A further series found psychiatric disturbance in 7 of 10 CTX patients, predominantly agitation and psychosis [99]. Some of these psychoses developed in the absence of cognitive impairment. Other authors have reported depression in CTX sufferers [100, 101], and more recently a fronto-temporal dementia picture in a compound heterozygote [102]. Because of the exceptional rarity of CTX and the small number of case reports, definitive conclusions are difficult to draw. However, it should be noted that 10 patients have been reported as suffering psychosis in an illness that has perhaps been diagnosed in only 200 patients worldwide [103]. This suggests that it occurs in up to 5% of patients, a rate five to ten times higher than the base rate of schizophrenia in the population. The early axonal dysfunction in CTX may be reflected in a preponderance toward psychotic (and other psychiatric) symptoms until gross neuronal loss (and dementia) supervenes, much like that seen in NPC.

Alpha mannosidosis

Alpha mannosidosis (AM) is a recessively inherited lysosomal storage disorder that results from deficiency of alpha mannosidase in lysosomes [104]. The illness is characterized by mild to moderate intellectual disability, hearing loss, skeletal changes, and recurrent infections [105]. Most sufferers develop illness early in childhood (type I) and die of severe infection. A more indolent form (type II) occurs in a minority of patients who survive to adulthood [106].

Alpha-mannosidase is coded by a gene on 19p13.2-q12 and functions in the normal lysosomal processing of N-linked oligosaccharides [107]. A range of splicing, mis-sense, and nonsense mutations to the gene have been described, although no clear genotype–phenotype correlations are evident [108]. Deficiency of alpha-mannosidase results in the intralysosomal accumulation of mannose-rich oligosaccharides and the formation of storage vacuoles in neuronal and glial cells [105]. This appears to impact significantly upon myelin formation in animal models and human neuropathological studies [109].

In type II AM, the predominant features are cerebellar ataxia, hearing loss, neuropsychological impairment, and retinopathy [110]. MRI scanning shows periventricular T2-hyperintensities in white matter [110, 111], which has been suggested as secondary to demyelination [112] although it is more likely to be an effect of myelin vacuolation [113]. Cortical and cerebellar atrophy is also not uncommon in type II patients [110, 114]. Diagnosis is established by the combination of a suggestive urinary pattern of oligosaccharides and demonstration of significantly reduced enzyme activity in leukocytes or cultured skin fibroblasts. The only treatment option is bone marrow transplantation [107].

Whereas some isolated case reports have suggested that, like NPC, some patients with type II AM may present as, and be diagnosed with, schizophrenia prior to the onset of frank neurological symptomatology [115], the most compelling evidence suggestive of a greater than expected rate of psychosis in the disorder comes from a few small series. Gutschalk and colleagues [110] described a trio of siblings, one of whom developed a psychosis characterized by delusions and hallucinations after the onset of sensorineural hearing loss. Malm and colleagues described a series of 45 patients over the age of 15, and found clearly diagnosable mental illness in 25%. The majority of these patients presented with a psychotic disorder characterized by delusions, hallucinations, confusion, and a prolonged period of postpsychotic somnolence [116]. Like the other disorders described in this chapter, psychosis in these patients had a distinctly "organic" feel, being accompanied by cognitive changes as well as significant neurological signs at the time of presentation. Like NPC, AM seems to initially affect myelinated structures before progressing to involve the whole neuronaxonal unit, and it may be this initial anatomical disconnection that predisposes adult individuals to psychosis prior to, or coincident with, the onset of their neurological and cognitive impairments.

Adult neuronal ceroid lipofuscinosis: Kufs' Disease

The neuronal ceroid lipofuscinoses (NCLs) are a group of neuronal storage disorders, one of which is Batten's Disease – the most common neurodegenerative disorder in childhood [117]. Eight different genetic forms of NCL are thought to exist, although at present only five genes have been discovered [118]. Most of the defective proteins in the NCLs are associated with lysosomal accumulation of mitochondrial ATP synthase subunit c [119]. Adult neuronal ceroid lipofuscinosis (ANCL, Kufs' Disease), was first described by Kufs in 1925 [120] and is thought to result from mutations in an as yet undiscovered gene, CLN4 [118].

ANCL is usually inherited recessively [121], although occasional dominant forms have been described [122, 123]. Symptoms most commonly appear at the beginning of the fourth decade but may be present early in the second. Neuropsychiatric disturbance in adolescent or adult-onset cases is very common [124]. Berkovic described two separate phenotypic groups of ANCL. The first group

219

(type A), was characterized clinically by progressive and treatment-refractory myoclonic epilepsy and dementia. Type B presented with neuropsychiatric disturbance, facial dyskinesia, and dementia [124, 125]. The visual signs commonly present in childhood onset-forms of NCL (known in the nineteenth and early twentieth centuries as "amaurotic idiocy") are absent in ANCL [118].

The characteristic neuropathology of ANCL is accumulation of lipofuscin-like material in lysosomes in neuronal and extraneuronal tissue, and diagnosis rests on identification of characteristic inclusions in skin punch biopsy or leukocytes [118]. The distribution of abnormal lysosomal inclusions in neurons is commonly diffuse through cortical and subcortical neurons, but may be localized to the cerebral cortex in a quarter of cases [125]. Hippocampal/enterorhinal cortex may be particularly susceptible [126]. Unlike most childhood forms, enzyme analysis or DNA testing is not available, as the presumed CLN4 gene has not been localized. MRI often shows cerebral and cerebellar atrophy, callosal thinning, and may show other features such as altered signal in subcortical nuclei, whereas SPECT commonly shows regional cortical hypoperfusion [127, 128, 129].

ANCL presents with psychosis in up to 20% of patients, with ages of onset between 13 and 41 [130, 131, 132, 133, 134, 135, 136, 137]. Backman and colleagues, in a series of juvenile NCL patients (mean age 15 years), described five adolescent patients with psychotic symptoms warranting psychotropic medication, although affective symptoms (predominantly depression) were more common [138]. Characteristic psychotic symptoms appear to be auditory hallucinations, delusions, and thought disorder [137], although occasionally catatonic motor changes are present [136]. Neuropsychological impairments are common, often with a mixed subcortical/cortical picture of psychomotor slowing, impaired new learning, and executive and attentional impairments [135]. An apparent sensitivity to the motor side effects of neuroleptic medication complicates the treatment of ACNL psychosis, including dystonia [131, 135] and neuroleptic malignant syndrome [136]. This sensitivity has been attributed to a combination of subcortical neuropathology and potentially muscle membrane pathology [136]. Treatment of psychosis, notwithstanding motor side effects, is usually with neuroleptic medication although electroconvulsive treatment has proven effective in a number of cases [130, 136].

A model for psychosis secondary to storage disorders: Niemann-Pick type C

As previously described in this book Chapter 6, much can be learned from the understanding of how organic diseases that present with schizophrenia-like psychosis produce psychotic symptoms, for this may inform the biological model and ultimately the treatment of schizophrenia. The core neuropathology of schizophrenia remains elusive, although it has been seen increasingly as a disorder of connectivity [139, 140, 141], particularly between frontal and temporal cortical regions and subcortical structures [3, 140]. Much evidence points to the role of dendritic and synaptic connections as anatomical substrates of this disconnectivity [142, 143, 144]. Myelinated axon structures are another key carrier of much CNS connectivity; hence, pathology in myelinated structures may also play a role [83, 145, 146]. The lipid-rich nature of myelinated axons, which is dependent on endogenous cholesterol [147], renders them highly vulnerable to disturbances of cholesterol or other lipid metabolism [55]. Given that disturbances in lipid biology may play some role in the pathology of schizophrenia [148], an understanding of how myelinated axons are functionally and structurally affected by NPC may provide a model for understanding how storage disorder-related psychosis develops in these disorders.

Using NPC as a model, its adolescent or early adulthood form may potentially disrupt key neurodevelopmental processes occurring during this period of CNS development, such as fronto-temporal myelination [6], impacting upon fronto-temporal connectivity and thus leading to psychosis [3, 140]. The initial cellular impact of NPC appears to occur at the axonal level, implicating the "macroconnectivity" that may underpin functional connectivity in the onset of psychotic symptoms in NPC [83]. Pathology in the striatum as described could also disrupt frontal-subcortical connectivity, which has also been linked to psychosis in schizophrenia [149]. The rates of psychosis in adult-onset NPC seem to approach those of adolescent/adult-onset metachromatic leukodystrophy (MLD), a disorder predominantly affecting white matter, where up to 50% of cases in this age group present with psychosis [2, 150]. In MLD, psychotic symptoms may be a result of impaired CNS function during a critical period of development of the CNS [151]. In adult-onset adrenoleukodystrophy,

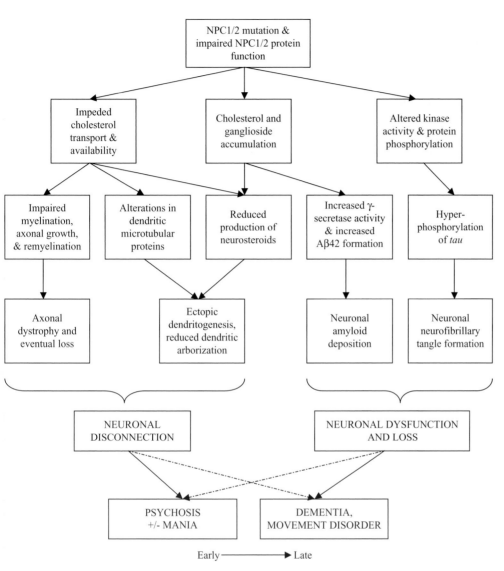

Figure 16.3 A model for the development of secondary schizophrenia based on the neuropathological findings in Niemann-Pick Disease type C. Initial impairment of connectivity through altered dendritic function and myelination results in functional disconnectivity and may lead to major mental illness prior to frank neuronal loss, whereby the clinical picture then shifts to one of frank motor and cognitive impairment.

where disruptions to myelination predominantly affect posterior zones, mania, or affective psychosis occurs more commonly than schizophrenia-like psychosis [152]. The reduced dendritic arborization that occurs in NPC also bears some homology to that seen in schizophrenia [142, 143] and may be an additional psychotogenic factor through its contribution to cortical disconnectivity at a "microconnectivity" level [153]. The progression of the clinical picture from psychosis to dementia and movement disorder in most cases may reflect an initial disconnectivity syndrome, resulting from dysfunction in axonal structures prior to degeneration, which is then followed by frank axonal loss and neurodegeneration in cortical and subcortical structures. This model, illustrated in Figure 16.3, may be applicable to storage disorders that affect axonal structures early before frank neuronal loss ensues.

In other disorders where predominantly grey-matter structures are affected, such as NCL, it may be that the connectivity impairments occur at a "microconnectivity" level (locally between proximally located neurons via synaptic connections) rather than through "macroconnectivity" (more distally located, but functionally interdependent, neural assemblies via axonal connections). Additionally, where neuronal pathology affects grey-matter regions known to be disproportionately affected in schizophrenia (frontal- and temporal-cortical regions, basal ganglia, and thalamus), this regional selectivity of pathology may be responsible for the psychotogenic effects of adult-onset disease. This model can be expanded to encompass other disorders, such as the mitochondrial disorders (Chapter 17). Here the regional effect on some regions of the brain (such as the basal ganglia), interact with the underlying state of the CNS at the time of maximal impact of the insult – where lower level neurodevelopmental systems are predominantly mature, but higher level systems are still undergoing significant plastic change. This results in a psychotic syndrome before the onset of more "frank" CNS impairment such as dementia or motor disturbance.

Laboratory diagnosis of storage disorders

The laboratory diagnosis for most storage disorders requires the alert clinician to think specifically about how the patient's clinical picture may be indicative of a storage disorder, as the confirmatory or exclusionary biochemical tests may be expensive and/or limited in accessibility (e.g. presence of a cherry red spot and VSO accompanying psychosis in GM2 gangliosidosis, or a history of neonatal jaundice and VSO accompanying psychosis in NPC).

GM2 gangliosidosis is generally diagnosed by the analysis of hexosaminadase A levels in peripheral blood[11] and referencing analysis against mutations to determine carrier or affected status, in addition to the detection of nonsignificant "pseudomutations" [154]. In particular, at-risk populations such as Ashkenazi Jewish individuals often are linked into screening programs during family planning or even rabbinical approval of unions[154]. In adult-onset patients, genetic analysis is often necessary due to residual enzyme levels and frequent heterozygosity[19].

With NPC, as a serum test is not currently available, skin fibroblasts from a punch biopsy are assessed for their rate of esterification, combined with filipin staining for lysosomal accumulation of free cholesterol [67]. In CTX, elevated plasma cholestanol and cholestanol:cholesterol ratio, is usually present, with the latter often increased 30-fold [103, 155], although urinary excretion of bile alcohols may be more sensitive [155]; molecular diagnosis of mutations in the CYP27A1 gene confirms diagnosis [156]. With AM, diagnosis can be made by a combination of an abnormal pattern of oligosaccharides in the urine [107], followed by testing for MANB levels in either peripheral leukocytes from venepuncture or skin fibroblasts from a punch biopsy, and analysis for mis-sense or nonsense mutations in the MANB gene [108].

In ACNL, because of the lack of a characteristic biochemical deficiency and molecular model, diagnosis rests on tissue diagnosis with microscopic identification of characteristic fingerprint inclusions and granular osmiophilic deposits (GRODs) at the ultrastructural level [118], using either cerebral or extracerebral (usually rectal mucosal) tissues [157]. Clinicians will rarely be at the point of tissue biopsy without having previously undertaken exhaustive biochemical and enzymatic analyses of blood and cerebrospinal fluid to exclude other, more readily identifiable causes of psychosis and neurological disturbance [136].

The treatment of psychosis in storage disorders

Some storage disorders show improvement in neurological symptoms when given definitive treatment, and given the neurobiological basis of psychotic symptoms, it seems likely that this would also result in a reduction in psychotic or other psychiatric symptomatology. Improvement in neurological symptoms has been reported with chenodeoxycholic acid treatment of CTX [158], and miglustat treatment of NPC [159, 160] but not yet Tay-Sachs Disease [161]. The mainstay of treatment for most psychotic disorders secondary to storage disorders remains antipsychotic medication, where a number of patients have been reported to respond to both typical and atypical antipsychotics [85, 86, 98]. Given that a number of patients with storage disorder-related psychosis are likely to have neurological and/or cognitive impairment, this is likely to render them vulnerable to the centrally mediated side effects of neuroleptic medication – including extrapyramidal motor side effects, sedation, cognitive dulling, and autonomic symptoms. In circumstances where treatment is limited by extrapyramidal or other side effects, ECT appears to be a safe and effective treatment in this group of patients.

References

1. Conzelmann E., Sandhoff K. Partial enzyme deficiencies: residual activities and the development of neurological disorders. *Dev Neurosci*, 1983. **6**:58–71.

2. Hyde T., Ziegler J., Weinberger D. Psychiatric disturbances in metachromatic leukodystrophy: insights into the neurobiology of psychosis. *Arch Neurol*, 1992. **49**:401–6.

3. Benes F. Why does psychosis develop during adolescence and early adulthood? *Curr Opin Psychiatry*, 2003. **16**:317–9.

4. Feinberg I. Schizophrenia: caused by a fault in programmed synaptic elimination during adolescence? *J Psychiatr Res*, 1982. **17**:319–34.

5. Huttenlocher P. (1994). Synaptogenesis in human cerebral cortex. In *Human Behavior and the Developing Brain*, Dawson G. and Fischer K. (Eds.). New York: The Guilford Press, pp. 137–52.

6. Benes F. Myelination of cortical hippocampal relays during late adolescence. *Schizophr Bull*, 1989. **15**:589–93.

7. Benes F., Vincent S., Molloy R. Dopamine-immunoreactive axon varicosities form nonrandom contacts with GABA-immunoreactive neurons of rat medial prefrontal cortex. *Synapse*, 1993. **15**:285–95.

8. Cunningham M., Bhattacharyya S., Benes F. Amygdalo-cortical sprouting continues into early adulthood: implications for the development of normal and abnormal function during adolescence. *J Comp Neurol*, 2002. **453**:116–30.

9. Sachs B. On amaurotic family idiocy. A disease chiefly of the grey matter of the central nervous system. *J Nerv Ment Dis*, 1903. **30**:1–13.

10. Sachs B. On arrested cerebral development, with special reference to its cortical pathology. *J Nerv Ment Dis*, 1887. **14**:541–53.

11. Gravel R., Clarke J., Kaback M., et al. (1995). The GM2 Gangliosidoses. In *The Metabolic and Molecular Basis of Inherited Disease*. Scriber C., Beaudet A., Sly W., and Valle D. (Eds.). New York: McGraw-Hill, pp. 2839–79.

12. Tay W. Symmetrical changes in the region of the yellow spot in each eye of an infant. *Trans Opthal Soc UK*, 1881. **1**:55.

13. Meek D., Wolfe L., Andermann E., et al. Juvenile progressive dystonia: a new phenotype of GM2 gangliosidosis. *Ann Neurol*, 1984. **15**:348–52.

14. Navon R., Padeh B., Adam A. Apparent deficiency of hexosaminidase A in healthy members of a family with Tay-Sachs disease. *Am J Hum Genet*, 1973. **25**:287–92.

15. Grebner E., Tomczak J. Distribution of three alpha-chain beta-hexosaminidase A mutations among Tay-Sachs carriers. *Am J Hum Genet*, 1991. **48**:604–7.

16. Chern C., Buetler E., Kuhl W., et al. Characterization of heteropolymeric hexosaminidase A in human x mouse hybrid cells. *Proc Natl Acad Sci USA*, 1976. **73**:3637–40.

17. Mahuran D. Biochemical consequences of mutations causing the GM2 gangliosidoses. *Biochim Biophys Acta*, 1999. **1455**:105–38.

18. Sandhoff K., Andreae U., Jatzkewitz H. Deficient hexosaminidase activity in an exceptional case of Tay-Sachs disease with additional storage of kidney globoside in visceral organs. *Life Sci*, 1968. **7**:283–8.

19. Neudorfer O., Pastores G. M., Zeng B. J., et al. Late-onset Tay-Sachs disease: phenotypic characterization and genotypic correlation in 21 affected patients. *Genet Med*, 2005. **7**:119–23.

20. Purpura D., Suzuki K. Distortion of neuronal geometry and formation of aberrant synopsis in neuronal storage disease. *Brain Res*, 1976. **116**:1–21.

21. Walkley S. Pathobiology of neuronal storage disease. *Int Rev Neurobiol*, 1988. **29**:191–244.

22. Suzuki K. Twenty five years of the "psychosine" hypothesis: a personal perspective of its history and present status. *Neurochem Res*, 1998. **23**:251–9.

23. Walkley S. Secondary accumulation of gangliosides in lysosomal storage disorders. *Semin Cell Dev Biol*, 2004. **15**:433–44.

24. Huang J., Trasler J., Igdoura S., et al. Apoptotic cell death in mouse models of GM2 gangliosidosis and observations on human Tay-Sachs and Sandhoff diseases. *Hum Mol Genet*, 1997. **6**:1879–85.

25. Jeyakumar M., Elliot-Smith E., Smith D., et al. Central nervous system inflammation is a hallmark of pathogenesis in mouse models of GM1 and GM2 gangliosidosis. *Brain Res*, 2003. **126**: 974–87.

26. Federico A., Palmeri S., Malandrini A. The clinical aspects of adult hexosaminidase deficiencies. *Dev Neurosci*, 1991. **13**:280–7.

27. MacQueen G., Rosebush P., Mazurek M. Neuropsychiatric aspects of the adult variant of Tay-Sachs disease. *J Neuro-psychiatry Clin Neurosci*, 1998. **10**:10–19.

28. Zaroff C., Neudorfer O. Morrison C., et al. Neuropsychological assessment of patients with late-onset GM2 gangliosidosis. *Neurology*, 2004. **62**:2283–6.

29. Frey L., Ringel S., Filley C. The natural history of cognitive dysfunction in late-onset GM2 gangliosidosis. *Arch Neurol*, 2005. **62**:989–94.

30. Streifler J., Golomb M., Gadoth N. Psychiatric features of adult GM2 gangliosidosis. *Br J Psychiatry*, 1989. **155**:410–3.

31. Jacobs J., Willemsen M., Groot-Loonen J., *et al.* Allogenic BMT followed by substrate reduction therapy in a child with subacute Tay-Sachs disease. *Bone Marrow Transplant*, 2005. **36**:925–6.

32. Navon R., Argov Z., Frisch A. Hexosaminidase deficiency in adults. *Am J Med Genet*, 1986. **24**:179–96.

33. Oates C., Bosch E., Hart M. Movement disorders associated with chronic GM2 gangliosidosis: case report and review of the literature. *Eur Neurol*, 1986. **25**:154–9.

34. Streifler J., Gornish M., Hadar H., *et al.* Brain imaging in late-onset GM2 gangliosidosis. *Neurology*, 1993. **43**:2055–8.

35. Renshaw P., Stern T., Welch C. Electroconvulsive therapy treatment of depression in a patient with adult GM2 gangliosidosis. *Ann Neurol*, 1992. **31**:342–4.

36. Rosebush P., MacQueen G., Mazurek M. Late-onset Tay-Sachs disease presenting as catatonic schizophrenia: diagnostic and treatment issues. *J Clin Psychiatry*, 1995. **56**:347–53.

37. Hurowitz G., Silver J., Brin M., *et al.* Neuropsychiatric aspects of adult-onset Tay-Sachs disease: two case reports with several new findings. *J Neuropsychiatry Clin Neurosci*, 1993. **5**:30–6.

38. Vanier M., Suzuki K. Recent advances in elucidating Niemann-Pick C disease. *Brain Pathol*, 1998. **8**:163–74.

39. Pentchev P., Vanier M., Suzuki K., *et al.* (1995). Niemann-Pick disease Type C: a cellular cholesterol lipidosis. In *The Metabolic and Molecular Bases of Inherited Disease*, 7th Ed. Scriver C., Beaudet A., Sly W., Valle D.,

(Eds.). New York: McGraw Hill, pp. 2625–39.

40. Spence M., Callahan J. (1989). The Niemann-Pick group of diseases. *The Metabolic Basis of Inherited Diseases*. 6th Ed. New York: McGraw-Hill, pp. 1655–76.

41. Crocker A. Niemann-Pick disease: A review of fifteen patients. *Medicine* (Baltimore), 1958. **37**:1–95.

42. Millat G., Marcais C., Rafi M., *et al.* Niemann-Pick C1 disease: the I1061T substitution is a frequent mutant allele in patients of Western European descent and correlates with a classic juvenile phenotype. *Am J Human Genet*, 1999. **65**:1321–9.

43. Kobayashi T., Beuchat M., Lindsay M., *et al.* Late endosomal membranes rich in lysobisphosphatidic acid regulate cholesterol transport. *Nat Cell Biol*, 1999. **1**:113–8.

44. Naureckiene S., Sleat D., Lackland H., *et al.* Identification of HE1 as the second gene of Niemann-Pick C disease. *Science*, 2000. **290**:2227–9.

45. Carstea E., Morris J., Coleman K., *et al.* Niemann-Pick C1 disease gene: homology to mediators of cholesterol homeostasis. *Science*, 1997. **277**:228–31.

46. Loftus S., Morris J., Carstea E., *et al.* Murine model of Niemann-Pick C disease: mutation in a cholesterol homeostasis gene. *Science*, 1997. **277**:232–5.

47. Vincent I., Bu B., Erickson R. Understanding of Niemann-Pick type C disease: a fat problem. *Curr Opin Neurol*, 2003. **16**:155–61.

48. Ory D. Niemann-Pick type C: A disorder of cellular cholesterol trafficking. *Biochim Biophys Acta*, 2000. **1529**:331–9.

49. Ioannou Y. The structure and function of the Niemann-Pick C1 protein. *Mol Genet Metab*, 2000. **71**:175–81.

50. Blom T., Linder M., Snow K., *et al.* Defective endocytic trafficking of NPC1 and NPC2 underlying infantile Niemann-Pick type C disease. *Hum Mol Genet*, 2003. **12**:257–72.

51. Zervas M., Dobrenis K., Walkley S. Neurons in Niemann-Pick type C accumulate gangliosides as well as unesterified cholesterol and undergo dendritic and axonal alterations. *J Neuropathol Exp Neurol*, 2001. **60**:49–64.

52. Suzuki K., Parker C., Pentchev P., *et al.* Neurofibrillary tangles in Niemann-Pick disease type C. *Acta Neuropathol* (Berl), 1995. **89**:227–38.

53. Saito Y., Suzuki K., Nanba E., *et al.* Niemann-Pick type C disease: accelerated neurofibrillary tangle formation and amyloid B deposition associated with apolipoprotein E4 homozygosity. *Ann Neurol*, 2002. **52**:351–5.

54. Liscum L. Niemann-Pick type C mutations cause lipid traffic jam. *Traffic*, 2000. **1**:218–25.

55. Nixon R. Niemann-Pick type C disease and Alzheimer's disease: the APP endosome connection fattens up. *Am J Pathol*, 2004. **164**:757–61.

56. Goodrum J., Pentchev P. Cholesterol reutilization during myelination of regenerating PNS axons is impaired in Niemann-Pick disease type C mice. *J Neurosci Res*, 1997. **49**:389–92.

57. Karten B., Vance D., Campenot R., *et al.* Trafficking of cholesterol from cell bodies to distal axons in Niemann Pick C1-deficiant neurons. *J Biol Chem*, 2003. **278**:4168–75.

58. Palmeri S., Battisti C., Federico A., *et al.* Hypoplasia of the corpus callosum in Niemann-Pick type C disease. *Neuroradiology*, 1994. **36**:20–2.

59. Ong W., Kumar U., Switzer R., *et al.* Neurodegeneration in Niemann-Pick type C disease

mice. *Exp Brain Res*, 2001. **141**: 218–31.

60. German D. C., Liang C. L., Song T., *et al.* Neurodegeneration in the Niemann-Pick C mouse: glial involvement. *Neuroscience*, 2002. **109**:437–50.

61. Harzer K., Schlote W., Peiffer J., *et al.* Neurovisceral lipidosis compatible with Niemann-Pick disease type C: morphological and biochemical studies of a late infantile case and enzyme and lipid assays in a prenatal case of the same family. *Acta Neuropathol*, 1978. **43**:97–104.

62. Elleder M., Jirasek A., Smid F., *et al.* Niemann-Pick disease type C. Study on the nature of the cerebral storage process. *Acta Neuropathol*, 1985. **66**:325–66.

63. March P., Thrall M., Brown D., *et al.* GABAergic neuroaxonal dystrophy and other cytopathological alterations in feline Niemann-Pick disease type C. *Acta Neuropathol*, 1997. **94**:164–72.

64. Paul C., Boegle A., Maue R. Before the loss: neuronal dysfunction in Niemann-Pick type C disease. *Biochim Biophys Acta*, 2004. **1685**:63–76.

65. Fan Q.-W., Yu W., Gong J-S., *et al.* Cholesterol-dependent modulation of dendrite outgrowth and microtubule stability in cultured neurons. *J Neurochem*, 2002. **80**:178–90.

66. Sakamoto H., Ukena K., Tsutsu K. Effects of progesterone synthesized de novo in the developing Purkinje cell on its dendritic growth and synaptogenesis. *J Neurosci*, 2001. **16**:6221–32.

67. Vanier M., Rodriguez-Lafrasse C., Rousson R., *et al.* Typc C Niemann-Pick disease: biochemical aspects and phenotypic heterogeneity. *Dev Neurosci*, 1991. **13**:307–14.

68. Fink J., Filling-Katz M., Sokal J. Clinical spectrum of

Niemann-Pick disease type C. *Neurology*, 1989. **39**:1040–9.

69. Brady R. O., Filling-Katz M. R., Barton N. W., *et al.* Niemann-Pick disease types C and D. *Neurol Clin*, 1989. **7**:75–88.

70. Millat G., Chikh K., Naureckienne S., *et al.* Niemann-Pick disease type C: spectrum of HE1 mutations and genotype/phenotype correlations in the NPC2 group. *Am J Human Genet*, 2001. **69**:1013–21.

71. Shulman L., Lang A., Jankovic J., *et al.* Case 1, 1995: psychosis, dementia, chorea, ataxia and supranuclear gaze dysfunction. *Mov Disord*, 1995. **10**(3):257–62.

72. Schiffman R. Niemann-Pick disease type C: from bench to bedside. *JAMA*, 1996. **276**(7):561–4.

73. Lossos A., Schlesigner I., Okon E., *et al.* Adult-onset Niemann-Pick type C disease: clinical, biochemical and genetic study. *Arch Neurol*, 1997. **54**:1536–41.

74. Tedeschi G., Bonavita S., Barton N., *et al.* Proton magnetic resonance spectroscopic imaging in the clinical evaluation of patients with Niemann-Pick type C disease. *J Neurol Neurosurg Psychiatry*, 1998. **65**:72–9.

75. Grau A., Brandt T., Weisbrod M., *et al.* Adult Niemann-Pick disease type C mimicking features of multiple sclerosis. *J Neurol Neurosurg Psychiatr*, 1997. **63**:522–5.

76. Uc E., Wenger D., Jankovic J. Niemann Pick disease type C: two cases and an update. *Mov Disord*, 2000. **15**:1199–202.

77. Battisti C., Tarugi P., Dotti M., *et al.* Adult-onset Niemann-Pick type C disease: a clinical, neuroimaging, and molecular genetic study. *Mov Disord*, 2003. **18**:1405–9.

78. Cataldo A., Peterhoff C., Troncoo J., *et al.* Endocytic pathway abnormalities precede amyloid

beta deposition in sporadic Alzheimer's disease and Down syndrome: differential effects of APOE genotype and presenelin mutations. *Am J Pathol*, 2000. **157**:277–86.

79. Hulette C., Earl N., Anthony D., *et al.* Adult onset Niemann-Pick disease type C presenting with dementia and absent organomegaly. *Clin Neuropathol*, 1992. **11**:293–7.

80. Campo J., Stowe R., Slomka G., *et al.* Psychosis as a presentation of physical disease in adolescence: a case of Niemann-Pick disease type C. *Dev Med Child Neurol*, 1998. **40**:126–9.

81. Velakoulis D., Pantelis C. What have we learned from functional imaging studies in schizophrenia? The role of frontal, striatal and temporal areas. *Aust NZ J Psychiatry*, 1996. **30**:195–209.

82. Heckers S. Neuropathology of schizophrenia: cortex, thalamus, basal ganglia, and neurotransmitter-specific projection systems. *Schizophr Bull*, 1997. **23**:403–21.

83. Walterfang M., Wood S., Velakoulis D., *et al.* Neuropathological, neurogenetic and neuroimaging evidence for white matter pathology in schizophrenia. *Neurosci Biobehav Rev*, 2006. **30**:918–48.

84. Shulman L., David N., Weiner W. Psychosis as the initial manifestation of adult-onset Niemann-Pick disease type C. *Neurology*, 1995. **45**: 1739–43.

85. Josephs K., Van Gerpen M., Van Gerpen J. Adult-onset Niemann-Pick disease type C presenting with psychosis. *J Neurol Neurosierg Psychiatry*, 2003. **74**:528–9.

86. Walterfang M., Feitz M., Sullivan D., *et al.* The neuropsychiatry of adult-onset Niemann-Pick type C disease. *J Neuropsychiatr Clin Neurosci*, 2006. **18**:158–70.

87. Breen L., Morris H., Alperin J., *et al.* Juvenile Niemann-Pick disease with vertical supranuclear opthalmoplegia. *Arch Neurol*, 1981. **38**:388–90.

88. Turpin J., Goas N., Masson M., *et al.* Type C Niemann-Pick disease: supranuclear opthalmoplegia associated with deficient biosynthesis of cholesterol esters. *Rev Neurol* (Paris), 1991. **147**(1):28–34.

89. Vanier M. Lipid changes in Niemann-Pick disease type C brain: personal experience and review of the literature. *Neurochem Res*, 1999. B(4):481–9.

90. Sullivan D., Walterfang M., Velakoulis D. Bipolar disorder and Niemann-Pick disease type C. *Am J Psychiatry*, 2005. **165**:1021–2.

91. Lee M., Hazard S., Carpten J., *et al.* Fine-mapping, mutation analyses, and structural mapping of cerebrotendinous xanthomatosis in U.S. pedigrees. *J Lipid Res*, 2001. **42**:159–69.

92. Salen G., Grundy S. The metabolism of cholestanol, cholesterol and bile acids in cerebrotendinous xanthomatosis. *J Clin Invest*, 1973. **52**:2822–35.

93. Moghadasian M., Salen G., Frohlich J., *et al.* Cerebro-tendinous xanthomatosis: a rare disease with diverse manifestations. *Arch Neurol*, 2002. **59**:527–9.

94. Berginer V., Berginer J., Korczyn A., *et al.* Magnetic resonance imaging in cerebrotendinous xanthomatosis: a prospective clinical and neuroradiological study. *Neurol Sci*, 1994. **122**: 102–8.

95. Dotti M., Federico A., Signorini E., *et al.* Cerebrotendinous xanthomatosis (van Bogaert-Scherer-Epstein disease): CT and MR findings. *AJNR Am J Neuroradiol*, 1994. **15**:1721–6.

96. Swanson P., Cromwell L. Magnetic resonance imaging in cerebrotendinous xanthomatosis. *Neurology*, 1986. **36**:124–6.

97. De Stefano N., Matthews P., Arnold D. Reversible decreases in N-acetyl aspartate after acute brain injury. *Mag Reson Med*, 1995. **34**:721–7.

98. Berginer V., Foster N., Sadowsky M., *et al.* Psychiatric disorders in patients with cerebrotendinous xanthomatosus. *Am J Psychiatry*, 1988. **145**:354–7.

99. Dotti M., Salen G., Federico A. Cerebrotendinous xanthomatosis as a multisystem disease mimicking premature ageing. *Dev Neurosci*, 1991. **13**:371–6.

100. Shapiro S. Depression in a patient with dementia secondary to cerebrotendinous xanthomato-sis. *J Nerv Ment Dis*, 1983. **171**:568–71.

101. Lee Y., Lin P., Chiu N., *et al.* Cerebrotendinous xanthomatosis with psychiatric disorder: report of three siblings and literature review. *Chang Gung Med J*, 2002. **25**:334–40.

102. Guyant-Marechal L., Verrip A., Girard C., *et al.* Unusual cerebrotendinous xanthomatosis with fronto-temporal dementia phenotype. *Am J Med Genet*, 2005. **139**:114–7.

103. Moghadasian M. Cerebro-tendinous xanthomatosis: clinical course, genotypes and metabolic backgrounds. *Clin Invest Med*, 2004. **27**:42–50.

104. Nilssen O., Berg T., Riise H., *et al.* Alpha-mannosidosis: functional cloning of the lysosomal alpha-mannosidase cDNA and identification of a mutation in two affected siblings. *Hum Mol Genet*, 1997. **6**:717–26.

105. Thomas G. (2001). Disorders of glycoprotein degradation: alpha mannosidosis, beta mannosidosis, fucosidosis and sialidosis.. In *The Metabolic and Molecular Bases of Inherited Disease*, 8th ed. Scriver C., Beaudet A., Valle D., and Sly W. (Eds.). New York: McGraw-Hill, pp. 3507–33.

106. Bennett J., Dembure P., Elsas L. Clinical and biochemical analysis of two families with type I and type II mannosidosis. *Am J Med Genet*, 1995. **55**:21–6.

107. Sun H., Wolfe J. Recent progress in lysosomal alpha mannosidase and its deficiency. *Exp Mol Med*, 2001. **33**:1–7.

108. Berg T., Riise H., Hensen G., *et al.* Spectrum of mutations in alpha mannosidosis. *Am J Hum Genet*, 1999. **64**:77–88.

109. Vandevelole M., Fankhauser R., Bichsel P., *et al.* Hereditary neurovisceral mannosidosis associated with alpha mannosidase deficiency in a family of Persian cats. *Acta Neuropathol*, 1982. **58**:64–8.

110. Gutschalk A., Harting I., Cantz M., *et al.* Adult alpha mannosidosis: clinical progression in the absence of demyelination. *Neurology*, 2004. **63**:1744–6.

111. Vite C., McGowan J., Braund K. Histopathology, electrodiagnostic testing and magnetic resonance imaging show significant peripheral and central nervous system myelin abnormalities in the cat model of alpha mannosidosis. *J Neuropathol Exp Neurol*, 2001. **60**:817–28.

112. Dietemann J., Flippi de la Palavesa M., Tranchant C., *et al.* MR findings in mannosidosis. *Neuroradiology*, 1990. **33**:485–7.

113. Sung J., YHayano M., Desnick R. Mannosidosis: pathology of the nervous system. *J Neuropathol Exp Neurol*, 1977. **36**:807–20.

114. Ara J., Mayayo E., Marzo M., *et al.* Neurological impairment in alpha mannosidosis: a longitudinal clinical and MRI study of a brother and sister. *Childs Nerv Syst*, 1999. **15**:369–71.

115. Seidl U., Giesel F., Cantz M., *et al.* Unusual course of alpha

mannosidosis with symptoms of paranoid-hallucinatory psychosis. *Nervenarzt*, 2004. **76**:335–8.

116. Malm D., Pantel J., Linaker O. Psychiatric symptoms in mannosidosis. *J Intell Dis Res*, 2005. **49**:865–71.

117. Mole S. Batten's disease: eight genes and still counting. *Lancet*, 1999. **354**:443–4.

118. Wisniewski K., Kida E., Golabek A., *et al.* Neruonal ceoid lipofuscinoses: classification and diagnosis. *Adv Genet*, 2001. **45**:1–34.

119. Ezaki J., Kominami E. The intracellular location and function of proteins of neuronal ceroid lipofuscinoses. *Brain Pathol*, 2004. **14**:77–85.

120. Kufs H. Uber eine spatform der amaurotischen idiotie und ihre heredofamiliaren grundlagen. *Z Ges Neurol Psychiatr.*, 1925. **95**:169–88.

121. Donnet A., Habib M., Pellissier J., *et al.* Kuf's disease presenting as progressive dementia with late-onset generalized seizures: a clinicopathological and electrophysiological study. *Epilepsia*, 1992. **33**:65–74.

122. Boehme D., Cottrell J., Leonberg S., *et al.* A dominant form of neuronal ceroid lipofuscinosis. *Brain*, 1971. **94**:745–60.

123. Nijssen P., Brusse E., Leyten A., *et al.* Autosomal dominant adult neuronal ceroid lipofuscinosis: parkinsonism due to both striatal and nigral dysfunction. *Mov Disord*, 2002. **17**:482–7.

124. Berkovic S., Carpenter S., Andermann F., *et al.* Kuf's disease: a critical re-appraisal. *Brain*, 1988. **111**:27–62.

125. Constantinidis J., Wisniewski K., Wisniewski T. The adult and a new late adult forms of neuronal ceroid lipofuscinosis. *Acta Neuropathol*, 1992. **83**:461–8.

126. Braak H., Braak E. Pathoarchitectonic pattern of iso- and allocortical lesions in juvenile and adult neuronal ceroid lipofuscinoses. *J Inherit Metabol Dis*, 1993. **16**:259–62.

127. D'Incerti L. MRI in neuronal ceroid lipofuscinosis. *Neurol Sci*, 2000. **21**:S71–S3.

128. Schreiner R., Becker I., Wiegand M. Kuf's disease: a rare cause of early-onset dementia. *Nervenarzt*, 2000. **71**:411–5.

129. Sayit E., Yorulmaz I., Bekis R., *et al.* Comparison of brain perfusion SPECT and MRI findings in children with neuronal ceroid-lipofuscinosis and in their families. *Ann Nucl Med*, 2002. **16**:201–6.

130. Tobo M., Mitsuyama Y., *et al.* Familial occurrence of adult-type neuronal ceroid lipofuscinosis. *Arch Neurol*, 1984. **41**:1091–4.

131. Gospe S. J., Jankovic J. Drug-induced dystonia in neuronal ceroid lipofuscinosis. *Pediatr Neurol*, 1986. **2**:236–7.

132. Charles N., Vighetto A., Pialat J., *et al.* Dementia and psychiatric disorders in Kufs disease. *Rev Neurol* (Paris), 1990. **146**:752–6.

133. Waldman A. Sometimes when you hear hoofbeats … two cases of inherited metabolic diseases with initial presentation of psychiatric symptoms. *J Neuropsychiatry Clin Neurosci*, 1992. **4**:113–4.

134. Augustine A., Fricchione G., Wiznicki R., *et al.* Adult neuronal ceroid lipofuscinosis presenting with psychiatric symptoms: a case report. *Int J Psychiatr Med*, 1993. **23**:315–22.

135. Hinkebein J., Callahan C. The neuropsychology of Kuf's disease: a case of atypical early onset dementia. *Arch Clin Neuropsychol*, 1997. **12**:81–9.

136. Reif A., Schneider M., Hoyer A., *et al.* Neuroleptic malignant syndrome in Kuf's disease. *J Neurol Neurosurg Psychiatry*, 2003. **74**:385–7.

137. Callagy C., O'Neill G., Murphy S., *et al.* Adult neuronal ceroid lipofuscinosis (Kufs' disease) in two siblings of an Irish family. *Clin Neuropathol*, 2000. **19**:109–18.

138. Backman M., Santavuori P., Aberg L., *et al.* Psychiatric symptoms of children and adolescents with juvenile neuronal ceroid lipofuscinosis. *J Intell Dis Res*, 2005. **49**:25–32.

139. Friston K. Schizophrenia and the disconnection hypothesis. *Acta Psychiatrica Scand Suppl*, 1999. **99**:68–79.

140. Friston K., Frith C. Schizophrenia: a disconnection syndrome? *Clin Neurosci*, 1995. **3**:89–97.

141. McGuire P., Frith C. Disordered functional connectivity in schizophrenia. *Psychol Med*, 1996. **26**:663–7.

142. Kalus P., Muller T., Zuschratter W., *et al.* The dendritic architecture of prefrontal pyramidal neurons in schizophrenic patients. *Neuroreport*, 2000. **11**:3621–5.

143. Rosoklija G., Toomayan G., Ellis S., *et al.* Structural abnormalities of subicular dendrites in subjects with schizophrenia and mood disorders – preliminary findings. *Arch Gen Psychiatry*, 2000. **57**:349–56.

144. Honer W., Young C. Presynaptic proteins and schizophrenia. *Int Rev Neurobiol*, 2004. **59**:175–99.

145. Bartzokis G. Schizophrenia: breakdown in the well-regulated lifelong process of brain development and maturation. *Neuropsychopharmacology*, 2002. **27**:672–83.

146. Davis K., Stewart D., Friedman J., *et al.* White matter changes in schizophrenia: evidence for myelin-related dysfunction. *Arch Gen Psychiatry*, 2003. **60**:443–56.

147. Morell P., Jurevics H. Origin of cholesterol in myelin. *Neurochem Res*, 1996. **21**:463–70.

148. Berger G., Wood S., Pantelis C., *et al.* Implications of lipid biology for the pathogenesis of schizophrenia. *Aust NZ J Psychiatry*, 2002. **36**:355–66.

149. Pantelis C., Barnes T., Nelson H., *et al.* Frontal-striatal cognitive deficits in patients with chronic schizophrenia. *Brain*, 1997. **120**:1823–43.

150. Weinberger D., Lipska B. Cortical maldevelopment, anti-psychotic drugs, and schizophrenia: a search for commonground. *Schizophr Res*, 1995. **16**:87–110.

151. Weinberger D. Implications of normal brain development for the pathogenesis of schizophrenia. *Arch Gen Psychiatry*, 1987. **44**:660–9.

152. Rosebush P., Garside S., Levinson A., *et al.* The neuropsychiatry of adult-onset adrenoleukodystrophy. *J Neuropsychiatry Clin Neurosci*, 1999. **11**:315–27.

153. Selemon L., Goldman-Rakic P. The reduced neuropil hypothesis: a circuit based model of schizophrenia. *Biol Psychiatry*, 1999. **45**:17–25.

154. Kaback M. Population-based genetic screening for reproductive counseling: the Tay-Sachs disease model. *Eur J Pediatr*, 2000. **159**: S192–5.

155. Koopman B., Wolthers B., Van Der Molen J., *et al.* Cerebrotendinous xanthomatosis: a review of biochemical findings of the patient population in the Netherlands. *J Inherit Metabol Dis*, 1988. **11**:56–75.

156. Gallus G., Dotti M., Federico A. Clinical and molecular diagnosis of cerebrotendinous xanthomatosis with a review of the mutations in the CYP27A1 gene. *Neurol Sci*, 2006. **27**:143–9.

157. Pasquinelli G., Cenacchi G., Piane E., *et al.* The problematic issue of Kufs disease diagnosis as performed on rectal biopsies: a case report. *Ultrastruct Pathol*, 2004. **28**:43–8.

158. Berginer V., Salen G., Shefer S. Long-term treatment of cerebrotendinous xanthomatosis with chenodeoxycholic acid. *N Engl J Med*, 1984. **311**:1649–52.

159. Patterson M., Platt F. Therapy of Niemann-Pick disease, type C. *Biochim Biophys Acta*, 2004. **1685**:77–82.

160. Chien Y., Lee N., Tsai L., *et al.* Treatment of Niemann-Pick disease type C in two children with miglustat: initial responses and maintenance of effects over 1 year. *J Inherit Metabol Dis*, 2007. **30**: 826.

161. Bembi B., Marchetti F., Guerci V., *et al.* Substrate reduction therapy in the infantile form of Tay-Sachs disease. *Neurology*, 2006. **66**:278–80.

17

Mitochondrial disorders and psychosis

Dennis Velakoulis and Mark Walterfang

Facts box

- A primary mitochondrial function is that of cellular energy metabolism through the respiratory chain.

- Four important concepts in relation to mitochondrial genetics are those of maternal inheritance, heteroplasmy/homoplasmy, mitotic segregation, and the role of autosomal genes that code for mitochondrial products.

- More than 100 disease-associated point mutations of mitochondrial DNA have been identified.

- Several lines of investigation point to potential mitochondrial involvement in patients with schizophrenia.

- The association of mitochondrial disorders with schizophrenia-like psychosis (SLP) relies on case reports. SLP has been described in some cases. In others, psychosis occurs in the setting of delirium or dementia. A family history of schizophrenia has been described in some cases.

- High rates of psychosis have been described in Wolfram Disease, an autosomal recessive disorder with a mutation on chromosome 4.

- In mitochondrial disorders, psychosis occurs in the setting of a wide range of medical comorbidities.

Mitochondrial functions

A primary mitochondrial function is that of cellular energy metabolism through the respiratory chain, the final common pathway for adenosine triphosphate (ATP) production. The mitochondrial/respiratory chain is a group of five enzyme complexes made up of polypeptides encoded by nuclear and mitochondrial genes, except for Complex II, which is entirely encoded in the cell nucleus. These complexes participate in a chain of metabolic processes, the overall process being referred to as oxidative phosphorylation (OXPHOS), which result in the production of ATP. ATP is used in the vast majority of cellular metabolic processes as an energy source and must be transported out of the mitochondrion by adenine nucleotide translocator. The respiratory chain responds to the energy needs of cells, which in some cases may be quite stable, whereas in others, for example, in the muscle, they may vary dramatically over time. Other functions of the mitochondria include cellular homeostasis, fatty acid oxidation, the urea cycle, intracellular signaling, apoptosis, and the metabolism of amino acids, lipids, cholesterol, steroids, and nucleotides [1, 2].

Mitochondrial genetics

Four important concepts are those of maternal inheritance, heteroplasmy/homoplasmy, mitotic segregation, and the role of autosomal genes that code for mitochondrial products.

Maternal inheritance

It is widely but not absolutely accepted that mitochondria are inherited through the maternal line. A mother will pass her mitochondria on to all her children, but only her daughters will pass on their mitochondria [3]. This is considered a consequence of the large imbalance between the number of mitochondria in the female oocyte (100,000) compared to the few mitochondria in the male sperm. Furthermore, it is now known that male mitochondria are destroyed in the zygote as if they were a foreign antigen [1, 4].

Heteroplasmy/homoplasmy

Mitochondrial DNA is identical (homoplasmic) within the cells of any one individual at birth. Mitochondrial DNA is not protected by repair mechanisms or histones and mutation rates are ten times greater than for nuclear DNA. Mutations may either be point mutations, which are usually maternally inherited, or sporadic partial deletions or duplications [5]. The occurrence of a mitochondrial DNA mutation may lead to a mixture of normal and mutated mitochondrial DNA within the one cell (heteroplasmic cell). The proportion of mutated and normal mitochondrial DNA can vary from cell to cell, including maternal oocytes. As a result, children of the same mother may inherit very different mitochondrial DNA. Further adding to the complexity of mitochondrial disorders caused by mutations, it is known that a threshold of mutant DNA is required within a cell before oxidative dysfunction will occur. This threshold will be determined by cell type, the cells' oxidative needs, and the mutation itself [6, 7].

Mitotic segregation

Mitochondrial numbers will vary from cell to cell within and between tissues and at different times within the development of cells. The division of a heteroplasmic cell may lead to different amounts of mutated mitochondrial DNA in the daughter cells. The variations in mitochondrial number will also be determined by tissue type and the metabolic needs of the cells. Mitochondrial DNA replication occurs at a much greater rate than nuclear DNA replication, is independent of the cell cycle, and is occurring continuously even in nondividing cells, such as muscle or brain [2].

Role of autosomal genes on mitochondrial function

As discussed earlier, mitochondrial function is also determined by cell nuclei genes. Mitochondrial disorders can therefore be inherited in a Mendelian pattern, that is, autosomal dominant or recessive inheritance.

Several broad clinical implications follow from the previous discussion of genetics [7]:

1 Mitochondrial disorders may be sporadic, maternally inherited, or inherited in an autosomal pattern.
2 Siblings may show a very broad range of clinical variability due to differences in the inheritance of heteroplasmic mitochondria.
3 Mitochondrial respiratory chain disorders will most affect tissues with high metabolic needs, for example, muscle, central and peripheral nervous system, heart, endocrine, and eye.
4 The clinical expression of mitochondrial disorders may vary widely from individual to individual with the same mutation depending on the proportion of mitochondria affected in different tissues and the interaction of that individual with the environment and the differential metabolic energy needs of different tissues within the one individual.

Clinical consequences of mitochondrial disorders

More than 100 disease-associated point mutations of mitochondrial DNA have been identified [8]. The exact number of identified mitochondrial DNA deletions and nuclear DNA mutations, however, remains unclear. These mutations may impair the respiratory chain or any other mitochondrial processes through effects on: respiratory chain complex structure, assembly proteins, mitochondrial membranes, mitochondrial division or intramitochondrial metabolism of lipids, cholesterol, amino acids, the urea cycle, or apoptosis. Whereas the type of tissues most commonly affected are well known, the exact mechanisms through which mutations lead to the spectrum of clinical symptoms in any one individual remain unclear.

Disorders due to mutations in the nuclear genome tend to have a more consistent clinical pattern and to present at a younger age compared to mitochondrial genome disorder. A number of these disorders such as Leigh Syndrome, infantile myoclonic epilepsy, mitochondrial neurogastrointestinal encephalomyopathy and Coenzyme Q10 deficiency are associated with mental retardation, seizures, and either white-matter disease or basal ganglia disease. The relatively early involvement of the central nervous system, the occurrence of seizures, and mental retardation usually lead to a diagnosis in childhood.

Disorders related to mutations in the mitochondrial genome on the other hand often present in early adulthood and can vary significantly in their clinical phenotype due to heteroplasmy, differential tissue distribution, and potentially greater environmental interaction [9]. It is this latter group that is of greatest relevance to the current discussion given schizophrenia often begins in early adulthood after relatively normal development, can present in a variety of ways even within the same family, and displays clinical variation during the course of illness. The "consistent" inconsistency of mitochondrial genomic disorders at a genetic and clinical level mirrors what schizophrenia clinicians and researchers have long observed, that is, that the presentations and course of illness is consistently inconsistent. In this regard, schizophrenia shares some of the characteristics of mitochondrial disorders:

1. Strong genetic heritability
2. Siblings and twins show a wide variability in expression of disease
3. Within the one individual there will be variability in the clinical picture over time
4. Expression of illness is influenced by environmental factors

Several lines of investigation point to potential mitochondrial involvement in patients with schizophrenia. A higher rate of maternal transmission has been identified in patients with schizophrenia[10, 11]. Altered mitochondrial gene expression [12, 13] and reduced mitochondrial numbers [14] have been identified in postmortem studies of brains from patients with schizophrenia. In a postmortem study, Cavelier and colleagues [13] identified a 63% reduction in cytochrome-c oxidase activity in the caudate nucleus and a 43% reduction of COX in the frontal gyrus compared to control subjects. Patients with Alzheimer's Disease did not exhibit these changes. Martorell and colleagues [15] investigated 6 mother–child schizophrenia pairs and compared their mitochondrial genome to 97 control subjects. They identified previously unreported mis-sense variants in mother–child pairs that were not seen in the normal controls. Two of these mis-sense variants had been previously identified in patients with bipolar disorder. The authors propose these variants that encode Complex 1 subunits are associated with psychotic disorders. In contrast to these findings suggestive of mitochondrial abnormalities in schizophrenia, a study of 300 patients found no one to have the mitochondrial mutation that is most common in MELAS (discussed later) [16].

To further examine the relationship between mitochondrial disorders and schizophrenia, a review of cases of schizophrenia in patients with documented mitochondrial disorders is warranted. A discussion

Table 17.1 Clinical features of mitochondrial disorders

Exercise intolerance
Short stature
Ptsosis with progressive ophthalmoplegia
Sensorineural hearing loss
Pigmented retinopathy
Optic atrophy
Seizures
Basal ganglia lesions
Diabetes
Cardiac conduction abnormalities
Cardiomyopathy

of the major features of the mitochondrial disorders will be followed by a review of cases that have been reported in association with a psychotic illness or schizophrenia.

Mitochondrial disorders due to mitochondrial genome mutations

Diseases caused by mitochondrial oxidative phosphorylation are the commonest inborn errors of metabolism accounting for 1 in 5,000 live births [17]. For the reasons outlined above, there is no clear genotype–phenotype relationship, especially for the mitochondrial genome disorders. The patterns of clinical presentation will vary significantly with regard to age of onset, the temporal order of symptoms and conditions, and the prognosis of the disorders. Clinical features common to mitochondrial disorders are summarized in Table 17.1. The majority of these clinical feature disorders have been described in patients with each of the named mitochondrial syndromes described below. Only those clinical features considered to be typical of the various syndromes will be discussed, although "overlap" syndromes have also been described.

Mitochondrial encephalomyopathy, lactic acidosis, stroke-like episodes syndrome

Mitochondrial encephalomyopathy, lactic acidosis, stroke-like episodes syndrome (MELAS) is the commonest of the mitochondrial disorders and will usually first present before early adulthood after a period of normal development. An A to G substitution at nucleotide 3243 of tRNA leucine (A3243G tRNA$^{Leu(UUR)}$) is one of the commonest disorders and accounts for about 80% of MELAS cases [8]. A further 10% of mutations are in other parts of this same gene, the remaining 10% of mutations occur in 6 other mitochondrial genes [5, 7]. Stroke-like episodes are the hallmark of MELAS and lead to hemiparesis, hemianopia, and cortical blindness. Vomiting and migraine-like headaches are often associated clinical symptoms [5]. Lactic acid level is elevated and has been correlated with the level of neurological symptoms [18]. The course of the disorder is highly variable, ranging from single stroke-like episodes through to combinations of the conditions outlined in Table 17.1, although optic atrophy and retinopathy are relatively rare in MELAS. The diagnosis is based on the clinical syndrome, muscle biopsy showing ragged red fibers, and elevated serum lactic acid levels. Ragged red fibers represent muscle fibers with mitochondrial proliferation, presumably a response to mitochondrial failure, treated with a particular stain.

The stroke-like episodes result in lesions that do not conform to vascular territories and are found in tempero-parieto-occipital regions, basal ganglia, brainstem, and cerebellum. MRI will show stroke-like lesions in these regions involving grey and white matter [7]. The etiology of these lesions remains unclear with the two main hypotheses being that the lesions represent the end result of either vascular damage "mitochondrial angiopathy" or cellular damage "mitochondrial cytopathy." A recent model proposes that mitochondrial dysfunction in endothelial cells or neurons leads to neuronal excitability, which triggers a cascade of epileptic activity, angiopathic capillary failure, and neuronal loss [19]. There is currently no available treatment for MELAS although antioxidants, respiratory chain substrates, and cofactors have been trialed with varying results [20].

Myoclonic epilepsy with ragged red fibers

Myoclonic epilepsy with ragged red fibers (MERRF) is most commonly caused by a A8344G tRNA^{lys} mutation and usually presents before middle adulthood. Typically, the disorder begins with photosensitive myoclonic seizures and is associated with limb-girdle weakness, dementia, and cerebellar ataxia. Muscle biopsy reveals ragged red fibers and the EEG is usu-

ally abnormal. There is no specific treatment, although appropriate management of the epilepsy is crucial.

Kearns-Sayre Syndrome

Kearns-Sayre Syndrome (KSS) is a sporadic single mutation disorder characterized by a relatively well-recognized triad of progressive external ophthalmoplegia, pigmentary retinopathy, plus one of: heart block, cerebellar ataxia, or elevated cerebrospinal fluid (CSF) protein. Muscle biopsy reveals ragged red fibers and serum lactate is often elevated. MRI will often show diffuse central white-matter abnormalities and basal ganglia calcification [7].

Other mitochondrial disorders

Maternally inherited Leigh syndrome (MILS) is an infantile encephalomyopathy with seizures, dystonia, heart block, and optic atrophy. Leber hereditary optic neuropathy (LHON) is a maternally inherited cause of bilateral visual neuropathy in young adults. Although usually confined to the optic nerve, it has been described together with white-matter pathology [21]. "Overlap syndromes" have been described that include features typical of MELAS plus one of the other syndromes, for example, LHON/MELAS, MELAS/MERRF, or Leigh/MELAS [17].

Mitochondrial disorders and schizophrenia-like psychosis

Mitochondrial disorders are rare and the clinical literature relies largely on case reports or case series. Psychiatric symptoms are usually embedded within a panoply of other somatic symptoms so that case reports focused on psychiatric symptoms are relatively rare and specific reports regarding psychosis or schizophrenia are even less common [22]. A literature review for "mitochondria or mitochondrial disorders" and "schizophrenia or psychosis" was used as the starting base for a search of cases. Further cases were identified through the reference lists of identified articles. Case reports were included if there was a confirmed diagnosis of a mitochondrial disorder by muscle biopsy or genetic mutation analysis and if there was sufficient information regarding the psychiatric history. Fifteen reports and two case series were selected and grouped into one of five categories:

1. Mitochondrial disease with a psychotic illness suggestive of schizophrenia (10 cases)

2. Mitochondrial disorders with psychiatric symptoms that were related to a delirium or dementia (3 cases)
3. Mitochondrial disorders with a strong family history of schizophrenia (2 cases)
4. Wolfram Disease (case series)
5. Other (review series)

Mitochondrial disease with a psychotic illness suggestive of schizophrenia

1. Mizukami and colleagues have described a patient with MELAS in three separate case reports at different stages of the man's illness [23, 24, 25]. The final report describes the postmortem findings in this man. He had presented at age 19 with generalized muscle atrophy and abdominal pain. He developed a medication-responsive schizophrenic illness, characterized by auditory hallucinations, persecutory delusions, and disorganized behavior with relapses at the ages of 28 and 30. He subsequently developed a progressive dementia. At age 35, he had a 3-week period of akinetic mutism and myoclonus. During this period, he was found to have sensorineural hearing loss, hypertrophic cardiomyopathy, and seizures. Over the next 3 years, he displayed disinhibited behavior, transient ischemic attacks, progressive muscle atrophy, nephrotic syndrome, and paralytic ileus. He died of heart failure aged 38. Postmortem revealed widespread cortical infarct-like lesions, cerebral and cerebellar white-matter gliosis, demyelinating lesions, and posterior column and spinocerebellar tract degeneration. Electron microscopy revealed abnormal mitochondrial aggregates in smooth muscle cells and cerebral/cerebellar vascular endothelium. The authors postulated that the pathogenic basis of the lesions was consistent with a mitochondrial angiopathy.

2. Yamazaki and colleagues [26] (English abstract only available) reported on a 37-year-old man with an 8-year history of schizophrenic psychosis and dementia who developed neuroleptic malignant syndrome on haloperidol. Physical examination revealed muscle atrophy and weakness. Muscle biopsy showed ragged red fibers and focal cytochrome-c oxidase deficiency. MELAS was diagnosed and he was started on Coenzyme Q and idebenone (free radical scavenger drug), which improved his psychiatric state. His schizophrenic symptoms disappeared several months later.

3. A novel mutation was identified in a 27-year-old man who initially presented with psychotic symptoms, depression, and suicidal ideas [27]. He was noted to have bilateral deafness and cerebellar signs. MRI revealed cerebral/cerebellar atrophy and T2 hyperintensities of the left basal ganglia. By age 33, he was blind, had severe muscle weakness, ataxia, and cognitive deficits. MRI abnormalities had progressed and now included periventricular white-matter changes. Muscle biopsy revealed ragged red fibers and mutational analysis identified a novel heteroplasmic A3274G tRNA$^{Leu(UUR)}$ mutation. The mutation was not identified in any tested maternal family members.

4. Amemiya [28] describes a man with no family history of neurological disease diagnosed with a point mutation C3256T tRNA$^{Leu(UUR)}$ gene after presenting at age 36 with muscle atrophy and weakness. Prior to this, he had had a 7-year history of episodic psychiatric symptoms such as "delusions and confusion." The patient continued to have episodic psychiatric symptoms, exhibited a progressive dementia, myoclonus, ataxia, seizures, ophthalmoplegia, and paralytic ileus. Interestingly, the muscle weakness did not progress at the same rate as the central nervous system (CNS) symptoms and the authors noted a decline in the proportion of mitochondrial mutation in two muscle biopsies taken at the ages of 36 and 45. The patient died of heart failure aged 46. The authors speculate that the proportion of mutated mitochondria within a tissue type will influence the severity of illness in that tissue and highlight the different rates of illness progression in different tissue types within the one individual.

5. Inagaki [29] describes a 37-year-old man of short stature and poor school performance who was diagnosed with sensorineural hearing loss at 29, Wolff-Parkinson-White syndrome, and diabetes at 31 years of age. At around this time, he developed auditory hallucinations and persecutory delusions, which resolved within a week of treatment with haloperidol. Four years later, in the context of behavioral disturbance, he was further investigated and a point mutation was identified

at A3243G tRNA$^{Leu(UUR)}$. There was no evidence of muscle atrophy or weakness. A muscle biopsy, electromyography, and MRI scan were all normal. The clinical course progressively deteriorated with affective blunting, personality change, disinhibition, and abulia. He was admitted and treated with idebenone with good effect on behavior and affect. The authors describe this as a case of maternally inherited diabetes and deafness as opposed to MELAS, given the lack of strokes or myopathy. Both clinical syndromes, however, arise from the same point mutation.

6. Prayson and colleagues present a 47-year-old woman with MELAS who had presented with a seizure on the background of a 20-year history of schizophrenia, migraine, deafness, and a temporal lobe infarct [30]. Investigations revealed bilateral basal ganglia calcification, a left temporal infarct, and an EEG was reported to show evidence for a diffuse encephalopathy. The patient died 3 months later of septicemia. The postmortem muscle biopsy identified ragged red fibers and a partial cytochrome-c oxidase deficiency. The mutational screen identified a A3243G tRNA$^{Leu(UUR)}$ mutation.

7. Spellberg reports on a 36-year-old man [31] with a 15-year history of psychosis, seizures, and sensorineural hearing loss who had been referred for diagnostic clarification. The patient's mother and her twin brother both had a history of deafness, diabetes, and seizure. This maternal uncle also had a psychiatric history. The patient was found to have abnormal gait and muscle weakness. Genetic analysis revealed A3243G tRNA$^{Leu(UUR)}$ mutation and a diagnosis of MELAS was made.

8. Saijo [32] reports on a man diagnosed with MELAS who had first presented with seizures, paralytic ileus, and muscle atrophy aged 10. At the age of 19, the patient developed psychosis with auditory and visual hallucinations in association with high CSF and blood lactic acid levels. He was treated with sodium dichloroacetate and the hallucinations improved with normalization of the lactic acid levels.

9. Thomeer [33] reports on a patient with no personal or family history of neurological or psychiatric disease who was assessed at age 14 for short stature, with no abnormalities identified. At the age of 18, she had two stroke-like episodes involving the left tempero-parietal and right tempero-occipital regions within several months of each other and developed focal epileptic seizures. She was also diagnosed with Wolff-Parkinson White Syndrome and retrocochlear deafness. No definitive diagnosis was made at this time. At age 22, she developed paranoid delusions, affective instability, and disinhibition, which were treated over the ensuing years with antipsychotic medication. She was also found to exhibit progressive aphasia and apraxia. The diagnosis of MELAS was made at the age of 27 on the basis of the clinical history, ragged red fibers on muscle biopsy, and the identification of a A3243G tRNA$^{Leu(UUR)}$ point mutation. The patient's subsequent course was marked by ongoing psychiatric symptoms of psychosis, delusions of reference and influence, auditory hallucinations, and suicidal ideation. She required secure inpatient care due to the severity of her psychiatric illness. She died at 31 of putative heart failure. The authors comment on the presentation of this patient with a chronic schizophrenia-like illness and the possible contribution of the temporal lobe pathology and the focal seizures.

10. Odawara [34] reported a patient with MELAS who had first presented with diabetes, deafness, and muscle atrophy at 21. She developed schizophrenia at age 23 and her cognitive state declined over the ensuing years. The patient had a family history in her mother and maternal uncle. The diagnosis of MELAS was not made until the patient was 52 years old.

Although the above ten cases provide variable information regarding the psychiatric symptoms, there is a consistent theme of the onset of psychotic symptoms (with or without features of mitochondrial disorder) prior to the age of 31. Seven of the ten cases had a diagnosis of MELAS whereas in the other three cases there was no evidence of stroke-like episodes. The mean age of the patients at the time of onset of their psychotic disorder was 24.7 and the mean delay in years between the onset of psychosis and the confirmation of a mitochondrial disorder was 12.6 years. Despite the presence of physical symptoms that, in retrospect, were features of the mitochondrial disorder, there was a mean delay of 14.0 years from the first physical symptoms (mean age 23.3) until the diagnosis. In three cases (case 4/8/9), there was a large difference between the age of psychosis onset (29/19/22) and the first physical manifestation of the disorder (36/10/14). In all other cases, the psychiatric and physical presentations occurred within a year's period. Interestingly, the one patient in whom the psychosis preceded physical symptoms by many years exhibited a novel C3256T tRNA$^{Leu(UUR)}$ mutation and the authors speculated on the different temporal progression of the patient's symptoms as a reflection of differential mutation loads in different brain regions. Seven of the remaining 8 patients with an identified mutation possessed the A3243G tRNA$^{Leu(UUR)}$ point mutation.

Mitochondrial disorders with psychiatric symptoms that were related to a delirium or dementia

11. Kaido [35] describes a 53-year-old Japanese lady whose index presentation was with vomiting, anuresis, and clouded conscious state on a background of 6 months of apathy. She had two daughters with known diagnoses of MELAS. All three exhibited the A3243G tRNA$^{Leu(UUR)}$ point mutation. The patient's mother had been short but otherwise no medical history was provided. Medical management improved her medical condition but she developed a "psychosis" (shouting loudly, fearful hallucinations, and neuroleptic treatment) and died 4 months later. This is more likely to have been a delirium rather than a psychotic illness.

12. A 58-year-old woman [36] presented with cardiomyopathy and muscle weakness, initially in the upper limbs and rapidly progressing to the lower limbs. There was no family history of note. During the admission, she developed psychotic symptoms in the form of paranoia, agitation, and hallucinations and was found to have widespread cognitive deficits across memory, language, and executive functioning. MRI revealed deep white-matter hyperintensities in a watershed distribution and bilateral cerebellar white matter. These abnormalities had not been present on an earlier MRI scan. A diagnosis of MELAS was confirmed on muscle biopsy and an A3243G tRNA$^{Leu(UUR)}$ mutation was identified. The authors comment on this case as displaying unusually prominent deep white-matter involvement in patients with MELAS.

13. The role of coenzyme Q in improving psychiatric symptoms was also noted by Shinkai and colleagues who described a 48-year-old woman who presented with stroke-like episodes, followed by behavioral change, cognitive deterioration, and paranoid ideation over the course of several months. The patient had been diagnosed with diabetes at age 40 and hearing loss at age 30. There were no symptoms or signs of muscle weakness or atrophy. MRI revealed bilateral tempero-parietal T1 hyperintensities and bilateral caudate calcification. CSF lactic acid levels were increased. Her father, mother, and younger sister also had hearing loss. A point mutation was identified at A3243G tRNA$^{Leu(UUR)}$. The woman was treated with Coenzyme Q and no antipsychotic medications with improvement in her psychotic symptoms and reduction of elevated CSF lactic acid levels.

These cases occurred in older adults who had been previously well. The psychotic presentations occurred in the presence of what is likely to have been pronounced neurodegenerative disorder and are unlikely to have been symptoms characteristic of schizophrenia.

Mitochondrial disorders with a family history of schizophrenia

14. Campos and colleagues [37] report on a Spanish family with the mtDNA tRNALeu$^{(UUR)}$ 3303 > T mutation. The index case was a 6-year-old girl who presented with cardiomyopathy and myopathy. Muscle biopsy confirmed the presence of ragged red fibers and revealed defects in respiratory chain complexes I and IV. Investigation of the family identified that her mother, a maternal aunt, maternal grandmother, maternal great grandmother, and a maternal great-uncle had all suffered with psychiatric illness from early adult life. The features of the psychoses are not described for all family members but were very similar to those noted in the mother and maternal aunt. These included recurrent depressive episodes (mother), recurrent

manic-depressive episodes (maternal aunt), and psychotic episodes (mother and maternal aunt) since adolescence. It was known that the maternal grandmother had died of unknown cause aged 68 and the maternal great grandmother had died of early dementia aged 60. None of the maternal relatives of the index case had been known to have cardiac or muscle disease. Mutation analyses identified 95% mutant molecules in the proband's muscle and 75% mutant molecules in her blood cells. The maternal and maternal aunt's blood cells contained 25% and 20% mutant molecules, respectively.

15. Ueda [38] identified a 12-year-old boy with asymptomatic proteinuria who was found to carry a point mutation in the tRNALeu$^{(UUR)}$ gene renal, but not muscle tissue. The boy was otherwise healthy. The boy's mother had depression and epilepsy, two maternal aunts had schizophrenia or amyotrophic lateral sclerosis, and a maternal grandmother had diabetes. The family members did not consent to mutation analyses. There was no history of cardiac disease or myopathy in the family.

Wolfram Disease

Wolfram Disease is an autosomal recessive disorder caused by a mutation in the WFDS1 (wolframin) gene on the short arm of chromosome 4 [39, 40]. WFDS1 gene codes for a transmembrane protein found in the endoplasmic reticulum, whose function remains unclear. Wolfram disorder is also known as DID-MOAD, an acronym for the characteristic conditions that comprise the disease (Diabetes Insipidus, Diabetes Mellitus, Optic Atrophy, Deafness). The disease has been associated with multiple mitochondrial deletions in some but not all families with the disease [41]. A study of 68 homozygous patients revealed very high rates of psychiatric illness [42]. Forty-one of the 68 patients had had psychiatric symptoms and 17 (25%) were classified as showing severe mental illness. Eleven (16%) patients had a history of psychotic symptoms. Further assessment of heterozygous family members revealed a high rate of psychiatric illness, approximately eight times greater than for noncarriers of the Wolframin gene. The high rate of schizophrenia-like psychosis in this disorder is similar to that seen in some other adult-onset neurological disorders such as velocardiofacial syndrome, metachromatic leukodys-trophy, and Niemann-Pick Disease type C, each of which show rates of psychosis in the 25% range [43].

Other cases

Fattal [22] has recently reviewed the relationship between mitochondrial disorders and a broad range of psychiatric disorders. This review identified 19 case reports of psychiatric disorder in patients with mitochondrial disorders, nine of which had a psychotic illness. These cases overlapped with seven of the cases presented above (Cases 3–5, 7–10). The authors emphasize the importance of "red flag" physical signs such as muscle weakness and hearing loss in patients with atypical psychiatric presentations. The presence of seizures, short stature, diabetes, Wolff-Parkinson-White Syndrome, or migraines should alert clinicians to the possibility of mitochondrial disorders in their patients.

Conclusions

In the absence of evidence regarding the number of patients with mitochondrial disorders who do not have schizophrenia, it is problematic to draw causal conclusions from a case report literature regarding the relationship between these disorders – one exceedingly rare and the other uncommon. The case report approach provides important information for clinicians who care for patients with mitochondrial disorders and those who care for patients with schizophrenia. There are also some potential clues for schizophrenia researchers.

From a clinical perspective, a survey of patients with chronic schizophrenia would quickly detect a wide range of medical comorbidities. It is well established that the prevalence of diabetes, heart disease, cardiac arrhythmias, and poor exercise tolerance is higher in patients with schizophrenia than the general population [44]. As pointed out by Fattal [22], these case reports alert the clinician to the possibility that his/her patient with a well-defined schizophrenic illness or a schizophrenia-like psychosis, diabetes, and cardiac disease, who has a stroke, an unexplained seizure, or deafness, may have an undiagnosed mitochondrial disorder. The diagnosis will carry important implications for the patient's management and treatment and highlights the importance of a clinical understanding of the "secondary schizophrenias." A good understanding of disorders that cause schizophrenia-like psychosis allow for the recognition

Table 17.2 Mitochondrial disorders with psychotic symptoms: discrepancy between ages of onset of physical and psychotic symptoms and diagnosis

Case no.	Author	Mutation	Onset (years)			Delay between onset and diagnosis	
			Physical	Psychosis	Diagnosis	Psychosis	Physical
1	Mizukami [23]	A3243G tRNALeu(UUR)	19	19	35	16	16
2	Yamazaki [26]	N/A	29	29	37	8	8
3	Jaksch [27]	A3274G tRNALeu(UUR)	27	27	33	6	6
4	Amemiya [28]	C3256T tRNALeu(UUR)	36	29	36	7	0
5	Inagakai [29]	A3243G tRNALeu(UUR)	29	31	35	4	6
6	Prayson [30]	A3243G tRNALeu(UUR)	27	27	47	20	20
7	Spellberg [31]	A3243G tRNALeu(UUR)	21	21	36	15	15
8	Saijo [32]	n/a	10	19	35	16	25
9	Thomeer [33]	A3243G tRNALeu(UUR)	14	22	27	5	13
10	Odawara [34]	n/a	21	23	52	29	31
	Mean (yrs)		**23.3**	**24.7**	**37.3**	**12.6**	**14.0**

of core symptoms or signs that fall outside those that are usually associated with schizophrenia and that represent either an unassociated separate illness or a marker of a single underlying illness causing both psychotic and other physical symptoms. The apparently high prevalence of psychiatric disorders in patients with mitochondrial disorders similarly alerts these patients' physicians to the need to be aware of psychiatric symptoms and to appropriately manage them as they may be significantly disabling for patients and families – and may also confer significant risk. Psychoses will generally respond to antipsychotic treatment regardless of the etiology of the symptoms.

The observation that schizophrenia-like psychoses occur early in the course of subsequently identified neurodegenerative disorders is well recognized and may provide important information regarding the brain's response to insult, whether metabolic, infectious, or neurodegenerative, at different stages of its development (Chapter 16). Neurological disorders, particularly storage disorders such as the leukodystrophies, that present in late adolescence and early adulthood tend to present with major psychiatric disorders such as schizophrenia, mania, or major depression. The wide range of pathoplastic effects of these disorders and affected regions suggests that the underlying developmental maturity of the CNS (and the neurodevelopmental trajectories that are interrupted by illness)

may be more important than the pathology of the illness itself in predicting major mental illness. Furthermore, the subtle illness effects seen in neuropathological and neuroimaging studies in schizophrenia would predict that schizophrenia-like psychosis would occur early rather than late in a developing neurodegenerative disorder and be later supervened by more gross clinical syndromes (such as seizures, dementia, and movement disorder) as the illness load on the CNS progresses. As seen in Table 17.2, in the mitochondrial disorders associated with schizophrenia-like psychosis, a psychotic illness is often the harbinger of later physical and neurological illness, often by more than a decade.

The role of oxidative stress in schizophrenia has been the subject of several reviews, research studies, and the basis for treatment of schizophrenia with antioxidants [45]. Failure of the mitochondrial OXPHOS system allows the build up of intracellular reactive oxygen species, which can then trigger cell necrosis and apoptosis. Recent therapeutic efforts in neurodegenerative disorders such as Alzheimer's Disease have been targeted at the development of mitochondrially active antioxidants [46]. A disturbance of mitochondrial function could account for some of the most puzzling features of schizophrenia such as the nature of its heredity, the phenotypic variation of illness within individuals over time and between family members, the high prevalence of medical comorbidities, and the potential therapeutic role of antioxidants. The findings of mitochondrial disturbance in some schizophrenia sufferers and of an elevated rate of psychosis in mitochondrial disorders, in the absence of clear evidence from linkage studies that mitochondrial genes are affected in schizophrenia pedigrees, raises the possibility that mitochondrial function may act as an additional diathesis to the development of psychosis in individuals who carry other biological vulnerabilities for psychosis, such as environmental insult or schizophrenia vulnerability genes. An interaction of this nature may also explain the elevated rates of psychosis in some mitochondrial disorders, with those individuals developing schizophrenia-like psychosis possibly being those who carry other psychotogenic diatheses.

References

1. Schon E. A. (2003). The mitochondrial genome. In *The Molecular and Genetic Basis of Neurologic and Psychiatric Disease*, Rosenberg R. N., Prusiner S. B. and DiMauro S., *et al.* (Eds.). Philadelphia: Butterworth Heinemann.

2. Chinnery P. F., Schon E. A. Mitochondria. *J Neurol Neurosurg Psychiatry*, 2003. **74**:1188–99.

3. Giles R. E., Blanc H., Cann H. M., *et al.* Maternal inheritance of human mitochondrial-DNA. *Proc Natl Acad Sci USA*, 1980. **77**(11): 6715–19.

4. Sutovsky P., Moreno, R. D., Ramalho-Santos J., *et al.* Development – Ubiquitin tag for sperm mitochondria. *Nature*, 1999. **402**(6760):371–2.

5. Finsterer J. Central nervous system manifestations of mitochondrial disorders. *Acta Neurol Scand*, 2006. **114**: 217–38.

6. Chinnery P. E., Howell N., Lightowlers R. N., *et al.* MELAS and MERRF – The relationship between maternal mutation load and the frequency of clinically affected offspring. *Brain*, 1998. **121**:1889–94.

7. DiMauro S. E. B. (2003). Mitochondrial disorders due to mutations in the mitochondrial genome. In *The Molecular and Genetic Basis of Neurologic and Psychiatric Disease*, Rosenberg R. N., Prusiner S. B., and DiMauro S., *et al.* (Eds.). Philadelphia: Butterworth Heinemann.

8. Servidei S. Mitochondrial encephalomyopathies:gene mutation. *Neuromusc Disord: NMD*, 2002. **12**(5):524.

9. Hirano M. (2003). Mitochondrial disorders due to mutations in the nuclear genome. In *The Molecular and Genetic Basis of Neurologic and Psychiatric Disease*, Rosenberg R. N., Prusiner S. B., and DiMauro S., *et al.* (Eds.). Philadelphia: Butterworth Heinemann.

10. Goldstein J. M., Faraone S. V., Chen W. J., *et al.* Sex differences in the familial transmission of schizophrenia. *Br J Psychiatry*, 1990. **156**:819–26.

11. Shimizu A., Kurachi M., Yamaguchi N., *et al.* Morbidity risk of schizophrenia to parents and siblings of schizophrenic patients. *Jap J Psychiatr Neurol*, 1987. **41**(1):65–70.

12. Whatley S. A., Curti D., Marchbanks R. M. Mitochondrial involvement in schizophrenia and other functional psychoses. *Neurochem Res*, 1996. **21**(9): 995–1004.

13. Cavelier L., Jazin E. E., Eriksson I., *et al.* Decreased cytochrome-c oxidase activity and lack of age-related accumulation of mitochondrial DNA deletions in the brains of schizophrenics. *Genomics*, 1995. **29**(1):217–24.

14. King L., Roberts R. C. Mitochondrial pathology in human schizophrenic striatum: a postmortem ultrastructural study. *Synapse*, 1999. **31**(1):67–75.

15. Martorell L., Segues T., Folch G., *et al.* New variants in the mitochondrial genomes of schizophrenic patients. *Eur J Hum Genet*, 2006. **14**(5):520–8.

16. Odawara M., Arinami T., Tachi Y., *et al.* Absence of association between a mitochondrial DNA mutation at nucleotide position 3243 and schizophrenia in Japanese. *Hum Genet*, 1998. **102**(6):708–9.

17. Janssen R., Nijtmans L. G., Van Den Heuvel L. P., *et al.* Mitochondrial complex I: structure, function and pathology. *J Inherit Metab Dis*, 2006. **29**(4): 499–515.

18. Abe K. Cerebral lactic acidosis correlates with neurological impairment in MELAS. *Neurology*, 2004. **63**(12):2458.

19. Iizuka T., Sakai F. Pathogenesis of stroke-like episodes in MELAS: analysis of neurovascular cellular mechanisms. *Curr Neurovasc Res*, 2005. **2**(1):29–45.

20. Scaglia F., Northrop J. L. The mitochondrial myopathy encephalopathy, lactic acidosis with stroke-like episodes (MELAS) syndrome – a review of treatment options. *CNS Drugs*, 2006. **20**(6):443–64.

21. Kovacs G. G., Hoftberger R., Majtenyi K., *et al.* Neuropathology of white matter disease in Leber's hereditary optic neuropathy. *Brain*, 2005. **128**(Pt 1):35–41.

22. Fattal O., Budur K., Vaughan A. J., *et al.* Review of the literature on major mental disorders in adult patients with mitochondrial diseases. *Psychosomatics*, 2006. **47**(1):1–7.

23. Mizukami K., Sasaki M., Suzuki T., *et al.* Central nervous system changes in mitochondrial encephalomyopathy: light and electron microscopic study. *Acta Neuropathol (Berl)*, 1992. **83**(4):449–52.

24. Suzuki T., Koizumi J., Shiraishi H., *et al.* Psychiatric disturbance in mitochondrial encephalomyopathy. *J Neurol Neurosurg Psychiatry*, 1989. **52**(7):920–2.

25. Suzuki Y., Taniyama M., Muramatsu T., *et al.* Diabetes mellitus associated with 3243 mitochondrial tRNA(Leu(UUR)) mutation: clinical features and coenzyme Q10 treatment. *Mol Aspects Med*, 1997. **18** (Suppl): S181–8.

26. Yamazaki M., Igarashi H., Hamamoto M., *et al.* A case of mitochondrial encephalomyopathy with schizophrenic psychosis, dementia and neuroleptic malignant syndrome. *Rinsho Shinkeigaku*, 1991. **31**(11): 1219–23.

27. Jaksch M., Lochmuller H., Schmitt F., *et al.* A mutation in mt tRNALeu(UUR) causing a neuropsychiatric syndrome with depression and cataract. *Neurology*, 2001. **57**(10): 1930.

28. Amemiya S., Hamamoto M., Goto Y., *et al.* Psychosis and progressing dementia: presenting features of a mitochondriopathy. *Neurology*, 2000. **55**(4):600–1.

29. Inagaki T., Ishino H., Seno H., *et al.* Psychiatric symptoms in a patient with diabetes mellitus associated with point mutation in mitochondrial DNA. *Biol Psychiatry*, 1997. **42**(11):1067–9.

30. Prayson R. A., Wang N. Mitochondrial myopathy, encephalopathy, lactic acidosis, and strokelike episodes (MELAS) syndrome: an autopsy report. *Arch Pathol Lab Med*, 1998. **122**(11):978–81.

31. Spellberg B., Carroll R. M., Robinson E., *et al.* mtDNA disease in the primary care setting. *Arch Intern Med*, 2001. **161**(20): 2497–500.

32. Saijo T, Naito E, Ito M, *et al.* Therapeutic effect of sodium dichloroacetate on visual and auditory hallucinations in a patient with MELAS. *Neuropediatrics*, 1991. **22**(3):166–7.

33. Thomeer E. C., Verhoeven W. M. A., Van De Vlasakker C. J. W., *et al.* Psychiatric symptoms in MELAS; a case report. *J Neurol Neurosurg Psychiatry*, 1998. **64**(5):692–3.

34. Odawara M., Isaka M., Tada K., *et al.* Diabetes mellitus associated with mitochondrial myopathy and schizophrenia: a possible link between diabetes mellitus and schizophrenia. *Diabet Med*, 1997. **14**(6):503.

35. Kaido M., Fujimura H., Soga F., *et al.* Alzheimer-type pathology in a patient with mitochondrial myopathy, encephalopathy, lactic acidosis and stroke-like episodes (MELAS). *Acta Neuropathol (Berl)*, 1996. **92**(3):312–8.

36. Apostolova L. G., White M., Moore S. A., *et al.* Deep white matter pathologic features in watershed regions: a novel pattern of central nervous system involvement in MELAS. *Arch Neurol*, 2005. **62**(7): 1154–6.

37. Campos Y., Garcia A., Eiris J., *et al.* Mitochondrial myopathy, cardiomyopathy and psychiatric illness in a Spanish family harbouring the mtDNA 3303C > T mutation. *J Inherit Metab Dis*, 2001. **24**(6):685–7.

38. Ueda Y., Ando A., Nagata T., *et al.* A boy with mitochondrial disease: asymptomatic proteinuria without neuromyopathy. *Pediatr Nephrol*, 2004. **19**(1):107–10.

39. Polymeropoulos M. H., Swift R. G., Swift M. Linkage of the gene for Wolfram syndrome to markers on the short arm of chromosome 4. *Nat Genet*, 1994. **8**(1):95–7.

40. Domenech E., Gomez-Zaera M., Nunes V. Wolfram/DIDMOAD syndrome, a heterogenic and molecularly complex neurodegenerative disease. *Pediatr Endocrinol Rev*, 2006. **3**(3):249–57.

41. Barrientos A., Volpini V., Casademont J., *et al.* A nuclear defect in the 4p16 region predisposes to multiple mitochondrial DNA deletions in families with Wolfram syndrome. *J Clin Invest*, 1996. **97**(7):1570–6.

42. Swift R. G., Perkins D. O., Chase C. L., *et al.* Psychiatric disorders in 36 families with Wolfram syndrome. *Am J Psychiatry*, 1991. **148**(6):775–9.

43. Shinkai T., Nakashima M., Ohmori O., *et al.* Coenzyme Q10 improves psychiatric symptoms in adult-onset mitochondrial myopathy, encephalopathy, lactic acidosis and stroke-like episodes: a case report. *Aust NZ J Psychiatry*, 2000. **34**:1034–5.

44. Lambert T. J., Velakoulis D., Pantelis C. Medical comorbidity in schizophrenia. *Med J Aust*, 2003. 178 Suppl:S67–70.

45. Fendri C., Mechri A., Khiari G., *et al.* Oxidative stress involvement in schizophrenia pathophysiology: a review. *Encephale*, 2006. **32**(2 Pt 1):244–52.

46. Szeto H. H. Mitochondria-targeted peptide antioxidants: novel neuroprotective agents. *AAPS J*, 2006. **8**(3):E521–31.

18

Psychosis associated with leukodystrophies

Patricia I. Rosebush, Rebecca Anglin, and Michael Mazurek

Facts box

- Inherited leukodystrophies are under recognized and under diagnosed in psychiatric populations.
- Psychiatric illness in patients with leukodystrophies may be indistinguishable from primary psychiatric disorders.
- Individuals with later-onset forms of inherited metabolic disorders are more likely to develop – and may present solely with – psychiatric illness.
- The diagnosis of an inherited leukodystrophy should be considered in patients with psychiatric illness and concurrent seizures or cognitive decline.
- Individuals with psychiatric illness and an underlying inherited metabolic disorder are often treatment resistant.
- Failure to diagnose an inherited metabolic disorder can impede treatment and have fatal consequences for certain patients.
- Use of psychotropic medications in patients with inherited metabolic disorders has the potential to worsen the underlying disease process and produce serious side effects.

Introduction

The term leukodystrophy refers to diseases of the white matter, which results in a functional "disconnection" between parts of the nervous system that communicate through the affected white-matter tracts. The clinical consequences of this "disconnection" depend on the localization of the white-matter pathology, whether it is in the brain, spinal cord, or brain stem. What are the principal clinical consequences of lesions that interrupt the white-matter bundles involved in cortico–

cortical interactions? In this case, one might expect the result to be a disturbance of mental function. In other words, a leukodystrophy that targets the white matter of the brain will tend to produce psychiatric symptomatology.

In this chapter, we review the major inherited leukodystrophies, with attention to the psychiatric manifestations associated with each. The age of onset and ensuing clinical course with most of these disorders reflect the severity of the underlying metabolic defects. Cases that begin in infancy or early childhood typically run an aggressive course, with a host of systemic and neurological problems that make it difficult to discern the associated psychiatric symptoms that might be present. Adult-onset cases, however, follow a more protracted clinical course, allowing the neuropsychiatric consequences of the white-matter pathology to become manifest. These adult cases, by potentially allowing phenotype–genotype and clinical–pathological correlations, offer insight into the pathology of psychiatric disease. It is on these adult-onset forms that we focus in this review.

Metachromatic leukodystrophy

Metachromatic leukodystrophy (MLD) is an autosomal recessive disorder associated with a deficiency of the lysosomal enzyme, aryl sulfatase A (ASA). MLD has traditionally been classified into subtypes, according to age of onset and severity of clinical progression [1]. As is the case with many inherited metabolic disorders, the early-onset cases tend to be associated with an aggressive course of illness and early death. The late-onset form, however, follows a more protracted clinical course and is often associated with neuropsychiatric symptomatology. Indeed, it has been suggested that late-onset MLD might serve as a window on the underlying pathobiology of schizophrenia [2, 3].

241

Genetics and pathobiology

The gene responsible for MLD has been localized to the long arm of chromosome 22 and a range of mutations has been identified. Some encode inactive ASA (the so-called "O-alleles") and others encode ASA with residual enzyme activity ("R-alleles"). In general, the O-alleles are associated with the severe early-onset forms of MLD, whereas the R-alleles tend to produce the less aggressive late-onset cases [4].

In all subtypes of MLD, the ASA deficiency leads to impaired conversion of sulfatides to cerebrosides, resulting in sulfatide accumulation in tissues. The principal targets of this process are the myelinated axons of the central and peripheral nervous systems, the kidneys, and the gall bladder [1]. When stained with cresyl violet, the affected tissues turn brown, producing the "metachromatic" effect for which the disease is named.

The late-onset form of MLD is associated with two major phenotypic presentations: one in which the initial symptoms are related to sensorimotor problems and another that begins with neuropsychiatric disturbances. A recent study found that these phenotypic subtypes tend to be associated with specific genetic profiles [5]. Of particular interest is the observation that patients who are heterozygous for the I179S mutation almost invariably present with social and behavioral abnormalities that closely resemble those associated with schizophrenia.

Prevalence

Adult or late-onset MLD is estimated to affect 1 in 40,000 individuals [6, 7], although this is almost certainly an underestimation given that psychiatric disturbances [1, 2, 8, 9, 10] often occur before neurological features develop. Affected patients tend to be diagnosed according to traditional psychiatric categories and the later emergence of significant cognitive impairment or neurological features may be overlooked or misdiagnosed.

There has been no large-scale study of the prevalence of MLD in psychiatric populations and the results from smaller studies have been compromised by the failure to test for pseudodeficiency (PD) [11, 12]. In this state, clinically normal subjects have low ASA activity but not the genetic defect associated with MLD. PD can be identified through genetic analysis or by the *absence* of sulfatide excretion in the urine.

Clinical features and neuroimaging

A review of the English literature revealed 81 cases of late-onset MLD that provided some information about clinical findings [8, 13, 14, 15, 16, 17, 18, 19, 20, 21, 22, 23, 24, 25, 26, 27, 28, 29, 30, 31, 32, 33, 34, 35, 36, 37, 38, 39, 40, 41, 42, 43, 44, 45, 46, 47, 48, 49, 50, 51, 52, 53]. The clinical profile that emerges from these cases is described in this section.

Age of onset and course of illness

The approximate age of illness onset was 25.4 (SD = 11.04 years, range 10–62 years). Neurological symptoms typically presented 4.1 ± 7.0 years *after* the development of psychiatric symptomatology. In 23 cases that were followed until death, the duration of illness varied from 2 to 47 years with an average of 12.0 (SD = 11.8) years.

Psychiatric features

The prevalence of psychiatric illness in patients with adult-onset MLD is estimated to be high and psychosis has been reported in 53% of published cases, although the possible presence of PD was not addressed. Of the 81 cases we found in the English literature [8, 13, 14, 15, 16, 17, 18, 19, 20, 21, 22, 23, 24, 25, 26, 27, 28, 29, 30, 31, 32, 33, 34, 35, 36, 37, 38, 39, 40, 41, 42, 43, 44, 45, 46, 47, 48, 49, 50, 51, 52, 53], 65 (80%) experienced some form of psychiatric symptomatology, 29 (36%) developed psychosis, and 19 (23%) were diagnosed with schizophrenia. In many cases, the disinhibition, emotional lability, apathy, silliness, poor judgment, lack of insight, impulsivity, and perseveration were highly suggestive of a frontal lobe syndrome. It was difficult to discern the role of impaired cognition in the early presentation. Of note, 66% of adult-onset MLD patients eventually suffered cognitive decline, often resulting in profound dementia in the later stages of the illness.

Neurological features

Gait disturbance is the most common early neurological problem in late-onset MLD, followed by dysarthria, seizures, incontinence, and evidence of upper or lower motor neuron involvement. Cranial nerves are usually normal. Optic atrophy can occur and in the late stages, most patients are mute, blind, and unresponsive.

Neuroimaging

MRI reveals diffuse, symmetric, and confluent demyelination, which preferentially affects the frontal white matter and corpus callosum while sparing arcuate U fibers [54]. As the disease progresses, there is significant enlargement of the ventricles due to the extensive loss of white matter. Grey matter is typically only minimally affected and the brain stem and cerebellum are rarely involved. Advances in imaging technology such as diffusion tensor imaging (DTI) and tractography [55, 56] hold promise for more precisely delineating the disease process.

Investigations

Making the diagnosis

1. Determination of ASA activity can be carried out in leukocytes or cultured skin fibroblasts. A finding of low enzyme activity is not sufficient to confirm the diagnosis as low enzyme activity can also be found in the more common condition of PD.
2. Urine test for sulphatide excretion.
3. Genetic analysis for MLD gene mutations is specific and confirmatory for MLD.

Treatment

Currently, there is no treatment that will stop or slow the progression of MLD. Enzyme replacement therapy, although successful *in vitro*, was not successful in the two patients in whom it was attempted [57, 58, 59]. Despite transiently high levels of arylsulphatase activity in the liver in both cases, there were no comparable increases in the brain [58]. Bone marrow transplantation (BMT) has been carried out on several patients with generally poor results to date [60, 61, 62, 63]. The rationale for this approach is based on the presumption that enzymes, delivered by healthy cells to deficient cells, can be endocytosed and made available for processing the accumulated sulphatides. Additional treatments currently being studied include retroviral gene therapy [64], immunomodulation [65], and the use of thiol proteinase inhibitors to prevent the breakdown of available arylsulfatase [66].

Adrenoleukodystrophy

Adrenoleukodystrophy (ALD) is an X-linked disorder in which very-long-chain fatty acids (VLCFA), defined as those having greater than 22 carbon chains, accumulate as a result of defective beta-oxidation within the peroxisome [67, 68]. It classically afflicts young boys, leading to death before the age of 10. As with MLD, however, there are now recognized to be less severe forms of the illness, with onset in adolescence or even adulthood. It is these later or "adult-onset" forms of ALD that concern us here.

Genetics and pathobiology

The ALD gene has been mapped to the q28 region of the X chromosome. It codes for a protein that has been localized to the peroxisomal membrane [69, 70] and is a member of the ABC (adenosine triphospate binding cassette) transporter superfamily [71]. This transporter forms a "pathway" through which the enzyme VLCFA CoA synthetase moves from the cytosol into the intraperoxisomal membrane space [68, 70]. Mutations of the ALD gene alter the transporter, thereby impairing the ability of the peroxisome to catabolize VLCFAs. Three classes of tissue are preferentially targeted: (1) myelin-producing cells of the CNS and PNS leading to demyelination, (2) the adrenal cortex, resulting in adrenal insufficiency (Addison's Disease), and (3) the Leydig cells of the testes, producing hypogonadism.

This pattern of pathology can bring about psychiatric symptomatology in two ways. The first is through central demyelination, which disrupts or "disconnects" cortical circuits that subserve normal cognitive and emotional function. The second is through adrenal insufficiency, which can lead to impaired cerebral function and, in severe cases, produce outright psychosis, so-called "Addison's encephalopathy" [72].

Although ALD was long thought to affect only males, the discovery of X inactivation has focused attention on female "carriers." This process, by which one of the two X chromosomes becomes condensed and permanently inactive, occurs at random in the embryonic stage. If the defective allele is on the chromosome that has been inactivated, there will be no phenotypic manifestation of the disease. If, on the other hand, the defective allele is on the active X chromosome, the other having been inactivated, there can be clinical expression of the disorder [73]. As many as 20% to 50% of female heterozygotes have neurological signs and symptoms that resemble, and may be diagnosed as, multiple sclerosis [74, 75]. Only 3%, however, have cognitive decline and less than 1% of female carriers have evidence of adrenal insufficiency [74].

243

Prevalence

The incidence of ALD is unknown but an estimate of at least 1:17,000 has been cited [67, 76]. This figure would be most accurate for the severe infantile form, which is a rapidly progressive, fatal, neurodegenerative disease [77, 78, 79, 80] but is likely to be an underestimation for the milder, late-onset variants of adolescence and adulthood.

Psychiatric features

There is very little information on the incidence or prevalence of psychiatric symptomatology in patients with "adult-onset" ALD, and most published reports provide few details regarding patients' mental status. Of the 41 [81, 82, 83, 84, 85, 86, 87, 88, 89, 90, 91, 92, 93, 94, 95, 96, 97, 98, 99, 100, 101, 102, 103, 104, 105, 106, 107, 108, 109, 110, 111, 112, 113, 114] late-onset cases we identified in the English literature up to 2006, 24 (58%) were reported to have psychiatric features, and in 17 (Table 18.1) a detailed psychiatric assessment was provided. Behavioral disturbance or personality change was often the earliest reported finding. Features of mania were present in 9 (53%) of the 17 patients and 5 (30%) were psychotic. Many patients were treatment-resistant and appeared to have an aggressive course of illness. Eventual cognitive impairment was common.

Neurological features and endocrine abnormalities

Gait impairment was the most common initial neurological complaint in 91% of adult-onset cases followed by peripheral neuropathy (58%), visual impairment (21%), seizures (20%), and dysarthria (20%). Most patients developed upper motor neuron pathology, affecting the legs in particular. Twenty-five (60%) of the 41 cases had biochemical evidence of adrenal insufficiency. The average age at the time of diagnosis of Addison's Disease was 29 ± 6 years.

Neuroimaging

MRI scanning typically shows T2-weighted symmetrical hyperintensities involving the parieto-occipital regions. As the disease progresses, demyelination moves forward to involve the frontal lobes. Atypical findings include early frontal lobe involvement (in approximately 15% of patients), early cerebellar involvement, or an asymmetric mass lesion suggestive of a brain tumor [115, 116, 117, 118]. In three cases, the disease process appears to have been triggered by a head injury, with pathological changes beginning in the same location as the trauma [99, 119].

Investigations

Young men with a schizophrenic syndrome should be screened for ALD if they have a history of Addison's Disease, an earlier diagnosis of attention deficit disorder, a disorganized type of psychosis, cranial MRI showing symmetric white-matter pathology, cognitive decline, seizures, or a family history of multiple sclerosis in female relatives.

The definitive diagnostic test is measurement of VLCFA in serum, preferably when the patient is in a fasting state. Most laboratories measure the absolute concentration of C26:0, hexacosanoic acid, and the ratio of C26:0/C22:0 and C24:0/C22:0 [68]. Levels are identical across different forms of the disease [120]. In patients who test positive, baseline levels of ACTH and cortisol should be determined. In addition, an ACTH stimulation test should be performed to evaluate adrenal reserve. Adrenal insufficiency can be life-threatening and regular reassessment of adrenal function should be done.

Treatment

Although there is no definitive treatment for ALD, the following are being actively studied:

1. Lorenzo's oil (LO), a 4:1 mixture of glyceryl trioleate and glyceryl triurecate, when combined with reduction of other fats, has been shown to lower serum levels of VLCFA. Although the effect on course of illness has been disappointing, a recent study demonstrated that genetically affected boys with normal cranial MRIs had a reduced risk of developing the cerebral form of the disorder when treated with LO [121, 122].

2. Hematopoetic stem cell transplantation has been considered for adults with early cerebral involvement [76]. This intervention is, unfortunately, associated with considerable risk and is, therefore, not recommended for individuals without MRI evidence of inflammatory disease, given that only 50% of those with ALD will go on to develop this problem.

Table 18.1 Neuropsychiatric and adrenal findings in 17 cases of late-onset adrenoleukodystrophy

Age of onset	Reference	Psychiatric findings	Neurologic findings	Adrenal involvement	Neuroimaging	Course of illness
26	Gray [81]	At age 23: change in behavior, irresponsible, stealing. At age 26: disinhibition, emotional lability, distractible, hyperkinetic	Staggering and dragging left leg for 3 weeks; hyperreflexia, bilateral extensor plantars	Hyperpigmentation but normal ACTH level and normal stimulation test	None	1 year later, patient incontinent of urine, increasingly more facile, emotionally labile, and disinhibited; no progression of other neurologic symptoms
16	James et al. [91]	Withdrawn, inattentive, anxious, violent	Left extensor plantar, severe memory dysfunction	Hyperpigmentation; ACTH level markedly elevated	CT: dilation of posterior walls of lateral ventricle	By age 17, florid psychosis with auditory hallucinations, delusions of passivity, paranoia. At age 20 developed seizures. Decline in IQ from 75 at age 15 to 59 by age 28
21	Sereni et al. [92]	Withdrawn, inattentive, anxious, violent	Left extensor plantar, severe memory dysfunction	Hyperpigmentation; ACTH level markedly elevated	MRI: bilateral demyelination involving temporal, parietal and occipital regions, right > left	6 months after admission, developed ataxia, bilateral extensor plantars; left homonymous hemianopia; constructive apraxia; death 8 months after presentation
31	Menza et al. [95]	Began at age 26: substance abuse; agitated, irritable, intrusive, hyperactive, sexually inappropriate, loud pressured speech, euphoric. Diagnosis: bipolar affective disorder	Urinary and fecal incontinence; bilateral extensor plantars	Adrenal insufficiency (on replacement therapy)	CT: some ventricular enlargement	Developed cognitive impairment 6 months later
33	Menza et al. [95]	Numerous hospitalizations, alcohol abuse; depression, multiple suicide attempts, auditory hallucinations, poor impulse control, irritability, paranoid delusions, pressured speech. Diagnosis: schizophrenia	None at presentation	None	CT: ventricular enlargement with periventricular WM lucencies	Memory impairment 2 years later; incontinent, ataxic, bilateral extensor plantars; progressive dementia
48	Panegyres et al. [98]	Personality changes, depression, increasingly uncommunicative, abusive, sexually aggressive, several suicide attempts	Incontinence, bilateral extensor plantars	None	CT: widespread WMD with contrast enhancement of corpus callosum, occipital and temporal lobes	At age 53, developed seizures and dementia and died soon after from pulmonary embolism
57	Weller et al. [99]	Disoriented, hypomanic, marked disinhibition	Slow apraxic gait, fluent asphasia, alexia, dysgraphia, dyscalculia, right	None	MRI: diffuse left hemispheric demyelination involving left frontotemporal and occipital regions,	One year later, severe dementia, global apraxia, right hemiparesis, and urinary incontinence

(cont.)

Table 18.1 (*cont.*)

Age of onset	Reference	Psychiatric findings	Neurologic findings	Adrenal involvement	Neuroimaging	Course of illness
			homonymous hemianopia, right extensor plantar response		corpus callosum and cerebral peduncle	
28	Angus *et al.* [100]	Disturbed personality; disinhibited, loud; self-neglect	Mild spastic paraparesis	None	MRI: increased periventricular T2-weighted signal	Unknown
24	Angus *et al.* [100]	At age 24: diagnosed with schizophrenia with delusional thoughts, hallucinations, anhedonia, self neglect, disinhibition; treatment-resistant	None	None initially; elevated ACTH at age 34	MRI: multiple T2-weighted hyperintensities in trigone and splenium of corpus callosum	At age 34, developed orofacial dyskinesia, choreoathetosis; by age 37, emaciated, deeply pigmented, with primitive reflexes, bilateral extensor plantars, disinhibition, and dementia
20	Angus *et al.* [100]	Personality changes, alcohol abuse, self-mutilation, and suicide attempts. Diagnosis: bipolar affective disorder	None	Adrenal insufficiency	CT: normal; MRI: symmetrical diffuse increase in T1 and T2 signal around temporal and occipital horns of lateral ventricles	Developed tonic-clonic seizures at age 25; by age 26, demented, mild spastic paraparesis, gait ataxia, peripheral neuropathy; functionally totally dependent; death 10 months after onset of seizures
33	Sobue *et al.* [101] (monozygotic twins)	Mania: irritability, aggression, increased spending, restlessness; verbal outbursts, disinhibition	Fatigability, anorexia, hyperreflexia, bilateral extensor plantars	ACTH level markedly elevated; significant adrenal insufficiency; hyperpigmentation	MRI: minor periventricular T2-weighted signals	At age 31, intellectually normal; age 33, progressive cognitive impairment
32	Sobue *et al.* [101] (monozygotic twins)	Anxiety, somatic preoccupation; quick-tempered, grandiose, profligate, belligerent, followed by depression Diagnosis: bipolar affective disorder	None at presentation	ACTH level mildly elevated	MRI: extensive T2 high intensity signal in occipital, parietal and temporal areas; also involvement of hippocampus and cerebellum	Initially trained as a dentist; by age 36, IQ = 65; developed spastic ataxic gait, urinary incontinence, horizontal nystagmus, dysarthria, hyperreflexia, bilateral extensor plantars, and loss of vibration and proprioception in both legs
30	Garside *et al.* [107]	Extensive history predating neurologic symptoms including substance abuse, psychosis with paranoid delusions, aggression, perseveration, marked disinhibition, distractibility	Wide-based, spastic ataxic gait, right/left confusion, apraxia, aphasia, hyperreflexia, bilateral extensor plantars, primitive reflexes, urinary incontinence, peripheral neuropathy	ACTH level markedly elevated; abnormal ACTH stimulation test	CT and MRI revealed extensive WMD involving left and right centrum semiovale, corona radiata, and parietal regions; pinpoint signal abnormality in basal ganglia and pons bilaterally	Cognitive decline; mute, wheelchair bound; death two years later from sepsis

Table 18.1 (cont.)

Age of onset	Reference	Psychiatric findings	Neurologic findings	Adrenal involvement	Neuroimaging	Course of illness
32	Gothelf et al. [109]	Age 32: first presentation with acute onset, markedly disorganized behavior, "manic psychotic" episodes, poor social judgment	Age 25: EEG – diffuse slowing; gait disturbance	Addison's Disease age 11	Age 25 and 30: MRI normal. Age 32: MRI: asymmetric periventricular WMD involving pons	Gradual impairment of memory. Died 9 months after psychiatric presentation: complications of bulbar palsy
13	Kopala et al. [108]	Age 13: bizarre, disorganized behavior; eating chalk, setting fires, aggression, silly, giddy, auditory hallucinations	Normal	None	MRI: extensive WMD of frontal lobes; minor involvement of corpus callosum	Not included
25	Sakakibara et al. [111]	Age 25: emotional lability	At presentation: spastic paraparesis; erectile dysfunction; peripheral neuropathy	Low cortisol response to ACTH stimulation	Age 34: MRI T2 weighted images showed small lesions in internal capsule bilaterally	Age 38: wheelchair bound. Age 41: died of respiratory infection
37	Luda et al. [110]	Age 32: hypomanic, character change. Age 38: circumstantial; poor insight, perseveration, impulsivity	Age 37: lower limb spasticity, bilateral Babinski, incontinence, sensory-motor neuropathy	Hypoadrenalism	MRI: diffuse WMD of centrum semiovale and corpus collosum	Age 32–38: progressive memory disturbance, constructional apraxia. Age 40: died of sepsis

Abbreviations: ACTH = corticotropin, WM = white matter, WMD = white matter disease.

Mitochondrial disorders

Mitochochondria are considered the "power-plants" of the cell, and generate the majority of cellular energy through a process known as oxidative phosphorylation (OXPHOS) [123]. Impairment of OXPHOS leads to the formation of reaction oxygen species that cause lipid peroxidation and oxidative damage to the cell. Oligodendrocytes and axons are particularly vulnerable to oxidative stress, resulting in significant pathology in white matter [124, 125] – hence, the designation of inherited mitochondrial disorders as leukodystrophies [126]. A recent study found that 90% of patients with mitochondrial disorders had wide-spread white matter hyperintensities, making this the most frequent abnormality [127].

Despite the recognition that mitochondrial disorders frequently affect the brain and produce white matter abnormalities, there has been little attention to the psychiatric manifestations of the disorders. We assessed and treated 23 patients who presented with primary psychiatric symptomatology, and who were eventually found to have a mitochondrial disorder [128], suggesting that this is an under-recognized feature of mitochondrial disease. We found an additional 38 cases in the literature [129, 130, 131, 132, 133, 134, 135, 136, 137, 138] which, combined with our series of 23 patients, gives a total of 61 cases. Psychosis was a very commonly reported symptom, being present in more than 50% of cases, and patients were often initially diagnosed with schizophrenia. In the majority of cases in which psychosis was reported, positive symptoms were described but there was little mention of negative symptoms. The majority of cases were associated with MELAS, particularly the A3243G mutation.

It is likely that the leukodystrophy associated with mitochondrial disorders plays an important role in the development of psychosis and other psychiatric symptoms. This may occur through disruption of important pathways that connect different parts of the brain involved in the control of emotion, thought, and behavior. In addition, the brain is especially energy-dependent, and any compromise in ATP production may lower the threshold and reduce the safety margin for the development of psychiatric illness. Finally, patients with mitochondrial disorders frequently experience chronic fatigue and cognitive dysfunction that may ultimately lead to an axis II or perhaps axis I disorder.

Currently, there is no curative treatment for mitochondrial disorders. Although clear evidence from randomized trials is lacking, supportive treatment with supplements, including creatine and co-enzyme Q10, is often initiated [139].

The reader is referred to the Chapter 17 by Velakoulis and Walterfang, in which mitochondrial disorders are discussed more fully.

Krabbe's Disease

Krabbe's Disease, also known as globoid cell leukodystrophy, is an autosomal recessive disorder caused by a deficiency in the lysosomal enzyme galactosylceramidase. This deficiency impairs degradation of galactolipids, including psychosine and galatosylceramide, which accumulate in central and peripheral nervous system myelin [140]. Psychosine is toxic to white matter and causes rapid loss of oligodendrocytes, demyelination, and secondary axonal degeneration [141]. Globoid cells are seen on pathology and likely reflect phagocytosis of galactolipids by macrophages. Findings on MRI include white-matter lesions that may be seen in the periventricular parieto-occipital regions and then become more diffuse [142]. Diagnosis is made by measuring galactocerebrosidase activity in peripheral leukocytes and by molecular analysis of the galacto-sylceramidase gene. The incidence of Krabbe's Disease varies geographically, and is approximately 1 in 100,000 in the United States and as high as 1 in 6,000 in a Druze kindred in Israel [143].

Krabbe's Disease most commonly presents before 6 months of age with irritability, spasticity, blindness, hearing loss, seizures, and rapid motor and mental deterioration, culminating in death within a few years. Onset after 6 months of age is termed late-onset Krabbe's Disease and has a variable but less severe course often characterized by intellectual decline, dementia, and spasticity [142]. Peripheral nervous system involvement is less common in late-onset disease, and patients are often clinically heterogeneous [143]. Although adult-onset forms have been identified, there are no reports of psychosis or other psychiatric symptoms in these patients. However, given its clinical and pathological similarity to more common leukodystrophies such as MLD and the involvement of CNS white matter in the late-onset form, it is most likely that psychosis can occur but may be unrecognized. Treatment involves bone marrow or umbilical cord blood transplantation to restore galactocerebrosidase levels [145, 146].

Pelizaeus-Merzbacher Disease

Pelizaeus-Merzbacher Disease (PMD) is a rare X-linked recessive dysmyelinating disorder caused by mutations in the proteolipid (PLP) gene [147]. PLP is a major constituent of myelin in the CNS, and affected patients demonstrate a classic "tigroid" appearance of white matter with areas of total loss of myelin interspersed with areas of relative preservation. The frequency of PMD is unknown but is estimated to be at least 1 in 500,000 in the United States. Diagnosis is often suggested by diffuse white-matter abnormalities on MRI indicating hypomyelination and confirmed by molecular analysis of the PLP gene. PMD generally presents in infancy with intellectual delay, nystagmus, stridor, cerebellar dysfunction, and a progressive upper motor neuron pattern of disease [148]. However, it may also present in adulthood with dementia or psychosis [149]. The prevalence of psychosis in PMD is unknown. Treatment remains supportive.

Cerebrotendinous Xanthomatosis

Cerebrotendinous xanthomatosis is an autosomal recessive disorder of bile acid synthesis. It is caused by deficiency in the mitochondrial enzyme sterol 27-hydroxylase (CYP27), resulting in an inability to convert cholesterol to cholic and chenodeoxycholic acids and the accumulation of bile alcohols in various organs, including the nervous system and cholestanol which can be toxic to oligodendiocytes [150]. In the brain, cerebral xanthomas can form, and there is loss of myelin, resulting in diffuse white-matter abnormalities. While previously thought to be a rare disorder, it is now considered to be one of the main causes of leukoencephalopathies in adults. Diagnosis is confirmed by measurement of elevated plasma and bile cholestanol and increased urinary excretion of bile alcohol glucuronides in association with clinical features of the disorder.

Clinical manifestations include chronic diarrhea, bilateral cataracts, Achilles tendon xanthomas, premature atherosclerosis, osteoporosis, and progressive neurological symptoms, including ataxia, pyramidal signs, and dementia [151]. Psychiatric symptoms were reported in 4 of 35 patients in a series by Berginer and colleagues [152]. Two patients were psychotic with auditory hallucinations and delusions, one patient presented with catatonia, and one patient developed agitation, aggression, and negativistic behavior. All patients in the series had diffuse white-matter abnormalities and no focal lesions. Treatment with chenodeoxycholic acid reduces cholestanol levels and generally results in marked clinical improvement, particularly if started prior to significant neurological deterioration [150]. Therefore, it is essential that patients with psychosis and features of cerebrotendinous xanthomatosis be appropriately investigated for this potentially treatable disorder.

Alexander's Disease

Alexander's Disease is a sporadic leukodystrophy associated with the accumulation of glial fibrillary acidic protein (GFAP) and heat shock proteins in astrocytes, forming characteristic inclusions termed Rosenthal fibers [153, 154]. There is associated diffuse myelin loss, with white-matter abnormalities most prominent in the frontal lobes. The prevalence is unknown, with approximately 450 cases reported in the world literature. Diagnosis is generally based on MRI findings, although genetic testing of the GFAP gene is now available. Alexander's Disease typically presents in infancy with megalencephaly, seizures, mental retardation, spasticity, and rapid death. Rarely, it may present in adolescence and adulthood with ataxia, spasticity, bulbar signs, and dementia [154]. Typically, there is less myelin loss in adult forms of the disease. Psychosis has not been reported in Alexander's Disease. This may be a result of underrecognition or the relative preservation of myelin in adult forms. There is no effective treatment for the disease.

Membranous lipodystrophy

Membranous lipodystrophy, also known as polycystic lipomembranous osteodysplasia with sclerosing leukoencephalopathy or Nasu-Hakola Disease, is a rare, recessive disorder associated with bone cysts and neuropsychiatric symptoms. Patients generally present in their second to third decade of life with pain in their ankles and wrists and associated pathological fractures [155]. This is followed by psychosis, progressive dementia, myoclonus, seizures, or gait disturbances in the third to fourth decade of life. The true incidence of psychosis is unknown. The disease is generally fatal by age 50. The disease has recently been linked to mutations in the gene encoding a tyrosine kinase binding protein [155], although the molecular and cellular pathogenesis remains unknown. In the brain, there is loss of myelin particularly in the frontal lobes, astrocytic gliosis, enlarged ventricles, calcifications and atrophy of basal ganglia, and atrophy of the corpus callosum [156]. There is no known treatment.

Principles of management for patients with inherited leukodystrophies

Monitoring the course of illness

Once the diagnosis of an inherited leukodystrophy has been made, it becomes important to monitor the progress of the underlying pathology. The following investigations are useful in this regard:

1. Cranial MRI at regular intervals, every 2–5 years or as clinically indicated
2. An EEG at baseline and as clinically indicated thereafter, given the common complication of seizures and the need to rule out seizure activity as a cause of psychiatric decompensation
3. Cognitive testing at baseline and at regular intervals
4. EMG and nerve conduction studies to assess peripheral nerve function
5. Regular neurological examinations

Treatment of psychiatric illness

Patients with leukodystrophies frequently prove refractory to traditional medication regimens. This indeed may be what prompts the initial investigation for an underlying metabolic disorder. They may also be especially vulnerable to developing medication side effects [107], necessitating regular reassessment of the risk:benefit ratio of any treatment regimen. Many psychotropic agents interfere with mitochondrial function. Specifically, many antipsychotic agents, both typical and atypical, have been shown to inhibit complex 1 of the respiratory chain and, therefore, may worsen symptoms [157]. In addition, the inhibition of oxidative phosphorylation and increased production of free radicals [157, 158] could worsen the underlying disease process, particularly in those with mitochondrial diseases. Certain psychotropic medications known as amphiphilic agents have been shown, *in vitro* and *in vivo*, to accelerate lipid deposition and promote lysosomal excretion of certain enzymes [159]. These effects have been implicated in a worsening of the underlying pathological process in certain metabolic disorders, such as the gangliosidoses [160, 161] and might also be relevant in the treatment of patients with other inherited metabolic diseases.

Extrapyramidal side effects (EPS) can exacerbate the functional impairment associated with upper motor neuron pathology and the anticholinergic properties of many psychotropic agents will tend to exacerbate cognitive impairment. Anticholinergic medications may be particularly problematic in the case of patients with ALD who may also have Addison's Disease, and prone to develop hypotension.

Benzodiazepines have the potential to exacerbate problems of dysarthria, gait disturbance, and short-term memory impairment to which these patients are vulnerable.

Patients with leukodystrophies frequently develop seizures, and status epilepticus is a leading cause of death in patients with mitochondrial disease. Unfortunately, most psychotropic agents, other than benzodiazepines, lower the seizure threshold. For this reason, when mood symptoms are prominent, anti-seizure medications may be preferable to lithium. Valproic acid, however, can cause a secondary impairment of mitochondrial function through the induction of carnitine deficiency [162]. The atypical antipsychotic, clozapine, which might otherwise be chosen to treat refractory psychotic symptoms, is associated with a lifetime cumulative risk of seizures: 10% after 3.8 years of treatment [163], even among those without a pre-existing epileptic disorder. One would imagine the risk to be much higher when used in the context of an underlying neurometabolic condition.

Several of the newer antipsychotic drugs such as olanzapine and clozapine are associated with a metabolic syndrome and may compound the risk of patients with mitochondrial disorders developing diabetes.

Summary and future directions

Patients with adult-onset forms of the inherited leukodystrophies have a very high prevalence of neuropsychiatric disturbances, many of which closely resemble the clinical features of schizophrenia. This is of interest for two reasons. For one, there are obvious therapeutic implications. Many medications used to treat psychiatric symptoms have the potential to exacerbate the clinical consequences of neurometabolic disorders and, in some cases, may worsen the underlying disease process. A substantial proportion of patients with schizophrenia are refractory to treatment. Might these individuals harbor an unrecognized leukodystrophy or other neurometabolic disorder?

There is another reason to note the high prevalence of psychiatric illness in patients with inherited leukodystrophies. At the present time, we do not understand the pathological processes that give rise to the clinical syndrome we call schizophrenia. The key feature common to all central leukodystrophies is the disconnection of brain regions from one another. Careful attention to the precise localization of the white-matter lesions may help us understand the pathobiology of particular psychiatric symptoms, and advances in the identification of genotype-phenotype relationships may illuminate why some patients develop psychiatric illness and others do not.

Finally, as treatments for inherited leukodystrophies develop, it will be imperative to accurately identify affected individuals who may benefit from these new approaches [164].

Acknowledgments

We wish to thank Mary Wilson for her expert and careful assistance in preparing this chapter.

References

1. Von Figura K., Gieselmann V., Jaekew J. (2001). Metachromatic leukodystrophy. In *The Metabolic Basis of Inherited Disease*, Scriver C. R., Beaudet A. L., Sly W. S., *et al.* (Eds.). Eighth Ed., vol 3. New York: McGraw-Hill, pp. 3695–724.

2. Hyde T. M., Ziegler J. C., Weinberger D. R. Psychiatric disturbances in metachromatic leukodystrophy. Insights into the neurobiology of psychosis. *Arch Neurol*, 1992. **49**:401–6.

3. Black D. N., Taber K. H., Hurley R. A. Metachromatic leukodystrophy: a model for the study of psychosis. *J Neuropsychiatr Clin Neurosci*, 2003. **15**:289–93.

4. Polten A., Fluharty A. L., Fluharty C. B., *et al.* Molecular basis of different forms of metachromatic leukodystrophy. *N Engl J Med*, 1991. **324**:18–22.

5. Rauschka H., Colsch B., Baumann N., *et al.* Late-onset metachromatic leukodystrophy: genotype strongly influences phenotype. *Neurology*, 2006. **67**:859–63.

6. Hreidarsson S. J., Thomas G. H., Kihara H., *et al.* Impaired cerebroside sulfate hydrolysis in fibroblasts of sibs with "pseudo" arylsulfatase A deficiency without metachromatic leukodystrophy. *Pediatr Res*, 1983. **17**:701–4.

7. Schipper H. I., Seidel D. Computed tomography in late-onset metachromatic leucodystrophy. *Neuroradiology*, 1984. **26**:39–44.

8. Betts T. A., Smith W. T., Kelly R. E. Adult metachromatic leukodystrophy (sulphatide lipidosis) simulating acute schizophrenia: report of a case. *Neurology*, 1968. **18**:1140–2.

9. Shapiro E. G., Lockman L. A., Knopman D., *et al.* Characteristics of the dementia in late-onset metachromatic leukodystrophy. *Neurology*, 1994. **44**:662–5.

10. Baumann N., Masson M., Carreau V., *et al.* Adult forms of metachromatic leukodystrophy: clinical and biochemical approach. *Dev Neurosci*, 1991. **13**:211–15.

11. Mahon-Haft H., Stone R. K., Johnson R., *et al.* Biochemical abnormalities of metachromatic leukodystrophy in an adult psychiatric population. *Am J Psychiatry*, 1981. **138**:1372–4.

12. Alvarez L. M., Castillo S. T., Perez Z. J. A., *et al.* Activity of aryl sulfatase A enzyme in patients with schizophrenic disorders. [English translation]. Rev *Invest Clin*, 1995. **47**:387–92.

13. Hohenschutz C., Friedl W., Schlor K. H., *et al.* Probable metachromatic leukodystrophy/pseudodeficiency compound heterozygote at the arylsulfatase A locus with neurological and psychiatric symptomatology. *Am J Med Genet*, 1988. **31**:169–75.

14. Ferraro A. Familiar form of encephalitis periaxialis diffusa. *J Nerv Ment Dis*, 1927. **66**:329–54.

15. van Bogaert L., Dewulf A. Diffuse progressive leukodystrophy in the adult. *Arch Neurol Psychiatry*, 1939. 1083–97.

16. Norman R. M. Diffuse progressive metachromatic leucoencephalopathy: a form of Schilder's disease related to the lipoidoses. *Brain*, 1947. **70**:234–50.

17. Sourander P., Svennerholm L. Sulphatide lipidosis in the adult with the clinical picture of progressive organic dementia with epileptic seizures. *Acta Neuropathol*, 1962. **1**:384–96.

18. Austin J., Armstrong D., Fouch S., *et al.* Metachromatic leukodystrophy (MLD). VIII. MLD in adults; diagnosis and pathogenesis. *Arch Neurol*, 1968. **18**:225–40.

19. Müller D., Pilz H., Ter Meulen V. Studies on adult metachromatic leukodystrophy. Part 1. Clinical, morphological and histochemical observations in two cases. *J Neurol Sci*, 1969. **9**:567–84.

20. Hirose G., Bass N. H. Metachromatic leukodystrophy in the adult: a biochemical study. *Neurology*, 1972. **22**:312–20.

21. Joosten E., Hoes M., Gabreels-Festen A., *et al.* Electron microscopic investigation of inclusion material in a case of adult metachromatic leukodystrophy; observations on kidney biopsy, peripheral nerve and cerebral white matter. *Acta Neuropathol*, 1975. **33**:165–71.

22. Guseo A., Deak G., Szirmai I. An adult case of metachromatic leukodystrophy. Light, polarization and electron microscopic study. *Acta Neuropathol*, 1975. **32**:333–9.

23. Quigley H. A., Green W. R. Clinical and ultrastructural ocular histopathologic studies of adult-onset metachromatic leukodystrophy. *Am J Ophthalmol*, 1976. **82**:472–9.

24. Percy A. K., Kaback M. M., Herndon R. M. Metachromatic leukodystrophy: comparison of early and late-onset forms. *Neurology*, 1977. **27**:933–41.

25. Pilz H., Duensing I., Heipertz R., *et al.* Adult metachromatic leukodystrophy. I. Clinical manifestation in a female aged 44 years, previously diagnosed in the preclinical state. *Eur Neurol*, 1977. **15**:301–7.

26. Manowitz P., Kling A., Kohn H. Clinical course of adult metachromatic leukodystrophy presenting as schizophrenia. A report of two living cases in siblings. *J Nerv Ment Dis*, 1978. **166**:500–6.

27. Bosch E. P., Hart M. N. Late adult-onset metachromatic leukodystrophy. Dementia and

polyneuropathy in a 63-year-old man. *Arch Neurol*, 1978. **35**:475–7.

28. Tagliavini F., Pietrini V., Pilleri G., *et al*. Adult metachromatic leucodystrophy: clinico-pathological report of two familial cases with slow course. *Neuropath Appl Neurobiol*, 1979. **5**:233–43.

29. Hoes M. J., Lamers K. J., Hommes O. R., *et al*. Adult metachromatic leukodystrophy. Arylsulphatase-A values in four generations of one family and some reflections about the genetics. *Clin Neurol Neurosurg*, 1978. **80**:174–88.

30. Besson J. A. A diagnostic pointer to adult metachromatic leucodystrophy. *Br J Psychiatry*, 1980. **137**:186–7.

31. Seidel D., Goebel H. H., Scholz W. Late-onset metachromatic leukodystrophy: diagnostic problems elucidated by a case report. *J Neurol*, 1981. **226**:119–24.

32. Skomer C., Stears J., Austin J. Metachromatic leukodystrophy (MLD). XV. Adult MLD with focal lesions by computed tomography. *Arch Neurol*, 1983. **40**:354–5.

33. Scully R. E., Mark E. J., McNeely B. U., *et al*. Case records of the Massachusetts General Hospital. Weekly clinicopathological exercises. Case 7–1984. A 34-year old man with progressive quadriparesis and mental deterioration. *New Engl J Med*, 1984. **310**:445–55.

34. Finelli P. F. Metachromatic leukodystrophy manifesting as a schizophrenic disorder: computed tomographic correlation. *Ann Neurol*, 1985. **18**:94–5.

35. Wulff C. H., Trojaborg W. Adult metachromatic leukodystrophy: neurophysiologic findings. *Neurology*, 1985. **35**:1776–8.

36. Alves D., Pires M. M., Guimaraes A., *et al*. Four cases of late onset metachromatic leucodystrophy in a family: clinical, biochemical and neuropathological studies.

J Neurol Neurosurg Psychiatry, 1986. **49**:1417–22.

37. Cerizza M., Nemni R., Tamma F. Adult metachromatic leucodystrophy: an under-diagnosed disease? (letter). *J Neurol Neurosurg Psychiatry*, 1987. **50**:1710–12.

38. Waltz G., Harik S. I., Kaufman B. Adult metachromatic leukodystrophy. Value of computed tomographic scanning and magnetic resonance imaging of the brain. *Arch Neurol*, 1987. **44**:225–7.

39. Sadeh M., Kuritzky A., Ben-David E., *et al*. Adult metachromatic leukodystrophy with an unusual relapsing-remitting course. *Postgrad Med J*, 1992. **68**:192–5.

40. Waldman A. J. Sometimes when you hear hoofbeats…two cases of inherited metabolic diseases with initial presentation of psychiatric symptoms (Letter). *J Neuro-psychiatr Clin Neurosci*, 1992. **4**:113–14.

41. Sadovnick A. D., Tuokko H., Applegarth D. A., *et al*. The differential diagnosis of adult onset metachromatic leukodystrophy and early onset familial Alzheimer disease in an Alzheimer clinic population. *Can J Neurol Sci*, 1993. **20**: 312–18.

42. Duyff R. F., Weinstein H. C. Late-presenting metachromatic leukodystrophy. *Lancet*, 1996. **348**:1382–3.

43. Navarro C., Fernandez J. M., Dominguez C., *et al*. Late juvenile metachromatic leukodystrophy treated with bone marrow transplantation; a 4-year follow-up study. *Neurology*, 1996. **46**:254–6.

44. Coulter-Mackie M. B., Gagnier L., Beis M. J., *et al*. Metachromatic leucodystrophy in three families from Nova Scotia, Canada: a recurring mutation in the arylsulphatase A gene. *J Med Genet*, 1997. **34**:493–8.

45. Vella G., Loriedo C., Raccah R., *et al*. Successful paroxetine treatment of major depression in an adult form of metachromatic leukodystrophy with cognitive disturbances (letter). *Can J Psychiatr*, 1998. **43**:748–9.

46. Fukutani Y., Noriki Y., Sasaki K., *et al*. Adult-type metachromatic leukodystrophy with a compound heterozygote mutation showing character change and dementia. *Psychiatry Clin Neurosci*, 1999. **53**:425–8.

47. Gallo S., Randi D., Bertelli M., *et al*. Late onset MLD with normal nerve conduction associated with two novel missense mutations in the ASA gene. *J Neurol Neurosurg Psychiatry*, 2004. **75**:655–7.

48. Fressinaud C., Vallat J. M., Masson M., *et al*. Adult onset metachromatic leukodystrophy presenting as isolated peripheral neuropathy. *Neurology*, 1992. **42**:1396–8.

49. Felice K. J., Lira G. M., Natowicz M. Adult onset metachromatic leukodystrophy: a gene mutation with isolated polyneuropathy. *Neurology*, 2000. **55**:1036–9.

50. Cengiz N., Osbenli T., Onar M., *et al*. Adult metachromatic leukodystrophy: three cases with normal nerve conduction velocities in a family. *Acta Neurol Scand*, 2002. **105**:454–7.

51. Tylki-Szymanska A., Berger J., Loschl B., *et al*. Late juvenile metachromatic leukodystrophy (MLD) in three patients with similar clinical course and identical mutation on one allele. *Clin Genet*, 1996. **50**:287–92.

52. Kumperscak H. G., Paschke E., Gradisnik P., *et al*. Adult metachromatic leukodystrophy: disorganized schizophrenia-like symptoms and postpartum depression in 2 sisters. *J Psychiatry Neurosci*, 2005. **30**: 33–6.

53. Kumperscak H. G., Plesinar B. K., Zalar B., *et al*. Adult metachromatic leukodystrophy: a

new mutation in the schizophrenia- like phenotype with early neurological signs. *Psychiatr Genet*, 2007. **17**:85–91.

54. Reider-Grosswasser I., Bornstein N. CT and MRI in late-onset metachromatic leukodystrophy. *Acta Neurol Scand*, 1987. **75**:64–9.

55. Taylor W. D., Hsu E., Krishnan K. R. R., *et al.* Diffusion tensor imaging: background, potential and utility in psychiatric research. *Biol Psychiatry*, 2004. **55**:201–7.

56. Patay Z. Diffusion-weighted MR imaging in leukodystrophies. *Eur Radiol*, 2005. **15**:2284–303.

57. Porter M. T., Fluharty A. L., Kihara H. Correction of abnormal cerebroside sulfate metabolism in cultured metachromatic leukodystrophy fibroblasts. *Science*, 1971. **172**:1263–5.

58. Greene H. L., Hug G., Schubert W. K. Metachromatic leukodystrophy. Treatment with arylsulfatase-A. *Arch Neurol*, 1969. **20**:147–53.

59. Austin J. H. Studies in metachromatic leukodystrophy XI. Therapeutic considerations, 1972. *Birth Defects: Original Article Series*, 1973. **9**:125–9.

60. Bayever E., Ladisch S., Philippart M., *et al.* Bone-marrow transplantation for metachromatic leucodystrophy. *Lancet*, 1985. **2**:471–3.

61. Krivit W., Lipton M. E., Lockman L. A., *et al.* Prevention of deterioration in metachromatic leukodystrophy by bone marrow transplantation. *Am J Med Sci*, 1987. **294**:80–5.

62. Dhuna A., Toro C., Torres F., *et al.* Longitudinal neurophysiologic studies in a patient with metachromatic leukodystrophy following bone marrow transplantation. *Arch Neurol*, 1992. **49**:1088–92.

63. Kapaun P., Dittmann R. W., Granitzny B., *et al.* Slow progression of juvenile metachromatic leukodystrophy 6 years after bone marrow transplantation. *J Child Neurol*, 1999. **14**:222–8.

64. Learish R., Ohashi T., Robbins P. A., *et al.* Retroviral gene transfer and sustained expression of human arylsulfatase A. *Gene Therapy*, 1996. **3**:343–9.

65. Nevo Y., Pestronk A., Lopate G., *et al.* Neuropathy of metachromatic leukodystrophy: improvement with immunomodulation. *Pediatr Neurol*, 1996. **15**:237–9.

66. von Figura K., Steckel F., Hasilik A. Juvenile and adult metachromatic leukodystrophy: partial restoration of arylsulfatase A (cerebroside sulfatase) activity by inhibitors of thiol proteinases. *Proc Natl Acad Sci*, 1983. **80**:6066–70.

67. Moser H. W., Smith K. D., Moser A. (1995). X-linked adrenoleukodystrophy. In *The Metabolic and Molecular Basis of Inherited Diseases*, 7th ed., Scriver C. R., Beaudet A. L., Sly W. S., *et al.* (Eds). New York: McGraw-Hill, pp. 2325–49.

68. Moser H. W. Adrenoleukodystrophy: phenotype, genetics, pathogenesis and therapy. *Brain*, 1997. **120**:1485–508.

69. Aubourg P., Mosser J., Douar A. M., *et al.* Adrenoleukodystrophy gene: unexpected homology to a protein involved in peroxisome biogenesis. *Biochimie* 1993. **75**:293–302.

70. Mosser J., Lutz Y., Stoeckel M. E., *et al.* The gene responsible for adrenoleukodystrophy encodes a peroxisomal membrane protein. *Hum Mol Genet*, 1994. **3**:265–71.

71. Higgins C. F. ABC transporters: from microorganisms to man. *Ann Rev Cell Biol*, 1992. **8**:67–113.

72. Anglin R. E., Rosebush P. I., Mazurek M. F. The neuropsychiatric profile of Addison's disease: revisiting a forgotten phenomenon. *J Neuropsychiatr Clin Neurosci*, 2006. **18**:450–9.

73. Puck J. M., Willard H. F. X-inactivation in females with X-linked disease. *N Engl J Med*, 1998. **338**:325–8.

74. Schmidt S., Traber F., Block W., *et al.* Phenotype assignment in symptomatic female carriers of X-linked adrenoleukodystrophy. *J Neurol*, 2001. **248**:36–44.

75. Moser H. W., Raymond G. V., Dubey P. Adrenoleukodystrophy: new approaches to a neurogenetive disease. *JAMA*, 2005. **294**:3131–4.

76. Mahmood A., Dubey P., Moser H. W., *et al.* X-linked adrenoleukodystrophy: therapeutic approaches to distinct phenotypes. *Pediatr Transplant*, 2005. **9**(Suppl 7):55–62.

77. Moser H. W., Moser A. E., Singh I., *et al.* Adrenoleukodystrophy: survey of 303 cases: biochemistry, diagnosis, and therapy. *Ann Neurol*, 1984. **16**:628–41.

78. Moser H. W., Moser A. B., Naidu S., *et al.* Clinical aspects of adrenoleukodystrophy and adrenomyeloneuropathy. *Dev Neurosci*, 1991. **13**:254–61.

79. Schaumburg H. H., Powers J. M., Raine C. S., *et al.* Adrenoleukodystrophy: a clinical and pathological study of 17 cases. *Arch Neurol*, 1975. **32**:577–91.

80. Van Geel B. M., Assies J., Wanders J. A. *et al.* X linked adrenoleukodystrophy: clinical presentation, diagnosis, and therapy. *J Neurol Neurosurg Psychiatry*, 1997. **63**:4–14.

81. Gray A. M. Addison's disease and diffuse cerebral sclerosis. *J Neurol Neurosurg Psychiatry*, 1969. **32**:344–7.

82. Budka H., Sluga E., Heiss W. D. Spastic paraplegia associated with Addison's disease: adult variant of adreno-leukodystrophy. *J Neurol*, 1976. **213**:237–50.

83. Scully R. E., Galdabini J. J., McNeely B. U. Case 18–1979: Case records of the Massachusetts General Hospital. *N Engl J Med*, 1979. **300**:1037–45.

84. Davis L. E., Snyder R. D., Orth D. N., *et al.* Adrenoleukodystrophy and adrenomyeloneuropathy associated with partial adrenal insufficiency in three generations of a kindred. *Am J Med*, 1979. **66**:342–7.

85. Weiss G. M., Nelson R. L., O'Neill B. P., *et al.* Use of adrenal biopsy in diagnosing adrenoleukomyelo-neuropathy. *Arch Neurol*, 1980. **37**:634–6.

86. Probst A., Ulrich J., Heitz U., *et al.* Adrenomyeloneuropathy: a protracted pseudosystemic variant of adrenoleukodystrophy. *Acta Neuropathol*, 1980. **49**:105–15.

87. O'Neill B. P., Marmion L. C., Feringa E. R. The adrenoleuko-myeloneuropathy complex: expression in four generations. *Neurology*, 1981. **31**:151–6.

88. Peckham R. S., Marshall M. C., Rosman P. M., *et al.* A variant of adrenomyeloneuropathy with hypothalamic-pituitary dysfunction and neurologic remission after glucocorticoid replacement therapy. *Am J Med*, 1982. **72**:173–6.

89. Kuroda S., Hirano A., Yuasa S. Adrenoleukodystrophy-cerebello-brainstem dominant case. *Acta Neuropathol*, 1983. **60**: 149–52.

90. Ohno T., Tsuchiya H., Fukuhara N., *et al.* Adrenoleukodystrophy: a clinical variant presenting as olivopontocerebellar atrophy. *J Neurol*, 1984. **231**:167–9.

91. James A. C., Kaplan P., Lees A., *et al.* Schizophreniform psychosis and adrenomyeloneuropathy. *J R Soc Med*, 1984. **77**:882–4.

92. Sereni C., Ruel M., Iba-zizen T., *et al.* Adult adrenoleuko-dystrophy: a sporadic case? *J Neurol Sci*, 1987. **80**:121–8.

93. Simpson R. H., Rodda J., Reinecke C. J. Adrenoleukodystrophy in a mother and son. *J Neurol Neurosurg Psychiatry* 1987. **50**:1165–72.

94. Jeffcoate W. J., McGivern D., Cotton R. E., *et al.* Late-onset adrenoleukodystrophy (Letter). *J Neurol Neurosurg Psychiatry*, 1987. **50**:1238–9.

95. Menza M. A., Blake J., Goldberg L. Affective symptoms and adrenoleukodystrophy: a report of two cases. *Psychosomatics*, 1988. **29**:442–5.

96. Ladenson P. W. Adrenoleuko-dystrophy. *JAMA*, 1989. **262**:1504–6.

97. Elrington G. M., Bateman D. E., Jeffrey M. J., *et al.* Adrenoleukodystrophy: heterogeneity in two brothers. *J Neurol Neurosurg Psychiatry*, 1989. **52**:310–13.

98. Panegyres P. K., Goldswain P., Kakulas B. A. Adult-onset adrenoleukodystrophy manifesting as dementia. *Am J Med*, 1989. **87**:481–3.

99. Weller M., Liedtke W., Peterson D., *et al.* Very-late-onset adrenoleukodystrophy: possible precipitation of demyelination by cerebral contusion. *Neurology*, 1992. **42**:367–70.

100. Angus B., de Silva R., Davidson R., *et al.* A family with adult-onset cerebral adrenoleucodystrophy. *J Neurol*, 1994. **241**:497–9.

101. Sobue G., Ueno-Natsukari I., Okamoto H., *et al.* Phenotypic heterogeneity of an adult form of adrenoleukodystrophy in monozygotic twins. *Ann Neurol*, 1994. **36**:912–15.

102. Maris T., Androulidakis E. J., Tzagournissakis M., *et al.* X-linked adrenoleukodystrophy presenting as neurologically pure familial spastic paraparesis. *Neurology*, 1995. **45**: 1101–4.

103. Schwankhaus J. D., Katz D. A., Eldridge R., *et al.* Clinical and pathological features of an autosomal dominant, adult-onset leukodystrophy simulating chronic progressive multiple sclerosis. *Arch Neurol*, 1994. **51**:757–66.

104. Afifi A. K., Menezes A. H., Reed L. A., *et al.* Atypical presentation of X-linked adrenoleukodystrophy with an unusual magnetic resonance imaging pattern. *J Child Neurol*, 1996. **11**:497–9.

105. Crum B. A., Carter J. L. 26 year old man with hyperpigmentation of skin and lower extremity spasticity. *Mayo Clin Proc*, 1997. **72**:479–82.

106. Munchau A., Hagel C., Vogel P. Adrenoleukodystrophy of very late onset. *J Neurol*, 1997. **244**:595–9.

107. Garside S., Rosebush P. I., Levinson A. J., *et al.* Late-onset adrenoleukodystrophy associated with long-standing psychiatric symptoms. *J Clin Psychiatry*, 1999. **60**:460–8.

108. Kopala L. C., Tan S., Shea C., *et al.* Adrednoleukodystrophy associated with psychosis (Letter). *Schizophr Res*, 2000. **45**:263–5.

109. Gothelf D., Levite R., Gadoth N. Bipolar affective disorder heralding cerebral demyelination in adreno-myelo-leukodystrophy. *Brain Dev*, 2000. **22**:184–7.

110. Luda E., Barisone M. G. Adult-onset adrenoleukodystrophy: a clinical and neuropsychological study. *Neurol Sci*, 2001. **22**:21–5.

111. Sakakibara R., Fukutake T., Arai K., *et al.* Unilateral caudate head lesion simulating brain tumour in X-linked adult onset adrenoleukodystrophy (Letter). *J Neurol Neurosurg Psychiatry*, 2001. **70**:3:414–15.

112. Hitomi T., Mezaki T., Tsujii T., *et al.* Improvement of central motor conduction after bone marrow transplantation in adrenoleukodystrophy. J Neurol *Neurosurg Psychiatry*, 2003. **74**:3:373–5.

113. Spurek M., Taylor-Gjevre R., Van Uum S., *et al.* Adrenomyelo-neuropathy as a cause of primary adrenal insufficiency and spastic paraparesis. *Can Med Assoc J*, 2004. **171**(9): 1073–7.

114. Mukherjee S., Newby E., Harvey J. N. Adrenomyeloneuropathy in patients with 'Addison's disease': genetic case analysis. *J R Soc Med*, 2006. **99**:245–9.

115. Castellote A., Vera J., Vasquez E., *et al.* MR in adrenoleuko-dystrophy: atypical presentation as bilateral frontal demyelination. *AJNR Am J Neuroradiol*, 1995. **16**(Suppl 4):814–15.

116. Close P. J., Sinnott S. J., Nolan K. T. Adrenoleukodystrophy: a case report demonstrating unilateral abnormalities. *Pediatr Radiol*, 1993. **23**:400–1.

117. MacDonald J. T., Stauffer A. E., Heitoff K. Adrenoleukodystrophy: early frontal lobe involvement on computed tomography. *J Comput Assist Tomogr*, 1984. **8**:128–30.

118. Young R. S., Ramer J. C., Towfighi J., *et al.* Adrenoleukodystrophy: unusual computed tomographic appearance. *Arch Neurol*, 1982. **39**:782–3.

119. Farrell D. F., Hamilton S. R., Krauss T. A., *et al.* X-linked adrenoleukodystrophy: adult cerebral variant. *Neurology*, 1993. **43**:1518–22.

120. Moser A. B., Kreiter N., Bezman L., *et al.* Plasma very long chain fatty acids in 3,000 peroxisome disease patients and 29,000 controls. *Ann Neurol*, 1999. **45**:100–10.

121. Moser H. W., Raymond G. V., Lu S. E., *et al.* Followup of 89 asymptomatic patients with adrenoleukodystrophy treated with Lorenzo's oil. *Arch Neurol*, 2005. **62**:1073–80.

122. Siva N. Positive effects with Lorenzo's oil (Letter). *Lancet*, 2005. **4**:529.

123. Saraste M. Oxidative phosphorylation at the fin de siecle. *Science*, 1999. **283**:1488–93.

124. Lerman-Sagie T., Leshinsky-Silver E., Watemberg N., *et al.* White matter involvement in mitochondrial diseases. *Mol Genet and Metab*, 2005. **84**:127–36.

125. Kovacs G. G., Hoftberger R., Majtenyi K., *et al.* Neuropathology of white matter disease in Leber's hereditary optic neuropathy. *Brain*, 2005. **128**:35–41.

126. Sedel F., Tourbah A., Fontaine B., *et al.* Leukoencephalopathies associated with inborn errors of metabolism in adults. *J Inherit Metab Dis*, 2008. **31**:295–307.

127. Barragan-Campos H. M., Vallee J. N., Lo D., Barrera-Ramirez C. F., *et al.* Brain magnetic resonance imaging findings in patients with mitochondrial cytopathies. *Arch Neurol*, 2005. **62**:737–42.

128. Anglin R., Mazurek M. F., Noseworthy M., *et al.* The psychiatric profile of mitochondrial disorders: clinical presentation and MR spectroscopy findings. *Society for Neuroscience Annual Meeting*, San Diego, November 2007.

129. Fattal O., Budur K., Vaughan A. J., *et al.* Review of the Literature on Major Mental Disorders in Adult Patients with Mitochondrial Diseases. *Psychosomatics*, 2006. **47**:1–7.

130. Ahn M. S., Sims K. B., Frazier J. A. Risperidone-induced psychosis and depression in a child with a mitochondrial disorder. *J Child Adolesc Psychopharmacol*, 2005. **15**:520–5.

131. Apostolova L. G., White M., Moore S. A., *et al.* Deep white matter pathologic features in watershed regions: a novel of central nervous system involvement in MELAS. *Arch Neurol*, 2005. **62**:1154–6.

132. Ban S., Mori N., Saito K., *et al.* An autopsy case of mitochondrial encephalomyopathy (MELAS) with special reference to extra-neuromuscular abnormalities. *Acta Pathol Jpn*, 1992. **42**:818–25.

133. Clark J. M., Marks M. P., Adalsteinsson E., *et al.* MELAS: Clinical and pathologic correlations with MRI, xenon/CT, and MR spectroscopy. *Neurology*, 1996. **46**:223–7.

134. Campos Y., Garcia A., Eiris J., *et al.* Mitochondrial myopathy, cardiomyopathy and psychiatric illness in a Spanish family harbouring the mtDNA 3303C>T mutation. *J Inherit Metab Dis*, 2001. **24**:685–7.

135. Desnuelle C., Pellissier J. F., Serratrice G., *et al.* Kearns-Sayre syndrome: mitochondrial encephalomyopathy caused by deficiency of the repiratory chain. *Rev Neurol*, 1989. **145**:842–50.

136. Prayson R. A., Wang N. Mitochondrial myopathy, encephalopathy, lactic acidosis, and strokelike episodes (MELAS) syndrome: an autopsy report. *Arch Pathol Lab Med*, 1998. **122**:978–81.

137. Sartor H., Loose R., Tucha O., *et al.* MELAS: a neuropsychological and radiological follow-up study. Mitochondrial encephalo-myopathy, lactic acidosis and stroke. *Acta Neurol Scand*, 2002. **106**:309–13.

138. Lacey C. J., Salzberg M. R. Obsessive-compulsive disorder with mitochondrial disease *Psychosomatics*, 2008. **49**:540–2.

139. Chinnery P., Majamaa K., Turnbull D., *et al.* Treatment for mitochondrial disorders. *Cochrane Database Syst Rev*, 2006. 1:CD004426.

140. Brockmann K., Dechent P., Wilken B., *et al.* Proton MRS profile of cerebral metabolic abnormalities in Krabbe disease. *Neurology*, 2003. **60**:819–25.

141. Suzuki K. Twenty five years of the "Psychosine Hypothesis": a personal perspective of its history

and present status. *Neurochem Res*, 1998. **23**:251–9.

142. Suzuki K., Suzuki Y., Suzuki K. (1995). Galactosylceramide lipidosis: globoid-cell leukodystrophy (Krabbe disease). In *The Metabolic Basis of Inherited Disease*, Scriver C. R., Beaudet A. L., Sly W. S., *et al.* (Eds.). Eighth Ed., vol 2. New York: McGraw-Hill, pp. 2671–92.

143. Husain A. M., Altuwaijri M., Aldosari M. Krabbe disease: neurophysiologic studies and MRI correlations. *Neurology*, 2004. **63**:617–20.

144. Lyon G., Hagberg B., Evrard P., *et al.* Symptomatology of late onset Krabbe's leukodystrophy: the European experience. *Dev Neurosci*, 1991. **13**(4–5): 240–4.

145. Escolar M. L., Poe M. D., Provenzale J. M., *et al.* Transplantation of umbilical-cord blood in babies with infantile Krabbe's disease. *N Eng J Med*, 2005. **352**:2069–81.

146. Krivit W., Shapiro E. G., Peters C., *et al.* Hematopoietic stem-cell transplantation in globoid-cell leukodystrophy. *N Eng J Med*, 1998. **338**:1119–26.

147. Koeppen A. H. A brief history of Pelizaeus-Merzbacher disease and proteolipid protein. *J Neurol Sci*, 2005. **228**:198–200.

148. Koeppen A. H., Robitaille Y. Pelizaeus-Merzbacher disease. *J Neuropathol Exp Neurol*, 2002. **61**:747–59.

149. Sasaki A., Miyanaga K., Ototsuji M., *et al.* Two autopsy cases with Pelizaeus-Merzbacher disease phenotype of adult onset, without mutation of proteolipid protein gene. *Acta Neuropathol*, 2000. **99**:7–13.

150. Moghadasian M. H., Salen G., Frohlich J. J., *et al.* Cerebrotendinous xanthomatosis: a rare disease with diverse manifestations. *Arch Neurol*, 2002. **59**:527–9.

151. Moghadasian M. H. Cerebrotendinous xanthomatosis: clinical course, genotypes and metabolic backgrounds. *Clin Invest Med*, 2004. **27**:42–50.

152. Berginer V. M., Foster N. L., Sadowsky M., *et al.* Psychiatric disorders in patients with cerebrotendinous xanthomatosis. *Am J Psychiatry*, 1988. **145**:354–7.

153. Brenner M., Johnson A. B., Boespflug-Tanguy O., *et al.* Mutations in GFAP, encoding glial fibrillary acidic protein, are associated with Alexander disease. *Nat Genet*, 2001. **27**:117–20.

154. Berger J., Moser H. W., Forss-Petter S. Leukodystrophies: recent developments in genetics, molecular biology, pathogenesis and treatment. *Curr Opin Neurol*, 2001. **14**:305–12.

155. Paloneva J., Kestila M., Wu J., *et al.* Loss-of-function mutations in TYROBP (DAP12) result in a presenile dementia with bone cyst. *Nat Genet*, 2000. **25**:357–61.

156. Araki T., Ohba H., Monzawa S., *et al.* Membranous lipodystrophy: MR imaging appearance of the brain. *Radiology*, 1991. **180**:793–7.

157. Maurer I., Moller H. G. Inhibition of complex 1 by neuroleptics in normal human brain cortex parallels the extrapyramidal toxicity of neuroleptics. *Mol Cell Biochem*, 1997. **174**:255–9.

158. Burkhardt C., Kelly J. P., Lim Y., *et al.* Neuroleptic medications inhibit complex I of the electron transport chain. *Ann Neurol*, 1993. **33**:512–17.

159. Lullman H., Lullman-Ranch R., Wassermann D. Lipidosis induced by amphiphilic cationic drugs. *Biochem Pharmacol*, 1978. **27**:1103–8.

160. Shapiro B. E., Hatters-Friedman S., Fernandes-Filho J. A., *et al.* Late-onset Tay-Sachs disease: adverse effects of medications and implications for treatment. *Neurology*, 2006. **67**: 875–7.

161. MacQueen G. M., Rosebush P. I., Mazurek M. F. Neuropsychiatric aspects of the adult-onset variant of Tay-Sachs disease. *J Neuropsychiatry Clin Neurosci*, 1998. **10**:10–19.

162. Neustadt J., Pieczenik S. R. Medication-induced mitochondrial damage and disease. *Mol Nutr Food Re*, 2008. **52**:780–8.

163. Pacia S. V., Devinsky O. Clozapine-related seizures: experience with 5,629 patients. *Neurology*, 1994. **44**:2247–9.

164. Sevin C., Aubourg P., Cartier N. Enzyme, cell and gene based therapies for metachromatic leukodystrophy. *J Inherit Metab Dis*, 2007. **30**:175–83.

Normal pressure hydrocephalus

Julian Trollor

Facts box

- Normal pressure hydrocephalus (NPH) presents as a progressive syndrome of gait disturbance, impaired cognition, and loss of bladder control.
- Noncognitive psychiatric and behavioral manifestations of NPH appear common but have not been systematically studied.
- A number of reports suggest that NPH can induce schizophrenia-like symptoms, and these appear more likely in cases of secondary NPH.
- Case reports indicate that when presenting as a manifestation of NPH, psychotic symptoms may improve with appropriate surgical management of NPH.
- There is potential for delayed recognition of NPH in situations where psychiatric and behavioral symptoms dominate the presentation.
- The pathogenesis of psychotic symptoms in NPH has not been examined but symptoms are assumed to arise in part from the impact of NPH on fronto-subcortical and basal forebrain networks.

Introduction

The capacity of normal pressure hydrocephalus (NPH) to induce a reversible dementia syndrome is well known. There is a less well-defined relationship between NPH and schizophrenia-like psychosis. Although evidence supporting a link between the two disorders is limited, available data supports an association. The specificity of the relationship between the two disorders is, however, confounded by the impact of etiological factors intrinsic to NPH itself. These factors may in themselves contribute vulnerability to psychotic disorder, and their effects on brain function

cannot be easily separated out from the impact of NPH alone.

History of the association

The father of medicine, Hippocrates (460–370 BC), first coined the term "hydrocephalus" but believed it to be a manifestation of fluid collection external to the brain. This thinking dominated the approach of our physician ancestors for the next 1,000 years, until the description of infantile hydrocephalus by the founder of surgery, Abul Qasim Al-Zahravi, also known as Albucasis (AD 936–1013). More recently, hydrocephalus has been divided broadly into three key categories, relating to disorders of cerebrospinal fluid production, circulation, and absorption. Although the precise mechanism underpinning the development of NPH is obscure in many cases, NPH is generally included in the latter group. It is further classified as either primary (idiopathic), or secondary (most commonly following intracranial hemorrhage, infection, or trauma). Hakim and Adams' [1] original description of the clinical presentation and surgical treatment of NPH began a focus on the classical triad of symptoms that continues to the present day. However, this narrow focus has meant that other aspects of the disorder, including broader psychiatric and behavioral aspects, have largely been ignored.

Schizophrenia and ventricular enlargement

Schizophrenia has a long-established association with ventricular enlargement. To the contemporary reader, the distinction between schizophrenia and NPH is clear. However, historically this boundary has not always been so well defined. Early air encephalographic studies of patients had shown an association between schizophrenia and enlargement of the ventricular system [2]. Later, the clinical triad of gait disturbance, incontinence, and dementia associated with NPH was described [1], as was the favorable response to insertion of a ventricular shunt [3]. An association between schizophrenia and ventricular enlargement was later confirmed by computerized tomography studies [4, 5]. However, the significance of the ventricular enlargement to the pathophysiology of schizophrenia remained uncertain. Nyback and colleagues [6] postulated an association between acute schizophrenic psychoses and disturbance in cerebrospinal fluid (CSF) circulation. The observation of abnormal CSF flows in 10 of 30 patients with schizophrenia studied using isotope cysternography [7] threatened to confuse the distinction between hydrocephalus per se and ventricular enlargement associated with schizophrenia. This was further compounded by the early reports of a favorable response to shunting observed in some individuals with both psychotic symptoms and NPH [8] or aqueduct stenosis [9]. However, with time and further clarification of the concepts, the distinction between subtle, nonprogressive ventricular enlargement seen in association schizophrenia and that observed in NPH became more apparent.

Clinical presentation of normal pressure hydrocephalus

Normal pressure hydrocephalus is considered the "quintessential" reversible dementia and is characterized by the clinical triad of gait disturbance, incontinence, and dementia [1]. A number of behavioral and psychiatric symptoms have been observed accompanying, or preceding NPH diagnosis. These include aggression [10], affective disorders including depression [11] and mania [12], and schizophreniform psychosis [8]. However, systematic study of the range of behavioral and psychiatric manifestations of NPH has not yet been undertaken.

A number of barriers to effective assessment and treatment of NPH exist. These include a lack of consensus on assessment methods, lack of systematic data on prevalence and treatment outcomes, variability in clinical presentation, and disparity of clinician approach in diagnosis and treatment. Evidence-based guidelines for classification of probable and possible idiopathic NPH have been proposed [13] and encompass specific aspects of history (including insidious onset with progression of symptoms with time in individuals over 40 years of age, minimum symptoms duration 3 months, no clear antecedent, and no alternative medical or psy-

chiatric causation); brain imaging findings (including computerized tomography or MRI of the brain demonstrating ventricular enlargement without evidence of CSF obstruction), and clinical findings (gait or balance disturbance plus either disturbed cognition or incontinence). With the removal of the specific exclusion clause for antecedent events, these criteria could also provide a guide for diagnosis in secondary NPH. Behavioral and personality changes are noted in this diagnostic system but are de-emphasized by their inclusion under cognitive manifestations.

Schizophrenia-like psychosis and hydrocephalus

A small literature exists in which hydrocephalus appears associated with symptoms of schizophrenia. A distinction appears in the literature between individuals with stenosis of the Sylvian aqueduct and those with NPH. Non-tumoral stenosis of the aqueduct usually presents in infancy or childhood, where it may be associated with specific genetic syndromes [14], perinatal insult, or developmental anomaly. Less commonly, aqueduct stenosis may present in early adulthood [9]. Psychotic symptoms have been reported in individuals with aqueduct stenosis [9, 15, 16, 17]. For some adult patients, the presentation with psychotic symptoms may be the trigger for the discovery of previously occult aqueduct stenosis [9]. The distinction of the latter cases from NPH is clear where, in retrospect, a neurodevelopmental insult or delayed developmental trajectory suggests decompensation of longstanding compensated occult hydrocephalus. However, in other situations, the distinction of cases of late aqueduct stenosis from NPH may be less clear. It has been proposed that aqueduct stenosis could occur as a late consequence of a communicating hydrocephalus such as NPH [18]. Smith [19] summarized the possible mechanisms that could relate to mechanical compression of the midbrain as the ventricular system expands [20] or proliferative gliosis of the aqueduct [21].

There are a small number of reported cases of psychotic symptoms arising in the context of idiopathic [8, 11, 22, 23, 24] and secondary [8, 10, 22, 25, 26] NPH in the literature. The temporal association between psychotic symptoms and clinical signs of NPH is remarkably variable in these case reports. A clear temporal relationship between onset of psychosis and classical signs and symptoms of NPH is more likely to reflect a specific association between the two disorders. Of particular interest are cases in which psychotic symptoms are a close antecedent to definitive manifestations of NPH [10, 22, 23, 26]. The complete elimination of psychotic symptoms with shunting in these cases also argues for a specific etiological contribution of NPH to psychosis. However, in a number of cases the specificity of the association is clouded by other vulnerability factors for psychosis, including recent traumatic brain injury [10, 26]. With few exceptions [23], there is very limited data to suggest idiopathic NPH as a clear and immediate precipitant of psychotic symptoms. This suggests that in the absence of other vulnerability factors, idiopathic NPH is rarely associated with psychotic symptoms.

In contrast to the above, cases have been reported in which psychotic symptoms precede obvious clinical signs and symptoms of NPH by many months [11], or even years [8]. The long lag between onset of psychosis and definitive signs of NPH in some of these cases would suggest it was unlikely that the psychotic symptoms experienced were a direct manifestation of hydrocephalus. However, both authors report resolution of psychotic symptoms with appropriate surgical management of NPH, suggesting at least a permissive role of emerging NPH in production of psychotic symptoms. Schizophrenia-like psychosis may arise decades after identification of NPH [27]. Such cases are atypical and, in this setting, the two disorders are less likely to be specifically associated.

Amelioration of psychotic symptoms following ventricular shunting for NPH has been reported in a number of contexts, including where both a short and a long delay is noted between onset of psychosis and obvious manifestations of NPH. Although case reports lack detail, the time course of improvement of psychosis following shunting for NPH is generally swift, and in most cases mirrors resolution of core symptoms of NPH [8, 11, 23, 26]. In the absence of surgical intervention (for example where hydrocephalus is said to be "compensated") positive response of psychotic symptoms to antipsychotic treatment has been reported [27]. The long-term outcome of psychotic symptoms following successful shunting for NPH is unknown.

Delayed or missed diagnoses

Delay in diagnosis of NPH has been reported in situations where psychotic symptoms have preceded classical signs and symptoms of NPH [11]. Given the clinical implications of delayed diagnosis of NPH, it is important to examine the possible contributors to this phenomenon. Motor and cognitive manifestations of NPH may be misattributed as side effects of neuroleptic treatment. Cognitive deterioration may be attributed solely to other physical treatments (such as electroconvulsive therapy). Other physical manifestations such as bladder instability or neurological signs may not be so readily assessed in the context of treatment within a psychiatric facility. However, the accessibility of neuroimaging facilities, and their almost routine use in first-episode psychosis mean that the majority of patients with close temporal association between NPH and psychotic symptoms can be readily identified. Because the likelihood of NPH rises with advancing age, it is particularly important that clinicians be aware of the manifestations of NPH in those presenting with an index episode of psychiatric disorder later in life. In those with chronic mental disorders, NPH may be suggested by a change in clinical presentation associated with abnormality of gait, cognitive disturbance, or incontinence.

Pathogenesis of psychotic symptoms in normal pressure hydrocephalus

NPH is a syndrome dominated by subcortical and basal forebrain impairments that appear to arise as a direct consequence of the compressive effects of ventricular expansion. Neuropsychological testing of individuals with NPH most commonly reveals slowed information processing, reduced psychomotor speed, and a "frontal" pattern of memory dysfunction characterized by reduced retrieval efficiency [28, 29, 30]. Variable patterns of CBF deficits have been reported, the most prominent of these being reduction in thalamic and basal ganglia CBF, which is reversed following successful surgical intervention [31]. The precise mechanism of development of psychotic symptoms in NPH is unclear but is likely to relate to impairment of subcortical and basal forebrain circuits. Psychotic symptoms are seen in a wide variety of "subcortical" disorders [32], including vascular dementia [33] and multiple sclerosis [34]. Furthermore, subcortical [35] and basal forebrain [36] regions are considered pivotal regions in the pathogenesis of schizophrenia. The manifestation of psychosis in only a small proportion of NPH cases suggests that NPH itself is one of many variables influencing the development of psychosis. It is likely that the manifestation of such symptoms is itself an end manifestation of an inter-action of a number of genetic, environmental, and medical variables in any given case. In support of this notion, the limited literature available suggests psychosis and NPH are more likely to coexist in cases of secondary NPH.

Summary and conclusions

Despite the long recognized presentation of NPH with cognitive symptoms, other behavioral and psychiatric manifestations of the disorder have been relatively neglected. Schizophrenia-like symptoms have been reported in association with NPH, most commonly with secondary NPH. However, the unique contribution of NPH to psychotic symptoms is difficult to establish in the latter group because of the presence of potentially shared antecedents for both disorders. Various temporal relationships have been reported between psychotic symptoms and definitive manifestations of NPH. Although there are case reports of improvement in psychotic symptoms following surgical treatment of NPH, predictors of improvement in psychosis remain unclear, and the long-term outcome of individuals so treated has not been reported. Clinician vigilance is required in order to minimize the likelihood of delayed or missed NPH diagnoses in cases where the initial presentation is with psychiatric or behavioral symptoms. The knowledge in this area would be augmented by large studies that include detailed evaluation of behavioral and psychiatric symptoms.

References

1. Hakim S., Adams R. D. The special clinical problem of symptomatic hydrocephalus with normal cerebrospinal fluid pressure. Observations on cerebrospinal fluid hydrodynamics. *J Neurol Sci*, 1965. Jul–Aug. **2**(4):307–27.

2. Jacobi W., Winkler H. Encephalograpische Studien am chronisch Schizophrenen. *Arch Psychiat Nervenkr*, 1927. **81**:299–332.

3. Adams R. D., Fisher C. M., Hakim S., *et al.* Symptomatic occult hydrocephalus with "normal" cerebrospinal-fluid pressure a treatable syndrome. *New Engl J Med*, 1965. **273**:117–26.

4. Johnstone E. C., Crow T. J., Frith C. D., *et al.* Cerebral ventricular size and cognitive impairment in chronic schizophrenia. *Lancet*, 1976. **2**(7992):924–6.

5. Weinberger D. R., Torrey E. F., Neophytides A. N., *et al.* Lateral cerebral ventricular enlargement in chronic schizophrenia. *Arch Gen Psychiatry*, 1979. **36**(7):735–9.

6. Nyback H., Wiesel F. A., Berggren B. M., *et al.* Computed tomography of the brain in patients with acute psychosis and in healthy volunteers. *Acta Psychiatr Scand*, 1982. **65**(6):403–14.

7. Oxenstierna G., Bergstrand G., Bjerkenstedt L., *et al.* Evidence of disturbed CSF circulation and brain atrophy in cases of schizophrenic psychosis. *Br J Psychiatry*, 1984. **144**:654–61.

8. Lying-Tunell U. Psychotic symptoms in normal-pressure hydrocephalus. *Acta Psychiatr Scand*, 1979. **59**(4):415–9.

9. Roberts J. K., Trimble M. R., Robertson M. Schizophrenic psychosis associated with aqueduct stenosis in adults. *J Neurol Neurosurg Psychiatry*, 1983. **46**(10):892–8.

10. Crowell R. M., Tew J. M., Jr., Mark V. H. Aggressive dementia associated with normal pressure hydrocephalus. Report of two unusual cases. *Neurology*, 1973. **23**(5):461–4.

11. Price T. R., Tucker G. J. Psychiatric and behavioral manifestations of normal pressure hydrocephalus. A case report and brief review. *J Nerv Ment Disease*, 1977. **164**(1):51–5.

12. Thienhaus O. J., Khosla N. Meningeal cryptococcosis misdiagnosed as a manic episode. *Am J Psychiatry*, 1984. **141**(11): 1459–60.

13. Relkin N., Marmarou A., Klinge P., *et al.* Diagnosing idiopathic normal-pressure hydrocephalus. *Neurosurgery*, 2005. **57**(3 Suppl): S4–16; ii–v.

14. Zhang J., Williams M. A., Rigamonti D. Genetics of human hydrocephalus. *J Neurol*, 2006. **253**(10):1255–66.

15. Reveley A. M., Reveley M. A. Aqueduct stenosis and schizophrenia. *J Neurol Neurosurg Psychiatry*, 1983. **46**(1):18–22.

16. Smith K. H. Aqueduct stenosis and schizophrenia. *Austr & NZ J Psychiatry*, 1990. Jun. **24**(2):158.

17. O'Flaithbheartaigh S., Williams P. A., Jones G. H. Schizophrenic psychosis and associated aqueduct stenosis. *Br J Psychiatry*, 1994. **164**(5):684–6.

18. Borit A. Communicating hydrocephalus causing aqueductal stenosis. *Neuropaediatrie*, 1976. **7**(4):416–22.

19. Smith K. H. Aqueduct stenosis and schizophrenia. *Austr NZ J Psychiatry*, 1990. **24**(2):158–64.

20. Nugent G. R., Al-Mefty O., Chou S. Communicating hydrocephalus as a cause of aqueductal stenosis. *J Neurosurg*, 1979. Dec. **51**(6): 812–8.

21. Vanneste J., Hyman R. Non-tumoural aqueduct stenosis and normal pressure hydrocephalus in the elderly. *J Neurol Neurosurg Psychiatry*, 1986. **49**(5):529–35.

22. Bret P., Chazal J. Chronic ("normal pressure") hydrocephalus in childhood and adolescence. A review of 16 cases and reappraisal of the syndrome. *Childs Nerv Syst*, 1995. **11**(12):687–91.

23. Pinner G., Johnson H., Bouman W. P., *et al.* Psychiatric manifestations of normal-pressure hydrocephalus: a short review and unusual case. *Int Psychogeriatrics*, 1997. **9**(4):465–70.

24. Larsson A., Stephensen H., Wikkelso C. Adult patients with "asymptomatic" and "compensated" hydrocephalus benefit from surgery. *Acta Neurol Scand*, 1999. **99**(2):81–90.

25. Kaiser G. L., Burke C. E. Schizophrenia like syndrome following chronic hydrocephalus in a teenager. *Eur J Pediatr Surg*, 1996. **6**(Suppl 1):39–40.

26. Bloom K. K., Kraft W. A. Paranoia – an unusual presentation of hydrocephalus. *Am J Phys Med Rehabil*, 1998. **77**(2):157–9.

27. Alao A. O., Naprawa S. A. Psychiatric complications of hydrocephalus. *Intl J Psychiatry Med*, 2001. **31**(3):337–40.

28. Ogino A., Kazui H., Miyoshi N., *et al.* Cognitive impairment in patients with idiopathic normal pressure hydrocephalus. *Dement Geriatr Cogn Disord*, 2006. **21**(2):113–9.

29. Raftopoulos C., Deleval J., Chaskis C., *et al.* Cognitive recovery in idiopathic normal pressure hydrocephalus: a prospective study. *Neurosurgery*, 1994. **35**(3):397–404; discussion 404–5.

30. Thomas G., McGirt M. J., Woodworth G., *et al.* Baseline neuropsychological profile and cognitive response to cerebrospinal fluid shunting for idiopathic normal pressure

hydrocephalus. *Dement Geriatr Cogn Disord*, 2005. **20**(2–3): 163–8.

31. Takeuchi T., Goto H., Izaki K., *et al.* Pathophysiology of cerebral circulatory disorders in idiopathic normal pressure hydrocephalus. *Neurol Med Chir (Tokyo)*, 2007. **47**(7):299–306; discussion.

32. Walterfang M., Wood S. J., Velakoulis D., *et al.* Diseases of white matter and schizophrenia-

like psychosis. *Aust NZ J Psychiatry*, 2005. **39**(9): 746–56.

33. Ballard C., Neill D., O'Brien J., *et al.* Anxiety, depression and psychosis in vascular dementia: prevalence and associations. *J Affect Disord*, 2000. **59**(2):97–106.

34. Feinstein A., du Boulay G., Ron M. A. Psychotic illness in multiple sclerosis. A clinical and magnetic

resonance imaging study. (See comment.) *Br J Psychiatry*, 1992. **161**:680–5.

35. Middleton F. A., Strick P. L. Basal ganglia and cerebellar loops: motor and cognitive circuits. *Brain Res Rev*, 2000. **31**(2–3):236–50.

36. Heimer L. Basal forebrain in the context of schizophrenia. *Brain Res Rev*, 2000. **31**(2–3): 205–35.

20 Brain tumors

Malcolm Hopwood and Lyn-May Lim

Facts box

- Although rare, psychosis secondary to brain tumors, including as the primary presentation, is well recognized.
- The prevalence of brain tumors in psychiatric patients is about 3% (range 1.7%–13.5%) from autopsy series, relative to 1% to 1.5% in the general population.
- The presentation may be indistinguishable from primary schizophrenia, or more typically involve nonauditory hallucinations, neurological signs, and prominent cognitive impairment.
- Tumors presenting with psychotic symptoms are most likely to be in the frontal or temporal lobes or in the pituitary.
- The most common association is with low-grade, slow-growing tumors such as meningiomas and low-grade gliomas.
- Treatment directed at the tumors, such as the use of steroids, may sometimes provoke psychotic symptoms.
- It is important for psychiatrists to be "brain-tumor conscious."

Introduction

Brain tumors most commonly present with features of raised intracranial pressure, focal neurological signs, or seizures [1]. However, the earliest manifestation of some intracranial tumors may consist of psychiatric symptoms or behavioral disturbance alone [2]. More specifically, psychosis may be the sole presenting feature, increasing the likelihood of such patients coming to the attention of a psychiatrist. Although psychosis secondary to brain tumor is relatively rare [3], this subgroup is at risk of misdiagnosis and delayed treatment, potentially resulting in increased morbidity and mortality. A 30-year retrospective study of psychi-atric inpatients [4] showed that the diagnosis of brain tumor was usually made only after the presence of definite neurological symptoms with the presenting psychotic symptoms in the majority presumed to be due to a functional disorder. McIntyre [3] has emphasized the need for psychiatrists to be more "brain-tumor conscious."

Despite the high prevalence of psychiatric symptomatology in patients with brain tumors, the prevalence of brain tumors in psychiatric patients is only about 3% as compiled from autopsy series from psychiatric hospitals [5]. In fact, the existing literature is inconsistent as to whether the prevalence of brain tumors is greater among psychiatric or general hospital patients [6]. Nonetheless, the presence of a brain tumor in this group of patients with an established psychotic disorder appears to be important to recognize given its potential to confound the presentation, management, and outcome of the primary psychotic disorder.

Definitions and diagnostic criteria

Tumor classification

Brain tumors may be classified according to whether they are primary or metastatic or according to their neuroanatomical site or histopathology. Primary tumors comprise about 80% of these, whereas metastatic tumors contribute to the remaining 20% [7]. Seventy percent of all intracranial tumors are located supratentorially, with most situated in the posterior fossa and temporal and frontal lobes [7].

The commonest primary tumors are gliomas with meningiomas; pituitary adenomas are the next most frequent [7]. Low-grade gliomas (grade I–II) are slow growing and generally benign whereas glioblastomas (grade IV) are rapidly growing and aggressive [1]. Metastases occur most frequently secondary to primary lesions in the lung and breast [7]. Brain metastases, especially if multiple, are associated with a poor prognosis with average survival rates between 1 to 2 years [7].

Diagnostic criteria

Psychosis secondary to brain tumor is included within the broader classification of "psychosis due to a general medical condition" according to the Diagnostic and Statistical Manual of Mental Disorders (DSMMD) [8]. This stipulates that psychotic symptoms must be identified as a direct physiologic consequence of the medical condition. The challenge emerges in demonstrating this causality in the context of confounding factors such as the presence of a pre-existing psychiatric or neurodegenerative condition and specific treatment for the brain tumor (e.g., steroids, radiotherapy). This diagnosis necessitates the exclusion of a primary psychotic disorder, substance-induced psychosis, dementia, and delirium as better diagnoses to account for the psychotic symptoms. The clinical features of the psychoses concerned are similar to the research diagnostic criteria for schizophrenia proposed by Spitzer and colleagues [9].

More broadly, psychosis secondary to a brain tumor has been accepted as an "organic psychosis," as opposed to a "functional psychosis" [10]. However, the term "organic" is problematic as it implies the presence of "identifiable structural brain disease or toxic-metabolic brain dysfunction," which has been shown to be the case in schizophrenia also. Hence, the most recent alternative classification proposes "primary and secondary schizophrenias" [11].

Epidemiology

The prevalence of intracranial tumors associated with psychiatric symptoms is difficult to estimate, with the existing literature yielding inconsistent findings. There are a number of methodological problems with many of the studies, including the high variability and poor sensitivity of screening methods. The nature of the populations studied has been highly variable (e.g., autopsy vs. living patients, psychiatric vs. general hospital patients). Furthermore, the conceptualization of both psychiatric and neurological illnesses has changed over the period these studies have been done. Older studies were more likely to combine all brain lesions associated with mental symptoms, including those of nonneoplastic etiology such as subdural hematomas and infectious lesions. The characterization of psychotic symptoms was also variable, with older studies often grouping together psychotic, affective, and acutely confused states.

With most studies adopting a retrospective study design, it has been difficult to establish causality between brain tumors and psychotic symptoms. Autopsy studies have typically not differentiated between brain tumors producing psychiatric symptoms and tumors developing in patients with pre-existing psychiatric illness, increasing the likelihood that a coincidental finding may be misattributed as causation.

Despite the limitations of the existing epidemiological data, some general conclusions may be drawn from the heterogeneous case material.

The prevalence of cerebral tumor in the general population is 0.16% [12], whereas the prevalence of intracranial tumors at autopsy is 1 to 1.5% [13]. This significant difference is presumably because many tumors remain neurologically silent throughout life and may only be discovered at autopsy. Despite some variation in figures, the prevalence of intracranial tumors in psychiatric patients is consistently reported to be higher. A review of nine mental hospital autopsy studies between 1909 and 1949 quoted figures of 1.7 to 11.2% [14], whereas other studies reported figures of up to 13.5% [15, 16].

In comparison, it is extremely common for patients with cerebral tumors to display psychiatric symptoms. The largest series of tumor patients studied by Keschner and colleagues [17] reported mental symptoms in 78% of 530 cases. However, very few studies solely reported the incidence of psychotic symptoms.

In their study of the literature, Lisanby and colleagues [6] found that tumors presenting with psychiatric symptoms tend to be more common among the elderly. The peak age of diagnosis was the seventh decade, with 27.6% of cases falling into this age range.

An excess of meningiomas in particular appear to be found in psychiatric patients compared to the general population in autopsy studies [18, 19]. Patton and Sheppard [18] found meningiomas constituted 33.2% of tumors in psychiatric hospitals compared with 13.7% in general hospitals. Rapidly progressive gliomas are more likely to present with focal neurological signs whereas slowly progressive meningiomas may be more likely to present with psychiatric symptoms in advance of any neurological signs. In a 5-year retrospective data analysis of benign brain tumors, Gupta and colleagues [20] found 21% of meningioma cases presented with psychiatric symptoms in the absence of neurological symptoms.

Clinical manifestations

Association with tumor location and laterality

The significance of tumor location in relation to mental symptoms has been much debated. Although tumors in many areas have been implicated in the causation of psychosis, no areas, when lesioned, have reliably produced psychotic symptoms [21].

Psychosis has been reported to be associated with intracranial tumors in a wide variety of locations, including the temporal lobes [22, 23, 24, 25, 26, 27, 28, 29, 30, 31], frontal lobes [31, 32], suprasellar region [26, 28, 31, 33], diencephalons [25, 26, 34, 35, 36, 37, 38, 39, 40, 41], corpus callosum [22], pituitary [3, 26, 28, 31, 42], and posterior fossa [22, 43].

Frontal- and temporal-lobe tumors have consistently shown a higher incidence of psychiatric disturbance compared with parietal, occipital, and infratentorial tumors [2, 17, 25, 26, 44, 45]. More specifically, psychosis is most common with tumors affecting temporal lobe and limbic structures [21, 46]. Mulder and Daly [23] reported that 20% of tumors affecting the temporal lobes were associated with schizophrenia-like psychosis. In a series by Malamud [25], schizophrenia-like psychosis was found to be associated with tumors in the hippocampus, amygdalae, and cingulate gyrus. Davison and Bagley [26] found that schizophrenia was significantly associated with pituitary tumors and that temporal lobe and suprasellar tumors were specifically associated with hallucinations.

In terms of laterality, case reports, although not larger series, show a preponderance of left limbic tumors [27, 29]. Some of these reports have suggested that psychosis may remit when left-temporal tumors have been excised.

Association with tumor type

There is no consistent evidence to suggest that the histological type of the tumor is linked to the presence or nature of psychotic symptoms [6, 17]. Consistent with the above-quoted literature related to broader psychiatric symptomatology, early reports suggested that meningiomas produced neuropsychiatric symptoms more often than other tumors [3]. More recently, Davison and Bagley [26] specifically reviewed the literature on patients with psychosis secondary to brain tumors and found no predominance of one tumor type over another. Lishman [2] has suggested that meningiomas and low-grade gliomas are more likely to produce behavioral and psychiatric symptoms because of their slow-growing nature, which may delay earlier neurological signs. Mostly, however, it appears that tumor histology is less significant than other factors in determining the presence and nature of psychiatric symptoms.

Other tumor features influencing symptom formation

Price and colleagues [45] list the extent of tumor involvement, the rapidity of its growth, and the propensity to cause raised intracranial pressure as the most significant factors influencing symptom formation. Other reports, however, suggest increased intracranial pressure as less likely to be a consistent major factor [2, 28].

In addition, the patient's psychiatric history, level of functioning, premorbid personality, and coping mechanisms may contribute to the nature of an individual's response to a cerebral tumor and the development of psychotic symptoms [45]. These highly individual host factors may modify the psychiatric effects of an intracranial tumor wherever it is situated.

Nature of psychotic symptoms

Psychotic symptoms secondary to brain tumor may be indistinguishable from symptoms due to a functional psychotic disorder. In particular, patients with temporal lobe tumors have been noted to have a high frequency of schizophrenia-like psychotic features [23, 24, 25].

However, some general differences have been noted when comparing the psychotic symptoms secondary to brain tumor to those of schizophrenia. Cummings [47] emphasized that delusions secondary to brain tumor tend to be simpler in nature than the systematized delusions of schizophrenia [47]. These delusions are most commonly persecutory or paranoid in nature [6, 28]. Visual hallucinations are the commonest type of hallucination secondary to brain tumor, followed by auditory hallucinations [28]. This is in contrast to functional psychotic disorders where auditory hallucinations are the commonest. Visual hallucinations may be brief, unformed, and stereotypical or they may be complex and well formed. Auditory hallucinations may occur with temporal-lobe tumors and are usually simpler in nature, consisting of ringing, whistling, hissing, or buzzing noises [17]. Other types of hallucinations are rare, although there have been isolated reports of olfactory and tactile hallucinations [48, 49].

Formal thought disorder has not commonly been described in case series of psychosis secondary to brain tumor [24, 50], but there are isolated reports of cases with loosening of associations [34].

Catatonia is rarely caused by an underlying brain tumor, although rare cases have been reported [24, 51, 52, 53].

Other psychiatric symptoms may occur along with psychotic symptoms in the context of a brain tumor. These include depression [17, 50, 54, 55], mania [50, 56, 57, 58, 59], and personality changes [50, 54, 60, 61] and may predate the diagnosis of the tumor.

Diagnostic evaluation

Although a brain tumor remains a relatively rare cause of psychosis, some patients warrant a higher index of suspicion for this diagnosis. Psychiatrists require some awareness of the clinical features that may heighten the possibility of a brain tumor in order to guide their practice in determining an appropriate diagnostic workup for a suspected intracranial mass lesion.

History and examination

The yield of diagnostic evaluation is increased by careful history taking and a thorough physical examination, bearing in mind that the neurological examination may be entirely normal. Price and colleagues [45] suggest that the following clinical features in a known psychiatric patient or a patient with an index presentation of psychiatric symptoms should heighten the clinician's index of suspicion of a brain tumor:

1. Seizures, especially if new onset in an adult or if they are focal or partial seizures
2. Headaches, especially if new onset, generalized, and dull (i.e. nonspecific), of increasing severity and/or frequency, positional or nocturnal, or present immediately on awakening
3. Nausea and vomiting

4. Sensory changes, especially if visual
5. Other focal neurological signs and symptoms, such as localized weakness or sensory loss, ataxia, or incoordination

Many of these signs, however, occur in the later stages of a brain tumor and may not be evident, especially with "silent" indolent-growing tumors.

Older patients and those with late-onset psychosis require a higher index of suspicion as brain tumors occur more frequently in this group [6].

Neuroimaging

Computer tomography (CT) and MRI scans have largely replaced plain skull X-ray, electroencephalography (EEG), pneumoencephalography, echoencephalography, and radioisotope brain scans as the standard diagnostic tests to detect the presence of a brain tumor. Both CT and MRI provide greater resolution of anatomic brain structures and are able to distinguish normality from pathology.

The capacity of CT scans to detect neoplasms is increased by the use of intravenous contrast, enhancing the presence of such lesions. Other radiological features that may indicate the presence of a brain tumor include calcification, cerebral edema, obstructive hydrocephalus, and midline shift. CT scanning may fail to detect very small tumors, masses located in the posterior fossa, tumors that are isodense with respect to brain tissue, and tumors diffusely involving the meninges.

MRI is superior to CT scanning due to its higher resolution, greater sensitivity for detecting very small lesions, and lesser exposure to radiation for the patient; however, it is vastly more expensive and is contraindicated in patients with ferrometallic objects (e.g. pacemakers). Enhancement of tumor masses is possible with gadolinium.

Hollister and Boutros [62] reviewed the clinical use of CT and MRI scans in psychiatric patients, concluding that the onset of psychotic symptoms or personality change after the age of 50 years or the presence of focal neurological signs are sound indications for ordering one of these scans in a psychiatric patient.

Other

Given that noninvasive radiography has high sensitivity and specificity in detecting brain tumors, other more invasive tests have a minimal role in the investigation of a suspected brain tumor. A lumbar puncture may be done for other reasons and may be associated with a brain tumor if elevated cerebrospinal fluid (CSF) protein and increased intracranial pressure (ICP) are found, although these findings are nonspecific. Furthermore, in the presence of raised ICP, there is a risk of cerebral herniation following lumbar puncture and, hence, this is not recommended practice when a brain tumor is suspected.

The EEG in patients with brain tumors may show nonspecific abnormalities such as spikes and slow waves; however, in the majority, the EEG is reported as unremarkable. This investigation has poor sensitivity and specificity in detecting brain tumors but may have an important role in the evaluation of seizures associated with an intracranial tumor.

Neuropsychological testing may show localizing cognitive deficits but has a low diagnostic yield for identifying brain tumors. Such testing has a greater role in determining a baseline of tumor-associated cognitive dysfunction compared with serial test results in the post-treatment setting.

Interrelationships

Psychosis is a phenomenon with a variety of differing etiologies found in many conditions. Secondary presentations of psychosis may account for approximately 3% of new cases of schizophrenia [63]. Although secondary schizophrenias may sometimes be discernible from primary psychotic disorders [26, 64], many have clinically identical presentations [65]. Even though the terminology has changed, Ferraro [66] posed the conceptual dilemma that continues to plague psychiatrists: "What should our attitude be in the presence of organic cerebral changes found in cases clinically diagnosed as functional psychosis? Must we adhere to the concept that a diagnosis of schizophrenia is incompatible with the presence of cerebral pathology? Must we, every time that organic changes are found in the brain of a supposedly schizophrenia patient, change our diagnosis to one of organic psychosis simulating dementia praecox? Must we talk in such cases of schizophrenia-like condition? Must we, on the other hand, maintain the diagnosis of schizophrenia and qualify it as being precipitated by such and such organic disease?" This dilemma is perhaps most poignantly expressed in the patient with a diagnosis of schizophrenia in whom a slow-growing cerebral tumor is identified.

Current neuroanatomical models of schizophrenia propose that the etiology of psychosis relates to a "disconnectivity syndrome" with aberrant integration of complex, interdependent neural mechanisms underlying perception and cognition, in particular affecting limbic and other subcortical structures [67]. In a recent review of diseases of white matter and schizophrenia-like psychosis, Walterfang and colleagues [68] emphasize that diffuse, rather than discrete lesions, particularly in the fronto-temporal zones, have been most strongly associated with schizophrenia-like psychosis. The involvement of limbic and limbic-related areas is thought to be highly significant and may produce defective integration of perceptual information and its relevance [21]. Hence, it is not surprising that the preponderance of brain tumors contributing to psychosis is situated in the frontal and temporal lobes.

Focal lesions do not precisely define the neurotransmitters involved in psychosis but areas containing dopaminergic or cholinergic circuits are frequently involved [31, 69]. The dopaminergic/cholinergic balance may also be important in the genesis of psychosis [69].

Pituitary tumors often produce hormones; however, the similarity of psychiatric presentation of secretory and nonsecretory adenomas suggests that the intracerebral extension of the tumor may be more important than endocrine dysfunction in the induction of psychosis [60, 70].

Treatment of psychosis in setting of brain tumor

Literature guiding the treatment of psychosis in association with brain tumors is relatively sparse. In some cases, active medical and surgical treatment of the brain tumor will ameliorate the psychotic symptoms [6, 32, 33, 36, 39, 41, 55, 71, 72, 73] although it was not always clear if the patients were continued on psychotropic medication.

In other cases, psychotic symptoms persisted or even worsened despite treatment of the underlying brain tumor [3, 29, 40, 43]. Given the potential of these symptoms to cause subjective distress, functional impairment, and disability, it is important for these psychotic symptoms to be treated in their own right. The treatment of these psychiatric symptoms may enhance the patient's quality of life regardless of the curability of the tumor [57].

The psychopharmacological management of psychosis in patients with an intracerebral tumor follows the same general therapeutic principles that apply to tumor-free patients. Antipsychotic medications remain the cornerstone of treatment. Low-potency typical antipsychotics may produce significant anticholinergic side effects and potentiate the risk of delirium, while high-potency agents may result in unwanted extrapyramidal side effects. Although there is a paucity of controlled research on the efficacy of the newer atypical antipsychotics in the treatment of brain tumor patients, it is noteworthy that they have been reported to be effective in the treatment of psychosis associated with other neurological disorders [45]. Given their improved adverse effect profile, they may be considered in preference to typical antipsychotic agents. It is important to be cognizant of the need to "start low and go slow," especially given the therapeutically effective dose of antipsychotic is often lower than in the treatment of primary schizophrenia and also that brain tumor patients generally would appear to have a greater susceptibility to side effects of psychotropic medication. This is especially true of patients who are in the immediate postoperative period or are receiving chemotherapy or radiotherapy.

Although the focus of a separate chapter, it is worth noting that seizures secondary to a brain tumor may also be a contributing factor, or on occasion, the main factor leading to psychotic symptoms. The latter is most likely to be true in patients with partial seizures secondary to a temporal lobe tumor. Effective seizure treatment with anticonvulsant medication may thus be an effective treatment for psychotic symptoms in such a case. Given the high frequency of seizures in patients with high-grade tumors, it is also worthy to bear in mind the possible role of some anticonvulsants in the induction of psychotic symptoms.

Psychiatric complications may arise from specific treatment directed against the brain tumor. In particular, steroids used to control peritumor edema may result in psychosis. Psychotic symptoms may be a clinical manifestation of delirium resulting from chemotherapeutic agents, intracranial irradiation, or metabolic or electrolyte disturbances related to the cerebral tumor. In this case, the underlying cause of delirium needs to be identified and addressed.

Summary and conclusions

Brain tumors occur with greater frequency in individuals with mental illness than the general population and are an uncommon but important cause of secondary schizophrenia. The symptomatic presentation of psychosis associated with brain tumors appears to vary from those indistinguishable from primary schizophrenia to more typical "organic" presentations involving nonauditory hallucinations, neurological signs, and prominent cognitive impairment. The nature of brain tumors presenting with psychotic symptoms may vary markedly, but it would appear that tumors in frontal and temporal regions, together with the pituitary, are most frequently associated with psychosis. Presentations have been reported in association with increasing age and the presence of other neurological symptoms, but not exclusively so. The associated tumor type has varied greatly within reports. Rapidly growing, high-grade tumors appear more likely to present with other neurological features as well as psychosis. Probably more common is the association with low-grade, slow-growing tumors such as meningiomas. The nature of the etiological association in this setting is complex and, in the case of slow-growing tumors, possibly unclear.

Implications for clinical practice

The clinical implications of this association can be divided into those related to assessment and those related to management. The role of structural neuroimaging as a screening measure in patients presenting with psychosis remains controversial in some quarters. Specifically in relation to brain tumors, further investigation appears to be warranted in any patient presenting with the onset of psychosis later than the usual age range, in the presence of atypical features or other neurological symptoms, including persistent headache. However, relying on such indicators alone may result in the failure to diagnose some of the more slowly growing tumors such as meningiomas. Ultimately, the decision to utilize neuroimaging needs to take into account both the current presentation and all the possible organic factors contributing to the presentation. Equally important is the retention of clinical vigilance in the patient with established psychotic symptoms who now presents with a changed clinical picture.

The treatment literature available to clinicians specific to this setting is poor. Evidence relating to the influence of treatment of the underlying tumor on the psychotic symptoms is conflicting, probably reflecting the diversity of tumor types, tumor treatments, and other risk factors present in any given case. Treatment needs to be appropriately tailored given the likely higher sensitivity to side effects in this population. Careful consideration also must be given to the most appropriate locus of treatment – the presence of psychotic symptoms can cause great alarm on the neurosurgical ward and the presence of a patient with a brain tumor can equally cause great anxiety on the psychiatric unit!

Suggestions for future research

Future research in this area could usefully examine a number of issues. Although many previous studies have focused on the broad relationship between psychiatric symptomatology, including psychosis, and brain tumors, the literature is still relatively poor in examining the specifics of this relationship utilizing modern diagnostic criteria. A more precise epidemiologic survey would give clinicians more information on which to base their decisions to investigate and how to investigate looking for the presence of a brain tumor. This same methodology may provide more accurate understanding of the complexities of the relationship between brain tumors and psychosis, leading to hypothesis-driven exploration of the etiologic link. It would appear unlikely that a broad survey of this diverse area is likely to lead to greater understanding of how a tumor in an individual leads to psychosis. Finally, greater research into the treatment of psychosis in this setting is required. Although sufficient data to provide a full evidence base would be difficult to accumulate, greater direction to management is sorely needed. For patients and their families, the combination of psychosis and a brain tumor is likely to present unique emotional challenges – challenges clinicians would prefer to face armed with adequate information to assist in their response.

References

1. Brain W. (1985). Intracranial tumour. In *Brain's Clinical Neurology*, Bannister R. (Ed.). London: Oxford University Press. pp. 223–55.

2. Lishman W. (2004). Cerebral tumours. In *Organic Psychiatry: the Psychological Consequences of Cerebral Disorders*, Lishman W. (Ed.). Melbourne: Blackwell Scientific Publications, pp. 218–36.

3. McIntyre H., McIntyre A. The problem of brain tumour in psychiatric diagnosis. *Am J Psychiatry*, 1942. **98**:720–6.

4. Remington F., Rubert S. Why patients with brain tumours come to a psychiatric hospital: a thirty-year survey. *Am J Psychiatry*, 1962. **119**:256–7.

5. Yudovsky S., Hales R. (2002). *The American Psychiatric Publishing Textbook of Neuropsychiatry and Clinical Neurosciences*. 4th ed. Washington, DC: American Psychiatric Publishing Inc.

6. Lisanby S., *et al.* Psychosis secondary to brain tumour. *Semin Clinical Neuropsychiatry*, 1998. **3**(1):12–22.

7. Lohr J., Cadet J. (1987). Neuropsychiatric aspects of brain tumours. In *The American Psychiatric Press Textbook of Neuropsychiatry*, Talbott J., Hales R., and Yudovsky S. (Eds.). Washington, DC: American Psychiatric Press, p. 356.

8. American Psychiatric Association (2000). *Diagnostic and Statistical Manual of Mental Disorders*. IV Ed. Washington, DC: APA.

9. Spitzer R., Endicott J., Robins E. (1975). *Research Diagnostic Criteria*, Division B. 2nd ed. New York: New York State Psychiatric Institute.

10. Cummings J. Organic psychosis. *Psychosomatics*, 1996. **29**:16–26.

11. Hyde T., Lewis S. (2003). The secondary schizophrenias. In *Schizophrenia*, Weinberger D. (Ed.). Oxford: Blackwell Science, pp. 187–202.

12. Davis F., *et al.* Prevalence estimates for primary brain tumours in the United States by behaviour and major histology groups. *Neuro-oncology*, 2001. **3**(3):152–8.

13. Russell D., Rubinstein L. (1963). *Pathology of Tumours of the Nervous System*. 2nd ed. London: Arnold Publishers.

14. Waggoner R., Bagchi B. Initial masking of organic brain changes by psychic symptoms. *Am J Psychiatry*, 1954. **110**:904–10.

15. Klotz M. Incidence of brain tumours in patients hospitalized for chronic mental disorders. *Psychiatr Q*, 1957. **31**:669–80.

16. Larson C. Intracranial tumours in mental hospital patients. A statistical study. *Am J Psychiatry*, 1940. **97**:49–54.

17. Keschner M. Bender M., Strauss I. Mental symptoms associated with brain tumours. *JAMA*, 1938. **100**:714–8.

18. Patton R. Sheppard J. Intracranial tumours found at autopsy in mental patients. *Am Psychiatry*, 1956. **113**:319–24.

19. Raskin N. Intracranial neoplasms in psychotic patients. *Am J Psychiatry*, 1956. **112**:481–4.

20. Gupta R., Kumar R. Benign brain tumours and psychiatric morbidity: a 5 year retrospective data analysis. *Aust and NZ J Psychiatry*, 2004. **38**:316–9.

21. Edwards-Lee T., Cummings J. (2000). Focal lesions and psychosis, In *Behaviour and Mood Disorders in Focal Brain Lesions*, Bogovsslavsky J. and Cummings J. (Eds.). Cambridge: Cambridge University Press, pp. 419–36.

22. Adelstein L., Carter M. Psychosis: its importance as a presenting symptom of brain tumour. *Am J Psychiatry*, 1932. **12**:317–29.

23. Mulder D., Daly D. Psychiatric symptoms associated with lesions of temporal lobes. *JAMA*, 1952. **150**:173–6.

24. Selecki B. Intracranial space-occupying lesions among patients admitted to mental hospitals. *Med J Aust*, 1965. **1**:383–90.

25. Malamud N. Psychiatric disorders with intracranial tumours of limbic system. *Arch Neurol*, 1967. **17**:113–23.

26. Davison K., Bagley C. Schizophrenia-like psychosis associated with organic disorders of the central nervous system: review of the literature. *Br J Psychiatry*, 1969. **113**(Suppl 1):18–69.

27. Uribe V. Psychiatric symptoms and brain tumour. *Am Family Physician*, 1986. **34**:95–8.

28. Galasko D., Kwo-on-yuen P., Thal L. Intracranial mass lesions associated with late-onset psychosis and depression. *Psychiatr Clin North Am*, 1988. **11**:151–66.

29. Kan R., *et al.* A case of temporal lobe astrocytoma associated with epileptic seizures and schizophrenia-like psychosis. *J Psychiatr Neurol*, 1989. **43**(1): 97–103.

30. Roberts G., *et al.* A 'mock up' of schizophrenia: temporal lobe epilepsy and schizophrenia-like psychosis. *Biol Psychiatry*, 1990. **28**:127–43.

31. Stevens J. (1991). *Psychosis and the Temporal Lobe*, Smith D., Treiman D. and Trimble, M. (Eds.). Vol 55. New York: Raven Press.

32. Sato T., *et al.* Frontal lobe tumour associated with late-onset seizure and psychosis: a case report. *Jap J Psychiatry Neurol*, 1993. **47**(3): 541–4.

33. Mordecai D., *et al.* Case study: suprasellar germinoma presenting with psychotic and obsessive-compulsive symptoms.

J Am Acad Child Adolesc Psychiatry, 2000. **39**(1):116–9.

34. Buchanan D., Abram H. Psychotic behaviour resulting from a lateral ventricle meningioma: a case report. *Disease Nerv Syst*, 1975. **36**(7):400–1.

35. Cramond W. Organic Psychosis. *Br Med J*, 1968. **30**(4):561–4.

36. Okada F., Aida T., Abe H. Schizophrenic symptoms induced by a tumour of the left basal ganglia with ipsilateral cerebral hemiatrophy. *Ann Clin Psychiatry*, 1992. **4**(2):105–9.

37. Neuman E., *et al.* Schizophreniform catatonia on 6 cases secondary to hydrocephalus with subthalamic mesencephalic tumour associated with hypodopaminrgia. *Neuropsychobiology*, 1996. **34**(2):76–81.

38. Carson B., *et al.* Third ventricular choroid plexus papilloma with psychosis: case report. *J Neurosurg*. 1997. **87**(1):103–5.

39. Mahendran R. Intraventricular tumour (astrocytoma) associated with an organic psychosis (letter). *Can J Psychiatry*, 1998. **43**(4):423.

40. Izci Y., Karlidere T., Caliskan U. Diencephalic tumours presenting as psychosis. *Acta Neuro-psychiatrica*, 2003. **15**(2):97–101.

41. Ouma J. Psychotic manifestations in brain tumour patients: 2 case reports from South Africa. *Afr Health Science*, 2004. **4**(3):189–93.

42. Sandyk R., Bergsneider M., Iacono R. Acute psychosis in a woman with a prolactinoma. *Intl J Neurosci*, 1987. **37**(4):187–90.

43. Pollak L., *et al.* Posterior fossa lesions associated with neuropsychiatric symptoma-tology. *Intl J Neurosci*, 1996. **87**(3–4):119–26.

44. Davison K. Schizophrenia-like psychoses associated with organic cerebral lesions: a review. *Psychiatr Dev*, 1983. **1**:1–34.

45. Price T., Goetz K., Lovell M. (2002). Neuropsychiatric aspects of brain tumours. In *The American Psychiatry Publishing Textbook of Neuropsychiatry and Clinical Neurosciences*, Yudovsky S. and Hales R. (Eds.). Washington, DC: American Psychiatric Publishing Inc. pp. 753–81.

46. Jeste D., *et al.* (1996). Neuropsychiatric aspects of the schizophrenias. In *Neuro-psychiatry*, Fogel B., Schiffer R. and Rao S. (Eds.). Baltimore: Williams and Wilkins. pp. 325–44.

47. Cummings J. Organic delusions. *Br J Psychiatry*, 1985. **146**:184–97.

48. Howe J., Gibson J. Uncinate seizures and tumours, a myth re-examined. *Ann Neurol*, 1982. **12**:227.

49. Takeda M., Tamino S., Nishinuma K. A case of hypophyseal prolactinoma with treatable delusions of dermatozoiasis. *Acta Psychiatr Scand*, 1985. **72**:470–5.

50. Minski L. The mental symptoms associated with 58 cases of cerebral tumour. *J Neurol Psychopathology*, 1933. **13**:313–30.

51. Newmann M. Periventricular diffuse pinealoma. *J Nerv Ment Dis*, 1955. **121**:193–204.

52. Abrams R., Taylor M. Catatonia: a prospective clinical study. *Arch Gen Psychiatry*, 1976. **33**:579–81.

53. Gelenberg A. The catatonic syndrome. *Lancet*, 1976. **1**:1339–41.

54. Moersch F., Graig W., Kernohan J. W. Tumours of the brain in aged persons. *Arch Neurol Psychiatry*, 1941. **45**:235–45.

55. Carlson R. Frontal lobe lesions masquerading as psychiatric disturbances. *Can Psychiatr Assoc*, 1977. **22**:315–8.

56. Krauthammer C., Klerman G. Secondary mania. *Arch Gen Psychiatry*, 1978. **35**:1333–9.

57. Jamieson R., Wells C. Manic psychosis in a patient with multiple metastatic brain tumours. *J Clin Psychiatry*, 1979. **40**:280–3.

58. Greenberg D., Brown G. Mania resulting from brainstem tumour. *J Nerv Ment Disorders*, 1985. **173**:434–6.

59. Starkstein S., *et al.* Mania after brain injury. *Arch Neurol*, 1987. **44**:1069–73.

60. Bleuler M. Psychiatry of cerebral diseases. *Br Med J*, 1951. **24**:1233–8.

61. Mulder D., Swenson W. (1974). Psychologic and psychiatric aspects of brain tumours. In *Handbook of Clinical Neurology*, Vinken P., Buryn B. (Eds.). Elsevier: New York: pp. 727–40.

62. Hollister L., Boutros N. Clinical use of CT and MR scans in psychiatric patients. *J Psychiatr Neurosci*, 1991. **16**:194–8.

63. Lewis S. (1995). The secondary schizophrenias. In *Schizophrenia*, Weinberger D. (Ed.). Blackwell Science: Oxford.

64. Cutting J. The phenomenology of acute organic psychosis. Comparison with acute schizophrenia. *Br J Psychiatry*, 1987. **151**:324–32.

65. Feinstein A., Ron M. Psychosis associated with demonstrable brain disease. *Psychiatr Med*, 1990. **20**:793–803.

66. Ferraro A. Pathological changes in the brain of a case clinically diagnosed dementia praecox. *J Neuropath Exp Neurol*, 1943. **2**:84–94.

67. Pearlson G. Neurobiology of schizophrenia. *Ann Neurol*, 2000. **48**:556–66.

68. Walterfang M., *et al.* Diseases of white matter and schizophrenia-like psychosis. *Aust NZ J Psychiatry*, 2005. **39**:746–56.

69. Cummings J. Psychosis in neurologic disease: neurobiology and pathogenesis. *Neuropsychiatr Neuropsychol Behav Neurol*, 1992. **5**:144–50.

70. White J., Cobb S. Psychological changes associated with giant pituitary neoplasms. *Arch Neurol Psychiatry*, 1955. **74**:383–96.

71. Oppler Q. Manic psychosis in a case of parasagittal meningioma. *Arch Neurolog Psychiatry*, 1950. **64**:417–30.

72. Binder R. Neurologically silent brain tumours in psychiatric hospital admissions: three cases and a review. *J Clin Psychiatry*, 1983. **44**:94–7.

73. Alee A., Knesevich M. Schizophrenia-like psychosis associated with vein of Galen malformation: a case report. *Canad J Psychiatry*, 1987. **32**:226–7.

21

Demyelinating disease and psychosis

Anthony Feinstein

Facts box

- The major demyelinating disorder is multiple sclerosis (MS) with three other conditions: neuromyelitis optica (Devic's Disease), acute disseminated encephalomyelitis, and acute and subacute necrotizing hemorrhagic encephalomyelitis making up the quartet.
- Although the data have been inconsistent, recent evidence suggests that psychosis is more likely to occur in MS than by chance association.
- A shared etiology is unlikely to explain the association of demyelinating disorders and schizophrenia.
- Brain lesions superimposed on a premorbid vulnerability (genetic, developmental, premorbid psychiatric history) offer a more plausible explanation for the association.
- There are no empirically based treatment studies of psychosis associated with MS.
- The increased prevalence of psychosis in demyelination challenges the notion of psychosis as a primarily cortical phenomenon.

Demyelinating disorders

Before discussing psychotic disorders that may arise from demyelination, it is important to comment briefly on the classification of demyelinating disorders, a topic not without controversy. To satisfy the descriptor "demyelinating," three criteria should be met:

1. Destruction of the myelin sheaths of nerve fibers with *relative* sparing of other elements of the nervous tissue, that is, axons and nerve cells, a consequence of which is a *relative* lack of Wallerian degeneration of fiber tracts
2. Infiltration of inflammatory cells in a perivascular distribution
3. Distribution of lesions that are primarily in the white matter [1]

If these three principles are obeyed, the classification is dominated by multiple sclerosis (MS) with three other conditions: neuromyelitis optica (Devic's Disease), acute disseminated encephalomyelitis, and acute and subacute necrotizing hemorrhagic encephalomyelitis making up the quartet. Absent from the list are disorders in which myelin loss is prominent, for example, anoxic encephalopathy, vascular occlusion as in Binswanger's Disease, progressive multifocal leukoencephalopathy, central pontine myelinolysis, Marchiafava Bignami Disease, and human immune virus HIV-associated encephalopathy. These disorders have been removed from the classification because their etiology has been established. Perhaps more controversial is the omission of the chronic progressive leukodystrophies of childhood and adolescence, on the basis that their cardinal pathological feature is not so much a loss (demyelination) but rather an abnormality (dysmyelination) of myelin [1]. Putting aside the debate over the choice of a correct prefix, it is germane to note that one of these disorders, metachromatic leukodystrophy, is associated with a rate of psychosis that may exceed all other neuropsychiatric disorders [2] – this association is discussed elsewhere in this book.

This brief introduction to taxonomy helps frame the content of this chapter, which consists primarily of a review of the literature pertaining to psychosis associated with MS and a shorter discussion on psychosis secondary to metachromatic leukodystrophy. The chapter concludes with some thoughts on the pathogenesis of psychosis in relation to pathology affecting the cerebral white matter.

Behavioral abnormalities in multiple sclerosis

Multiple sclerosis is the most common cause of neurological disability in young and middle-aged adults. Behavioral sequelae are frequent. The lifetime prevalence of major depression approaches 50%, bipolar affective disorder occurs twice as often than in the general population, and pathological laughter and crying affects up to 10% of patients. In addition, approximately 40% of community-living MS patients are cognitively impaired [3].

The association between MS and psychosis has until recently been considered uncommon, which helps explain the paucity of research devoted to the topic. Given that the lifetime prevalence for a psychotic illness such as schizophrenia is approximately 1% and for MS 0.1 to .01% (varying according to latitude), the two disorders can be expected to appear together by chance every 0.5 to 1 in 100,000 cases. Therefore, to support the specific notion of an MS psychosis that is distinct from schizophrenia, factors regarding descriptive, predictive, and constructive validity should be present.

Psychosis secondary to multiple sclerosis

Prevalence

Most reports of MS and psychosis are single case studies, with the earliest dating from the nineteenth century. In their comprehensive review of "schizophrenia-like psychoses associated with organic disorders of the central nervous system (CNS)," Davison and Bagley [4] devoted a section to demyelinating disease. They reviewed every published report (irrespective of language) of multiple sclerosis that occurred concurrently with a psychotic illness that fulfilled the 1957 World Health Organization (WHO) criteria for schizophrenia. Given their belief that the presence of coarse cerebral pathology would render some signs and symptoms invalid, they excluded catatonia, autism, and change in personality from the WHO guidelines and were left with the following: the presence of an unequivocal disorder of the central nervous system (CNS); the presence at some stage of shallow, incongruous affect, thought disorder, hallucinations, and delusions; and the absence, when psychotic, of features suggesting a delirium, dementia, dysmnesic syndrome, and affective psychosis. Applying these criteria to their literature review, they came across 39 reports, a frequency judged not to exceed chance expectation.

The view that psychosis seldom occurs with MS has been cautiously supported by studies investigating the number of MS patients found in large, inpatient psychiatric populations. Percentages from state hospitals in Massachusetts (.07%), Manhattan (.05%), and Queensland (.06%) are similar and do not exceed chance probability, but may be misleadingly low because of a greater community tolerance for mental disturbance in the presence of MS or alternative admissions to hospitals caring for the physically disabled [4].

A more recent study has, however, challenged prevailing assumptions. Population-based evidence from Alberta, Canada suggests psychosis in MS patients is more common than was previously thought [5]. As part of universal health care insurance in Alberta, all subjects seen by physicians are given diagnoses coded by the International Classification of Diseases, Ninth Edition Clinical Modification (ICD-9-CM). In 2002, 10,367 of the 2.45 million residents of this Canadian province over 15 years of age were found to have multiple sclerosis, giving an estimated prevalence of 330 per 100,000, in keeping with Alberta's historically high prevalence rate. The authors also looked for the co-occurrence of two ICD-9-CM psychiatric diagnoses in these MS patients. The first was "nonorganic/nonaffective psychoses" (which included schizophrenia-spectrum disorders, delusional disorders, and other nonorganic psychoses) and the second category was broadly defined as organic psychotic disorders (which comprised drug-induced psychotic disorders, other transient organic psychotic disorders, and other organic psychotic disorders). Care was taken to exclude patients with dementia and alcohol-related psychoses.

Results were given separately for each of these two large categories and were stratified according to the following age groups: 15 to 24; 25 to 44; 45 to 64; and 65+. Consistent findings emerged across all age groups and in both psychiatric categories, namely, that the prevalence of psychosis in MS patients significantly exceeded that reported in patients without MS.

The main weakness of this study was an offshoot of its greatest strength. The large sample size precluded detailed psychiatric data being collected, so the ICD-9-CM categories provide only bare bones phenomenology. Nevertheless, under the very broad descriptive rubric of psychosis, an unequivocal picture emerged of elevated rates of psychosis, in the order of 2% to 3%, occurring in patients with MS. This study provides the most compelling evidence to date that psychosis in MS occurs more frequently than chance dictates.

Distinguishing characteristics

Temporal association

Davison and Bagley's MS review [4] revealed that in 36% of cases, the neurological and psychiatric symptoms appeared at approximately the same time. Furthermore, in 61.5% of cases, the psychosis appeared either 2 years before the onset of neurological symptoms or after the onset. This temporal association in approximately two-thirds of cases led the authors to conclude that although psychosis secondary to MS was rare, when it did occur, demyelination was most likely implicated in the pathogenesis. This result was not, however, replicated by Feinstein and colleagues [6] in a case control study of 10 psychotic MS patients. The mean duration of neurological symptoms before the onset of psychosis was 8.5 years (range 0–19 years). In only one case was the diagnosis of MS made at the time of psychosis onset.

Clinical features

Feinstein and colleagues [6] examined the case notes of 10 psychotic MS patients treated at a tertiary referral center. Mental state was assessed retrospectively using the symptom checklist (SCL) derived from the Present State Examination (PSE) [7]. From the SCL, half the subjects were given a diagnosis of schizophrenia and the other half an affective psychosis. Lack of insight characterized all the patients' presentations. Persecutory delusions occurred in more than two-thirds of cases and was the commonest psychotic feature. Nonspecific evidence of psychosis (which included heightened or changed perception, "minor" hallucinations, viz. music, noises) was recorded in 60% of patients. Delusions of control (passivity) and delusions with a sexual or fantastic content were present in a third of patients, and delusions of reference noted in 1 in 5 patients. The symptom profile was notable for the relative infrequency of well-formed hallucinations. Second-person auditory hallucinations were present in 20% of patients as were visual hallucinations. Third-person auditory hallucinations (two or more voices commenting on the person) were found in only one case. Thus, delusions in various forms, but particularly with a persecutory content, predominated. The findings lend support to the ICD-10 notion of the psychosis being more akin to an "organic delusional disorder," with perceptual disturbances less noticeable and of secondary import.

Another frequently cited clinical observation in the literature of secondary psychosis, namely, the preservation of affective responses, also received empirical support [6]. Thus, it would appear that when patients with MS become psychotic, the predominant presentation is one of "positive" psychotic symptoms (delusions, less often hallucinations) with relative preservation of affective responses. The "negative" or "defect" state associated with schizophrenia, that is, apathy, impoverished speech and thought, together with blunted affect, is seldom seen. Notwithstanding this well-documented group profile that demarcates the clinical picture of MS psychosis from schizophrenia, it needs to be emphasized that on an individual level, it is frequently difficult to tell the conditions apart [8, 9].

Age of presentation

The mean age of first presentation of psychosis in schizophrenic patients is 23 years [10], which is considerably younger than that reported in two studies of MS patients with psychosis. Thus, Davison and Bagley's review [4] noted a mean age of onset of psychosis a decade older and in Feinstein and colleagues' study [6], the average age was 36.6 years. A similar picture emerges from studies of other CNS disorders [11, 12, 13] and the relatively later age of presentation is therefore further evidence that sets psychosis secondary to MS apart from schizophrenia.

The Alberta population-based study [5] does not specifically address the age of onset of psychosis. But the prevalence figures stratified by age are nevertheless informative. For example, the prevalence of "organic" psychosis was found to increase with age with peak prevalence in the 65 years and over group. But the strongest relative effect (i.e., highest odds ratio) was found in the 15- to 24-year age group. Although this observation can be explained by the fact that "organic" psychosis is extremely rare in young patients without MS, it cannot obscure the fact that even young MS patients still have a heightened risk of psychosis.

Gender ratio

It is unclear whether the gender ratio noted in psychotic MS patients differs from that found in either MS or late-onset schizophrenia. For example, Davison and Bagley [4] reported 21 of 39 cases were male, which is at odds with the 1.5:1 female to male ratio in MS and the equal gender ratio in schizophrenia (see Lewis, 1992 [14] for a dissenting view). On the other hand, the Alberta study did not find that gender modified the association between psychosis and MS [5].

Etiology

Genetic links

If the psychosis associated with MS were simply the chance co-occurrence of schizophrenia, then one would expect to find increased evidence of schizophrenia in the relatives of the affected proband. Evidence is scanty on this point, but does not support a familial link [4].

Viral hypothesis

It has been postulated that similarities in disease course, age of onset, geographical distribution, and immunological response of patients with schizophrenia and MS imply some overlap with respect to pathogenesis [15]. In particular, exposure to a virus at a crucial developmental stage (in utero, childbirth, childhood) may be the common thread linking what are clinically two very different conditions. This viewpoint fits well with theories of schizophrenia as a neurodevelopmental disorder triggered by insult to the fetal brain [16]. It has also been reported that infection during childhood with the herpes virus may leave some patients prone to develop MS in later life. Migration studies have shown that for those who emigrate after adolescence, the risk of developing MS does not change from that of their country of origin [17].

Although theorizing offers intriguing possibilities, the marked differences in clinical presentations between the two disorders outweigh any similarities, making a shared pathogen unlikely.

MRI brain changes

Compelling evidence linking brain changes in MS to psychosis comes from a case-control MRI study of 10 MS patients with psychosis and 10 without psychosis [6], who were matched for age, sex, duration of illness, and physical disability. The following PSE [7] diagnoses were assigned: schizophrenia (2), schizoaffective psychosis (2), paranoid disorder (1), psychotic depression (1), and mania with psychotic features (4).

Subjects and controls underwent contiguous, multislice axial MRI of the brain. All scanning protocols included T_2 weighted images that optimized lesion detection.

Subjects were compared with controls with respect to site and extent of lesions. MRI analysis was undertaken by a neuroradiologist blind to psychiatric diagnosis. The psychotic patients had a greater total lesion and periventricular lesion score, but these were not statistically significant. Trends emerged for a higher lesion score in the psychotic group for areas surrounding the temporal horns bilaterally. A similar result was also obtained in the left trigone. Combining the left temporal horn and adjacent left trigone area scores produced a statistically significant difference between the psychotic and control groups.

A clearer picture of the difference in the distribution of lesion scores between the psychotic and control MS patients was demonstrated by observing what percentage of the total lesion score was present in each particular area. In the controls, the total lesion score was distributed equally between periventricular and other brain areas whereas in the psychotic patients the periventricular lesion score contributed more than 60% of the total lesion score. This difference was not, however, statistically significant. The most marked differences were present around the temporal horns where the "percentage score" in the psychotic patients was almost double that of the control group. Thus, not only did the psychotic patients have a greater lesion score, but also lesions were differentially distributed in periventricular areas and in particular around the temporal horns of the lateral ventricles. A closer look at the individual patient data demonstrated that in all but one case control pair, the psychotic patient had a greater temporal horn lesion score than the matched control.

Although the MRI data fit with findings from the primary [18, 19] and secondary [4, 11] psychosis literature, it could not answer why only certain patients with temporal lobe involvement became psychotic. Whereas the study suggested a "threshold" lesion volume had to be exceeded before psychosis ensued, this did not invariably apply, as some patients with a large temporal lesion score did not become delusional. One can therefore posit that the presence of brain plaques in the temporal lobes is unlikely to fully explain the development of psychosis in all cases. Rather, brain lesions superimposed on a premorbid vulnerability (genetic, developmental, premorbid psychiatric history) seems a more plausible explanation.

Treatment

There are no empirically based treatment studies of psychosis associated with MS. Early reports found electroconvulsive treatment [8] and insulin coma [9] to be ineffective in individual cases. The mainstay of present treatment is antipsychotic medication [6] and, given the often severe nature of the behavioral disturbance, psychiatric hospitalization is often required in the acute stages.

In an analogous situation to that encountered with the floridly manic patient, treatment can present a considerable therapeutic challenge. Experience has taught that MS patients are frequently sensitive to the side effects of antipsychotic medication. Thus, high-potency drugs such as the butyrophenones (e.g. haloperidol), which are associated with extrapyramidal side effects (EPS), may further compromise patients' mobility and balance, resulting in falls that prove distressing to patients, family, and nursing staff. A choice of less potent antipsychotics, such as the phenothiazine groups of compounds, lessens the risk of EPS, but anticholinergic difficulties are more prominent, which may aggravate other difficulties such as bladder and bowel control and impaired vision. The associated dry mouth may add to dysarthric difficulties. All antipsychotic medication, irrespective of class, can produce excessive sedation, which may similarly affect already impaired coordination and balance.

Newer atypical antipsychotic drugs offer fewer side effects. Furmaga and colleagues [20] have reported that risperidone was helpful in 10 patients with a heterogenous mix of medical conditions who became psychotic and who had not previously responded to a conventional antipsychotic drug. Olanzapine, a thiobenzodiazepine, has less EPS than risperidone, although weight gain and sedation can be problematic, the latter magnified in a disease where fatigue is ubiquitous. It also has the advantage of a convenient once–a–day dose (recommended dose of 10 mg per day) that can be started immediately. Similarly, Seroquel (quetiapine fumarate), a psychotropic agent belonging to a chemical class, the dibenzothiazepine derivatives, potentially offers the same benefits, albeit in a slightly less-friendly dosing schedule. Adverse side effects with both olanzapine and quetiapine have been reported in one psychotic MS patient whereas ziprasidone (a member of the benzothiazolylpiperazine class of antipsychotics) was well tolerated and effective [21].

Should behavioral control still be required despite adequate antipsychotic dosage, benzodiazepines may be added. Lorazepam has the advantage of being given either via the oral or intramuscular route. Oral dosages rarely exceed 8 mg per day and the clinician should bear in mind that the intramuscular dose is equivalent to 2 to $2\frac{1}{2}$ times the oral dose, because it avoids the first-pass metabolism.

Outcome

Earlier literature, much of it predating the appearance of antipsychotic medication in the early 1950s, reported that psychotic MS patients either recovered spontaneously, progressed from psychosis to dementia, or ran a relapsing-remitting course with respect to psychosis and MS that ultimately went on to dementia. More recent data demonstrates that antipsychotic medication has substantially altered this outlook. Of 10 psychotic patients followed for approximately 6 years, the median duration of their first psychotic episode was 5 weeks (range 1–72 weeks). Six (60%) of the patients did not experience another psychotic episode, three patients had one further relapse, and a single patient had multiple recurrences. Overall, the psychosis remitted in 90% of cases, with a chronic, paranoid psychosis ensuing in a single patient. In general, patients did not require long-term oral or depot antipsychotic use. If a relapse occurred, short-term antipsychotic medication was reintroduced and subsequently discontinued after improvement in the mental state [6].

Summary

Psychosis data have been presented in relation to demyelination, in particular, multiple sclerosis. The fact that psychosis occurs more often than by chance challenges prevailing theories of psychosis as a mainly cortical phenomenon. Defining the neuroanatomy of the human cerebral white-matter tracts and assigning functional relevance to each offers the prospect of novel insights into a complex pathogenesis [22].

References

1. Ropper A. H., Brown R. H. (2005). *Adam's and Victor's Principles of Neurology.* 8th Ed. New York: McGraw Hill, p. 771.

2. Hyde T. M., Ziegler J. C., Weinberger D. R. Psychiatric disturbances in metachromatic leukodystrophy. *Arch Neurol*, 1992. **49**:401–6.

3. Feinstein A. The neuropsychiatry of multiple sclerosis. *Can J Psychiatry*, 2004. **49**:157–63.

4. Davison K., Bagley C. R. (1969). Schizophrenia-like psychoses associated with organic disorders of the central nervous system. A review of the literature. In *Current Problems in Neuropsychiatry*, Herrington R. N. (Ed.). Ashford, Kent: Hedley, pp. 113–84.

5. Patten S. B., Svenson L. W., Metz L. M. Psychotic disorders in MS: population-based evidence of an association. *Neurology*, 2005. **65**:1123–5.

6. Feinstein A., du Boulay G., Ron M. A. Psychotic illness in multiple sclerosis. A clinical and magnetic resonance imaging study. *Br J Psychiatry*, 1992. **161**:680–5.

7. Wing J. K., Cooper J. E., Sartorius N. (1974). *The Measurement and Classification of Psychiatric Symptoms. An Instruction Manual for the Present State Examination and CATEGO Programme.*

Cambridge: Cambridge University Press.

8. Schmalzbach O. Disseminated sclerosis in schizophrenia. *Med J Australia*, 1954. **1**:451–2.

9. Parker N. Disseminated sclerosis presenting as schizophrenia. *Med J Australia*, 1956. **1**:405–7.

10. Lieberman J. A., Alvir A., Woerner M., *et al.* Prospective study of psychopathology in first episode schizophrenia at Hillside Hospital. *Schizophr Bull*, 1992. **18**:351–71.

11. Slater E., Beard A. W., Glithero E. The schizophrenia-like psychoses of epilepsy. *Br J Psychiatry*, 1963. **109**:95–150.

12. Cummings J. L. Organic delusions: phenomenology, anatomical correlations and review. *Br J Psychiatry*, 1985. **146**:184–97.

13. Feinstein A., Ron M. A. Psychosis associated with demonstrable brain disease. *Psychol Med*, 1990. **20**:793–803.

14. Lewis S. Sex and schizophrenia: vive la difference. *Br J Psychiatry*, 1992. **161**:445–50.

15. Stevens J. R. Schizophr and multiple sclerosis. *Schizophr Bull*, 1988. **14**:231–41.

16. Torrey E. F., Taylor E., Bracha H. S., *et al.* Prenatal origin of

schizophrenia in a subgroup discordant monozygotic twins. *Schizophr Bull*, 1994. **20**: 423–32.

17. Dean G. Annual incidence, prevalence and morbidity of multiple sclerosis in white South African-born and in white immigrants to South Africa. *Br Med J*, 1967. **2**:724–30.

18. Suddath R. L., Casanova M. F., Goldberg T. E., *et al.* Temporal lobe pathology in schizophrenia: a quantitative magnetic resonance imaging study. *Am J Psychiatry*, 1989. **146**:464–72.

19. Suddath R. L., Christison G. W., Torrey E. F., *et al.* Anatomical abnormalities in the brains of monozygotic twins discordant for schizophrenia. *N Engl J Med*, 1990. **322**:789–94.

20. Furmaga K. M., DeLeon O., Sinha S., *et al.* Risperidone response in refractory psychosis due to a general medical condition. *J Neuropsychiatry and Clin Neurosci*, 1995. **7**:417 (Abstract).

21. Davids E., Hartwig U., Gastpar M. Antipsychotic treatment for psychosis associated with multiple sclerosis. *Prog Neuropsychopharmacol Biol Psychiatry*, 2004. **28**:743–4.

22. Schmahman J., Pandya D. (2006). *Fiber Pathways of the Brain.* New York: Oxford University Press.

Organic syndromes of schizophrenia: *systemic disorders*

Infection and schizophrenia

Alan S. Brown and Ezra S. Susser

Facts box

- Accumulating evidence supports prenatal infections as potential risk factors for schizophrenia.
- Early evidence consisted of proxy measures of in utero infection such as epidemics in populations.
- Using documentation of infection based on maternal serologic measures, investigators have confirmed previous associations and extended the range of infections examined.
- Prenatal infections associated with schizophrenia in offspring include influenza, toxoplasmosis, rubella, and maternal/genital reproductive infections. Elevated prenatal cytokines have also been related to an increased risk of schizophrenia.
- Studies have also revealed associations between seroprevalence of toxoplasmosis and schizophrenia in adult patients, although the direction of cause and effect is inconclusive given that most of these studies are cross-sectional in design.
- Future studies are warranted to replicate these findings, identify susceptibility genes that may interact with these infections, and identify pathogenic mechanisms by which these agents might increase the risk of schizophrenia.

Introduction

In this chapter, we review accumulating evidence that supports prenatal infection in the etiology of schizophrenia. There is a considerable amount of data from diverse fields of inquiry that schizophrenia results in part from a disruption in neurodevelopment. Given that many, if not most, of the critical neurodevelopmental events occur during fetal life, and in utero

exposure to infection is a known cause of many congenital central nervous system (CNS) anomalies, it has been hypothesized that in utero exposure to infection is a risk factor for schizophrenia.

Early clues

In the earliest work in this area, investigators assessed proxy measures of in utero infection. Season of birth, which covaries with fluctuations in the incidence of many infections, especially influenza and other respiratory pathogens, has been examined in relation to risk of schizophrenia. These studies have demonstrated a 5% to 15% excess risk of schizophrenia for births during January and March [1]. Urban birth has also been associated with a greater risk of schizophrenia [2, 3]. Although there are several potential explanations for this finding, one compelling interpretation is that increased crowding present in urban areas enhances the likelihood of transmission of pathogenic microbes. Both season of birth and urbanicity of birth contribute significantly to the population attributable risk for development of schizophrenia [2, 3].

Ecologic studies

Following on these initial clues, a series of investigations were conducted on the relationship between influenza epidemics in large populations and schizophrenia among those who were in utero at the time of the epidemics. The initial studies focused on the 1957 type A2 influenza epidemic, and additional studies examined influenza epidemics over periods of many years. The incidence of these infections varies by year but is generally believed to be from 15% to 30%. Although several studies yielded positive associations between influenza epidemics and schizophrenia among individuals who would have been in utero during the second trimester, there have been a number of failures to replicate these results [4]. These discrepancies may be due in large part to misclassification of

Table 22.1 Summary table of research findings in prenatal infections and schizophrenia

Citation	Prenatal risk factor	Cohort/sample	Findings*
Brown et al., 2000 [26]	Rubella	RBDEP	RR = 5.2, 95% CI = 1.9–14.3, p < .001
Brown et al., 2001 [27]		RBDEP	20.4% prevalence of schizophrenia
Brown et al., 2000 [56]	Maternal exposure to respiratory infections, second trimester	CHDS/PDS	RR = 2.1, 95% CI = 1.1–4.4, p = .04
Brown et al., 2004 [13]	Maternal influenza exposure, first half pregnancy	CHDS/PDS	OR = 3.0, 95% CI = 0.98–10.1, p = .05
Brown et al., 2005 [18] Mortensen et al., 2007 [19]	Elevated maternal toxoplasma IgG antibody titre (1:128–1:1024) Elevated neonatal toxoplasma IgG antibody titre (>75th percentile)	CHDS/PDS	OR = 2.6, 95% CI = 1.0–4.8, p = .05, OR = 1.8, 95% CI = 1.0–3.2, p = .05
Brown et al., 2004 [41]	Elevated maternal interleukin-8, second trimester	CHDS/PDS	p = .04
Buka et al., 2001 [21]	Herpesvirus type 2 (HSV2) IgG antibody, at delivery of neonate	NCPP**	p = .02***
Babulas et al., 2006 [25]	Maternal genital/ reproductive infections, periconceptional	CHDS/PDS	RR = 5.0, 95% CI = 2.0–3.7, p = .001

* OR = Odds ratio, RR = Rate ratio. P-values are provided when no OR or RR are reported; ** National Collaborative Perinatal Project; *** Outcome is psychosis.

the exposure, since the majority of individuals who were in utero during influenza epidemics would not have been exposed to this virus; such misclassification would bias any association toward the null [5]. Further methodological limitations included the sole reliance on hospital registry diagnoses, which could result in diagnostic misclassification, and selection biases from loss to follow-up. Similar study designs have been used to assess relationships between other infections and risk of schizophrenia. These studies suggest that exposure to epidemics of certain respiratory infections [6, 7], measles, varicella-zoster [8], and polio [9] were associated with later schizophrenia, mostly in the second trimester.

Serologic studies

In order to surmount the limitations of previous studies, our group and others have capitalized on several methodological advantages made possible by the use of large birth cohorts that have been followed up for schizophrenia in adulthood. These advantages include the use of maternal sera acquired during pregnancy, permitting the use of biomarkers to define exposure status, prospectively collected data on infectious exposures, and, in most cases, rigorous diagnoses using research-based interviews and psychiatric

records. Below, we review the findings of these studies. These findings are summarized in Table 22.1.

Influenza

Our group examined the relationship between maternal influenza and risk of schizophrenia utilizing archived maternal serum samples from mothers in the cohort of the Child Health and Development Study (CHDS) [10, 11], which enrolled pregnant women who were members of the Kaiser Permanente Medicare Care Plan (KPMCP) from 1959 to 1967 in Alameda County, California. In the Prenatal Determinants of Schizophrenia (PDS) study, we ascertained and diagnosed schizophrenia using a structured diagnostic interview and longitudinal psychiatric records among members of this birth cohort [12]. (This cohort was also used in our studies of toxoplasmosis, cytokines, maternal genital/reproductive infection, and maternal respiratory infection, described below).

To characterize influenza infection in the cohort, we analyzed the maternal sera corresponding to cases and matched controls in the cohort for influenza antibody. Because the gestational timing of the availability of serum samples in each pregnancy did not permit the assessment of a fourfold rise in antibody titer between serial samples (the "gold standard" for diagnosis of influenza infection), we utilized a method to characterize the presence of influenza using only a single serum sample. For this purpose we validated an antibody titer of > 20 against known influenza infection in the cohort using serial samples from pregnancies that had serum samples from each trimester, and who were neither cases nor controls in the study. The validity parameters, including sensitivity, specificity, and positive predictive value, were excellent (see [13] for description). We found that maternal exposure during the first half of pregnancy was associated with an increased risk of schizophrenia in adult offspring ($OR = 3.0$, 95% $CI = 0.98$–10.1, $\chi^2 = 3.8$, $p = .052$). For first trimester exposure to influenza, we observed a sevenfold increased risk of schizophrenia in offspring ($OR = 7.0$, 95% $CI = 0.7$–75.3, $\chi^2 = 3.0$, $p = .08$) [13]. There was no increased risk of schizophrenia for exposures occurring in the second half of pregnancy, for the second trimester as a whole, or for the third trimester [13].

In gestational influenza exposure, the mechanism of teratogenesis is not clearly understood because the virus does not appear to cross the placenta or blood-brain barrier and invade the fetal brain [14]. One possible mechanism is that maternal IgG antibodies elicited by influenza, rather than the infection itself, cross the placenta and react with fetal brain antigens by molecular mimicry, thereby disturbing fetal brain development and increasing vulnerability to schizophrenia [15]. Another plausible mechanism is that the effect is mediated by maternal cytokines (discussed later), which have been associated with periventricular leukomalacia, cerebral palsy, and preterm birth.

Toxoplasmosis

The plausibility of Toxoplasma gondii (*T. gondii*) as a risk factor for neurodevelopmental schizophrenia is supported by its association with CNS anomalies and both subtle and severe fetal and childhood neurocognitive disturbances [16, 17]. Using bioassays on archived maternal sera, we demonstrated that elevated toxoplasma IgG antibody titer (> 1:128) was associated with an increased risk of schizophrenia in adult offspring ($OR = 2.6$, 95% $CI = 1.0$–4.8, $\chi^2 = 3.8$, $p = .05$) [18]. For toxoplasma IgM, there was no elevation in maternal sera for any of the cases or controls, suggesting that active infection is unlikely. This work has recently been replicated in a Danish sample with neonatal blood from filter paper samples [19].

Although that study differed from our work in that prenatal sera were not available, the source of IgG to toxoplasma in neonatal blood should have been infection that occurred in the mother either during or prior to pregnancy, as would have been the case in our study.

Toxoplasma may increase liability to schizophrenia via reactivation of toxoplasma oocysts. After acute infection, toxoplasma oocysts exist in a dormant state in which they are sequestered in affected organs, including the brain [16, 17]. Host immunosuppression or other factors can lead these cysts to rupture and become transformed from the inactive bradyzoite form to the active tachyzoite form. Tachyzoites proliferate and invade cells and potentially cross the placenta and infect the fetus [16, 20]. Another possibility is that elevated toxoplasma IgG may itself be teratogenic, or that the cytokine response which suppresses toxoplasma from becoming reactivated may damage the fetal brain [18].

Herpes simplex virus

In a study from the Collaborative Perinatal Project (CPP), an association was observed between IgG levels to herpes simplex virus type 2 (HSV-2) and risk of psychotic illness in 27 offspring ($p = .04$) [21]. These offspring had diagnoses of schizophrenia, affective psychoses, and other psychotic disorders. No association was observed in this study between psychotic disorders and IgG antibody to herpes simplex virus type 1 (HSV-1), cytomegalovirus (CMV), rubella virus, human parvovirus B19, chlamydia trachomatis, or human papillomavirus type 16. We were not able to replicate this finding, however, in a larger investigation on schizophrenia and other schizophrenia spectrum disorders, the vast majority (85%) of whom had either schizophrenia or schizoaffective disorder based on the PDS study [22]. This negative finding persisted whether HSV-2 IgG antibody was categorized as a dichotomous ($OR = 1.13$, 95% $CI = 0.51$–2.55, $p = 0.76$) or as a continuous variable ($OR = 0.82$, 95% $CI = 0.09$–7.75, $p = 0.86$) for subjects who were seropositive to HSV-2. For the latter analysis, we also analyzed the IgG levels in both seropositive and in seronegative subjects, as in the study from the CPP cohort; again, no effects were observed. Differences between the findings of the two studies may have resulted from the fact that our study focused on schizophrenia and schizophrenia spectrum disorders, and had a considerably larger sample, which may have provided greater stability of odds ratios and confidence intervals. However, an even larger study of HSV-2 IgG antibody in neonatal filter paper blood samples from Denmark, which utilized assay methodology identical to that in the CPP study, also did not report an association with "schizophrenia and related disorders," although no measures of effect were reported in that paper [19]. Because this work is ongoing in each of the birth cohorts described above, it would be premature to conclude at this time that there is no association between prenatal herpes viruses and the risk of schizophrenia.

Maternal genital/reproductive infections

It has long been known that maternal genital/reproductive (G/R) infections during pregnancy increase the risk of congenital neurological disorders in offspring [23, 24]. We demonstrated that periconceptional genital/reproductive infection was related to a marked elevation in schizophrenia risk among offspring ($RR = 5.0$, 95% $CI = 2.0–3.7$, $p = .001$) [25]. Unlike the infections previously described, these microbes directly infect the uterus and an effect on schizophrenia may arise from infection of the early embryo. In that study, HSV was not reported in any of the mothers of cases who later developed schizophrenia.

Rubella

Like *T. gondii*, rubella is a known central nervous system teratogen. In the Rubella Birth Defects Evaluation Project (RBDEP) we had a unique opportunity to relate in utero rubella infection to adult schizophrenia [26, 27]. A key advantage of the RBDEP cohort was that all mothers and offspring in the cohort were prospectively documented with prenatal rubella infection by clinical examination [26, 27, 28, 29] and serologic testing [28]. Such a cohort was ideal for investigating the role of a prenatal infection and risk of schizophrenia. Hence, we administered a psychiatric diagnostic assessment on members of this cohort during early-middle adulthood [27]. We found that the prevalence of schizophrenia and other spectrum disorders was 20.4%, which suggested a *15 to 20-fold increased risk* of these disorders given population-based estimates for this broader diagnostic outcome [30, 31]. The effect appeared strongest for the first

two months of pregnancy [27]. We also capitalized on prospective data collected in childhood and adolescence in nearly every subject in the cohort, which allowed us to demonstrate a marked decline in IQ in nearly every subject who later developed schizophrenia spectrum disorders; in contrast, only one-third of exposed subjects who remained free of the disorder at the time of follow-up [27] exhibited a decline in IQ. This finding provides validation of the strong association between prenatal rubella and schizophrenia, which has since been associated with premorbid cognitive decline in population-based samples [32]. Whereas the mechanisms that may increase the risk of schizophrenia are unclear, rubella has long been documented to cross the placenta, enter the fetal brain, and disrupt development of the central nervous sytem [33], resulting in inhibition of mitosis, which leads to diminished neurons and total brain size [34, 35], diminished replication of oligodendrocytes, and a consequent deficit of myelin [36], as well as a pro-inflammatory response, which increases levels of cytokines and other immune-mediating molecules, leading to ischemic damage [35, 37].

Cytokines

The cytokines are a family of soluble, polypeptide proteins that are known to mediate host responses to a broad array of infections [38] and are known to lead to adverse reproductive outcomes [39, 40]. We found a marked and significant increase in the mean level of serum interleukin-8 (IL-8) in the mothers of schizophrenia cases, as compared to mothers of controls ($p = 0.02$); levels of this cytokine were nearly twice as high in mothers of schizophrenia offspring than controls [41]. There were no differences with regard to maternal IL-1β, IL-6, and TNF-α between schizophrenia cases and controls. Unlike other cytokines, interleukin-8 (IL-8) has been associated with chorioamnionitis in infants born at term, and maternal and neonatal serum IL-8 levels are significantly correlated with one another [39]. IL-8 belongs to a subclass of the cytokine superfamily known as chemokines [42, 43] and is especially important for neutrophil attraction and activation [42, 44, 45]. Increased IL-8 has been associated with some autoimmune disorders including psoriasis [46].

For each of the infections and immune abnormalities discussed above, we must also consider the possibility that nonspecific pathogenic mechanisms might account for the findings. These include hyperthermia, a known cause of neural tube defects in animal studies [47], cold, flu, or analgesic remedies, which may have teratogenic effects [47], and stress, which induces hypothalamo-pituitary-adrenal axis activation that causes maldevelopment of the hippocampus and other brain structures and functions implicated in the pathogenesis of schizophrenia [48].

Studies of infection and schizophrenia in adult patients

Although not the focus of this chapter, it is worth noting that a considerable number of studies have demonstrated increased seroprevalence of toxoplasmosis in patients with schizophrenia [49]. In a recent meta-analysis, the *combined odds ratio* was 2.73 (*95% CI =* 2.1–3.6). The finding was similar for both first-episode patients and chronically ill patients. Although intriguing, the studies reviewed are characterized by substantial variability in methodological design, and rigorous epidemiologic methods were generally not used with regard to case and control ascertainment. Of note, among the 23 studies reviewed, controls were variously defined as "general population," "hospital employees," and "normal persons." The use of individuals who are screened out for all psychiatric disorders and hospital employees is prone to the selection of a "super-normal," control group, characterized by better lifestyle habits than a control group that represented the source population from which the cases were derived. Moreover, given that all of these studies are cross-sectional, the direction of cause and effect cannot be definitively determined. Lifestyle differences secondary to the illness that could predispose to toxoplasma infection may even have occurred among first-episode patients, who may have been ill for some time before the diagnosis of schizophrenia.

Implications for clinical practice

Research on prenatal etiologies of schizophrenia may have important implications for prevention of this disorder, through the institution of public health measures. This work has the potential of identifying at-risk individuals who experienced in utero insults, or their sequelae, and who possess genetic vulnerability to schizophrenia.

Suggestions for future research

First, we believe it is essential to replicate these findings in independent samples and to identify additional infections that may play etiologic roles in schizophrenia. In order to accomplish this, we believe it is essential to employ larger samples utilizing newer technologies to identify a wider array of infectious pathogens than currently exist, for example, high throughput assays that can delineate the microbial genome. Several large cohort studies are under way that will permit the application of these approaches. Second, it is unlikely that prenatal environmental exposures are sufficient in and of themselves to result in schizophrenia in most cases. Thus, we believe that future work is necessary to examine whether these infectious exposures interact with susceptibility genes to increase vulnerability to this disorder. Intriguingly, several susceptibility genes for schizophrenia that have been replicated in several studies appear to play important roles in fetal brain development [50, 51]. Given the relatively small effects of individual genes in previous association studies, the modest effect sizes observed in the positive studies of prenatal infection, and the large samples necessary for studies of gene–environment interaction to achieve adequate statistical power, we anticipate that the numbers of cases for these studies will need to be in the hundreds or perhaps thousands in order to reveal meaningful interactions; thus, the same large cohorts alluded to above should be highly suitable for this purpose.

Translational approaches

Translational research approaches hold the promise of identifying pathogenic mechanisms by which these exposures increase schizophrenia risk. Animal models have provided evidence that offspring of mice that were infected with influenza at day 9 of gestation exhibit deficits in prepulse inhibition (PPI) in the acoustic startle response, alterations in open-field, novel object, and social interaction tests, and improvement in PPI disruptions following administration of psychotomimetic and antipsychotic medications [52]. PPI and other deficits were also observed when poly I:C, a potent immune activator, was administered at this time in fetal development in the absence of I infection, suggesting that these aberrations were secondary to the maternal immune response. In another study, prenatal influenza appeared to disrupt neuronal migration, as evidenced by decreased reelin-positive Cajal-Retzius cells in the cortex and hippocampus [53]. Translational approaches may also facilitate the identification of new molecular targets for psychopharmacologic intervention. In addition to the correction of prenatal immune-mediated neurophysiologic and behavioral abnormalities, activation of the maternal immune response was associated with the postpubertal emergence of increased sensitivity to locomotor stimulation following amphetamine administration and increased amphetamine-induced striatal dopamine release [54].

Summary and conclusions

Despite a considerable amount of research on the underpinnings of schizophrenia, its etiology and pathogenesis remain unknown. In utero infections are emerging as potentially important risk factors for schizophrenia, in which neurodevelopmental influences likely play an important role. Our group and others have embarked on investigations aimed at identifying these infectious risk factors and examining the mechanisms by which they increase vulnerability to this disorder.

This work has the potential to lead to strategies aimed at preventing this disorder. Most of the prenatal infections identified to date are relatively common during pregnancy, and these factors confer at least a twofold, and as high as a fivefold, increase in risk of schizophrenia. Hence, the combined population attributable risk (PAR) (the proportion of cases in the population that could be prevented if these exposures were eliminated) is potentially substantial. For influenza alone, the PAR for early to mid-gestational exposure may be as high as 10% to 15% [13]. Many of these exposures can be prevented by relatively inexpensive public health measures; for example, influenza is preventable by vaccination of women of childbearing age; the incidence of *T. gondii* can be markedly reduced by standard hygienic practices such as avoidance of direct contact with cat feces and ingestion of undercooked meat [55]; several maternal/genital reproductive infections can be minimized by condom use and early identification and treatment; and homocysteine levels can be normalized by ingestion of folate from the diet or vitamin supplements. Although rubella has been virtually eliminated in the industrialized world, it remains a significant problem in the developing world, where the vaccine is not routinely administered. Some of our greatest successes in global medicine in the twentieth century have been achieved by the elimination of infectious diseases through vaccination programs and improved sanitation. We believe that similar public health initiatives have the potential to reap similar rewards with regard to a reduction in the incidence of schizophrenia and potentially reveal new molecular targets for pharmacotherapeutic intervention.

Acknowledgments

This manuscript was supported by the following grants: NIMH 1K02MH65422–01 (A.S.B.), NIMH 1R01MH 63264–01A1 (A.S.B.), an NARSAD Independent Investigator Award (A.S.B.), NICHD N01-HD-1–3334 (B. Cohn), and NICHD NO1-HD-6–3258 (B. Cohn). We wish to thank Catherine Schaefer, PhD, Barbara Cohn, PhD, Barbara van den Berg, MD, Michaeline Bresnahan, PhD, and Justin Penner, MA, for their contributions to this work.

References

1. Bradbury T. N., Miller G. A. Season of birth in schizophrenia: a review of evidence, methodology, and etiology. *Psychol Bull*, 1985. **98**(3):569–94.

2. Lewis G., David A, Andréasson S., Allebeck P. Schizophrenia and city life. *Lancet*, 1992. **340**(8812):137–40.

3. Mortensen P. B., Pedersen C. B., Westergaard T., *et al*. Effects of family history and place and season of birth on the risk of schizophrenia. *N Engl J Med*, 1999. **340**(8):603–8.

4. Bagalkote H. Maternal influenza and schizophrenia in the offspring. *Int J Ment Health*, 2001. **29**(4):3–21.

5. Brown A. S., Susser E. S. In utero infection and adult schizophrenia. *Ment Retard Dev Disabil Res Rev*, 2002. **8**(1):51–7.

6. Watson C. G., Kucala T., Tilleskjor C., Jacobs L. Schizophrenic birth seasonality in relation to the incidence of infectious diseases and temperature extremes. *Arch Gen Psychiatry*, 1984. **41**(1): 85–90.

7. O'Callaghan E., Sham P. C., Takei N., *et al*. The relationship of schizophrenic births to 16 infectious diseases. *Br J Psychiatry*, 1994. **165**(3):353–6.

8. Torrey E. F., Rawlings R., Waldman I. N. Schizophrenic births and viral diseases in two states. *Schizophr Res*, 1988. **1**(1):73–7.

9. Suvisaari J., Haukka J., Tanskanen A., Hovi T., Lönnqvist J., Association between prenatal exposure to poliovirus infection and adult schizophrenia. *Am J Psychiatry*, 1999. **156**(7):1100–2.

10. Van Den Berg B. J. The California child health and development studies: twenty years of research. *World Health Stat Q*, 1979. **32**(4):269–86.

11. Van Den Berg B. J. (1984). The California child health and development studies. In *Handbook of Longitudinal Research*, Mednick S. A., Harway M., and Finello K. (Eds.). New York: Praeger, pp. 166–79.

12. Susser E. S., Schaefer C. A., Brown A. S., Begg M. D., Wyatt R. J. The design of the prenatal determinants of schizophrenia study. *Schizophr Bull*, 2000. **26**(2):257–73.

13. Brown A. S., Begg M. D., Gravenstein S., *et al*. Serologic evidence for prenatal influenza in the etiology of schizophrenia. *Arch Gen Psychiatry*, 2004. **61**:774–80.

14. DeLisi L. E. Is there a viral or immune dysfunction etiology to schizophrenia? Re-evaluation a decade later. *Schizophr Res*, 1996. **22**(1):1–4.

15. Wright P., Takei N., Murray R. M., Sham P. C. (1999). Seasonality, prenatal influenza exposure, and schizophrenia. In *Prenatal Exposures in Schizophrenia*, Susser E. S., Brown A. S., and Gorman J. M. (Eds.). Washington, DC: American Psychiatric Press, Inc., pp. 89–112.

16. Remington J. S., McLeod R., Thulliez P., Desmonts G. (2001). Toxoplasmosis. In *Infectious Diseases of the Fetus and Newborn Infant*, Remington J. S. and Klein J. O. (Eds.). Philadelphia: W.B. Saunders Company, pp. 205–346.

17. Dukes C. S., Luft B. J., Durak D. T. (1997). Toxoplasmosis. In *Infections of the Central Nervous System*, Scheld W. M., Whitley R. J., and Durack D. T. (Eds). Philadelphia: Lippincott-Raven, pp. 785–806.

18. Brown A. S., Schaefer C. A., Quesenberry C. P. Jr., *et al*. Maternal exposure to toxoplasmosis and risk of schizophrenia in adult offspring.

Am J Psychiatry, 2005. **162**(4): 767–73.

19. Mortensen P. B., Nergaard-Pedersen B., Waltoft B. L., *et al*. Toxoplasma gondii as a risk factor for early-onset schizophrenia: analysis of filter paper blood samples obtained at birth. *Biol Psychiatry*, 2007. **61**(5): 688–93.

20. Frenkel J. K., Nelson B. M., Arias-Stella J. Immuno-suppression and toxoplasmic encephalitis – clinical and experimental aspects. *Hum Pathol*, 1975. **6**(1):97–111.

21. Buka S. L., Tsuang M. T., Torrey E. F., *et al*. Maternal infections and subsequent psychosis among offspring. *Arch Gen Psychiatry*, 2001. **58**(11):1032–7.

22. Brown A. S., Schaefer C. A., Quesenberry C. P. Jr., Shen L., Susser E. S. No evidence of relation between maternal exposure to herpes simplex virus type 2 and risk of schizophrenia. *Am J Psychiatry*, 2006. **163**(12): 2178–80.

23. Corey L., Whitley R. J., Stone E. F., Mohan K. Difference between herpes simplex virus type 1 and type 2 neonatal encephalitis in neurological outcome. *Lancet*, 1988. **1**(8575–6):1–4.

24. Ingall D., Sanchez P. J. (1995). Syphilis. In *Infectious Diseases of the Fetus and Newborn*, Remington J. S. and Klein J. O. (Eds.). Philadelphia: WB Saunders. p. 652.

25. Babulas V., Factor-Litvak P., Goetz R., Schaefer C. A., Brown A. S. Prenatal exposure to maternal genital and reproductive infections and adult schizophrenia. *Am J Psychiatry*, 2006. **163**(5):927–9.

26. Brown A. S., Cohen P., Greenwald S., Susser E. Nonaffective psychosis after prenatal exposure to rubella. *Am J Psychiatry*, 2000. **157**(3):438–43.

27. Brown A. S., Cohen P., Harkavy-Friedman J., *et al.* A.E. Bennett Research Award. Prenatal rubella, premorbid abnormalities, and adult schizophrenia. *Biol Psychiatry*, 2001. **49**(6): 473–86.

28. Chess S., Korn S., Fernandez P. (1971). *Psychiatric Disorders of Children with Congenital Rubella.* New York: Brunner/Mazel.

29. Chess S. Follow-up report on autism in congenital rubella. *J Autism Child Schizophr*, 1977. 7(1):69–81.

30. Eaton W. W. Epidemiology of schizophrenia. *Epidemiol Rev*, 1985. 7:105–26.

31. Kendler K. S., MacLean C. J., O'Neill F. A., *et al.* Evidence for a schizophrenia vulnerability locus on chromosome 8p in the Irish Study of High-Density Schizophrenia Families. *Am J Psychiatry*, 1996. **153**(12): 1534–40.

32. Reichenberg A., Weiser M., Rapp M. A., *et al.* Elaboration on premorbid intellectual performance in schizophrenia: premorbid intellectual decline and risk for schizophrenia. *Arch Gen Psychiatry*, 2005. **62**(12): 1297–304.

33. Whitley R. J., Stagno S. (1997). Perinatal infections. In *Infections of the Central Nervous System*, Scheld W. M., Whitley R. J., and Durack D. T. (Eds.). Philadelphia: Lippincott-Raven Press, pp. 223–53.

34. Boue J. G., Boue A. Effects of rubella virus infection on the division of human cells. *Am J Dis Child*, 1969. **118**(1):45–8.

35. Rorke L. B. Nervous system lesions in the congenital rubella syndrome. *Arch Otolaryngol*, 1973. **98**(4):249–51.

36. Kemper T. L., Lecours A. R., Gates M. J., Yakoviev P. I. Retardation of the myelo- and cytoarchitectonic maturation of the brain in the congenital rubella syndrome. *Res Publ Assoc Res Nerv Ment Dis*, 1973. **51**:23–62.

37. Townsend J. J. (1994). Rubella virus disease. In *Handbook of Neurovirology*, McKendall R. R. and Stropp W. G. (Eds.). New York: Marcel Dekker, pp. 603–11.

38. Weizman R., Bessler H. (1999). Cytokines: Stress and Immunity. In *Cytokines: Stress and Immunity*, Plotnikoff N. P., Faith R. E., and Murgo A. J., *et al.* (Eds.). Boca Raton, FL: CRC Press, pp. 1–15.

39. Shimoya K., Matsuzaki, N., Taniguchi T., *et al.* Interleukin-8 level in maternal serum as a marker for screening of histological chorioamnionitis at term. *Int J Gynaecol Obstet*, 1997. **57**(2):153–9.

40. Gilmore J. H., Jarskog L. F. Exposure to infection and brain development: Cytokines in the pathogenesis of schizophrenia. *Schizophr Res*, 1997. **24**(3):365–7.

41. Brown A. S., Hooton J., Schaefer C. A., *et al.* Elevated maternal interleukin-8 levels and risk of schizophrenia in adult offspring. *Am J Psychiatry*, 2004. **161**(5): 889–95.

42. Atta-ur-Rahman, Harvey K., Siddiqui R. A. Interleukin-8: an autocrine inflammatory mediator. *Curr Pharm Des*, 1999. **5**(4): 241–53.

43. Mukaida N. The roles of cytokine receptors in diseases. *Rinsho Byori*, 2000. **48**(5):409–15.

44. Detmers P. A., La S. K., Olsen-Egbert E., *et al.* Neutrophil-activating protein 1/interleukin 8 stimulates the binding activity of the leukocyte adhesion receptor CD11b/CD18 on human neutrophils. *J Exp Med*, 1990. **171**(4):1155–62.

45. Huber A. R., Kunkel S. L., Todd R. F., 3rd, Weiss S. J. Regulation of transendothelial neutrophil migration by endogenous interleukin-8. *Science*, 1991. **254**(5028):99–102.

46. Zalewska A., Glowacka E., Wyczolkowska J., *et al.* Interleukin 6 and 8 levels in plasma and fibroblast cultures in psoriasis. *Mediators Inflamm*, 2006. **2006**: 81767.

47. Brown A. S., Susser E. (1999). Plausibility of prenatal rubella, influenza, and other viral infections as risk factors for schizophrenia. In *Prenatal Exposures in Schizophrenia*, Susser E., Brown A. S., and Gorman J. M. (Eds.). Washington, DC: American Psychiatric Press, Inc., pp. 113–31.

48. Koenig J. I., Kirkpatrick B., Lee P. Glucocorticoid hormones and early brain development in schizophrenia. *Neuropsychopharmacology*, 2002. **27**(2): 309–18.

49. Torrey E. F., Bartko J. J., Lun Z. R., Yolken R. H. Antibodies to toxoplasma gondii in patients with schizophrenia: a meta-analysis. *Schizophr Bull*, 2007. **33**(3):729–36.

50. Anton E. S., Marchionni M. A., Lee K. F., *et al.* Role of GGF/neuregulin signaling in interactions between migrating neurons and radial glia in the developing cerebral cortex. *Development*, 1997. **124**(18): 3501–10.

51. Kamiya A., Kubo K., Tomoda T., *et al.* A schizophrenia-associated mutation of DISC1 perturbs cerebral cortex development. *Nat Cell Biol*, 2005. 7(12):1167–78.

52. Shi L., Fatemi S. H., Sidwell R. W., Patterson P. H. Maternal influenza infection causes marked behavioral and pharmacological changes in the offspring. *J Neurosci*, 2003. **23**(1):297–302.

53. Fatemi S. H., Emamian E. S., Kist D., *et al.* Defective corticogenesis and reduction in reelin immunoreactivity in cortex and hippocampus of prenatally infected neonatal mice. *Mol Psychiatry*, 1999. 4(2):145–54.

54. Zuckerman L., Rehavi M., Nachman R., Weiner I. Immune activation during pregnancy in rats leads to a postpubertal emergence of disrupted latent inhibition, dopaminergic hyperfunction, and altered limbic morphology in the offspring: a novel neurodevelop- mental model of schizophrenia. *Neuropsychopharmacology*, 2003. **28**(10):1778–89.

55. Centers for Disease Control and Prevention. CDC recommendations regarding selected conditions affecting women's health. *MMWR Morb Mortal Wkly Rep*, **49**(RR-2): 57–75. 2000.

56. Brown A. S., Schaefer C. A., Wyatt R. J., *et al.* Maternal exposure to respiratory infections and adult schizophrenia spectrum disorders: a prospective birth cohort study. *Schizophr Bull*, 2000. **26**(2):287–95.

23

The status of genetic investigations of schizophrenia

Bryan Mowry

Facts box

- Schizophrenia (SZ) has a substantial genetic predisposition.
- The inheritance pattern is complex, likely involving multiple, commonly occurring risk variants, each exerting a modest effect on overall disease risk.
- Significant progress has recently occurred with consensus chromosomal regions being linked to SZ and specific candidate genes, often located within these linkage regions, being associated with SZ in multiple populations with variable ancestry.
- However, indisputable evidence of association is lacking and no allele/haplotype has yet been conclusively implicated for any candidate gene.
- Further progress will depend on rigorous phenotyping (including the use of alternative phenotypes) and comprehensive LD mapping of large, ethnically homogeneous samples.
- To guard against false-positive findings, replication is essential.
- Functional studies of replicated variants should help clarify underlying molecular mechanisms that may lead to the development of targeted molecular treatments for SZ.

Genetic complexity of schizophrenia

Psychiatry has always suspected that schizophrenia (SZ) has a genetic predisposition. Kraepelin wrote in 1919 that "dementia praecox not at all infrequently is familial, often appearing in brothers and sisters" [1]; in 1916, Schulz used the family study method to evaluate the validity of Kraepelin's subtyping system for

SZ [2], and in 1946, Kallmann analyzed 691 SZ twin families [3]. Decades of family [4], twin [5, 6], and adoption studies [7, 8] have substantiated these early views indicating a substantial genetic component to SZ risk, with an 80% heritability (the proportion of the total phenotypic variance explained by genetic factors) [9, 10], a 50% concordance rate in monozygotic twins, and a 10% risk to siblings relative to a 1% general population risk [11]. The inheritance pattern is complex (i.e. non-Mendelian), and there are no known familial subtypes [12]. Available data suggest multiple, common SZ variants, each exerting small to moderate effect on overall disease risk [12], possibly interacting with environmental factors [13] and epigenetic processes [14] in a neurodevelopmental context to confer vulnerability [15]. An alternative view is that multiple genes are certainly implicated, but that each is highly penetrant (and hence of large effect) and rare in the population, being specific to individual cases or single families [16]. It is probably better to assume that there is a spectrum of risk variants of varying effect sizes, including both common and rare alleles [17]. In any case, the exact number of alleles, the degree of allelic interaction, and each allele's contribution to overall disease risk remain unknown [18]. Moreover, there may be individual differences in disease allele frequency within a gene (allelic heterogeneity), between genes (locus heterogeneity), between samples (population heterogeneity), and within phenotypes (clinical heterogeneity), making initial detection and replication difficult [19].

Despite such formidable challenges, after 20 years of intensive international effort, progress is occurring. Replicated SZ linkages are accumulating and converging on a modest number of loci across the genome, and association studies have identified and confirmed a number of susceptibility genes. Before discussing these findings, it is important to mention the clinical, molecular, and analytic developments that have triggered this progress.

Clinical phenotype

Diagnostic categories

Phenotype definition and measurement are fundamentally important for the success of gene identification [20]. This represents a challenge for psychiatric genetics, given the lack of biologically valid measures currently available [21].

Since its initial description, SZ has been defined on the basis of clinical criteria. In the fifth edition of his textbook *Psychiatrie*, Kraepelin described "dementia praecox" as a syndrome of psychotic symptoms and chronic deterioration and contrasted it with manic-depressive insanity, characterized by remission between periods of mood disturbance [1]. In 1911, Bleuler coined the term "schizophrenia" denoting a "split between thinking and perception," emphasizing blunted emotions, abnormal association of ideas, and impaired volition [22], and in 1933 Kasanin introduced "schizoaffective psychosis" [23]. Schneider's "first rank" symptoms such as delusions of control, thought broadcast, and commentary hallucinations were also influential [24]. These concepts, combined with a landmark study demonstrating significant international (US–UK) differences in SZ diagnosis [25], contributed to the development of more specific diagnostic criteria to increase reliability. Successive waves of progress have produced the current sets of diagnostic criteria, DSM-IV [26] and ICD-10 [27]. Parallel advances have included: (i) semistructured, standardized interviews such as the Diagnostic Interview for Genetic Studies [28] and the Family Interview for Genetic Studies [29, 30]; and (ii) comprehensive diagnostic approaches such as the Best Estimate Final Diagnosis (BEFD) procedure [31] in which two experienced research diagnosticians independently review all available data and then meet to determine a consensus BEFD [32].

Alternative clinical phenotypes

A comprehensive approach to the SZ phenotype has served the psychiatric genetics community well, as evidenced by the progress outlined later. Nevertheless, it lacks precision and may represent, as Bleuler suggested, a group of diseases [22]. In addition, quantitative traits may have greater power than categorical diagnoses in genetic analyses, especially if analyses only include individuals with extreme phenotypic values [33, 34]; moreover, evidence suggests that susceptibility variants may not respect diagnostic boundaries [35]. Thus, efforts to refine the SZ phenotype are justified. These include: (i) the application of alternative diagnostic systems, for example, Leonhard's classification [36] with the catatonic SZ phenotype attracting some support from genetic studies [37, 38]; (ii) the derivation of symptom dimensions using instruments such as the Operational Criteria Checklist for Psychotic and Affective Illness (OPCRIT) [39] and the Lifetime Dimensions of Psychosis Scale (LDPS), a 21-item scale for rating the lifetime duration and severity of positive, bizarre, negative, disorganized, and mood symptoms of psychotic disorders [40]; (iii) identifying clinical characteristics shared by clusters of related individuals, using techniques such as latent class analysis (LCA); and (iv) the study of SZ endophenotypes.

Statistical studies provide support for several alternative phenotypes. A recent factor analysis of OPCRIT symptoms identified five factors (mania, reality distortion, depression, disorganization, and negativity) that explained more of the disease characteristics than diagnosis but the explanatory power of diagnosis was also high [41]. A prominent latent class analysis found six latent classes (classic SZ, major depression, schizophreniform disorder, bipolar-schizomania, schizodepression, and hebephrenia), all of which, except for depression, showed increased risks for SZ in relatives [42]; the most marked risk occurred in hebephrenic probands who were linked to chromosome 8p significantly more often than others [43]. There is also some support for endophenotypes, quantitatively measurable traits situated along the pathway between the clinical phenotype and the distal genotype [44]. Candidate endophenotypes for SZ [45, 46] include (i) neurophysiological markers [47], for example, sustained attention deficits [48], P50 suppression deficits associated with the alpha7 nicotinic acetylcholine receptor gene, *CHRNA7* [49]; (ii) neuroimaging results [50], for example, bilateral fronto-striato-thalamic and left lateral temporal grey-matter volume deficits [51]; and (iii) neurocognitive markers [52], for example, spatial working memory [53], and a pervasive cognitive deficit linked to chromosome 6p25–24 [54]. One large-scale application of the endophenotype paradigm is the multisite Consortium on the Genetics of Endophenotypes in Schizophrenia (COGS) study [55]. However, the endophenotype paradigm is not without difficulties [56], with little convincing evidence for any candidate showing a simpler genetic architecture than SZ, the requirement for special measurement procedures constraining sample size, and the need to address the challenges of interlaboratory variation [57].

Molecular genetics

The molecular genetic revolution has greatly accelerated the ability to search for disease-associated variants. Before the mid-1970s, the only genetic markers available for mapping diseases were blood groups, serum proteins, and HLA tissue types relating to only a handful of chromosomal locations. With the discovery of restriction enzymes, which cut double-stranded DNA at specific recognition sequences, restriction fragment length polymorphisms (RFLPs) were used as genome-wide markers for mapping disease genes. Polymerase chain reaction (PCR) methodology subsequently made it possible to amplify highly polymorphic microsatellite markers (STRPs), which superseded RFLPs. With the completion of the human genome sequence [58], gene mapping now increasingly utilizes single nucleotide polymorphisms (SNPs) involving a single base change. Compared with RFLPs and STRPs, SNPs are: (i) easily detectable; (ii) amenable to high throughput, automated typing, with low error rates; (iii) abundant, occurring one in every 1000 base pairs, with several million, well-characterized SNPs now available for disease studies [59]; (iv) uniformly distributed across the genome and present within exons, introns, promoters, enhancers, and intergenic regions; and (v) stable, being less prone to mutation than other types of polymorphism [60].

In the wake of the Human Genome Project, other projects are making substantial contributions to clarifying the genetic basis of disease. The National Human Genome Research Institute's ENCODE (Encyclopedia of DNA Elements) was launched in 2003 to identify all functional elements in the human genome sequence [61]. The International HapMap Consortium is developing a map of common patterns of DNA sequence variation by determining the genotypes of more than one million SNPs, their frequencies, and the degree of association between them, in DNA samples from populations with African, Asian, and European ancestry [62]. This exploits: (i) the concept of the "haplotype" (the linear arrangement of closely linked alleles inherited as a unit on one member of a chromosome pair), which may provide statistical power advantages over the single locus approach to identify genetic variants associated with disease [63, 64, 65]; and (ii) the

underlying haplotype structure of the human genome consisting of discrete haplotype blocks (of tens to hundreds of kilobases) disrupted by sites of ancestral recombination [66, 67, 68]. These data have revealed profound variation in haplotype block length across the genome, reflecting regional differences in the frequency of recombination events. The HapMap consortium has also generated a vast and growing set of genetically validated markers for use in disease studies, together with bioinformatics tools such as Haploview [69], which provides a visual representation of LD – the nonrandom association of alleles at neighboring markers – in regions of interest. Moreover, by utilizing LD, the HapMap enables the representation of the majority of genomic variation in a region by typing only a subset of "tagSNPs" – SNPs that are highly correlated with untyped SNPs in the same LD block and provide similar information – thus reducing the substantial cost of conducting such experiments.

One of the assumptions underlying the HapMap approach is the common variant/common disease hypothesis, which proposes that most risk variants for common diseases are relatively common (frequency $> 0.01–0.10$) in the general population and are of modest effect size [70, 71]. This hypothesis is supported by a meta-analysis of genetic association studies [72] and by multiple recent large-scale studies identifying susceptibility variants in a range of common diseases (discussed later).

In addition to SNPs, previously unrecognized larger-sized (non-SNP) structural variants (size range: $\sim$1kb – 3Mb) have recently been identified [73]. These include copy number variations (CNVs), inversions, and insertion/deletion variants (InDels). CNVs, for example, can contain entire genes and may influence nearby genes, making them important candidates for disease gene investigations.

Statistical genetics

Linkage analysis

Linkage describes the nonrandom segregation of disease and marker loci, leading to co-inheritance of the same marker allele by multiple affected family members; the linked marker allele is consistent within families but can differ across families [20, 74]. Linkage has been widely applied in complex genetic disorders such as SZ, following its success in identifying the variants underlying many Mendelian disorders. Another impetus for employing linkage in psychiatric genetics is that it does not require a priori knowledge about the location of disease genes. Linkage has been widely applied for genome-wide screening – typically using several hundred STRP markers (and more recently, panels of several thousand SNP markers) of known location. The goal of such studies is to identify one or more chromosomal regions showing convincing evidence of linkage to SZ (criteria provided later). Substantial sample sizes are required to detect variants of modest effect [70, 75] and the identified region(s) are often very large, that is, > 20cM [20 million base pairs]. Follow-up studies with a higher density of markers may then be conducted to extract maximal linkage information from the implicated region(s) and sufficiently constrain the region to allow fine-scale LD mapping (discussed later).

Stimulated by the feasibility of genome-wide linkage scans of pedigree cohorts, analytic methods were developed to meet the need for (i) multipoint linkage analysis with many markers across the genome; and (ii) robustness in the face of uncertainty about mode of inheritance in non-Mendelian diseases. Guidelines for the interpretation of results have been another critical development. Specific statistical criteria have been proposed [76], based on the number of times one would expect a result by chance in a genome-wide scan (GWS). Standard thresholds are suggestive, significant, and highly significant linkage, which are expected to occur by chance once, 0.05 times, and 0.001 times, respectively, in a GWS. For sib pair studies, these categories correspond to pointwise significance levels of 7×10^{-4}, 2×10^{-5}, and 3×10^{-7}, and LOD scores of 2.2, 3.6, and 5.4. It has been widely suggested that these guidelines are overly stringent, due to potentially unrealistic assumptions underlying their derivation [77]. For these reasons, research groups often use simulation to empirically determine type I error (i.e. false-positive) rates in their own dataset, thereby assigning empirical significance levels that may be evaluated for study-wide significance [78].

Association analysis

Whereas linkage identifies broad genetic regions (that may contain hundreds of genes) linked with disease, association aims to identify a specific associated risk allele. Association detects correlation between disease and marker allele(s)/haplotype(s) in a population, which may be seen as one very large pedi-

gree that has undergone thousands of meioses (generations) and displays LD (usually within distances < 0.2 cM) between an associated marker allele and the untyped causative allele(s). Thus, association studies appear to be more powerful than linkage studies for identifying common genetic variants of small to modest effect on overall disease risk [19, 70, 79]. The power of a primary association study is influenced by sample size, true effect size of the disease-causing allele, disease allele versus control allele frequency, and the extent of LD between marker and disease allele [80]. To detect variants of small effect (odds ratio: 1.3–1.5), similar to those anticipated in SZ, thousands of cases and controls would be required [70, 81].

Association analysis is conducted in either case-control samples or nuclear families [19, 82]. In case-control studies, the presence of population stratification – arising when case and control groups differ in the prevalence of distinct ethnic groups – can increase the type I error rate, as any trait more common in one group will show association with alleles having higher frequency in that same group [83]. Careful selection of cases and controls from relatively homogeneous populations, especially prospective cohorts, can reduce this bias [84] as can the use of analytic methods that correct for population structure [85, 86, 87, 88]. Family-based methods such as the transmission disequilibrium test (TDT) are robust to population stratification, as control alleles are determined from family members (usually parents) of the affected individual [89]. The use of trios (both parents plus affected offspring) also increases the accuracy of haplotype inference [90].

Association studies have typically been used for evaluating defined candidate regions and/or disease susceptibility genes. However, the public availability of millions of well-characterized SNPs [59, 62], and rapid improvements in SNP genotyping technology have ushered in the era of genome-wide association studies (GWA), which utilize hundreds of thousands of SNPs so that there is an increased chance of a genotyped marker being either: (i) a risk variant itself or (ii) close enough to a risk variant so that they stay together through many generations (i.e., in strong LD with one another) [91]. The first wave of GWA studies for complex diseases has reported statistically significant evidence for a number of variants. Strongly associated SNPs have been identified and replicated for Crohn's Disease [92, 93, 94], type 1 diabetes [93, 95], type 2 diabetes [93, 96, 97], and prostate cancer [98]; for prostate cancer, three new studies [99, 100, 101] have replicated multiple independent variants strongly associated with disease within a consensus linkage region on chromosome 8q24 [98]. These findings highlight the value of undertaking large-scale, complementary GWA studies across multiple populations [98] and underline the importance of common variants of modest effect contributing to overall disease risk in complex disease. The first published GWA for SZ [102] examined more than 500,000 markers in a case-control study of 178 SZ spectrum cases and reported a significant association with SNP rs4129148 ($p = 3.7 \times 10^{-7}$), near the colony stimulating factor receptor 2 alpha (*CSF2RA*) gene in the pseudoautosomal region. This association surpassed the threshold for genome-wide significance based on a Bayesian formula [103]. This result awaits replication in larger samples.

Given the huge number of tests performed in large-scale association studies, a critical issue is appropriate control of the type I error rate. A common approach to multiple testing correction is Bonferroni correction [70, 104], which assumes the independence of all tests performed. However, this approach is often overly conservative due to intermarker LD and nonindependence of the individual tests. Other methods for determining statistical significance include the false discovery rate and use of q-values [105], a Bayesian approach involving the prior odds and power [106], and permutation methods including the application of extreme value distributions to permuted data [107].

Schizophrenia linkage studies

After years of intensive international effort, linkage studies have achieved progress in identifying promising susceptibility regions for SZ. A number of regions have demonstrated statistical significance in at least one study or strong support from multiple independent studies. These are shown in Figure 23.1. To address the limitations of small samples, research groups have also combined their samples to conduct large (> 700 SZ pedigrees), multicenter, region-specific analyses that have provided support for some regions including 6p and 8p [108] and 6q [109] but no support for others such as 1q [110] and 22q [111]. Meta-analyses have highlighted somewhat different but overlapping regions, with Badner and Gershon [112] supporting 8p, 13q, and 22q, and a rank-based genome scan meta-analysis (GSMA) [113] supporting 2q plus a number of other regions including 3p, 8p, and 22q. Since the GSMA was published on data from

20 schizophrenia genome scans (1208 pedigrees, 2,945 affected), 12 additional studies have been reported in over 1,400 additional families from diverse populations, primarily supporting the linkages on 8p, 2q, 5p, 5q, 6p, 6q, and 10q.

Schizophrenia association studies

Biologically plausible SZ candidate genes have been identified primarily through their position in linkage candidate regions or near cytogenetic abnormalities (Disrupted-in-Schizophrenia 1, *DISC1*, catechol-o-methyltransferase, *COMT*). Additionally, candidates have been identified through (i) differential gene expression in postmortem brain (e.g. regulator of G-protein signaling 4 (RGS4) gene, *RGS4* [159]); (ii) psychopharmacological hypotheses regarding functional polymorphisms in monoaminergic receptor genes (e.g. the dopamine receptor, *DRD3* [160, 161]; 5-hydroxytryptamine (serotonin) receptor 2A, *HTR2A* [162, 163]); and (iii) specific hypotheses, for example, aberrant signal transduction (RAC-alpha serine/threonine-protein kinase *AKT1*, [164]. Table 23.1 lists SZ candidate genes currently attracting the most support. There have been a number of recent reviews of this literature [56, 165, 166, 167, 168, 169, 170]. In this paper, relevant issues in SZ genetics will be illustrated through an in-depth examination of one candidate gene, *DISC1*.

DISC1: an illustrative example

Cytogenetics, linkage, and association

Figure 23.2 shows the genomic position, structure, and published findings for DISC1 (and the neighboring gene, TSNAX). Jacobs originally reported a chromosomal-balanced translocation disrupting regions of chromosomes 1 and 11 (1;11)(q42;q14.3) [190] in the proband and other members of a four generational Scottish pedigree. Thirty-four of 77 pedigree members available for karyotyping carried this translocation [191], which generated a LOD score of 7.1 with a disease phenotype crossing traditional diagnostic boundaries (including recurrent major depression, bipolar disorder, and SZ); the SZ LOD score was 3.6, and the LOD score for affective disorders was 4.5 [115]. The translocation directly disrupts the function of two novel genes on 1q42, termed Disrupted-In-Schizophrenia 1 and 2 (DISC1, DISC2) [175]. DISC1 occupies $\sim$ 415 Kb

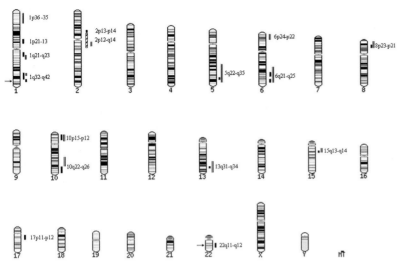

Figure 23.1 Locations of linkage findings and chromosomal abnormalities implicated in SZ

Notes. Genome-wide significant linkages (black line); consensus linkage regions attracting strong support from more than one independent study (parallel lines); best region (2p12-q24) from rank based genome scan meta-analysis (GMSA)(striped box); arrows mark the sites of chromosomal abnormalities: 1q42 [114, 115]; 22q11: [116, 117, 118, 119];
Linkage regions (asterisks indicate significant genome-wide evidence):
1p36-p35 [120], [121]
1p21-p13 [122]*
1q21-q24: [123]*, [124]
1q32-q42: [125]*, [115], [126]*, [127]
2p15-p13: [128]*, [129], [130]
2p12-q14: [113], [131]
5q22-q35: [120], [127], [128], [130], [132], [133], [134], [135]
6p24-p22: [135], [136], [137], [138], [139], [140]
6q21-q25: [141], [142], [143]*, [109], [144]*
8p23-p21: [145]*, [123], [127], [135], [146], [147]
10p15-p12: [132]*, [139], [148], [149]
10q22-q26: [137]*, [143], [150], [151]*, [152]
13q31-q34: [121], [145]*, [153]
15q13-q14: P50 inhibitory deficit [154]*; Periodic catatonia [155]*, [137], [141], [156], [157]
17p11-q25: [151], [158]*
22q11-q12: [132], [145], [151], [155], [158], [159]
Chromosome ideograms were adapted from Ensembl Genome Browser (August, 2006).

of genomic DNA, comprises a 13-exon transcript of ∼7.5 Kb, and encodes a novel protein of 854 AAs) [192]. DISC2 specifies an antisense noncoding RNA molecule believed to be involved in regulating DISC1 expression [193].

Multiple independent observations of a rearrangement affecting a particular gene would be strong evidence for the involvement of this gene in the pathophysiology of SZ [214]. This evidence is currently lacking. However, the original linkage finding has been extended to the general Scottish population [205, 208] and beyond. Linkage of this region of 1q to SZ has also been detected in an internal Finnish isolate [122] and families from across Finland [125]. The strongest evidence for linkage (LOD = 3.21) in the combined Finnish sample was observed for a marker located within DISC1, D1S2709. A follow-up study of 70 Finnish families [201] observed maximal linkage (LOD = 2.70) with an intragenic SNP, rs1000731.

Other populations have reported linkage of the DISC1 region to SZ [200], Schizoaffective Disorder (SA) [203], and Bipolar Disorder (BP) [198, 199, 215, 216], and associations for SZ, BP, SA, and Major Depressive Disorder [205, 208, 210, 211].

Since the initial linkage reports, numerous studies have shown association of DISC1 variants with SZ (Figure 23.2). Although some consistency has been observed across studies, the associated haplotypes vary widely in their location within DISC1 and their constituent alleles. In a study conducted in 458 Finnish

Table 23.1 Schizophrenia candidate genes and strength of evidence

		Strength of evidence (0 to 5)					
Gene	Location	Linkage to gene locus	Association with SZ	Cytogenetics	Biological plausibility	Altered expression in SZ	References: original report(s) / review(s)
DTNBP1	6p22	+ + + +	+ + + + +		+ +	Yes, + +	[171] / [172]
NRG1	8p12-21	+ + + +	+ + + + +		+ + +	Yes, +	[173] / [174]
DISC1	1q42	+ +	+ + + +	+ + + + +	+ + + +	Yes, +	[115], [175] / [176]
RGS4	1q21-22	+ + +	+ + +		+ +	Yes, + +	[177], [178] / [159], [179], [180]
COMT	22q11	+ + + +	+	+ + + + +	+ + + +	Yes, +	[181] / [118], [119]
DAOA (G72/G30)	13q32-34	+ +	+ + +		+ +	Not known	[182] /[183], [184]
PPP3CC	8p21	+ + + +	+		+ + + +	Yes, +	[185], [186] / [168]
CHRNA7	15q13-14	+	+ +		+ + +	Yes, + + +	[154], [155] / [49]
AKT1	14q22-32	+ +	+		+ +	Yes, + +	[164] / [187]
DRD3	3q13		+ +		+ + +	Yes, + +	[188] / [160], [161]
5HT2A	13q14.2		+ +		+ + +	Yes, + +	[189] / [162], [163]

Notes. Adapted from [167]; *DTNBP1*: dystrobrevin binding protein 1; *NRG1*: neuregulin 1; *DISC1*, disrupted in schizophrenia 1; *RGS4*, regulator of G-protein signaling 4; *COMT*, catechol-O-methyltransferase; *DAOA*, D-amino acid oxidase activator; *PPP3CC*, protein phosphatase 3 (formerly 2B), catalytic subunit, gamma isoform (calcineurin A gamma); *CHRNA7*, cholinergic receptor, nicotinic, alpha 7; *AKT1*, v-akt murine thymoma viral oncogene homolog 1; *DRD3*, dopamine receptor D3; *5HT2A*, 5-hydroxytryptamine (serotonin) receptor 2A.

SZ pedigrees, Hennah and colleagues [204] identified four DISC1 haplotypes (termed HEP 1 to 4) associated with a broad diagnostic model (SZ/SA/BP/MDD). Association of the HEP3 haplotype was only significant for affected females ($p = 0.00024$) but showed a trend with negative symptoms and hallucinations in both sexes. Other studies have reported association with the HEP3 haplotype [208] and larger haplotypes containing HEP3 [205, 206], although the associated haplotypes differ in their component alleles (Figure 23.2). These larger haplotypes also involve variants within the adjacent translin-associated factor X gene (*TSNAX*). Additionally, the largest associated haplotype (SNPs 1–8) demonstrated association with BP in females ($p = 0.00026$) [205]. Using 102 Taiwanese affected sib-pair families, Liu and colleagues [209] screened 12 genes within 1.5 megabases of D1S251 (within DISC1) to fine-map their chromosome 1 linkage peak [200]. Two haplotypes showed association with a subgroup of SZ with sustained attention deficits; one was in *DISC1*, 3′ of HEP3 (SNPs 10, 11: $p = 0.0008$), the other was located within glyceronephosphate O-acyltransferase (*GNPAT*) [209]. Even further 3′ of HEP3, near the translocation breakpoint, associ-

ation of HEP1 (SNPs 17–19) has been reported by two Finnish studies, for SZ $p = 0.0009$ [201] and semantic clustering ($p = 0.006$) [206]. A second cytogenetic abnormality has also been reported within exon12 (a four base-pair deletion at the 3' end of DISC1) in three affected siblings and their unaffected father [194], although involvement of this deletion with SZ has not yet been statistically supported. Negative reports include a large Japanese sample [217].

Endophenotypes

Initially, Blackwood [115] reported amplitude reduction and latency prolongation in the auditory P300 event-related potential in translocation carriers and those with SZ compared with noncarriers and controls. Apart from a recent SZ dimensional study of lifetime severity of delusions [213], other endophenotypic reports include impairments in spatial working memory [197, 206, 211, 218], short-term visual working memory and visual attention [207], verbal working memory [218], sustained attention deficits [209], and semantic processing in long-term memory [206]. Neuroimaging variables showing association with DISC1

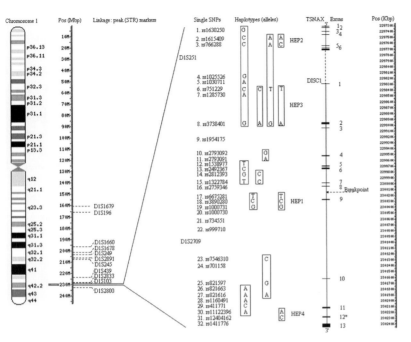

Figure 23.2 Genomic position, structure and published findings on DISC1 (and TSNAX)
Notes. Chromosome 1 ideogram, positions (Mbp = megabases; Kbp = kilobases), TSNAX = translin-associated factor X gene;
DISC1 = Disrupted in Schizophrenia 1; STR markers = simple tandem repeat markers; SNP = single nucleotide polymorphism; SNPs 1–31 are
taken from the DISC1 literature; Haplotypes = linear arrangement of closely linked alleles inherited as a unit on one member of a
chromosome pair; global *p* values incorporate multiple test correction; unless otherwise indicated, all scores are for the schizophrenia (SZ)
phenotype; BP = Bipolar Disorder; SA = Schizoaffective Disorder; MDD = Major Depressive Disorder;
Translocation breakpoint: LOD = 7.1 (SZ, BP, MDD) [115]
Exon 12*: Frameshift site(s) identified in single U.S. multiplex SZ pedigree [194]

Linkage STR markers:
D1S1679: LOD = 6.50 [123]
D1S196: LOD = 3.20 [127]; LOD = 2.40 [124]
D1S249: LOD = 2.00 [195]
D1S2891: LOD = 3.82 [125]; LOD = 2.67 [195]
D1S245: LOD = 3.46 [126]
D1S439: LOD = 2.62 [196]
D1S2833: *p* = 0.007 spatial working memory deficit in SZ [197]
D1S103: LOD = 2.63 BP [198]; LOD = 2.39 BP, SA, MDD [199]
D1S251(intragenic): LOD = 2.18 [200]
SNP 19 (rs1000731)(intragenic): LOD = 2.70 [201]
D1S2709 (intragenic): LOD = 3.21 [126]; 3.31 [202]
D1S2800: LOD = 3.54 [203] SA

SNP markers/haplotypes:
HEP1 (SNPs 17–19), HEP2 (SNPs 2, 3), HEP3 (SNPs 6, 8), HEP4 (SNPs 30, 31): haplotypes identified by Hennah *et al.*, 2003 [204]
SNPs 1–8 (global *p* = 0.0066: BP); SNPs 14–15 (C-C): (global *p* = 0.0044: SZ); SNPs 12–15 (global *p* = 0.00026: BP females; (global *p* = 0.0016): BP
males & females, 26–30 (global *p* = 0.0053) [205]
SNPs 2, 3, 6, 8 (A-A-T-G): *p* = 0.001; choice reaction time *p* = 0.002 [206]
SNPs 6, 8 (Arg264Gln) (T-A): males and females: (global *p* = 0.0031); affected females: (global *p* = 0.00024) [204]; short-term visual working
memory (*p* = 0.0013) and visual attention (*p* = 0.0079) deficits [207]
SNPs 6, 8 (C-A): *p* = 2.4 × 10^{-22} [208]
SNP 10: *p* = 0.0053; SNPs 10, 11 (G-A): *p* = 0.0008 SZ with sustained attention deficit [209]
SNP 17 (Leu607Pro): *p* = 0.2.3 × 10^{-6} [210]
SNPs 17–19: *p* = 0.0009 [201]; *p* = 0.02 [206]; *p* = 0.006 semantic clustering [206]
SNPs 23, 25, 27 (C-G-A) (Global *p* = 0.002); SNP 25 (A) (*p* = 0.004) [211]
SNP 27 (ser704cys)(G) (*p* = 0.005) MDD [212]; (*p* = 0.002) lifetime severity of delusions in SZ [213]
All STR and SNP marker positions are based on the NCBI Build 36 assembly of the human genome (November 2005).

genotypes include reduced hippocampal volume [206, 211], reduced prefrontal grey-matter density [206], reduced cingulate grey-matter volume [212], and altered engagement of the hippocampus during cognitive tasks assayed with functional MRI [211].

Functional studies

Expression studies: mRNA

As with many putative candidate genes, DISC1 is transcriptionally complex with evident multiple alternate splicing events, antisense transcription, and intergenic splicing [193]. DISC1 has eight coding transcripts, the longest containing 13 exons, a transcript length of 7,059 bp, and 854 amino acid (AA) residues (Figure 23.2) [193, 219]. The translocation breakpoint is located between exons 8 and 9 and may produce a truncated protein via loss of 257 amino acids at the C-terminus. SNP rs821616 is a major alternative splice site and is responsible for an AA change from serine to leucine at codon 704 (Ser704Cys), with a deletion of 22 AAs from exon 11. This results in two of the eight isoforms, DISC1^{ser} and DISC1^{cys}, which are widely expressed in the brain and other tissues. In the brain, the dentate gyrus of the hippocampus has the highest DISC1 mRNA expression levels in adult mouse [220] and primate brains [221]. DISC1 is conserved across primates, rodents, and fish, but it appears to have no insect or worm homologue [193, 222].

Expression studies: protein

Expression at the protein level is similarly complex, with antibodies against several portions of DISC1 detecting a variety of protein products [223, 224, 225, 226, 227, 228]. DISC1 expression occurs preferentially in the forebrain (hippocampus, cerebral cortex, olfactory bulbs) throughout life and is regulated developmentally, with the highest expression in rat cortex occurring during late embryonic and postnatal stages [223, 225], suggesting DISC1 has a crucial role in neurodevelopment and maturation [229]. Subcellular studies have revealed four major distribution sites: (i) microtubule-associated cytoskeletons and the centrosome [225, 226, 228, 230]; (ii) mitochondria in primary neurons [225, 226, 227, 228]; (iii) post-synaptic density of adult brains [231]; and (iv) the nucleus [231].

Protein interactors: Many yeast-2-hybrid screening studies have been conducted to further investigate DISC1 function [232]. A recent network analysis of these studies implicates DISC1 in cell-cycle/division, cytoskeletal organization, and intracellular transport, incorporating 127 proteins and 158 interactions in a "DISC1 interactome," providing evidence that DISC1 may be an essential synaptic protein [233]. Moreover, DISC1 and DTNBP1 appear to share interactions thus suggesting functional convergence of SZ candidate genes. Millar and colleagues [234] recently reported a balanced translocation in two affected family members that disrupted the gene encoding phosphodiesterase 4B (PDE4B), which inactivates adenosine 3',5'-monophosphate (cAMP), a second messenger implicated in learning, memory, and mood. It is proposed that DISC1 interacts with the UCR2 domain of PDE4B in a cAMP feedback loop.

Thus, DISC1 illustrates a number of issues characterizing most current candidate genes for SZ: (i) linkage and association evidence is present for several psychiatric disorders including SZ, BP, and SA; (ii) multiple populations with variable ancestry have been studied, with most but not all reporting positive findings; and (iii) the precise polymorphism(s) conferring risk and their functional implications remain unknown; most replication studies have been inconsistent with respect to the associated alleles, haplotypes, and conferred risks. This may reflect the low a priori probability of directly genotyping a causal variant, combined with population variation in LD patterns, such that different alleles show association in different populations [82].

Implications for clinical practice

It is likely that most SZ susceptibility genes will be found to individually exert small to modest effect on overall disease risk (with the possible exception of the t(1:11), with an effect size the equivalent of MZ inheritance). Thus, for any individual locus, its importance will lie not in its population-attributable risk (i.e. the proportion of disease that would be cured in the population if the allele were absent), but in contributing to understanding the molecular mechanisms and pathways involved in disease [235]. However, in combination with the discovery of other susceptibility loci and environmental exposures, impending clinical implications could include molecular diagnosis and personalized treatment.

Molecular diagnosis

The presence of risk alleles in an unaffected individual may motivate the detailed study of environmental risk factors and perhaps the application of preventative therapeutics [235]. However, the discovery of susceptibility alleles alone may not be sufficient to carve the complicated nature of psychiatric nosology "at its joints" [236].

Molecular treatment

With the availability of the reference human genome sequence and the International HapMap, pharmacogenetics (single-gene focus) and pharmacogenomics (multiple-gene focus) are set to yield valuable outcomes for psychiatric disorders [237]. Combinations of susceptibility alleles could help subclassify patients for inclusion in drug response trials [235]. For example, based on association between familial P50 auditory evoked potential suppression deficits and alpha7 nicotinic acetylcholine receptor gene (*CHRNA7*) variants [47], SZ patients who are poor P50 suppressors may be candidates for adjunctive therapy using *CHRNA7* agonists.

Suggestions for future research

Clinical

Further refinement of the SZ phenotype is warranted and could involve: (i) supplementing a comprehensive diagnostic approach (standardized individual and family diagnostic interviews, medical records collection) with psychopathological dimensions, to highlight clinical variability within categories and similarities across categories; (ii) addressing sources of clinical variability such as geographical origin (variable environmental exposures, sociocultural factors) and ascertainment methods (variable clinical settings producing different clinical profiles) [21]; and (iii) wherever feasible, incorporating neuroimaging, neurophysiological, and neuropsychological endophenotypes. This should help reduce phenotypic heterogeneity and thereby facilitate our investigations of genotype/phenotype relationships.

Population characteristics

It is important to undertake studies of sufficiently large, ethnically homogeneous samples across diverse populations. In addition, recruiting smaller-sized samples from population isolates could make a valuable contribution through reduced phenotypic variability, increased environmental homogeneity [82, 238], fewer distinct risk variants (decreasing genetic heterogeneity), and more extensive LD, improving the power to detect disease-associated variants [239, 240, 241, 242].

Laboratory

Systematic large-scale association studies, including LD mapping of candidate regions (including genes) and GWA approaches are needed. LD mapping of a disease-associated region will entail (i) exhaustive genotyping, including screening for submicroscopic structural variants such as CNVs, insertion/deletion variants, and inversions [73]; (ii) thorough resequencing in order to identify all known variation (both common and rare) [243]; and (iii) screening for sequence conservation across the entire region and the identification of highly conserved noncoding elements (CNEs) [244], which may be involved in gene regulation. The identified disease-associated variants will then require interrogation with functional studies in molecular, cellular, and animal models.

Functional studies could include (i) DNA microarray studies in postmortem brain tissue to discover genes whose altered expression contributes to disease [245]; (ii) cellular and molecular studies to identify mutations altering the expression of candidate gene mRNA and/or protein; (iii) epigenomic studies to investigate factors that alter gene expression in the absence of DNA mutation [246, 247]; (iv) microRNA studies to identify additional levels of regulation and to explore the downstream effects of altered gene expression [248]; and (v) the development of animal models, including knock-out and transgenic mice, to elucidate gene function.

Analytic

Given the large-scale datasets generated in GWA studies and expression studies, it is important that more robust methods are developed to deal with multiple comparisons [249]. New methods are also needed to reduce confounding by locus and allelic heterogeneity, and to detect gene-environment interactions. Population-specific HapMaps would be a welcome development given variability in LD block structure among populations, notwithstanding the conservation (and hence transferability) of tagSNP patterns across populations [250].

Replication

Replication is the gold standard of both linkage and association studies. The field must attempt to consistently replicate new and current findings across different studies and populations. The National Cancer Institute–National Human Genome Research Institute (NCI-NHGRI) Working Group on Replication in Association has recently published criteria for establishing replication in an effort to help separate "true associations from the blizzard of false positives" expected with the transition of the field to GWA studies [104]. Thus, replication studies should be of sufficient sample size to convincingly distinguish the proposed effect from no effect, conducted in independent data sets, analyzing the same phenotype with the same genetic model, and demonstrating a similar magnitude of effect and significance with the same SNP, or a SNP in perfect or very high LD with the prior SNP [104].

Summary and conclusions

Great advances have been made in the last 5 years. Based primarily on consensus linkage findings but also on associations with chromosomal abnormalities, a number of candidate genes are now implicated in SZ predisposition. Each has attracted support from multiple studies across a range of populations. These developments have been founded on improved consistency of phenotyping, molecular genetic advances such as completion of the human genome sequence, and the availability of the human HapMap and SNP databases, together with the evolution of statistical genetics theory and practice. For each gene, however, unequivocal evidence of association is lacking, and no allele/haplotype has been conclusively implicated. Rigorous phenotyping of large ethnically homogeneous samples and comprehensive LD mapping should facilitate identification and replication of risk variants for SZ. Functional studies of these variants should then help clarify underlying molecular mechanisms that may in turn lead to the development of targeted molecular treatments. The future certainly holds promise.

Acknowledgments
The author thanks Elizabeth Holliday, PhD, for her helpful comments. This work was supported in part by the Australian National Health and Medical Research Council grant 339454 and the US National Institute of Mental Health grant R01 MH59588.

References

1. Kraepelin E. (1919). Dementia praecox. In *The Clinical Roots of the Schizophrenia Syndrome*, Cutting J. and Shepherd M. (Eds.). Cambridge: Cambridge University Press, pp. 15–24.

2. Kendler K. S., Zerbin-Rudin E. Abstract and review of "Zur Erbpathologie der Schizophrenie" (Contribution to the genetics of schizophrenia). 1916. *Am J Med Genet*, 1996. **67**:343–6.

3. Kallmann F. J. The genetic theory of schizophrenia. An analysis of 691 schizophrenic twin index families. 1946. *Am J Psychiatry*, 1994. **151**:188–98.

4. Levinson D. F., Mowry B. J. (2000). Genetics of schizophrenia. In *Genetic Influences on Neural and Behavioural Functions*, Pfaff D., Berrettini W., and Maxson S., *et al.* (Eds.). New York: CRC Press, pp. 47–82.

5. Gottesman I. I., Shields J. (1982). *Schizophrenia: the Epigenetic Puzzle*. Cambridge: Cambridge University Press.

6. McGuffin P., Farmer A. E., Gottesman I. I., *et al.* Twin concordance for operationally defined schizophrenia. Confirmation of familiality and heritability. *Arch Gen Psychiatry*, 1984. **41**:541–5.

7. Rosenthal D., Wender P. H., Kety S. S., *et al.* The adopted-away offspring of schizophrenia. *Am J Psychiatry*, 1971. **128**:307.

8. Kety S. S. Schizophrenic illness in the families of schizophrenic adoptees: findings from the Danish national sample. *Schizophr Bull*, 1988. **14**:217–22.

9. Cardno A. G., Gottesman I. I. Twin studies of schizophrenia: from bow-and-arrow concordances to Star Wars Mx and functional genomics. *Am J Med Genet*, 2000. **97**:12–17.

10. Sullivan P. F., Kendler K. S., Neale M. C. Schizophrenia as a complex trait: evidence from a meta-analysis of twin studies. *Arch Gen Psychiatry*, 2003. **60**:1187–92.

11. Maier W., Lichtermann D., Minges J., *et al.* Continuity and discontinuity of affective disorders and schizophrenia. Results of a controlled family study. *Arch Gen Psychiatry*, 1993. **50**:871–83.

12. Risch N. Linkage strategies for genetically complex traits. I. Multilocus models. *Am J Hum Genet*, 1990. **46**:222–8.

13. Tsuang M. Schizophrenia: genes and environment. *Biol Psychiatry*, 2000. **47**:210–20.

14. Petronis A. Human morbid genetics revisited: relevance of epigenetics. *Trends Genet*, 2001. **17**:142–6.

15. Lewis D. A., Levitt P. Schizophrenia as a disorder of neurodevelopment. *Ann Rev Neurosci*, 2002. **25**:409–32.

16. McClellan J. M., Susser E., King M. C. Schizophrenia: a common disease caused by multiple rare alleles. *Br J Psychiatry*, 2007. **190**:194–9.

17. Wang W. Y., Barratt B. J., Clayton D. G., *et al.* Genome-wide association studies: theoretical and practical concerns. *Nat Rev Genet*, 2005. **6**:109–18.

18. Owen M. J., Williams N. M., O'Donovan M. C. The molecular genetics of schizophrenia: new findings promise new insights. *Mol Psychiatry*, 2004. **9**:14–27.

19. Cardon L. R., Bell J. I. Association study designs for complex diseases. *Nat Rev Genet*, 2001. **2**:91–9.

20. Lander E. S., Schork N. J. Genetic dissection of complex traits. *Science*, 1994. **265**:2037–48.

21. Craddock N., O'Donovan M. C., Owen M. J. Phenotypic and genetic complexity of psychosis. Invited commentary on … Schizophrenia: a common disease caused by multiple rare alleles. *Br J Psychiatry*, 2007. **190**:200–3.

22. Bleuler E. (1950). *Dementia Praecox or the Group of Schizophrenias*. 1911. New York: International Universities Press.

23. Kasanin J. The acute schizoaffective psychoses. 1933. *Am J Psychiatry*, 1994. **151**: 144–54.

24. Schneider K. (1959). *Clinical Psychopathology*. New York: Grune & Stratton.

25. Cooper J. E., Kendell R. E., Gurland B. J., *et al.* (1972). *Psychiatric Diagnosis in New York and London: a Comparative Study of Mental Hospital Admissions*. London: Oxford.

26. APA (1994). *Diagnostic and Statistical Manual of Mental Disorders*. Fourth ed. Washington, DC: American Psychiatric Association.

27. WHO (1993). *The ICD-10 classification of mental and behavioural disorders: diagnostic criteria for research*. Geneva: World Health Organization.

28. Nurnberger J. I., Jr., Blehar M. C., Kaufmann C. A., *et al.* Diagnostic interview for genetic studies. Rationale, unique features, and training. NIMH Genetics Initiative. *Arch Gen Psychiatry*, 1994. **51**:849–59.

29. Gershon E. S., DeLisi L. E., Hamovit J., *et al.* A controlled family study of chronic psychoses. Schizophrenia and schizoaffective disorder. *Arch Gen Psychiatry*, 1988. **45**:328–36.

30. Maxwell M. E. (1992). *Family interview for genetic studies (FIGS): a manual for FIGS*. Bethesda, Maryland: National Institute of Mental Health.

31. Leckman J. F., Sholomskas D., Thompson W. D., *et al.* Best estimate of lifetime psychiatric diagnosis: a methodological

study. *Arch Gen Psychiatry*, 1982. **39**:879–83.

32. Suarez B. K., Duan J., Sanders A. R., *et al.* Genomewide linkage scan of 409 European-ancestry and African-American families with schizophrenia: suggestive evidence of linkage at 8p23.3-p21.2 and 11p13.1-q14.1 in the combined sample. *Am J Hum Genet*, 2006. **78**:315–33.

33. Van Gestel S., Houwing-Duistermaat J. J., Adolfsson R., *et al.* Power of selective genotyping in genetic association analyses of quantitative traits. *Behav Genet*, 2000. **30**:141–6.

34. Huang B. E., Lin D. Y. Efficient association mapping of quantitative trait loci with selective genotyping. *Am J Hum Genet*, 2007. **80**:567–76.

35. Craddock N., Owen M. J. The beginning of the end for the Kraepelinian dichotomy. *Br J Psychiatry*, 2005. **186**:364–6.

36. Leonhard K. (1999). *Classification of Endogenous Psychoses and their Differentiated Etiology*. 2nd ed. Vienna and New York: Springer Verlag.

37. Franzek E., Schmidtke A., Beckmann H., *et al.* Evidence against unusual sex concordance and pseudoautosomal inheritance in the catatonic subtype of schizophrenia. *Psychiatry Res*, 1995. **59**:17–24.

38. Beckmann H., Franzek E., Stober G. Genetic heterogeneity in catatonic schizophrenia: a family study. *Am J Med Genet*, 1996. **67**:289–300.

39. McGuffin P., Farmer A., Harvey I. A polydiagnostic application of operational criteria in studies of psychotic illness. Development and reliability of the OPCRIT system. *Arch Gen Psychiatry*, 1991. **48**:764–70.

40. Levinson D. F., Mowry B. J., Escamilla M. A., *et al.* The Lifetime Dimensions of Psychosis Scale (LDPS): description and interrater reliability. *Schizophr Bull*, 2002. **28**:683–95.

41. Dikeos D. G., Wickham H., McDonald C., *et al.* Distribution of symptom dimensions across Kraepelinian divisions. *Br J Psychiatry*, 2006. **189**:346–53.

42. Kendler K. S., Karkowski L. M., Walsh D. The structure of psychosis: latent class analysis of probands from the Roscommon Family Study. *Arch Gen Psychiatry*, 1998. **55**:492–9.

43. Kendler K. S., Myers J. M., O'Neill F. A., *et al.* Clinical features of schizophrenia and linkage to chromosomes 5q, 6p, 8p, and 10p in the Irish Study of High-Density Schizophrenia Families. *Am J Psychiatry*, 2000. **157**:402–8.

44. Gottesman I. I., Gould T. D. The endophenotype concept in psychiatry: etymology and strategic intentions. *Am J Psychiatry*, 2003. **160**:1–10.

45. Braff D. L., Freedman R., Schork N. J., *et al.* Deconstructing schizophrenia: an overview of the use of endophenotypes in order to understand a complex disorder. *Schizophr Bull*, 2007. **33**:21–32.

46. Jablensky A. Subtyping schizophrenia: implications for genetic research. *Mol Psychiatry*, 2006. **11**:815–36.

47. Turetsky B. I., Calkins M. E., Light G. A., *et al.* Neurophysiological endophenotypes of schizophrenia: the viability of selected candidate measures. *Schizophr Bull*, 2007. **33**:69–94.

48. Chen W. J., Chang C. H., Liu S. K., *et al.* Sustained attention deficits in nonpsychotic relatives of schizophrenic patients: a recurrence risk ratio analysis. *Biol Psychiatry*, 2004. **55**:995–1000.

49. Leonard S., Freedman R. Genetics of chromosome 15q13-q14 in schizophrenia. *Biol Psychiatry*, 2006. **60**:115–22.

50. Glahn D. C., Thompson P. M., Blangero J. Neuroimaging endophenotypes: strategies for finding genes influencing brain structure and function. *Hum Brain Mapp*, 2007. **28**:488–501.

51. McDonald C., Bullmore E. T., Sham P. C., *et al.* Association of genetic risks for schizophrenia and bipolar disorder with specific and generic brain structural endophenotypes. *Arch Gen Psychiatry*, 2004. **61**:974–84.

52. Gur R. E., Calkins M. E., Gur R. C., *et al.* The consortium on the genetics of schizophrenia: neurocognitive endophenotypes. *Schizophr Bull*, 2007. **33**:49–68.

53. Glahn D. C., Therman S., Manninen M., *et al.* Spatial working memory as an endophenotype for schizophrenia. *Biol Psychiatry*, 2003. **53**:624–6.

54. Hallmayer J. F., Kalaydjieva L., Badcock J., *et al.* Genetic evidence for a distinct subtype of schizophrenia characterized by pervasive cognitive deficit. *Am J Hum Genet*, 2005. **77**:468–76.

55. Calkins M. E., Dobie D. J., Cadenhead K. S., *et al.* The Consortium on the Genetics of Endophenotypes in Schizophrenia: model recruitment, assessment, and endophenotyping methods for a multisite collaboration. *Schizophr Bull*, 2007. **33**:33–48.

56. Owen M. J., Craddock N., O'Donovan M. C. Schizophrenia: genes at last? *Trends Genet*, 2005. **21**:518–25.

57. Swerdlow N. R., Sprock J., Light G. A., *et al.* Multi-site studies of acoustic startle and prepulse inhibition in humans: initial experience and methodological considerations based on studies by the Consortium on the Genetics of Schizophrenia. *Schizophr Res*, 2007. **92**:237–51.

58. International Human Genome Sequencing Consortium. Finishing the euchromatic sequence of the human genome. *Nature*, 2004. **431**:931–45.

59. Sachidanandam R., Weissman D., Schmidt S. C., *et al.* A map of human genome sequence variation containing 1.42 million single nucleotide polymorphisms. *Nature*, 2001. **409**:928–33.

60. Palmer L. J., Cardon L. R. Shaking the tree: mapping complex disease genes with linkage disequilibrium. *Lancet*, 2005. **366**:1223–34.

61. Thomas D. J., Rosenbloom K. R., Clawson H., *et al.* The ENCODE Project at UC Santa Cruz. *Nucleic Acids Res*, 2007. **35**:D663–7.

62. International HapMap Consortium. The International HapMap Project. *Nature*, 2003. **426**:789–96.

63. Akey J., Jin L., Xiong M. Haplotypes vs single marker linkage disequilibrium tests: what do we gain? *Eur J Hum Genet*, 2001. **9**:291–300.

64. Schaid D. J. Evaluating associations of haplotypes with traits. *Genet Epidemiol*, 2004. **27**:348–64.

65. Clark A. G. The role of haplotypes in candidate gene studies. *Genet Epidemiol*, 2004. **27**:321–33.

66. Daly M. J., Rioux J. D., Schaffner S. F., *et al.* High-resolution haplotype structure in the human genome. *Nat Genet*, 2001. **29**:229–32.

67. Gabriel S. B., Schaffner S. F., Nguyen H., *et al.* The structure of haplotype blocks in the human genome. *Science*, 2002. **296**:2225–9.

68. Cardon L. R., Abecasis G. R. Using haplotype blocks to map human complex trait loci. *Trends Genet*, 2003. **19**:135–40.

69. Barrett J. C., Fry B., Maller J., *et al.* Haploview: analysis and visualization of LD and haplotype maps. *Bioinformatics*, 2005. **21**:263–5.

70. Risch N., Merikangas K. The future of genetic studies of complex human diseases. *Science*, 1996. **273**:1516–17.

71. Chakravarti A. Population genetics – making sense out of sequence. *Nat Genet*, 1999. **21**:56–60.

72. Lohmueller K. E., Pearce C. L., Pike M., *et al.* Meta-analysis of genetic association studies supports a contribution of common variants to susceptibility to common disease. *Nat Genet*, 2003. **33**:177–82.

73. Feuk L., Marshall C. R., Wintle R. F., *et al.* Structural variants: changing the landscape of chromosomes and design of disease studies. *Hum Mol Genet*, 2006. 15 Spec No **1**:R57–66.

74. Ott J. (1999). *Analysis of human genetic linkage*. 3rd ed. Baltimore: The Johns Hopkins University Press.

75. Altmuller J., Palmer L. J., Fischer G., *et al.* Genomewide scans of complex human diseases: true linkage is hard to find. *Am J Hum Genet*, 2001. **69**:936–50.

76. Lander E., Kruglyak L. Genetic dissection of complex traits: guidelines for interpreting and reporting linkage results. *Nat Genet*, 1995. **11**:241–7.

77. Bacanu S. A. Robust estimation of critical values for genome scans to detect linkage. *Genet Epidemiol*, 2005. **28**:24–32.

78. Sawcer S., Jones H. B., Judge D., *et al.* Empirical genomewide significance levels established by whole genome simulations. *Genet Epidemiol*, 1997. **14**:223–9.

79. Risch N. J. Searching for genetic determinants in the new millennium. *Nature*, 2000. **405**:847–56.

80. Risch N., Teng J. The relative power of family-based and case-control designs for linkage disequilibrium studies of complex human diseases I. DNA pooling. *Genome Res*, 1998. **8**:1273–88.

81. Zondervan K. T., Cardon L. R. The complex interplay among factors that influence allelic association. *Nat Rev Genet*, 2004. **5**:89–100.

82. Hirschhorn J. N., Daly M. J. Genome-wide association studies for common diseases and complex traits. *Nat Rev Genet*, 2005. **6**:95–108.

83. Laird N. M., Lange C. Family-based designs in the age of large-scale gene-association studies. *Nat Rev Genet*, 2006. **7**:385–94.

84. Manolio T. A., Bailey-Wilson J. E., Collins F. S. Genes, environment and the value of prospective cohort studies. *Nat Rev Genet*, 2006. **7**:812–20.

85. Devlin B., Roeder K., Wasserman L. Genomic control, a new approach to genetic-based association studies. *Theor Popul Biol*, 2001. **60**:155–66.

86. Zheng G., Freidlin B., Gastwirth J. L. Robust genomic control for association studies. *Am J Hum Genet*, 2006. **78**:350–6.

87. Gorroochurn P., Hodge S. E., Heiman G. A., *et al.* A unified approach for quantifying, testing and correcting population stratification in case-control association studies. I. *Hum Hered*, 2007. **64**:149–59.

88. Price A. L., Patterson N. J., Plenge R. M., *et al.* Principal components analysis corrects for stratification in genome-wide association studies. *Nat Genet*, 2006. **38**:904–9.

89. Spielman R. S., McGinnis R. E., Ewens W. J. Transmission test for linkage disequilibrium: the insulin gene region and insulin-dependent diabetes mellitus (IDDM). *Am J Hum Genet*, 1993. **52**:506–16.

90. Beckman K. B., Abel K. J., Braun A., *et al.* Using DNA pools for genotyping trios. *Nucleic Acids Res*, 2006. 34:e129.

91. McGuffin P., Cohen S., Knight J. Homing in on depression genes. *Am J Psychiatry*, 2007. **164**:195–7.

92. Duerr R. H., Taylor K. D., Brant S. R., *et al.* A genome-wide association study identifies IL23R as an inflammatory bowel disease gene. *Science*, 2006. **314**:1461–3.

93. Wellcome Trust Case Control Consortium. Genome-wide association study of 14,000 cases of seven common diseases and 3,000 shared controls. *Nature*, 2007. **447**:661–78.

94. Parkes M., Barrett J. C., Prescott N. J., *et al.* Sequence variants in the autophagy gene IRGM and multiple other replicating loci contribute to Crohn's disease susceptibility. *Nat Genet*, 2007. **39**:830–2. Epub 2007 Jun 6.

95. Todd J. A., Walker N. M., Cooper J. D., *et al.* Robust associations of four new chromosome regions from genome-wide analyses of type 1 diabetes. *Nat Genet*, 2007. **39**:857–64. [Epub Jun 6, 2007.]

96. Sladek R., Rocheleau G., Rung J., *et al.* A genome-wide association study identifies novel risk loci for type 2 diabetes. *Nature*, 2007. **445**:881–5.

97. Zeggini E., Weedon M. N., Lindgren C. M., *et al.* Replication of genome-wide association signals in UK samples reveals risk loci for type 2 diabetes. *Science*, 2007. **316**:1336–41.

98. Witte J. S. Multiple prostate cancer risk variants on 8q24. *Nat Genet*, 2007. **39**:579–80.

99. Gudmundsson J., Sulem P., Manolescu A., *et al.* Genome-wide association study identifies a second prostate cancer susceptibility variant at 8q24. *Nat Genet*, 2007. **39**:631–7.

100. Yeager M., Orr N., Hayes R. B., *et al.* Genome-wide association study of prostate cancer identifies a second risk locus at 8q24. *Nat Genet*, 2007. **39**:645–9.

101. Haiman C. A., Patterson N., Freedman M. L., *et al.* Multiple regions within 8q24 independently affect risk for prostate cancer. *Nat Genet*, 2007. **39**:638–44.

102. Lencz T., Morgan T. V., Athanasiou M., *et al.* Converging evidence for a pseudoautosomal cytokine receptor gene locus in schizophrenia. *Mol Psychiatry*, 2007. **12**:572–80.

103. Freimer N., Sabatti C. The use of pedigree, sib-pair and association studies of common diseases for genetic mapping and epidemiology. *Nat Genet*, 2004. **36**:1045–51.

104. Chanock S. J., Manolio T., Boehnke M., *et al.* Replicating genotype–phenotype associations. *Nature*, 2007. **447**:655–60.

105. Storey J. D., Tibshirani R. Statistical significance for genomewide studies. *Proc Natl Acad Sci USA*, 2003. **100**:9440–5.

106. Wacholder S., Chanock S., Garcia-Closas M., *et al.* Assessing the probability that a positive report is false: an approach for molecular epidemiology studies. *J Natl Cancer Inst*, 2004. **96**:434–42.

107. Dudbridge F., Koeleman B. P. Efficient computation of significance levels for multiple associations in large studies of correlated data, including genomewide association studies. *Am J Hum Genet*, 2004. **75**:424–35.

108. Schizophrenia L. C. G. Additional support for schizophrenia linkage on chromosomes 6 and 8: a multicenter study. Schizophrenia Linkage Collaborative Group for Chromosomes 3, 6 and 8. *Am J Med Genet*, 1996. **67**:580–94.

109. Levinson D. F., Holmans P., Straub R. E., *et al.* Multicenter linkage study of schizophrenia candidate regions on chromosomes 5q, 6q, 10p, and 13q: schizophrenia linkage collaborative group III. *Am J Hum Genet*, 2000. **67**:652–63.

110. Levinson D. F., Holmans P. A., Laurent C., *et al.* No major

111. Mowry B. J., Holmans P. A., Pulver A. E., *et al.* Multicenter linkage study of schizophrenia loci on chromosome 22q. *Mol Psychiatry*, 2004. **9**:784–95.

112. Badner J. A., Gershon E. S. Meta-analysis of whole-genome linkage scans of bipolar disorder and schizophrenia. *Mol Psychiatry*, 2002. 7:405–11.

113. Lewis C. M., Levinson D. F., Wise L. H., *et al.* Genome scan meta-analysis of schizophrenia and bipolar disorder, part II: schizophrenia. *Am J Hum Genet*, 2003. **73**:34–48.

114. Millar J. K., Wilson-Annan J. C., Anderson S., *et al.* Disruption of two novel genes by a translocation co-segregating with schizophrenia. *Hum Mol Genet*, 2000. **9**:1415–23.

115. Blackwood D. H., Fordyce A., Walker M. T., *et al.* Schizophrenia and affective disorders – cosegregation with a translocation at chromosome 1q42 that directly disrupts brain-expressed genes: clinical and P300 findings in a family. *Am J Hum Genet*, 2001. **69**:428–33.

116. Pulver A. E., Karayiorgou M., Lasseter V. K., *et al.* Follow-up of a report of a potential linkage for schizophrenia on chromosome 22q12-q13.1: Part 2. *Am J Med Genet*, 1994. **54**:44–50.

117. Bassett A. S., Chow E. W. 22q11 deletion syndrome: a genetic subtype of schizophrenia. *Biol Psychiatry*, 1999. **46**:882–91.

118. Williams H. J., Owen M. J., O'Donovan M. C. Is COMT a susceptibility gene for schizophrenia? *Schizophr Bull*, 2007. **33**:635–41.

119. Tunbridge E. M., Harrison P. J., Weinberger D. R. Catechol-o-methyltransferase, cognition, and psychosis: Val158Met and

schizophrenia locus detected on chromosome 1q in a large multicenter sample. *Science*, 2002. **296**:739–41.

beyond. *Biol Psychiatry*, 2006. **60**:141–51.

120. Sklar P., Pato M. T., Kirby A., *et al.* Genome-wide scan in Portuguese Island families identifies 5q31–5q35 as a susceptibility locus for schizophrenia and psychosis. *Mol Psychiatry*, 2004. **9**:213–18.

121. Abecasis G. R., Burt R. A., Hall D., *et al.* Genomewide scan in families with schizophrenia from the founder population of Afrikaners reveals evidence for linkage and uniparental disomy on chromosome 1. *Am J Hum Genet*, 2004. **74**:403–17.

122. Hovatta I., Varilo T., Suvisaari J., *et al.* A genomewide screen for schizophrenia genes in an isolated Finnish subpopulation, suggesting multiple susceptibility loci. *Am J Hum Genet*, 1999. **65**:1114–24.

123. Brzustowicz L. M., Hodgkinson K. A., Chow E. W., *et al.* Location of a major susceptibility locus for familial schizophrenia on chromosome 1q21-q22. *Science*, 2000. **288**:678–82.

124. Shaw S. H., Kelly M., Smith A. B., *et al.* A genome-wide search for schizophrenia susceptibility genes. *Am J Med Genet*, 1998. **81**:364–76.

125. Ekelund J., Hovatta I., Parker A., *et al.* Chromosome 1 loci in Finnish schizophrenia families. *Hum Mol Genet*, 2001. **10**:1611–17.

126. Gurling H. M., Kalsi G., Brynjolfson J., *et al.* Genomewide genetic linkage analysis confirms the presence of susceptibility loci for schizophrenia, on chromosomes 1q32.2, 5q33.2, and 8p21–22 and provides support for linkage to schizophrenia, on chromosomes 11q23.3–24 and 20q12.1–11.23. *Am J Hum Genet*, 2001. **68**:661–73.

127. Camp N. J., Neuhausen S. L., Tiobech J., *et al.* Genomewide multipoint linkage analysis of seven extended ocaliz pedigrees with schizophrenia, by a Markov-chain Monte Carlo method. *Am J Hum Genet*, 2001. **69**:1278–89.

128. Coon H., Myles-Worsley M., Tiobech J., *et al.* Evidence for a chromosome 2p13–14 schizophrenia susceptibility locus in families from Palau, Micronesia. *Mol Psychiatry*, 1998. **3**:521–7.

129. Devlin B., Bacanu S. A., Roeder K., *et al.* Genome-wide multipoint linkage analyses of multiplex schizophrenia pedigrees from the oceanic nation of Palau. *Mol Psychiatry*, 2002. **7**:689–94.

130. Levinson D. F., Mahtani M. M., Nancarrow D. J., *et al.* Genome scan of schizophrenia. *Am J Psychiatry*, 1998. **155**:741–50.

131. DeLisi L. E., Shaw S. H., Crow T. J., *et al.* A genome-wide scan for linkage to chromosomal regions in 382 sibling pairs with schizophrenia or schizoaffective disorder. *Am J Psychiatry*, 2002. **159**:803–12.

132. Paunio T., Ekelund J., Varilo T., *et al.* Genome-wide scan in a nationwide study sample of schizophrenia families in Finland reveals susceptibility loci on chromosomes 2q and 5q. *Hum Mol Genet*, 2001. **10**:3037–48.

133. Straub R. E., MacLean C. J., O'Neill F. A., *et al.* Support for a possible schizophrenia vulnerability locus in region 5q22–31 in Irish families. *Mol Psychiatry*, 1997. **2**:148–55.

134. Straub R. E., MacLean C. J., Ma Y., *et al.* Genome-wide scans of three independent sets of 90 Irish multiplex schizophrenia families and follow-up of selected regions in all families provides evidence for multiple susceptibility genes. *Mol Psychiatry*, 2002. **7**:542–59.

135. Straub R. E., MacLean C. J., O'Neill F. A., *et al.* A potential vulnerability locus for schizophrenia on chromosome 6p24–22: evidence for genetic heterogeneity. *Nat Genet*, 1995. **11**:287–93.

136. Fallin M. D., Lasseter V. K., Wolyniec P. S., *et al.* Genomewide linkage scan for schizophrenia susceptibility loci among Ashkenazi Jewish families shows evidence of linkage on chromosome 10q22. *Am J Hum Genet*, 2003. **73**:601–11.

137. Maziade M., Roy M. A., Chagnon Y. C., *et al.* Shared and specific susceptibility loci for schizophrenia and bipolar disorder: a dense genome scan in Eastern Quebec families. *Mol Psychiatry*, 2005. **10**:486–99.

138. Schwab S. G., Hallmayer J., Albus M., *et al.* A genome-wide autosomal screen for schizophrenia susceptibility loci in 71 families with affected siblings: support for loci on chromosome 10p and 6. *Mol Psychiatry*, 2000. **5**:638–49.

139. Maziade M., Roy M. A., Rouillard E., *et al.* A search for specific and common susceptibility loci for schizophrenia and bipolar disorder: a linkage study in 13 target chromosomes. *Mol Psychiatry*, 2001. **6**:684–93.

140. Kaufmann C. A., Suarez B., Malaspina D., *et al.* NIMH Genetics Initiative Millenium Schizophrenia Consortium: linkage analysis of African-American pedigrees. *Am J Med Genet*, 1998. **81**:282–9.

141. Cao Q., Martinez M., Zhang J., *et al.* Suggestive evidence for a schizophrenia susceptibility locus on chromosome 6q and a confirmation in an independent series of pedigrees. *Genomics*, 1997. **43**:1–8.

142. Lerer B., Segman R. H., Hamdan A., *et al.* Genome scan of Arab Israeli families maps a schizophrenia susceptibility gene to chromosome 6q23 and supports a locus at chromosome 10q24. *Mol Psychiatry*, 2003. **8**:488–98.

143. Lindholm E., Ekholm B., Shaw S., et al. A schizophrenia-susceptibility locus at 6q25, in one of the world's largest reported pedigrees. Am J Hum Genet, 2001. 69:96–105.

144. Blouin J. L., Dombroski B. A., Nath S. K., et al. Schizophrenia susceptibility loci on chromosomes 13q32 and 8p21. Nat Genet, 1998. 20:70–3.

145. Garver D. L., Holcomb J., Mapua F. M., et al. Schizophrenia spectrum disorders: an autosomal-wide scan in multiplex pedigrees. Schizophr Res, 2001. 52:145–60.

146. Kendler K. S., MacLean C. J., O'Neill F. A., et al. Evidence for a schizophrenia vulnerability locus on chromosome 8p in the Irish Study of High-Density Schizophrenia Families. Am J Psychiatry, 1996. 153:1534–40.

147. Faraone S. V., Matise T., Svrakic D., et al. Genome scan of European-American schizophrenia pedigrees: results of the NIMH Genetics Initiative and Millennium Consortium. Am J Med Genet, 1998. 81:290–5.

148. Schwab S. G., Hallmayer J., Albus M., et al. Further evidence for a susceptibility locus on chromosome 10p14-p11 in 72 families with schizophrenia by nonparametric linkage analysis. Am J Med Genet, 1998. 81:302–7.

149. Faraone S. V., Hwu H. G., Liu C. M., et al. Genome scan of Han Chinese schizophrenia families from Taiwan: confirmation of linkage to 10q22.3. Am J Psychiatry, 2006. 163:1760–6.

150. Williams N. M., Norton N., Williams H., et al. A systematic genomewide linkage study in 353 sib pairs with schizophrenia. Am J Hum Genet, 2003. 73:1355–67.

151. Mowry B. J., Ewen K. R., Nancarrow D. J., et al. Second stage of a genome scan of schizophrenia: study of five positive regions in an expanded sample. Am J Med Genet, 2000. 96:864–9.

152. Brzustowicz L. M., Honer W. G., Chow E. W., et al. Linkage of familial schizophrenia to chromosome 13q32. Am J Hum Genet, 1999. 65:1096–103.

153. Freedman R., Leonard S., Olincy A., et al. Evidence for the multigenic inheritance of schizophrenia. Am J Med Genet, 2001. 105:794–800.

154. Leonard S., Gault J., Moore T., et al. Further investigation of a chromosome 15 locus in schizophrenia: analysis of affected sibpairs from the NIMH Genetics Initiative. Am J Med Genet, 1998. 81:308–12.

155. Freedman R., Coon H., Myles-Worsley M., et al. Linkage of a neurophysiological deficit in schizophrenia to a chromosome 15 locus. Proc Natl Acad Sci USA, 1997. 94:587–92.

156. Stober G., Saar K., Ruschendorf F., et al. Splitting schizophrenia: periodic catatonia-susceptibility locus on chromosome 15q15. Am J Hum Genet, 2000. 67:1201–7.

157. Bulayeva K. B., Glatt S. J., Bulayev O. A., et al. Genome-wide linkage scan of schizophrenia: a cross-isolate study. Genomics, 2007. 89:167–77.

158. Coon H., Holik J., Hoff M., et al. Analysis of chromosome 22 markers in nine schizophrenia pedigrees. Am J Med Genet, 1994. 15:72–9.

159. Talkowski M. E., Chowdari K., Lewis D. A., et al. Can RGS4 polymorphisms be viewed as credible risk factors for schizophrenia? A critical review of the evidence. Schizophr Bull, 2006. 32:203–8.

160. Williams J., Spurlock G., Holmans P., et al. A meta-analysis and transmission disequilibrium study of association between the dopamine D3 receptor gene and schizophrenia. Mol Psychiatry, 1998. 3:141–9.

161. Leriche L., Diaz J., Sokoloff P. Dopamine and glutamate dysfunctions in schizophrenia: role of the dopamine D3 receptor. Neurotox Res, 2004. 6:63–71.

162. Abdolmaleky H. M., Faraone S. V., Glatt S. J., et al. Meta-analysis of association between the T102C polymorphism of the 5HT2a receptor gene and schizophrenia. Schizophr Res, 2004. 67:53–62.

163. Abi-Dargham A. Alterations of serotonin transmission in schizophrenia. Int Rev Neurobiol, 2007. 78:133–64.

164. Emamian E. S., Hall D., Birnbaum M. J., et al. Convergent evidence for impaired AKT1-GSK3beta signaling in schizophrenia. Nat Genet, 2004. 36:131–7.

165. Craddock N., O'Donovan M. C., Owen M. J. Genes for schizophrenia and bipolar disorder? Implications for psychiatric nosology. Schizophr Bull, 2006. 32:9–16.

166. Craddock N., O'Donovan M. C., Owen M. J. The genetics of schizophrenia and bipolar disorder: dissecting psychosis. J Med Genet, 2005. 42:193–204.

167. Straub R. E., Weinberger D. R. Schizophrenia genes – famine to feast. Biol Psychiatry, 2006. 60:81–3.

168. Riley B., Kendler K. S. Molecular genetic studies of schizophrenia. Eur J Hum Genet, 2006. 14:669–80.

169. Harrison P. J., Weinberger D. R. Schizophrenia genes, gene expression, and neuropathology: on the matter of their convergence. Mol Psychiatry, 2005. 10:40–68.

170. Karayiorgou M., Gogos J. A. Schizophrenia genetics: uncovering positional candidate genes. Eur J Hum Genet, 2006. 14:512–19.

171. Straub R. E., Jiang Y., MacLean C. J., et al. Genetic variation in the 6p22.3 gene DTNBP1, the human

ortholog of the mouse dysbindin gene, is associated with schizophrenia. *Am J Hum Genet*, 2002. **71**:337–48.

172. Williams N. M., O'Donovan M. C., Owen M. J. Is the dysbindin gene (DTNBP1) a susceptibility gene for schizophrenia? *Schizophr Bull*, 2005. **31**:800–5.

173. Stefansson H., Sigurdsson E., Steinthorsdottir V., *et al.* Neuregulin 1 and susceptibility to schizophrenia. *Am J Hum Genet*, 2002. **71**:877–92.

174. Tosato S., Dazzan P., Collier D. Association between the neuregulin 1 gene and schizophrenia: a systematic review. *Schizophr Bull*, 2005. **31**:613–17.

175. Millar J. K., Christie S., Semple C. A., *et al.* Chromosomal location and genomic structure of the human translin-associated factor X gene (TRAX; TSNAX) revealed by intergenic splicing to DISC1, a gene disrupted by a translocation segregating with schizophrenia. *Genomics*, 2000. **67**:69–77.

176. Porteous D. J., Millar J. K. Disrupted in schizophrenia 1: building brains and memories. *Trends Mol Med*, 2006. **12**:255–61.

177. Mirnics K., Middleton F. A., Stanwood G. D., et al. Disease-specific changes in regulator of G-protein signaling 4 (RGS4) expression in schizophrenia. *Mol Psychiatry*, 2001. **6**:293–301.

178. Chowdari K. V., Mirnics K., Semwal P., *et al.* Association and linkage analyses of RGS4 polymorphisms in schizophrenia. *Hum Mol Genet*, 2002. **11**:1373–80.

179. Talkowski M. E., Seltman H., Bassett A. S., *et al.* Evaluation of a susceptibility gene for schizophrenia: genotype based meta-analysis of RGS4 polymorphisms from thirteen

independent samples. *Biol Psychiatry*, 2006. **60**:152–62.

180. Levitt P., Ebert P., Mirnics K., *et al.* Making the case for a candidate vulnerability gene in schizophrenia: Convergent evidence for regulator of G-protein signaling 4 (RGS4). *Biol Psychiatry*, 2006. **60**:534–7.

181. Ohmori O., Shinkai T., Kojima H., *et al.* Association study of a functional catechol-O-methyltransferase gene polymorphism in Japanese schizophrenics. *Neurosci Lett.* 1998. **243**:109–12.

182. Chumakov I., Blumenfeld M., Guerassimenko O., *et al.* Genetic and physiological data implicating the new human gene G72 and the gene for D-amino acid oxidase in schizophrenia. *Proc Natl Acad Sci USA*, 2002. **99**:13675–80.

183. Detera-Wadleigh S. D., McMahon F. J. G72/G30 in schizophrenia and bipolar disorder: review and meta-analysis. *Biol Psychiatry*, 2006. **60**:106–14.

184. Li D., He L. G72/G30 genes and schizophrenia: a systematic meta-analysis of association studies. *Genetics*, 2007. **175**:917–922.

185. Gerber D. J., Hall D., Miyakawa T., *et al.* Evidence for association of schizophrenia with genetic variation in the 8p21.3 gene, PPP3CC, encoding the calcineurin gamma subunit. *Proc Natl Acad Sci USA*, 2003. **100**:8993–8.

186. Liu Y. L., Fann C. S., Liu C. M., *et al.* More evidence supports the association of PPP3CC with schizophrenia. *Mol Psychiatry*, 2007. **12**:966–74.

187. Norton N., Williams H. J., Owen M. J. An update on the genetics of schizophrenia. *Curr Opin Psychiatry.* 2006. **19**:158–64.

188. Crocq M.-A., Mant R., Asherson P. *et al.* Association between schizophrenia and homozygosity at the dopamine D3 receptor

gene. *Am J Med Genet*, 1992. **29**:858–60.

189. Inayama Y., Yoneda H., Sakai T., *et al.* Positive association between a DNA sequence variant in the serotonin 2A receptor gene and schizophrenia. *Am J Med Genet*, 1996. **67**:103–5.

190. Jacobs P. A., Brunton M., Frackiewicz A., *et al.* Studies on a family with three cytogenetic markers. *Ann Hum Genet*, 1970. **33**:325–36.

191. St Clair D., Blackwood D., Muir W., *et al.* Association within a family of a balanced autosomal translocation with major mental illness. *Lancet, 1990.* **336**:13–16.

192. Millar J. K., Christie S., Anderson S., *et al.* Genomic structure and localization within a linkage hotspot of Disrupted in Schizophrenia 1, a gene disrupted by a translocation segregating with schizophrenia. *Mol Psychiatry*, 2001. **6**:173–8.

193. Taylor M. S., Devon R. S., Millar J. K., *et al.* Evolutionary constraints on the Disrupted in Schizophrenia locus. *Genomics*, 2003. **81**:67–77.

194. Sachs N. A., Sawa A., Holmes S. E., *et al.* A frameshift mutation in Disrupted in Schizophrenia 1 in an American family with schizophrenia and schizoaffective disorder. *Mol Psychiatry*, 2005. **10**:758–64.

195. Jang Y. L., Kim J. W., Lee Y. S., *et al.* Linkage of schizophrenia with chromosome 1q32 in Korean multiplex families. *Am J Med Genet B Neuropsychiatr Genet*, 2007. **144**:279–84.

196. Ekelund J., Lichtermann D., Hovatta I., *et al.* Genome-wide scan for schizophrenia in the Finnish population: evidence for a locus on chromosome 7q22. *Hum Mol Genet*, 2000. **9**:1049–57.

197. Gasperoni T. L., Ekelund J., Huttunen M., *et al.* Genetic linkage and association between chromosome 1q and working memory function in

schizophrenia. *Am J Med Genet*, 2003. **116B**:8–16.

198. Macgregor S., Visscher P. M., Knott S. A., *et al.* A genome scan and follow-up study identify a bipolar disorder susceptibility locus on chromosome 1q42. *Mol Psychiatry*, 2004. **9**:1083–90.

199. Gejman P. V., Martinez M., Cao Q., *et al.* Linkage analysis of fifty-seven microsatellite loci to bipolar disorder. *Neuropsychopharmacology*, 1993. **9**:31–40.

200. Hwu H. G., Liu C. M., Fann C. S., *et al.* Linkage of schizophrenia with chromosome 1q loci in Taiwanese families. *Mol Psychiatry*, 2003. **8**:445–52.

201. Ekelund J., Hennah W., Hiekkalinna T., *et al.* Replication of 1q42 linkage in Finnish schizophrenia pedigrees. *Mol Psychiatry*, 2004. **9**:1037–41.

202. Hennah W., Tomppo L., Hiekkalinna T., *et al.* Families with the risk allele of DISC1 reveal a link between schizophrenia and another component of the same molecular pathway, NDE1. *Hum Mol Genet*, 2007. **16**:453–62.

203. Hamshere M. L., Bennett P., Williams N., *et al.* Genomewide linkage scan in schizoaffective disorder: significant evidence for linkage at 1q42 close to DISC1, and suggestive evidence at 22q11 and 19p13. *Arch Gen Psychiatry*, 2005. **62**:1081–8.

204. Hennah W., Varilo T., Kestila M., *et al.* Haplotype transmission analysis provides evidence of association for DISC1 to schizophrenia and suggests sex-dependent effects. *Hum Mol Genet*, 2003. **12**:3151–9.

205. Thomson P. A., Wray N. R., Millar J. K., *et al.* Association between the TRAX/DISC locus and both bipolar disorder and schizophrenia in the Scottish population. *Mol Psychiatry*, 2005. **10**:657–668, 616.

206. Cannon T. D., Hennah W., van Erp T. G., *et al.* Association of DISC1/TRAX haplotypes with schizophrenia, reduced prefrontal gray matter, and impaired short- and long-term memory. *Arch Gen Psychiatry*, 2005. **62**:1205–13.

207. Hennah W., Tuulio-Henriksson A., Paunio T., *et al.* A haplotype within the DISC1 gene is associated with visual memory functions in families with a high density of schizophrenia. *Mol Psychiatry*, 2005. **10**:1097–103.

208. Zhang F., Sarginson J., Crombie C., *et al.* Genetic association between schizophrenia and the DISC1 gene in the Scottish population. *Am J Med Genet B Neuropsychiatr Genet*, 2006. **141**:155–9.

209. Liu Y. L., Fann C. S., Liu C. M., *et al.* A single nucleotide polymorphism fine mapping study of chromosome 1q42.1 reveals the vulnerability genes for schizophrenia, GNPAT and DISC1: Association with impairment of sustained attention. *Biol Psychiatry*, 2006. **60**:554–62.

210. Hodgkinson C. A., Goldman D., Jaeger J., *et al.* Disrupted in schizophrenia 1 (DISC1): association with schizophrenia, schizoaffective disorder, and bipolar disorder. *Am J Hum Genet*, 2004. **75**:862–72.

211. Callicott J. H., Straub R. E., Pezawas L., *et al.* Variation in DISC1 affects hippocampal structure and function and increases risk for schizophrenia. *Proc Natl Acad Sci USA*, 2005. **102**:8627–32.

212. Hashimoto R., Numakawa T., Ohnishi T., *et al.* Impact of the DISC1 Ser704Cys polymorphism on risk for major depression, brain morphology and ERK signaling. *Hum Mol Genet*, 2006. **15**:3024–3033.

213. DeRosse P., Hodgkinson C. A., Lencz T., *et al.* Disrupted in

schizophrenia 1 genotype and positive symptoms in schizophrenia. *Biol Psychiatry*, 2007. **61**:1208–10.

214. Pickard B. S., Millar J. K., Porteous D. J., *et al.* Cytogenetics and gene discovery in psychiatric disorders. *Pharmacogenomics J*, 2005. **5**:81–8.

215. Curtis D., Kalsi G., Brynjolfsson J., *et al.* Genome scan of pedigrees multiply affected with bipolar disorder provides further support for the presence of a susceptibility locus on chromosome 12q23-q24, and suggests the presence of additional loci on 1p and 1q. *Psychiatr Genet*, 2003. **13**:77–84.

216. Detera-Wadleigh S. D., Badner J. A., *et al.* A high-density genome scan detects evidence for a bipolar-disorder susceptibility locus on 13q32 and other potential loci on 1q32 and 18p11.2. *Proc Natl Acad Sci USA*, 1999. **96**:5604–9.

217. Kockelkorn T. T., Arai M., Matsumoto H., *et al.* Association study of polymorphisms in the 5' upstream region of human DISC1 gene with schizophrenia. *Neurosci Lett*, 2004. **368**:41–5.

218. Burdick K. E., Hodgkinson C. A., Szeszko P. R., *et al.* DISC1 and neurocognitive function in schizophrenia. *Neuroreport*, 2005. **16**:1399–402.

219. Ishizuka K., Paek M., Kamiya A., *et al.* A review of Disrupted-In-Schizophrenia-1 (DISC1): neurodevelopment, cognition, and mental conditions. *Biol Psychiatry*, 2006. **59**:1189–97.

220. Austin C. P., Ky B., Ma L., *et al.* Expression of Disrupted-In-Schizophrenia-1, a schizophrenia-associated gene, is prominent in the mouse hippocampus throughout brain development. *NeuroScience*, 2004. **124**:3–10.

221. Austin C. P., Ma L., Ky B., *et al.* DISC1 (Disrupted in

Schizophrenia-1) is expressed in limbic regions of the primate brain. *Neuroreport*, 2003. **14**:951–4.

222. Porteous D. J., Thomson P., Brandon N. J., *et al.* The genetics and biology of DISC1 – an emerging role in psychosis and cognition. *Biol Psychiatry,* 2006. **60**:123–31.

223. Schurov I. L., Handford E. J., Brandon N. J., *et al.* Expression of disrupted in schizophrenia 1 (DISC1) protein in the adult and developing mouse brain indicates its role in neurodevelopment. *Mol Psychiatry,* 2004. **9**:1100–10.

224. Sawamura N., Sawamura-Yamamoto T., Ozeki Y., *et al.* A form of DISC1 enriched in nucleus: altered subcellular distribution in orbitofrontal cortex in psychosis and substance/alcohol abuse. *Proc Natl Acad Sci USA,* 2005. **102**:1187–92.

225. Ozeki Y., Tomoda T., Kleiderlein J., *et al.* Disrupted-in-Schizophrenia-1 (DISC-1): mutant truncation prevents binding to NudE-like (NUDEL) and inhibits neurite outgrowth. *Proc Natl Acad Sci USA,* 2003. **100**:289–94.

226. Miyoshi K., Honda A., Baba K., *et al.* Disrupted-In-Schizophrenia 1, a candidate gene for schizophrenia, participates in neurite outgrowth. *Mol Psychiatry,* 2003. **8**:685–94.

227. James R., Adams R. R., Christie S., *et al.* Disrupted in Schizophrenia 1 (DISC1) is a multicompartmentalized protein that predominantly localizes to mitochondria. *Mol Cell Neurosci,* 2004. **26**:112–22.

228. Brandon N. J., Handford E. J., Schurov I., *et al.* Disrupted in Schizophrenia 1 and Nudel form a neurodevelopmentally regulated protein complex: implications for schizophrenia and other major neurological disorders. *Mol Cell Neurosci,* 2004. **25**:42–55.

229. Mackie S., Millar J. K., Porteous D. J. Role of DISC1 in neural development and schizophrenia. *Curr Opin Neurobiol,* 2007. **17**:95–102.

230. Morris D. W., Rodgers A., McGhee K. A., *et al.* Confirming RGS4 as a susceptibility gene for schizophrenia. *Am J Med Genet B Neuropsychiatr Genet,* 2004. **125**:50–3.

231. Kirkpatrick B., Xu L., Cascella N., *et al.* DISC1 immunoreactivity at the light and ultrastructural level in the human neocortex. *J Comp Neurol,* 2006. **497**:436–50.

232. Millar J. K., James R., Brandon N. J., *et al.* DISC1 and DISC2: discovering and dissecting molecular mechanisms underlying psychiatric illness. *Ann Med,* 2004. **36**:367–78.

233. Camargo L. M., Collura V., Rain J. C., *et al.* Disrupted in Schizophrenia 1 Interactome: evidence for the close connectivity of risk genes and a potential synaptic basis for schizophrenia. *Mol Psychiatry,* 2007. **12**:74–86.

234. Millar J. K., Pickard B. S., Mackie S., *et al.* DISC1 and PDE4B are interacting genetic factors in schizophrenia that regulate cAMP signaling. *Science,* 2005. **310**:1187–91.

235. Todd J. A. Statistical false positive or true disease pathway? *Nat Genet,* 2006. **38**:731–3.

236. Kendler K. S. Reflections on the relationship between psychiatric genetics and psychiatric nosology. *Am J Psychiatry,* 2006. **163**:1138–46.

237. Shastry B. S. Pharmacogenetics and the concept of individualized medicine. *Pharmacogenomics J,* 2006. **6**:16–21.

238. Jorde L. B., Watkins W. S., Kere J., *et al.* Gene mapping in isolated populations: new roles for old friends? *Hum Hered.* 2000. **50**:57–65.

239. Service S., DeYoung J., Karayiorgou M., *et al.* Magnitude and distribution of linkage disequilibrium in population isolates and implications for genome-wide association studies. *Nat Genet,* 2006. **38**:556–60.

240. Varilo T., Peltonen L. Isolates and their potential use in complex gene mapping efforts. *Curr Opin Genet Dev,* 2004. **14**:316–23.

241. Botstein D., Risch N. Discovering genotypes underlying human phenotypes: past successes for mendelian disease, future approaches for complex disease. *Nat Genet,* 2003. **33**(Suppl):228–37.

242. Kaessmann H., Zollner S., Gustafsson A. C., *et al.* Extensive linkage disequilibrium in small human populations in Eurasia. *Am J Hum Genet,* 2002. **70**:673–85.

243. Topol E. J., Frazer K. A. The resequencing imperative. *Nat Genet,* 2007. **39**:439–40.

244. Vavouri T., Walter K., Gilks W. R., *et al.* Parallel evolution of conserved non-coding elements that target a common set of developmental regulatory genes from worms to humans. *Genome Biol,* 2007. **8**:R15.

245. Mirnics K., Levitt P., Lewis D. A. Critical appraisal of DNA microarrays in psychiatric genomics. *Biol Psychiatry,* 2006. **60**:163–76.

246. Callinan P. A., Feinberg A. P. The emerging science of epigenomics. *Hum Mol Genet,* 2006. 15 Spec No 1:R95–101.

247. Feinberg A. P. Phenotypic plasticity and the epigenetics of human disease. *Nature,* 2007. **447**:433–40.

248. Pillai R. S. MicroRNA function: multiple mechanisms for a tiny RNA? *RNA,* 2005. **11**:1753–61.

249. Roeder K., Bacanu S. A., Wasserman L., *et al.* Using linkage genome scans to improve power of association in genome scans. *Am J Hum Genet*, 2006. **78**:243–52.

250. Gu S., Pakstis A. J., Li H., *et al.* Significant variation in haplotype block structure but conservation in tag SNP patterns among global populations. *Eur J Hum Genet*, 2007. **15**:302–12.

24

Velocardiofacial syndrome (chromosome 22q11.2 deletion syndrome) as a model of schizophrenia

Vandana Shashi and Margaret N. Berry

Facts box

- Velocardiofacial syndrome (VCFS), caused by a heterozygous deletion of chromosome 22q11.2, is associated with congenital anomalies, medical complications, and cognitive impairment.

- VCFS is associated with an extraordinarily high risk (30%–40%) of major psychiatric illnesses, in late adolescence and early adulthood, mainly schizophrenia (25%–30%) but also schizotypy, bipolar illness, and major depression.

- It has been found that 1%–2% of individuals with schizophrenia in the general population have a 22q11.2 deletion, whereas 5% of patients with childhood-onset schizophrenia will have VCFS upon testing.

- The early neurocognitive manifestations in VCFS are similar to those that would be expected to occur on the pathway to schizophrenia.

- The brain structural abnormalities in VCFS have many parallels with those seen in schizophrenia.

- In individuals with VCFS, there is controversy about the relationship between the COMT genotype, the cognitive deficits, and schizophrenia. There are other genes of interest in the deletion region that may be of relevance to schizophrenia.

- Mouse models of VCFS have proven to be of limited value in understanding the mechanisms involved in psychosis.

Introduction

In recent years, schizophrenia has been viewed as a neurodevelopmental disorder [1, 2]. This neuro-developmental theory suggests that neurocognitive and neuroanatomical abnormalities often precede the development of overt psychosis. The delineation of the progression of these often subclinical neurocognitive and morphological brain anomalies provides an opportunity to identify at-risk individuals, improve the understanding of the pathogenesis of this complex disorder, and ultimately hasten the development of prophylactic interventions.

Numerous epidemiological and genetic linkage studies have provided incontrovertible evidence that genetic factors are important in the predisposition to schizophrenia spectrum disorders [3, 4, 5], with the heritability estimated to be 60%–90% [6]. However, gene identification has largely been unsuccessful, due to the complex nature of the inheritance of the genes and the probability that multiple genes of individual modest effect are involved. Identification of predisposing genetic markers would provide a model that would enable the prospective study of the factors contributing to psychosis in a high-risk group of individuals.

Velocardiofacial syndrome (VCFS), caused by a heterozygous deletion of chromosome 22q11.2, is associated with congenital anomalies, medical complications, and cognitive impairment. Since the early 1990s, retrospective studies have reported a markedly high incidence (~40%) of schizophrenia and mood psychoses in late adolescence and adulthood in individuals with the deletion [7, 8, 9, 10]. The risk of schizophrenia spectrum disorders in VCFS approaches that of a monozygotic twin of a patient with schizophrenia, or that of an individual with two parents with schizophrenia. *These observations provide the strongest known link between psychosis and an identified genetic condition.* In addition, because the signs, symptoms, and response to treatment of schizophrenia in this disorder are thought to be no different to that in the general population, it has been suggested that VCFS represents an ideal model for the study of schizophrenia [11]. This chapter delineates the

Table 24.1 Features that should warrant testing for VCFS in patients with schizophrenia (modified from [15])

Psychiatric	Dev/psychological	Medical history	Family history	Physical examination
Mental retardation	Developmental delay	Conotruncal heart anomalies*	VCFS in first degree relative*	Low anterior hairline
Borderline IQ	Hypernasal speech*	Hypoparathyroidism*	Conotruncal Heart Anomalies*	Hooded eyelids
Depression	Learning disability	VPI, submucous cleft*	Surgery for Palate Abnormalities	External ear anomalies*
Anxiety disorder		T cell immune deficiency*		Bulbous nasal tip, wide middle part of nose*
		Feeding difficulty with nasopharyngeal reflux*		Asymmetric crying facies*
		Renal anomalies* (including missing kidney)		Long slender fingers
		Autoimmune disease–vitiligo, Graves Disease, juvenile rheumatoid arthritis, idiopathic thrombocytopenic purpura		Hypospadius, polydactyly imperforate anus long, slender fingers

* Indicates that the presence of this feature alone is sufficient to consider FISH testing. Otherwise, the presence of two or more features should prompt a genetics referral and/or FISH testing.
Common heart anomalies seen in VCFS include tetralogy of fallot, interrupted aortic arch, truncus arteriosus, ventricular septal defect, atrial septal defect and a vascular ring.

psychological and psychiatric findings, brain morphometric abnormalities, and the genetic studies that underscore the importance of VCFS in understanding the neurodevelopmental trajectory of schizophrenia.

Velocardiofacial syndrome

Deletion of chromosome 22 at band q11.2 resulting in VCFS is the most common chromosome microdeletion syndrome in human beings, occurring with an incidence of 1/2000 to 1/6000 births [12, 13, 14]. Also known as chromosome 22q11.2 deletion syndrome, DiGeorge syndrome, or Cayler cardiofacial syndrome, it is commonly associated with learning disabilities (80%–100%), congenital heart disease (70%), palatal abnormalities (70%), immune deficiency (70%), hypoparathyroidism (60%), feeding problems (30%), and characteristic facial features. Mental retardation is seen in 50% of affected individuals. Although more than 180 manifestations have been reported, illustrating the extent of the clinical variability of the condition, the diagnosis should be suspected when one or more of the more common features are present in the individual patient (Table 24.1). It is to be emphasized that, undoubtedly, many individuals with VCFS, being evaluated and treated by mental health professionals, have not been diagnosed

with the condition and thus a high index of suspicion needs to be maintained. A history of a congenital abnormality or a host of medical and developmental problems should prompt referral to a clinical geneticist. The clinical diagnosis is made typically during one of the following time periods: (i) prenatally, when a conotruncal heart anomaly is detected with or without other structural organ abnormalities, (ii) in infancy, due to conotruncal heart abnormalities, hypocalcemia, immune deficiency, other medical problems, and developmental delays, (iii) during the childhood years, due to speech difficulties related to velopharyngeal insufficiency (often needing surgical repair) and cognitive problems, (iv) in adulthood, due to the occurrence of major psychiatric illnesses and/or having a child with the condition. At all ages, the typical facial features can be evident, including a low anterior hairline, hooded upper eyelids, widening of the middle part of the nose or a bulbous nasal tip, ear anomalies, and a small chin (Figure 24.1). However, as with all the other features in the condition, the facial abnormalities may be variable and can be subtle or not discernible (Figure 24.2) and thus the diagnosis may be missed, unless a high index of suspicion is maintained. The clinical suspicion is confirmed by the detection of the microdeletion by fluorescence in-situ hybridization (FISH) analysis (Figure 24.3). Most

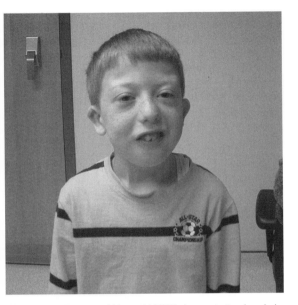

Figure 24.1 Ten year-old boy with VCFS, demonstrating hooded upper eyelids, widened middle part of the nose, and ear abnormalities.

(A)

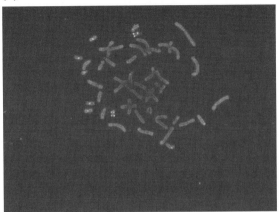

(B)

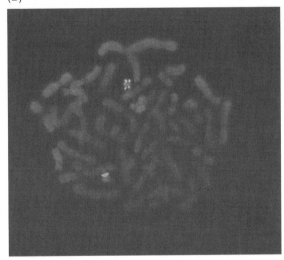

Figure 24.3 Fluorescence *in-situ* hybridization showing the presence of both 22q11.2 regions (a) and the deletion (b) with the commercially available probe (Vysis, Gaithersburg, MD. Courtesy: Mark Pettenati, PhD, Department of Pediatrics, Wake Forest University School of Medicine.) (See color plate section.)

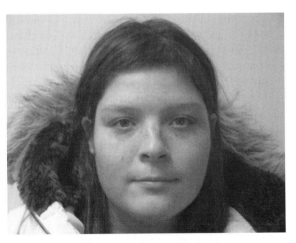

Figure 24.2 Sixteen year-old girl with VCFS who does not demonstrate the typical facial appearance, apart from small ears, illustrating the variability of these features. The practicing psychiatric health professional thus needs a high index of suspicion to make the diagnosis.

deletions are sporadic and occur *de novo* (> 90 %), but a small percentage are inherited from an affected parent (7%).

Relevance of VCFS to schizophrenia

Although the well-described intellectual disabilities in VCFS (discussed later) are findings that are common to many genetic conditions, it was in the early 1990s that it became clear that VCFS had an important distinguishing characteristic: an extraordinarily high risk (30%–40%) of major psychiatric illnesses in late adolescence and early adulthood, mainly schizophrenia (25%–30%) but also schizotypy, bipolar illness, and major depression [7, 8, 9, 10, 16]. Recent evidence indicates that the frequency of psychiatric diagnoses in adults with VCFS may be even higher (~60%) [17]. Overall, such an incredible risk of psychiatric illnesses has not been described in other conditions associated with mental retardation [18]. In addition, in individuals with schizophrenia, there is an increased prevalence of the 22q11.2 deletion (1%–5%) [19, 20, 21]. Thus, because schizophrenia risk is undoubtedly increased in VCFS and the incidence of VCFS is increased in individuals with schizophrenia in the general population and because genes in the 22q11.2 interval are likely to be involved in the causation of schizophrenia, VCFS offers a unique opportunity to examine the factors contributing to this catastrophic illness.

The neurodevelopmental hypothesis of schizophrenia

This hypothesis states that schizophrenia is the outcome of an aberration of neurodevelopment that begins long before the onset of clinical symptoms [22, 23]. A combination of genetic and environmental factors, including pre- and perinatal events, postnatal developmental processes, and environmental stressors are believed to result in the illness [1, 24, 25, 26]. Evidence of abnormal neurodevelopment is provided by the presence of neuropsychological and structural brain abnormalities before and at the onset of illness. Minor facial dysmorphisms [27, 28, 29] in these patients are also consistent with the abnormal development theory.

A number of studies have reported the occurrence of a high frequency of neuropsychological abnormalities, *prior to the onset of illness* in individuals with schizophrenia. These include motor delays, speech problems, cognitive difficulties, impaired social skills with poor peer relationships, social anxiety, and poor intellectual functioning in childhood between the ages of 2 and 15 years [23, 30, 31, 32]. However, the fairly high frequency of such cognitive problems in the general population of children (15%–30%) [33] decreases their predictive value for schizophrenia. Assessments of specific higher neurocognitive deficits such as poor executive function, sustained attention, and working memory show more promise as being more specific in predicting psychosis in individuals at high risk [34, 35, 36]. The recent National Institutes of Mental Health-Measurement and Treatment Research to Improve Cognition in Schizophrenia (NIMH-MATRICS) initiative has ranked executive functions, attention/vigilance, memory processes, and problem-solving ability as being the most valuable in assessing cognitive deficits in schizophrenia [37], lending credence to the supposition that detecting deficits in these domains in earlier life may have value in disease prediction.

Several structural brain abnormalities have been described at the onset of illness in patients with schizophrenia, such as cortical atrophy, ventricular enlargement, decreased gray matter, a small corpus callosum (CC) [38, 39, 40, 41], medial temporal and superior temporal gyri abnormalities, decreased dorsolateral prefrontal cortex and parietal lobes, cavum septum pellucidi, abnormal basal ganglia, small cerebellum [42, 43], and a decrease in the hippocampus, thalami [44, 45], and anterior cingulate gyrus volumes [46]. Family members of individuals with schizophrenia, whose vulnerability to the illness is believed to be increased due to genetic factors, manifest similar changes, of lesser severity, strengthening the neurodevelopmental hypothesis [47].

These brain aberrations in schizophrenia are thought to be due to an exaggeration of normal cortical development, such that normal development going awry may result in the illness. Normally, the cortical structures continue to develop well into adolescence [48, 49]. Gray matter increases in late childhood (peaks at 11.5 years in females and 14.5 years in males) and then decreases in adolescence in a "back to the front" pattern, believed to be related to early neuronal overproduction, followed by selective elimination and alteration of dendritic synapses – "synaptic pruning" [50, 51, 52]. The gray-matter reduction occurs first in the dorsal parietal cortices (primary sensorimotor areas) and then progresses to the other areas, with the dorso-prefrontal cortex being the last to mature, toward the end of the adolescent period. Such cortical thinning in the frontal and parietal lobes in adolescence is associated with improved verbal functioning [53]. On neuroimaging in childhood-onset schizophrenia, striking loss of gray matter is seen, first in the parietal lobe, progressing to the temporal lobe, and the dorsolateral prefrontal cortices, findings consistent with the supposition that excess synaptic pruning contributes to the illness [54]. Similar mechanisms involving exaggerated synaptic pruning have been proposed in schizophrenia with a typical onset in late adolescence/early adulthood [55].

Underlying such abnormal neurodevelopment, undoubtedly, are aberrations in the genes that contribute to the normal process, but the genetic factors operative in schizophrenia remain poorly understood. Linkage analyses have indicated various areas of the genome as being implicated, including the 22q11.2 region [56].

The central idea of the neurodevelopmental model of schizophrenia is strongly supported by the genetic, psychological, and brain morphometric findings in individuals with VCFS. The advantages of using VCFS as a model for schizophrenia are that: (i) the inevitable genetic heterogeneity that would occur in a high-risk group in the general population is minimized, because individuals with VCFS all have a known deletion, (ii) it allows for the study of specific etiological genes in the 22q11.2 interval that are known to contribute to schizophrenia in the general population, and (iii) the study of children and adolescents with VCFS provides the opportunity to study the trajectory of schizophrenia spectrum disorders in a population that is relatively untainted by the catastrophic consequences of psychotic disorders.

Prevalence of VCFS in schizophrenia

It has been found that 1%–2% of individuals with schizophrenia in the general population have a 22q11.2 deletion [19, 20], whereas 5% of patients with childhood-onset schizophrenia will have VCFS upon testing [21]. It is to be noted that the indication for testing for the deletion in these studies was the occurrence of schizophrenia alone. However, if genetic testing were to be offered to those with other abnormalities such as congenital heart disease or palatal problems, the incidence of the 22q11.2 deletion could be as high as 30% [15]. For the practicing clinician, Table 24.1 lists the features in association with schizophrenia that should warrant consideration of testing for the 22q11.2 deletion. The FISH test, using a commercial probe (Vysis, Gaithersburg, MD) is widely available through most cytogenetic laboratories.

Premorbid neuropsychological and brain morphometric findings in VCFS

This section describes the neuropsychological abnormalities and structural brain abnormalities that *predate psychosis* in individuals with VCFS.

Psychological abnormalities in children with VCFS

Cognitive deficits are common, with at least 80% of children experiencing developmental delays and learning disabilities [57, 58, 59, 60, 61]. The mean intelligence quotient (IQ) is 75. A complex and distinctive pattern of disabilities occurs with deficits in visual-spatial processing, arithmetic performance, language, reading comprehension, attention, working memory, and executive functioning; and relative strengths in reading and spelling skills. This results in a nonverbal learning disability [58, 59, 60, 62, 63]. This type of nonverbal disability is not unique to VCFS, because it is seen in other genetic conditions such as Turner syndrome [64].

Parallels between children with VCFS (prior to the onset of psychotic illness) and individuals in the premorbid stage of schizophrenia can be drawn, based on the similarities in early manifestations. Social and attention problems are common in VCFS [58] and are similar to those seen in the premorbid stage of schizophrenia. Additionally, children with VCFS in comparison to control subjects manifest less efficient sensorimotor gating in the form of reduced prepulse inhibition [65], easy distractibility, disinhibition, reduced mismatch negativity, and impaired sustained attention, executive function, and verbal working memory [66, 67, 68, 69]. Such significantly impaired sustained attention, executive function, and working memory are thought to be reliable indicators of psychosis risk and are suggestive of frontal and temporal dysfunction [69]. The fronto-temporal circuit is part of the heteromodal cortices, the dysfunction of which (particularly the prefrontal cortex) is believed to be central to the pathogenesis of schizophrenia [70]. Thus, the early neurocognitive manifestations in VCFS are similar to those that would be expected to occur on the pathway to schizophrenia.

Psychiatric diagnoses in childhood in VCFS

Children with VCFS seldom develop psychosis prior to the age of 15 years or so. Instead, a number of less dramatic abnormalities are seen in approximately 40%, such as attention deficit/hyperactivity disorder (AD/HD), oppositional defiant disorder (ODD), obsessive compulsive disorder (OCD) and anxiety disorders [71, 72, 73, 74]. Upon systematic psychiatric assessments of children with VCFS, mood disorders (40%–60%) and impairment in social skills [9, 75] are common, although at least one study found no differences in psychiatric diagnoses between VCFS children and control subjects [76]. It is widely hypothesized that the minor psychiatric disorders in childhood

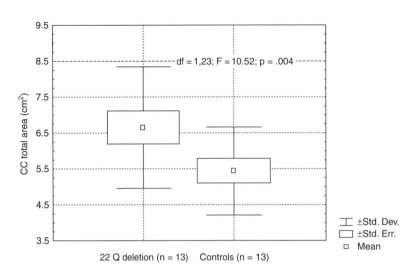

Figure 24.4 Representation of the corpus callosum area in children with VCFS, as compared to control subjects (From [87] with permission. Copyright © 2004 Elsevier Inc. All rights reserved.)

ultimately lead to full-blown schizophrenia [9, 77, 78]. A recent report of psychotic symptoms in 17% of children with VCFS below the age of 13 years, most commonly auditory hallucinations, reiterates the occurrence of a spectrum of psychiatric symptoms before the onset of overt psychosis [79]. Such psychotic symptoms increase in frequency with age, with reports of 28% by age 19 and up to 48% in the age range of 13–25 years [80] and are often associated with a decline in verbal abilities [79], a finding seen in the high-risk schizophrenia population as well [81, 82]. It is not yet known if aggressive treatment of such early psychotic symptoms would have an impact upon the progression to overt psychosis or upon the prognosis thereof.

Structural brain abnormalities in VCFS

On qualitative (routine) studies of brain anatomy in VCFS, midline anomalies (cavum septum pellucidum and a small cerebellar vermis), white-matter hyperdensities, and enlarged Sylvian fissures were reported [83, 84, 85, 86, 87]. A cavum septum pellucidum is thought to be indicative of maldevelopment of structures bordering it, such as the corpus callosum and the hippocampus, structures frequently reported to be abnormal in schizophrenia. It is seen in 45% of individuals with schizophrenia [42] and in a similar percentage of individuals with VCFS who have schizophrenia [88].

Quantitative MRI studies in children with VCFS

Morphometric MRI analyses in VCFS children *prior to the development of psychoses* have found a variety of abnormalities such as reduced total brain volume, white-matter reductions in nonfrontal areas, grey-matter reduction in the parietal and occipital lobes, relatively large frontal lobes, decreased right cerebellar tissue volume, and reductions in the cingulate gyrus, temporal lobe, superior temporal gyrus, and hippocampus [89, 90, 91, 92, 93, 94, 95]. A relative increase in the grey matter within the frontal lobes and the insula and an increase in the volume of the caudate body and the amygdala have been reported [96, 97, 98, 99, 100]. The area of the corpus callosum (CC) is also increased in children with VCFS, compared to control subjects (Figure 24.4) [87, 101]. The exact significance of such relative increases in brain volume is unclear, because this is in contradiction with the finding of volumetric reduction of these areas in most studies of individuals at high risk of schizophrenia in the general population [24, 40, 47, 102, 103]. However, it indirectly supports the hypothesis that neuronal dysmaturation occurs in subjects at high risk of schizophrenia, such as VCFS, due to an exaggeration of the normal cortical developmental processes in childhood, previously discussed. The regional increases in grey matter volume may reflect initial neuronal overgrowth and may be correlated with the early neurocognitive abnormalities that are seen in children with VCFS (see next paragraph). Grey-matter reductions seen in adults with VCFS who have schizophrenia (discussed later in this chapter) support the notion that this initial exaggerated neuronal overgrowth may be followed by excessive synaptic pruning in later life.

A few cross-sectional studies have attempted to correlate the morphological brain abnormalities with neuropsychological findings in VCFS children. Two studies have observed that increases in brain area/volume are associated with behavioral problems and minor psychiatric symptoms. In the first study, an increase in fronto-striatal grey-matter volume was associated with more severe social problems and an increase in grey matter in the temporo-occipital lobe with elevated schizotypal traits [99]. The second study found that there was a positive correlation between the volume of the amygdala and the internalizing, externalizing, anxiety, and aggression scores on the child behavior checklist [100]. Decreases in grey matter have also been correlated with behavioral problems in children with VCFS. Decreased temporal grey matter was associated with behavioral problems [104]; whereas children with VCFS had a larger area of the CC as a group, those with ADHD had a smaller CC, similar to the finding with ADHD in the general population [103]. The authors of the CC study postulated that an overall increase in the size of the CC was suggestive of delayed synaptic pruning in children with VCFS. These studies have provided preliminary data that suggest that relative increases/decreases in grey matter (possibly related to abnormal synaptic pruning) are associated with the minor psychiatric diagnoses in children with VCFS. An imbalance in synapses (too many or too few) has long been believed to be related to the symptoms of schizophrenia [24, 105]. Future research involving longitudinal studies throughout childhood and adolescence will be critical in determining the nature of such changes and their relevance to schizophrenia.

Schizophrenia phenotype in VCFS

When the first reports of schizophrenia in VCFS emerged in the early 1990s, initial reports were conflicting, reporting later age of onset and fewer negative symptoms [10], as well as younger age of onset [16, 106], due to small sample sizes and inclusion of VCFS individuals who were mentally retarded. Since then, a report of a series of VCFS patients indicates

that in VCFS subjects without mental retardation, the age of onset, lifetime or cross-sectional positive and negative symptoms and global functioning are similar to that seen in individuals with schizophrenia in the general population [107]. It is to be noted that this study needs to be replicated, because ascertainment bias may have occurred; the VCFS patients were identified after a diagnosis of schizophrenia had been already made and thus their features may not be representative of the VCFS population as a whole. However, further evidence for the similarity in the schizophrenia phenotype between the general population and VCFS is provided by the findings that in childhood schizophrenia associated with VCFS, the age of onset, premorbid functioning, or severity of psychosis were no different than that in the general population [21]. It is important to emphasize that schizophrenia represents the most severe of these manifestations and individuals with VCFS may frequently have symptoms that are less severe, such as major depression and schizotypy, and it is conceivable that a given individual may fluctuate within these diagnostic entities at different time points, as suggested for schizophrenia in the general population [108]. Further studies with larger sample sizes are needed to fully define the clinical phenotype of schizophrenia in VCFS.

The neurocognitive abnormalities (working memory and executive function) and motor skills of individuals with VCFS who have schizophrenia are similar to those that occur with schizophrenia in the general population [11]. Similarly, deficits in spatial working memory, strategy formation, visual recognition, and attention are worse in VCFS adults with psychosis than in those without psychosis [109]. This apparent lack of distinguishing features between VCFS related schizophrenia and that seen in the general population further bolsters the utility of VCFS as a model to study the neurodevelopmental hypothesis of schizophrenia.

Quantitative MRI studies in adults with VCFS

In adults with VCFS, the first quantitative study reported that compared to controls, there was loss of grey matter in frontal and temporal areas, including the insula and diffuse loss of white matter [88]. On diffusion tensor imaging, VCFS adolescents and adults had evidence of impaired fronto-temporal connectivity compared to control subjects [110]. High-lighting the differences between VCFS adults with schizophrenia and those without, Chow and colleagues reported a decrease in total grey matter, regional differences in grey and white matter in the frontal, temporal, and parietal lobes, and an increased volume of cerebrospinal fluid in those with schizophrenia [111]. A more recent study found that within VCFS adults, those with schizophrenia have reduced brain volumes affecting both grey and white matter and increased CSF volumes, compared to VCFS subjects without schizophrenia and control subjects [112]. Although these studies are few in numbers and involve small numbers of subjects, the decrease in grey matter in the heteromodal cortices in VCFS individuals with schizophrenia is consistent with the supposition that during the period of adolescence and early adulthood, the normal process of synaptic pruning may well be exaggerated in these individuals [111, 112]. Other findings in this group include loss of white matter, a smaller cerebellum, a cavum septum pellucidum, and large ventricles [86, 88, 110], findings similar to schizophrenia in the general population.

Treatment of VCFS-associated psychiatric illnesses

There is a paucity of clinical trials that have examined the efficacy of specific treatments (both behavioral and pharmacological interventions) in children and adults with VCFS. Although clinicians remain concerned about the possibility of unmasking psychosis by treating ADHD with methylphenidate, at least one study as well the clinical experience of psychiatrists familiar with VCFS seem to indicate that this medication is both safe and efficacious in VCFS individuals [78, 113]. The pharmacological treatment of schizophrenia in VCFS, based on the existing literature, appears similar to that in the general population, with newer atypical antipsychotic medications being effective [10, 21, 107]. There are no literature reports of systematic evaluations of behavioral interventions in the psychiatric manifestations in VCFS. In the future, controlled clinical trials examining the value of both the psychological and pharmacological treatments are essential to formulating better management strategies and to effectively evaluate the benefits of early intervention in this high-risk population.

Molecular genetics of schizophrenia as related to chromosome 22q11.2

Linkage studies in families with schizophrenia, unrelated to VCFS, are indicative of this region containing a gene(s) that predispose(s) to schizophrenia [3, 56, 114]. A few families with bipolar disorder have also been linked to the same interval [115, 116]. Although DNA studies thus far have failed to identify a specific gene(s) that is (are) etiologically related [117, 118], it is likely that a gene(s) in the 22q11.2 region is (are) contributory to the illness in the general population as well as in individuals with VCFS.

It is to be noted that because individuals with VCFS have a deletion encompassing ~35 genes on one chromosome 22 with the corresponding genes on the other chromosome 22 being present, they are haploinsufficient/hemizygous for these genes.

It is believed that decreased expression of this sequential group of genes due to the haploinsufficiency may be the cause of schizophrenia in VCFS [119, 120, 121]. In addition, it is possible that specific single nucleotide polymorphisms (SNPs) in the remaining allele of the genes in the 22q11.2 interval may contribute to psychosis risk in these individuals. The presence or absence of such polymorphisms in the hemizygous genes (remaining copy) could partly account for the variability seen in the occurrence of psychoses, because 60%–75% of VCFS individuals do not develop psychiatric illnesses, although the overwhelming majority of affected individuals have the same size deletion. Such polymorphisms in the "normal" allele have been postulated as accounting for the variability in manifestations in several genetic disorders, including VCFS [122, 123].

The deleted segment in individuals with VCFS is about 3 Mb in size. However, the region that is thought to be critical for the etiology of schizophrenia is about 1.5 Mb [19]. SNPs within one or more genes in this critical interval (Figure 24.5) may alter the abundance of the proteins (usually by decreasing transcription), thus contributing to the risk of schizophrenia [5, 124, 125, 126]. Detailed below are some of these genes, the most promising of which are the COMT and PRODH genes that are involved in dopaminergic and glutaminergic neurotransmission, respectively. Dopamine and glutamate are thought to be major mediators of schizophrenia in the general population.

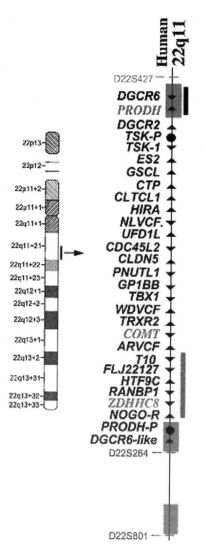

Figure 24.5 Ideogram of Chromosome 22, with a listing of all the genes in the 1.5 Mb interval in the q11.2 region, thought to be critical for schizophrenia. The genes denoted in red are thought to be most likely related to psychosis. (See color plate section.)

COMT

The COMT (catechol-O-methyl transferase) protein is the major enzyme responsible for the degradation of dopamine in the prefrontal cortex [127], unlike the striatum, where degradation of dopamine is largely due to the dopamine transporter gene [128]. A common SNP in the COMT gene, with the substitution of methionine (Met) for valine (Val) at codon 158, causes the Met allele to have one fourth the enzymatic activity of the Val allele [129], resulting in increased

availability of dopamine in the prefrontal cortex [130]. The prefrontal cortex is the seat of executive functioning and sustained attention and is contributory to working memory. Increased dopamine levels associated with the Met allele are thought to confer a cognitive advantage. In studies of healthy individuals, as well as patients with schizophrenia and schizotypy (unrelated to VCFS), individuals homozygous for the Met allele have been shown to perform better on tests of prefrontal cognition, as compared to those with Val homozygosity or heterozygosity for Met/Val [131, 132, 133]. Furthermore the Val allele occurred often in individuals with schizophrenia spectrum disorders [134, 135, 136]. Thus, there is considerable evidence that the Val/Met polymorphism is associated with the neurocognitive deficits observed in schizophrenia in the general population, especially those related to executive function and working memory, although some studies have been contradictory [137].

In individuals with VCFS, there is controversy about the relationship between the COMT genotype, the cognitive deficits, and schizophrenia. Initial studies that examined the association between the COMT polymorphism and neurocognition in children with VCFS found that children hemizygous for the low activity Met allele performed better on measures of executive function than Val hemizygous individuals [138, 139], a finding that was consistent with the reports in the general population with and without schizophrenia as discussed previously. Other studies have found that the Met allele is associated with poor neurocognitive functioning [66], minor psychiatric diagnoses, such as ADHD [140], and may predict longitudinal decline in verbal IQ as well as psychosis [141]. In a study of adults with VCFS, there was no association between the COMT genotype and schizophrenia [10]. A new study of adults with VCFS reported that the Met allele was associated with poor neurocognition, but the Val/Met polymorphism was not associated with schizophrenia [142]. This apparent contradiction in findings may in part be due to small sample sizes, different age groups, as well as issues related to methodology (selection of neurocognitive tests versus diagnostic psychiatric assessments) across the various studies. Also plausible is an unifying explanation that may help explain the controversial reports of the effects of the Val/Met polymorphism in VCFS: the concept that any deviation from the normal metabolism of dopamine in the form of excessive or defective clearance is likely to result in abnormal neurocognition, similar to that seen in schizophrenia [143]. However, given the relatively recent evidence that the cognitive deficits in schizophrenia are indeed associated with a hypoactive dopaminergic system in the prefrontal cortex as would be expected with the *Val* allele, further exploration of this issue in children with VCFS may yield important information [144, 145, 146].

Other SNPs in the *COMT* gene have been analyzed to determine a relationship to schizophrenia in the general population and of interest are rs737865 and rs165599 [147, 148]. The three marker haplotype consisting of genotypes at rs4680-rs737865-rs165599 (rs4680 = *Val/Met* polymorphism) is said to be associated with schizophrenia in the general population [149]. As yet, the impact of such haplotypes in individuals with VCFS has not been well delineated.

PRODH

The proline dehydrogenase (*PRODH*) gene product is responsible for the degradation of proline, an amino acid that functions as an inhibitory neurotransmitter and/or a metabolic precursor of glutamate [150, 151]. Proline enhances glutamate release, resulting in increased synaptic transmission. Reduced glutaminergic neurotransmission through the N-methyl-D-aspartate (NMDA) receptor, which is found in high concentrations in the prefrontal cortex, is believed to be related to schizophrenia, especially the deficits in working memory [152, 153]. A model implicating glutamate in the pathogenesis of schizophrenia proposes that reduced glutamate during the prenatal and adolescent periods accounts for the premorbid neurocognitive manifestations and the onset of illness, because reduced glutamate is believed to result in excessive synaptic elimination. After the onset of the illness, an increase in glutamate release occurs, secondary to elevated dopamine levels, causing increased neurotoxic cell loss, thus leading to disease progression [25]. In a mouse model with *PRODH* deficiency, locomotor deficits were attributed to elevated proline levels enhancing glutaminergic transmission [154]. These authors did not find any deficits in spatial working memory in *PRODH* deficient mice. It is possible that similar to dopamine, deficiency and excess of glutamate may have different effects in different areas of the brain at different stages of psychosis and further

work is needed before the role of *PRODH* in glutaminergic transmission is clear. The *PRODH* gene has also been implicated in apoptosis by supporting the generation of reactive oxygen species [155], but it is unclear if this property is related to schizophrenia. Examination of this function of *PRODH* and schizophrenia would be intriguing, because excessive apoptosis has been proposed as an additional mechanism in the pathogenesis of the disorder [25]. Several SNPs in the *PRODH* gene (rs2238731, rs2904551, rs3970559, rs450046) have been reported to be associated with schizophrenia in the general population, of which some are thought to be responsible for elevated proline levels [124, 126]. Thus, *PRODH* is regarded as an important candidate gene for schizophrenia, although not all studies have found such a link [156, 157].

In individuals with VCFS, there are not enough studies on *PRODH* thus far; a small study involving genotyping of two polymorphisms within the *PRODH* gene did not find any specific associations between these and psychiatric diagnoses [141]. Another study reported no association between the *PRODH* polymorphism and schizophrenia in 12 patients with VCFS and schizophrenia [158]. A recent study reported that hyperprolinemia was found in 37% of individuals with VCFS and that elevated proline levels were associated with lower IQ but not psychosis. Interestingly, these authors reported that elevated proline in combination with the *Met* allele in the *COMT* gene was associated with psychotic illnesses [159]. Thus, the *PRODH* and *COMT* genes in conjunction may modify psychosis risk, speculatively through the interaction between dopaminergic and glutaminergic transmission, as has been suggested in schizophrenia in the general population [128].

ZDHHC8

This gene lies at the distal end of the critical deleted segment and is involved in palmitoylation, a process that consists of modification of proteins with the lipid palmitate. *ZDHHC8* is highly expressed in the human brain [125] and is thought to be important for synaptic transmission, because palmitoylation is believed to modify neurotransmitters as well as other neuronal proteins [160]. A particular SNP rs175174 within the gene results in the production of a truncated protein and has been demonstrated to have an association with schizophrenia [125, 161]. There are no studies of an association between this gene and schizophrenia in humans with VCFS.

UFD1L

The ubiquitin fusion degradation 1 gene is believed to be important in embryogenesis. It is expressed in the medial telencephalon, which forms the hippocampus, in fetal life starting at 10 weeks of gestation and continuing into postnatal life. A functional SNP rs5992403 that results in upregulation of the gene has been studied and has been found to be associated with schizophrenia in the general population [162]. It is postulated that both upregulation and downregulation of the gene (the latter would be true of VCFS) is believed to result in neuronal dysfunction and apoptosis [163], but, thus far, there have been no reports of SNPs in this gene being linked to the cognitive or psychiatric abnormalities in individuals with VCFS.

TBX1

One of several transcription factors involved in developmental processes, the *TBX1* gene, has been shown to be responsible for several of the phenotypic features of VCFS, including the cardiac anomalies, facial features, thymic hypoplasia, and the parathyroid dysfunction [164]. Indirect evidence for a possible role of *TBX1* in the neurobehavioral manifestations of VCFS comes in the form of abnormal sensorimotor gating in mice models who are haploinsufficient for *TBX1* [165]. A mother and her two children (both with Asperger syndrome) with phenotypic features of VCFS, but no detectable 22q11.2 deletion, had a heterozygous deletion within the *TBX1* gene. This was cited as evidence that *TBX1* is involved in the behavioral abnormalities in VCFS [165]. There was no information regarding possible psychosis in this family and, although of interest, further studies are necessary to confirm this association.

Other genes of interest in the causation of schizophrenia in this interval could be identified in the future by expression patterns of these genes within the developing fetal and adult brain [166]. Because individuals with VCFS are hemizygous for genes in the 22q11.2 interval, genotype analysis and correlations with psychological and neuroanatomical findings would be more easily feasible than with traditional high-risk families.

Mouse models of VCFS: relevance to schizophrenia

Although the primary motive in creating a mouse model of the 22q11.2 deletion was to characterize the structural defects and the specific genes responsible for these, there has been considerable interest in determining the gene(s) that contribute to the psychiatric manifestations as well. A major challenge in using the mouse model for this purpose is that it is difficult to identify core human psychiatric traits that can be effectively studied in mice. Indeed, this will continue to pose limitations to the amount of information pertinent to schizophrenia that can be gleaned from the mouse model. This being said, traits that can be characterized are: anxiety, decreased sociability, and impaired working memory and sensorimotor gating (measured by prepulse inhibition). The most studied of these is the prepulse inhibition (PPI) of the acoustic startle reflex, considered a phenotypic marker for schizophrenia, although not a specific one, because it is also seen in obsessive-compulsive disorder, Tourette syndrome, and Asperger syndrome [167].

Various knockout mouse models have been utilized to study the genes responsible for the neuropsychiatric manifestations in VCFS. A region of the mouse chromosome 16 is homologous to the 22q11.2 interval in humans: the models created thus far include mice with heterozygous deletions of genes in the interval-(*Dfl/+*) [168] and *Lgdel/+* [169], as well as mice models with specific single gene mutations, as described later in this chapter.

In *Dfl/+* mice with a heterozygous deletion of a subset of 18 genes corresponding to the 22q11.2 interval, reduced PPI and reduced learning and difficulty in processing complex information were noted, compared to wild-type mice [170]. The authors pointed out the similarities to the neurocognitive abnormalities that have been described in schizophrenia in humans. In the *Lgdel/+* mice with a deletion of 27 genes, reduced PPI and an exaggerated startle were noticed [169]. Other studies have attempted to link these deficits, especially reduced PPI, to specific genes by creating point mutations/deletions of single genes using the mouse model. In the *COMT* knockout mice, there were no differences in PPI between the heterozygous and homozygous states [130]. Cognitive impairments in the *COMT* knockout mice have yet to be studied. In mice homozygous for a missense mutation in the *PRODH* gene, elevated proline levels and

319

reduced PPI were observed, whereas mice heterozygous for the mutation had near normal proline levels, but no observation was made on their behavior [171]. Intriguingly, mice that have a deletion of one *PRODH* gene in conjunction with deletions of contiguous genes in the 22q11.2 interval (including the *TBX1, COMT, PRODH,* and *ZDHHC8* genes), show more abnormal PPI, despite normal proline levels, as compared to mice homozygous for the missense mutation discussed previously [170], indicative of the possibility that mechanisms other than gene dosage are responsible for the association between *PRODH* and abnormal sensorimotor gating. One such plausible mechanism is the additive effect of the deletion of several genes in the 22q11DS interval. An interaction between *PRODH* and *COMT* has been suggested; *PRODH* deficient mice have increased dopamine levels in the frontal cortex, as a result of which there is compensatory upregulation of the *COMT* gene product normally [154]. Because individuals with VCFS may be unable to compensate in this manner for the *PRODH* heterozygosity due to the coexisting *COMT* deletion, they may be at an added disadvantage in combating the effects of decreased *PRODH* expression, thus exponentially increasing their vulnerability to psychosis.

The relationship between the *ZDHHC8* gene and sensorimotor gating has been addressed in one study in mice. Although there was a suggestion of a gender-specific effect on PPI, with females showing modestly reduced PPI, it appears, based on the available evidence, that *ZDHHC8* heterozygosity in and of itself is unlikely to cause behavioral abnormalities in the mouse model [125]. A role for the *TBX1* and *GNB1L* genes in causing reduced PPI in the mouse model has been suggested [165]; because *TBX1* is expressed in vascular tissue of the mouse brain, it has been postulated that disruption of the microvasculature may be responsible for the reduced PPI. However, other studies have not found behavioral abnormalities in mice that were haploinsufficient for *TBX1* [169, 172]. Thus, the role of *TBX1* in the psychiatric manifestations in the mouse model is yet to be fully defined. In general, the existing evidence in the mouse models of VCFS substantiates the supposition that the concomitant loss of several genes in the deleted interval is likely to cause the psychiatric

phenotype, rather than haploinsufficiency of a single gene.

Gene expression studies in mouse models are useful in identifying genes that could be involved in the pathogenesis of schizophrenia in VCFS. Profiling of gene expression within the hippocampus in mice with the heterozygous deletion of a subset of genes corresponding to the 22q11.2 interval demonstrated a 33% reduction in expression of 12 genes, including the *PRODH* and *COMT* genes. The *ZDHHC8* gene expression was not reduced [173]. However, illustrating once more the limitations of the mouse model in delineating schizophrenia pathogenesis in VCFS, this gene profile in the mouse model showed virtually no overlap with the profile seen in human hippocampal neurons [174].

In conclusion, VCFS represents an etiological subtype of schizophrenia spectrum disorders. Testing for VCFS should be considered in individuals with schizophrenia who have had congenital anomalies or dysmorphic features. Preliminary studies in VCFS individuals have shown that premorbid psychological and structural brain abnormalities are common in these individuals and overlap those seen in individuals with and at risk of schizophrenia. These data strongly support the notion that neuronal dysmaturation and disrupted synaptic pruning are likely involved in the pathogenesis of cognitive and behavioral abnormalities in childhood in VCFS, similar to the model proposed by proponents of the neurodevelopmental hypothesis of schizophrenia. Emerging correlations between the psychological and morphometric brain findings hold the promise that such changes may be beneficial in predicting psychosis in the future. Genes in the 22q11.2 interval are undoubtedly involved in the causation of schizophrenia in VCFS and are very likely to contribute to the illness in the general population. Thus, prospective studies of the psychological and brain morphometric changes and the genetics of the deleted interval in children and adolescents with VCFS offer the unparalleled opportunity to delineate the trajectory of events that occur on the pathway toward schizophrenia. Such an understanding of the neurodevelopmental basis of schizophrenia promises better understanding of the pathogenesis and potentially early identification and treatment of the most vulnerable individuals, thereby improving the chances of a better prognosis.

References

1. Weinberger D. R. Implications of normal brain development for the pathogenesis of schizophrenia. *Arch Gen Psychiatry*, 1987. **44**:660–9.

2. Andreasen N. C., Nopoulos P., O'Leary D. S., *et al.* Defining the phenotype of schizophrenia: cognitive dysmetria and its neural mechanisms. *Biol Psychiatry*, 1999. **46**:908–20.

3. Hovatta I., Lichtermann D., Juvonen H., *et al.* Linkage analysis of putative schizophrenia gene candidate regions on chromosomes 3p, 5q, 6p, 8p, 20p and 22q in a population-based sampled Finnish family set. *Mol Psychiatry*, 1998. **3**:452–7.

4. Shaw S. H., Kelly M., Smith A. B., *et al.* A genome-wide search for schizophrenia susceptibility genes. *Am J Med Genet*, 1998. **81**:364–76.

5. Liu H., Abecasis G. R., Heath S. C., *et al.* Genetic variation in the 22q11 locus and susceptibility to schizophrenia. *Proc Natl Acad Sci USA*, 2002. **99**:16859–64.

6. Kendler K. S. Hierarchy and heritability: the role of diagnosis and modeling in psychiatric genetics. *Am J Psychiatry*, 2002. **159**:515–18.

7. Shprintzen R. J., Goldberg R., Golding-Kushner K. J., *et al.* Late-onset psychosis in the velo-cardio-facial syndrome. *Am J Med Genet*, 1992. **42**: 141–2.

8. Pulver A. E., Nestadt G., Goldberg R., *et al.* Psychotic illness in patients diagnosed with velo-cardio-facial syndrome and their relatives. *J Nerv Ment Dis*, 1994. **182**:476–8.

9. Papolos D. F., Faedda G. L., Veit S., *et al.* Bipolar spectrum disorders in patients diagnosed with velo-cardio-facial syndrome: does a hemizygous deletion of chromosome 22q11 result in bipolar affective disorder? *Am J Psychiatry*, 1996. **153**:1541–7.

10. Murphy K. C., Jones L. A., Owen M. J. High rates of schizophrenia in adults with velo-cardio-facial syndrome. *Arch Gen Psychiatry*, 1999. **56**:940–5.

11. Chow E. W., Watson M., Young D. A., *et al.* Neurocognitive profile in 22q11 deletion syndrome and schizophrenia. *Schizophr Res*, 2006. **87**:270–78.

12. Wilson D. I.Cross I. E., Wren C. Minimum prevalence of chromosome 22q11 deletions. *Am J Hum Genet*, 1994. 55:A169.

13. Tezenas Du M. S., Mendizabai H., Ayme S., *et al.* (1996) Prevalence of 22q11 microdeletion. *J Med Genet*, 1996. **33**:719.

14. Shprintzen R. J. Velocardiofacial syndrome. *Otolaryngol Clin North Am*, 2000. 33:1217–40, vi.

15. Bassett A. S., Chow E. W. 22q11 deletion syndrome: a genetic subtype of schizophrenia. *Biol Psychiatry*, 1999. **46**:882–91.

16. Bassett A. S., Hodgkinson K., Chow E. W., *et al.* 22q11 deletion syndrome in adults with schizophrenia. *Am J Med Genet*, 1998. **81**:328–37.

17. Bassett A. S., Chow E. W., Husted J., *et al.* Clinical features of 78 adults with 22q11 Deletion Syndrome. *Am J Med Genet A*, 2005. **138**:307–13.

18. Fraser W., Nolan M. (1994) Psychiatric disorders in mental retardation. In *Mental Health in Mental Retardation*, Bouras N. (Ed.). Cambridge: Cambridge University Press, pp. 79–92.

19. Karayiorgou M., Morris M. A., Morrow B., *et al.* Schizophrenia susceptibility associated with interstitial deletions of chromosome 22q11. *Proc Natl Acad Sci USA*, 1995. **92**:7612–16.

20. Arinami T., Ohtsuki T., Takase K., *et al.* Screening for 22q11 deletions in a schizophrenia population. *Schizophr Res*, 2001. 52:167–70.

21. Sporn A., Addington A., Reiss A. L., *et al.* 22q11 deletion syndrome in childhood onset schizophrenia: an update. *Mol Psychiatry*, 2004. **9**:225–6.

22. Andreasen N. C. A unitary model of schizophrenia: Bleuler's "fragmented phrene" as schizencephaly. *Arch Gen Psychiatry*, 1999. **56**:781–7.

23. Rapoport J. L., Addington A. M., Frangou S., *et al.* The neuro-developmental model of schizophrenia: update 2005. *Mol Psychiatry*, 2005. **10**:434–49.

24. Keshavan M. S., Anderson S., Pettegrew J. W. Is schizophrenia due to excessive synaptic pruning in the prefrontal cortex? The Feinberg hypothesis revisited. *J Psychiatr Res*, 1994. **28**:239–65.

25. Keshavan M. S. Development, disease and degeneration in schizophrenia: a unitary pathophysiological model. *J Psychiatr Res*, 1999. **33**:513–21.

26. O'Callaghan E., Larkin C., Kinsella A., *et al.* Familial, obstetric, and other clinical correlates of minor physical anomalies in schizophrenia. *Am J Psychiatry*, 1991. **148**:479–83.

26. Pantelis C., Yucel M., Wood S. J., *et al.* Early and late neuro-developmental disturbances in schizophrenia and their functional consequences. *Aust NZ J Psychiatry*, 2003. **37**:399–406.

27. Green M. F., Satz P., Gaier D. J., *et al.* Minor physical anomalies in schizophrenia. *Schizophr Bull*, 1989. **15**:91–9.

28. Jones P., Rodgers B., Murray R., *et al.* Child development risk factors for adult schizophrenia in the British 1946 birth cohort. *Lancet*, 1994. **344**:1398–1402.

29. Scutt L. E., Chow E. W., Weksberg R., *et al.* Patterns of dysmorphic features in schizophrenia. *Am J Med Genet*, 2001. **105**:713–23.

30. Walker E. F., Savoie T., Davis D. Neuromotor precursors of schizophrenia. *Schizophr Bull*, 1994. **20**:441–51.

31. Hollis C. Child and adolescent (juvenile onset) schizophrenia. A case control study of premorbid developmental impairments. *Br J Psychiatry*, 1995. **166**:489–95.

32. Pantelis C., Maruff P. The cognitive neuropsychiatric approach to investigating the neurobiology of schizophrenia and other disorders. *J Psychosom Res*, 2002. **53**:655–64.

33. Kessler R. C., Demler O., Frank R. G., *et al.* Prevalence and treatment of mental disorders, 1990 to 2003. *N Engl J Med*, 2005. **352**: 2515–23.

34. Cornblatt B. A., Erlenmeyer-Kimling L. Global attentional deviance as a marker of risk for schizophrenia: specificity and predictive validity. *J Abnorm Psychol*, 1985. **94**:470–86.

35. Niemi L. T., Suvisaari J. M., Tuulio-Henriksson A., *et al.* Childhood developmental abnormalities in schizophrenia: evidence from high-risk studies. *Schizophr Res*, 2003. **60**:239–58.

36. Morey R. A., Inan S., Mitchell T. V., *et al.* Imaging frontostriatal function in ultra-high-risk, early, and chronic schizophrenia during executive processing. *Arch Gen Psychiatry*, 2005. **62**:254–62.

37. Kern R. S., Green M. F., Nuechterlein K. H., *et al.* NIMH-MATRICS survey on assessment of neurocognition in schizophrenia. *Schizophr Res*, 2004. **72**:11–19.

38. Degreef G., Ashtari M., Bogerts B., *et al.* Volumes of ventricular system subdivisions measured from magnetic resonance images in first-episode schizophrenic patients. *Arch Gen Psychiatry*, 1992. **49**:531–7.

39. Keshavan M. S., Rosenberg D., Sweeney J. A., *et al.* Decreased caudate volume in neuroleptic-naive psychotic patients. *Am J Psychiatry*, 1998. 155;774–8.

40. Zipursky R. B., Lambe E. K., Kapur S., *et al.* Cerebral gray matter volume deficits in first episode psychosis. *Arch Gen Psychiatry*, 1998. 55:540–6.

41. DeQuardo J. R., Keshavan M. S., Bookstein F. L., *et al.* Landmark-based morphometric analysis of first-episode schizophrenia. *Biol Psychiatry*, 1999. **45**:1321–8.

42. Shenton M. E., Dickey C. C., Frumin M., *et al.* A review of MRI findings in schizophrenia. *Schizophr Res*, 2001. **49**:1–52.

43. Molina V., Sanchez J., Reig S., *et al.* N-acetyl-aspartate levels in the dorsolateral prefrontal cortex in the early years of schizophrenia are inversely related to disease duration. *Schizophr Res*, 2005. **73**:209–19.

44. Nelson M. D., Saykin A. J., Flashman L. A., *et al.* Hippocampal volume reduction in schizophrenia as assessed by magnetic resonance imaging: a meta-analytic study. *Arch Gen Psychiatry*, 1998. **55**:433–40.

45. Konick L. C., Friedman L. Meta-analysis of thalamic size in schizophrenia. *Biol Psychiatry*, 2001. **49**:28–38.

46. Choi J. S., Kang D. H., Kim J. J., *et al.* Decreased caudal anterior cingulate gyrus volume and positive symptoms in schizophrenia. *Psychiatry Res*, 2005. **139**:239–47.

47. Keshavan M. S., Diwadkar V. A., Montrose D. M., *et al.* Premorbid indicators and risk for schizophrenia: a selective review and update. *Schizophr Res*, 2005. **79**:45–57.

48. Giedd J. N., Snell J. W., Lange N., *et al.* Quantitative magnetic resonance imaging of human brain development: ages 4–18. *Cereb Cortex*, 1996. **6**:551–60.

49. Rapoport J. L., Castellanos F. X., Gogate N., *et al.* Imaging normal and abnormal brain development: new perspectives for child psychiatry. *Aust N Z J Psychiatry*, 2001. **35**:272–81.

50. Zecevic N., Bourgeois J. P., Rakic P. Changes in synaptic density in motor cortex of rhesus monkey during fetal and postnatal life. *Brain Res Dev Brain Res*, 1989. **50**:11–32.

51. Huttenlocher P. R., Dabholkar A. S. Regional differences in synaptogenesis in human cerebral cortex. *J Comp Neurol*, 1997. **387**: 167–78.

52. Giedd J. N., Clasen L. S., Lenroot R., *et al.* (2006) Puberty-related influences on brain development. *Mol Cell Endocrinol*, 2006. 254–5:154–62.

53. Sowell E. R., Thompson P. M., Leonard C. M., *et al.* Longitudinal mapping of cortical thickness and brain growth in normal children. *J Neurosci*, 2004. **24**:8223–31.

54. Thompson P. M., Vidal C., Giedd J. N., *et al.* Mapping adolescent brain change reveals dynamic wave of accelerated grey matter loss in very early-onset schizophrenia. *Proc Natl Acad Sci USA*, 2001. **98**:11650–5.

55. McGlashan T. H., Hoffman R. E. Schizophrenia as a disorder of developmentally reduced synaptic connectivity. *Arch Gen Psychiatry*, 2000. **57**:637–48.

56. Gill M., Vallada H., Collier D., *et al.* A combined analysis of D22S278 marker alleles in affected sib-pairs: support for a susceptibility locus for schizophrenia at chromosome 22q12. Schizophrenia Collaborative Linkage Group (Chromosome 22). *Am J Med Genet*, 1996. **67**:40–5.

57. Shprintzen R. J., Goldberg R. B., Young D., *et al.* The velo-cardio-facial syndrome: a clinical and genetic analysis. *Pediatrics*, 1981. **67**:167–72.

58. Swillen A., Devriendt K., Legius E., *et al.* Intelligence and psychosocial adjustment in velocardiofacial syndrome: a study of 37 children and adolescents with VCFS. *J Med Genet*, 1997. **34**:453–8.

59. Moss E. M., Batshaw M. L., Solot C. B., *et al.* Psychoeducational profile of the 22q11.2 microdeletion: a complex pattern. *J Pediatr*, 1999. **134**:193–8.

60. Woodin M., Wang P. P., Aleman D., *et al.* Neuropsychological profile of children and adolescents with the 22q11.2 microdeletion. *Genet Med*, 2001. **3**:34–9.

61. Glaser B., Mumme D. L., Blasey C., *et al.* Language skills in children with velocardiofacial syndrome (deletion 22q11.*2*). *J Pediatr*, 2002. **140**:753–8.

62. Gerdes M., Solot C., Wang P. P., *et al.* Cognitive and behavior profile of preschool children with chromosome 22q11.2 deletion. *Am J Med Genet*, 1999 **85**:127–33.

63. Sobin C., Kiley-Brabeck K., Daniels S., *et al.* Neuropsychological characteristics of children with the 22q11 Deletion Syndrome: a descriptive analysis. *Child Neuropsychol*, 2005a. **11**:39–53.

64. Rovet J. F., Buchanan L. (1999) Turner syndrome: a cognitive neuroscience approach. In *Neurodevelopmental Disorders*, Tager F. (Ed.). Cambridge, Mass.: The MIT Press, pp. 223–50.

65. Sobin C., Kiley-Brabeck K., Karayiorgou M. Associations between prepulse inhibition and executive visual attention in children with the 22q11 deletion syndrome. *Mol Psychiatry*, 2005b. **10**:553–62.

66. Baker K., Baldeweg T., Sivagnanasundaram S., *et al.* COMT Val108/158 Met modifies mismatch negativity and cognitive function in 22q11 deletion syndrome. *Biol Psychiatry*, 2005. **58**:23–31.

67. Bish J. P., Ferrante S. M., Donald-McGinn D., *et al.* Maladaptive conflict monitoring as evidence for executive dysfunction in children with chromosome 22q11.2 deletion syndrome. *Dev Sci*, 2005. **8**:36–43.

68. Simon T. J., Bearden C. E., Mc-Ginn D. M., *et al.* Visuospatial and numerical cognitive deficits in children with chromosome 22q11.2 deletion syndrome. *Cortex*, 2005a. **41**:145–55.

69. Lewandowski K. E., Shashi V., Berry P. M., *et al.* Schizophrenic-like neurocognitive deficits in children and adolescents with 22q11 deletion syndrome. *Am J Med Genet, B Neuropsychiatr Genet*, 2007. **144**:27–36.

70. Buchanan R. W., Francis A., Arango C., *et al.* Morphometric assessment of the heteromodal association cortex in schizophrenia. *Am J Psychiatry*, 2004. **161**:322–31.

71. Swillen A., Devriendt K., Legius E., *et al.* The behavioural phenotype in velo-cardio-facial syndrome (VCFS): from infancy to adolescence. *Genet Couns*, 1999. **10**:79–88.

72. Swillen A., Vogels A., Devriendt K., *et al.* Chromosome 22q11 deletion syndrome: update and review of the clinical features, cognitive-behavioral spectrum, and psychiatric complications. *Am J Med Genet*, 2000. **97**:128–35.

73. Arnold P. D., Siegel-Bartelt J., Cytrynbaum C., *et al.* Velo-cardio-facial syndrome: implications of microdeletion 22q11 for schizophrenia and mood disorders. *Am J Med Genet*, 2001. **105**:354–62.

74. Gothelf D., Presburger G., Zohar A. H., *et al.* Obsessive-compulsive disorder in patients with velocardiofacial (22q11 deletion) syndrome. *Am J Med Genet, B Neuropsychiatr Genet*, 2004. **126**:99–105.

75. Heineman-de Boer J. A., Van Haelst M. J., Cordia-de H. M., *et al.* Behavior problems and personality aspects of 40 children with velo-cardio-facial syndrome. *Genet Couns*, 1999. **10**:89–93.

76. Feinstein C., Eliez S., Blasey C., *et al.* Psychiatric disorders and behavioral problems in children with velocardiofacial syndrome: usefulness as phenotypic indicators of schizophrenia risk. *Biol Psychiatry*, 2002. **51**:312–18.

77. Murphy K. C., Owen M. J. Velo-cardio-facial syndrome: a model for understanding the genetics and pathogenesis of schizophrenia. *Br J Psychiatry*, 2001. **179**:397–402.

78. Murphy K. C. Annotation: velo-cardio-facial syndrome. *J Child Psychol Psychiatry*, 2005. **46**:563–71.

79. Debbane M., Glaser B., David M. K., *et al.* (2006a) Psychotic symptoms in children and adolescents with 22q11.2 deletion syndrome: Neuropsychological and behavioral implications. *Schizophr Res*, 2006a. **84**:187–93.

80. Baker K. D., Skuse D. H. Adolescents and young adults with 22q11 deletion syndrome: psychopathology in an at-risk group. *Br J Psychiatry*, 2005. **186**:115–20.

81. Cannon M., Caspi A., Moffitt T. E., *et al.* Evidence for early-childhood, pan-developmental impairment specific to schizophreniform disorder: results from a longitudinal birth cohort. *Arch Gen Psychiatry*, 2002. **59**:449–56.

82. Davalos D. B., Compagnon N., Heinlein S., *et al.* Neuropsychological deficits in children associated with increased familial risk for schizophrenia. *Schizophr Res*, 2004. **67**:123–30.

83. Mitnick R. J., Bello J. A., Shprintzen R. J. Brain anomalies in velo-cardio-facial syndrome. *Am J Med Genet*, 1994. **54**:100–6.

84. Bingham P. M., Zimmerman R. A., Donald-McGinn D., *et al.* Enlarged Sylvian fissures in infants with interstitial deletion of chromosome 22q11. *Am J Med Genet*, 1997. **74**:538–43.

85. Vataja R., Elomaa E. Midline brain anomalies and schizophrenia in people with CATCH 22 syndrome. *Br J Psychiatry*, 1998. **172**:518–20.

86. Chow E. W., Mikulis D. J., Zipursky R. B., *et al.* Qualitative MRI findings in adults with 22q11 deletion syndrome and schizophrenia. *Biol Psychiatry*, 1999. **46**:1436–42.

87. Shashi V., Muddasani S., Santos C. C., *et al.* Abnormalities of the corpus callosum in nonpsychotic children with chromosome 22q11 deletion syndrome. *Neuroimage*, 2004. **21**:1399–406.

88. van A. T., Daly E., Robertson D., *et al.* Structural brain abnormalities associated with deletion at chromosome 22q11: quantitative neuroimaging study of adults with velo-cardio-facial syndrome. *Br J Psychiatry*, 2001. **178**:412–19.

89. Usiskin S. I., Nicolson R., Krasnewich D. M., *et al.* Velocardiofacial syndrome in childhood-onset schizophrenia. *J Am Acad Child Adolesc Psychiatry*, 1999. **38**:1536–43.

90. Eliez S., Schmitt J. E., White C. D., *et al.* Children and adolescents with velocardiofacial syndrome: a volumetric MRI study. *Am J Psychiatry*, 2000. **157**: 409–15.

91. Katesa W. R., Burnettea C. P. Posterior cortical white matter anomalies in velocardiofacial syndrome. pp 1S–173S *Biol Psychiatry*, 2000. 47(Suppl 1): S102–73S.

92. Eliez S., Blasey C. M., Schmitt E. J., *et al.* Velocardiofacial syndrome: are structural changes in the temporal and mesial temporal regions related to schizophrenia? *Am J Psychiatry*, 2001. **158**:447–53.

93. Simon T. J., Ding L., Bish J. P., *et al.* Volumetric, connective, and morphologic changes in the brains of children with chromosome 22q11.2 deletion syndrome: an integrative study. *Neuroimage*, 2005b. **25**:169–80.

94. Bearden C. E., van Erp T. G., Dutton R. A., *et al.* Mapping cortical thickness in children with 22q11.2 deletions. *Cereb Cortex*, 2007. **17**:1889–98. [Epub Oct 20, 2006.]

95. Debbane M., Schaer M., Farhoumand R., *et al.* Hippocampal volume reduction in 22q11.2 deletion syndrome. *Neuropsychologia*, 2006b. **44**:2360–5.

96. Sugama S., Bingham P. M., Wang P. P., *et al.* Morphometry of the head of the caudate nucleus in patients with velocardiofacial syndrome (del 22q11.2). *Acta Paediatr*, 2000. **89**:546–9.

97. Eliez S., Barnea-Goraly N., Schmitt J. E., *et al.* Increased basal ganglia volumes in velo-cardio-facial syndrome (deletion 22q11.2). *Biol Psychiatry*, 2002. **52**:68–70.

98. Kates W. R., Burnette C. P., Bessette B. A., *et al.* Frontal and caudate alterations in velocardiofacial syndrome (deletion at chromosome 22q11.2). *J Child Neurol*, 2004. **19**:337–42.

99. Campbell L. E., Daly E., Toal F., *et al.* Brain and behaviour in children with 22q11.2 deletion syndrome: a volumetric and voxel-based morphometry MRI study. *Brain*, 2006. **129**:1218–28.

100. Kates W. R., Miller A. M., AbdulSabur N., *et al.* Temporal lobe anatomy and psychiatric symptoms in velocardiofacial syndrome (22q11.2 deletion syndrome). *J Am Acad Child Adolesc Psychiatry*, 2006. **45**:587–95.

101. Antshel K. M., Conchelos J., Lanzetta G., *et al.* Behavior and corpus callosum morphology relationships in velocardiofacial syndrome (22q11.2 deletion syndrome). *Psychiatry Res*, 2005. **138**:235–45.

102. Keshavan M. S., Dick E., Mankowski I., *et al.* Decreased left amygdala and hippocampal volumes in young offspring at risk for schizophrenia *Schizophr Res*, 2002a. **58**:173–83.

103. Keshavan M. S., Diwadkar V. A., Harenski K., *et al.* Abnormalities of the corpus callosum in first episode, treatment naive schizophrenia. *J Neurol Neurosurg Psychiatry*, 2002b. **72**:757–60.

104. Bearden C. E., van Erp T. G., Monterosso J. R., *et al.* Regional brain abnormalities in 22q11.2 deletion syndrome: association with cognitive abilities and behavioral symptoms. *Neurocase*, 2004b. **10**:198–206.

105. Feinberg I. Schizophrenia: caused by a fault in programmed synaptic elimination during adolescence? *J Psychiatr Res*, 1982. **17**:319–34.

106. Gothelf D., Frisch A., Munitz H., *et al.* Clinical characteristics of schizophrenia associated with velo-cardio-facial syndrome. *Schizophr Res*, 1999. **35**:105–12.

107. Bassett A. S., Chow E. W., AbdelMalik P., *et al.* The schizophrenia phenotype in 22q11 deletion syndrome. *Am J Psychiatry*, 2003. **160**:1580–6.

108. Meehl P. E. Toward an integrated theory of schizotaxia, schizotypy and schizophrenia. J *Personality Disorders*, 1990. **4**:1–99.

109. van A. T., Henry J., Morris R., *et al.* Cognitive deficits associated with schizophrenia in velo-cardio-facial syndrome. *Schizophr Res*, 2004b. **70**:223–32.

110. Barnea-Goraly N., Menon V., Krasnow B., *et al.* Investigation of white matter structure in velocardiofacial syndrome: a diffusion tensor imaging study.

Am J Psychiatry, 2003. **160**:1863–9.

111. Chow E. W., Zipursky R. B., Mikulis D. J., et al. Structural brain abnormalities in patients with schizophrenia and 22q11 deletion syndrome. *Biol Psychiatry*, 2002. **51**:208–15.

112. van A. T., Daly E., Henry J., et al. Brain anatomy in adults with velocardiofacial syndrome with and without schizophrenia: preliminary results of a structural magnetic resonance imaging study. *Arch Gen Psychiatry*, 2004a. **61**:1085–96.

113. Gothelf D., Gruber R., Presburger G., et al. Methylphenidate treatment for attention-deficit/hyperactivity disorder in children and adolescents with velocardiofacial syndrome: an open-label study. *J Clin Psychiatry*, 2003. **64**: 1163–9.

114. Lasseter V. K., Pulver A. E., Wolyniec P. S., et al. (1995) Follow-up report of potential linkage for schizophrenia on chromosome 22q: Part 3. *Am J Med Genet*, 1995. **60**:172–3.

115. Lachman H. M., Kelsoe J. R., Remick R. A., et al. Linkage studies suggest a possible locus for bipolar disorder near the velo-cardio-facial syndrome region on chromosome 22. *Am J Med Genet*, 1997. **74**:121–8.

116. Kelsoe J. R., Spence M. A., Loetscher E., et al. A genome survey indicates a possible susceptibility locus for bipolar disorder on chromosome 22. *Proc Natl Acad Sci USA*, 2001. **98**:585–90.

117. Funke B., Saint-Jore B., Puech A., et al. Characterization and mutation analysis of goosecoid-like (GSCL), a homeodomain-containing gene that maps to the critical region for VCFS/DGS on 22q11. *Genomics*, 1997. **46**:364–72.

118. Sirotkin H., O'Donnell H., DasGupta R., et al. (1997) Identification of a new human catenin gene family member (ARVCF) from the region deleted in velo-cardio-facial syndrome. *Genomics*, 1997. **41**:75–83.

119. Kurahashi H., Nakayama T., Osugi Y., et al. Deletion mapping of 22q11 in CATCH22 syndrome: identification of a second critical region. *Am J Hum Genet*, 1996. **58**:1377–81.

120. Kurahashi H., Tsuda E., Kohama R., et al. Another critical region for deletion of 22q11: a study of 100 patients. *Am J Med Genet*, 1997. **72**:180–5.

121. Karayiorgou M., Gogos J. A. The molecular genetics of the 22q11-associated schizophrenia. *Brain Res Mol Brain Res*, 2004. **132**:95–104.

122. Carey J. C., Viskochil D. H. Neurofibromatosis type 1: a model condition for the study of the molecular basis of variable expressivity in human disorders. *Am J Med Genet*, 1999. **89**:7–13.

123. Breuning M. H. Phenotypic variability: genetics and chance–deletion 22q11 and schizophrenia. *Ned Tijdschr Geneeskd*, 2002. **146**:2016–19.

124. Li T., Ma X., Sham P. C., et al. Evidence for association between novel polymorphisms in the PRODH gene and schizophrenia in a Chinese population. *Am J Med Genet, B Neuropsychiatr Genet*, 2004. **129**:13–15.

125. Mukai J., Liu H., Burt R. A., et al. Evidence that the gene encoding ZDHHC8 contributes to the risk of schizophrenia. *Nat Genet*, 2004. **36**:725–31.

126. Bender H. U., Almashanu S., Steel G., et al. Functional consequences of PRODH missense mutations. *Am J Hum Genet*, 2005. **76**:409–20.

127. Karoum F., Chrapusta S. J., Egan M. F. 3-Methoxytyramine is the major metabolite of released

dopamine in the rat frontal cortex: reassessment of the effects of antipsychotics on the dynamics of dopamine release and metabolism in the frontal cortex, nucleus accumbens, and striatum by a simple two pool model. *J Neurochem*, 1994. **63**:972–9.

128. Weinberger D. R., Egan M. F., Bertolino A., et al. Prefrontal neurons and the genetics of schizophrenia. *Biol Psychiatry*, 2001. **50**:825–44.

129. Aksoy S. , Klener J., Weinshilboum R. M. Catechol O-methyltransferase pharmacogenetics: photoaffinity labelling and western blot analysis of human liver samples. *Pharmacogenetics*, 1993. **3**: 116–22.

130. Gogos J. A., Morgan M., Luine V., et al. Catechol-O-methyltransferase-deficient mice exhibit sexually dimorphic changes in catecholamine levels and behavior. *Proc Natl Acad Sci USA*, 1998. **95**:9991–6.

131. Egan M. F., Goldberg T. E., Kolachana B. S., et al. Effect of COMT Val108/158 Met genotype on frontal lobe function and risk for schizophrenia. *Proc Natl Acad Sci USA*, 2001. **98**:6917–22.

132. Bilder R. M., Volavka J., Czobor P., et al. Neurocognitive correlates of the COMT Val(158)Met polymorphism in chronic schizophrenia. *Biol Psychiatry*, 2002. **52**:701–7.

133. Malhotra A. K., Kestler L. J., Mazzanti C., et al. A functional polymorphism in the COMT gene and performance on a test of prefrontal cognition. *Am J Psychiatry*, 2002. **159**:652–4.

134. Li T., Sham P. C., Vallada H., et al. Preferential transmission of the high activity allele of COMT in schizophrenia. *Psychiatr Genet*, 1996. **6**:131–3.

135. Avramopoulos D., Stefanis N. C., Hantoumi I., et al. Higher scores of self reported schizotypy in

healthy young males carrying the COMT high activity allele. *Mol Psychiatry*, 2002. 7:706–11.

136. Wonodi I., Stine O. C., Mitchell B. D., *et al.* Association between Val108/158 Met polymorphism of the COMT gene and schizophrenia. *Am J Med Genet B Neuropsychiatr Genet*, 2003. **120**:47–50.

137. Munafo M. R., Bowes L., Clark T. G., *et al.* (2005) Lack of association of the COMT (Val158/108 Met) gene and schizophrenia: a meta-analysis of case-control studies. *Mol Psychiatry*, 2005. **10**:765–70.

138. Bearden C. E., Jawad A. F., Lynch D. R., *et al.* Effects of a functional COMT polymorphism on prefrontal cognitive function in patients with 22q11.2 deletion syndrome. *Am J Psychiatry*, 2004a. **161**:1700–2.

139. Shashi V., Keshavan M. S., Howard T. D., *et al.* Cognitive correlates of a functional COMT polymorphism in children with 22q11.2 deletion syndrome. *Clin Genet*, 2006. **69**:234–8.

140. Gothelf D., Michaelovsky E., Frisch A., *et al.* Association of the low-activity COMT 158Met allele with ADHD and OCD in subjects with velocardiofacial syndrome. *Int J Neuropsychopharmacol*, 2007. **10**:301–8. [Epub May 31, 2006.]

141. Gothelf D., Eliez S., Thompson T., *et al.* COMT genotype predicts longitudinal cognitive decline and psychosis in 22q11.2 deletion syndrome. *Nat Neurosci*, 2005. **8**:1500–2.

142. Bassett A. S., Caluseriu O., Weksberg R., *et al.* Catechol-O-methyl transferase and expression of schizophrenia in 73 adults with 22q11 deletion syndrome. *Biol Psychiatry*, 2007. **61**:1135–40. [Epub Jan 9, 2007.]

143. Goldman-Rakic P. S., Muly E. C. III, Williams G. V. D(1) receptors in prefrontal cells and circuits.

Brain Res Brain Res Rev, 2000. **31**:295–301.

144. Davis K. L., Kahn R. S., Ko G., *et al.* Dopamine in schizophrenia: a review and reconceptualization. *Am J Psychiatry*, 1991. **148**:1474–86.

145. Goldman-Rakic, P. S. (1991) Prefrontal cortical dysfunction in schizophrenia: the relevance of working memory. In *Psycho-pathology and the Brain*, Carroll B. J. and Barrett J. E. (Eds.). New York: Raven Press, pp. 1–23.

146. Braver T. S., Barch D. M., Cohen J. D. Cognition and control in schizophrenia: a computational model of dopamine and prefrontal function. *Biol Psychiatry*, 1999. **46**:312–28.

147. Chen X., Wang X., O'Neill A. F., *et al.* Variants in the catechol-o-methyltransferase (COMT) gene are associated with schizophrenia in Irish high-density families. *Mol Psychiatry*, 2004b. **9**:962–7.

148. Palmatier M. A., Pakstis A. J., Speed W., *et al.* COMT haplotypes suggest P2 promoter region relevance for schizophrenia. *Mol Psychiatry*, 2004. **9**:859–70.

149. Handoko H. Y., Nyholt D. R., Hayward N. K., *et al.* Separate and interacting effects within the catechol-O-methyltransferase (COMT) are associated with schizophrenia. *Mol Psychiatry*, 2005. **10**:589–97.

150. Fremeau R. T. Jr., Caron M. G., Blakely R. D. Molecular cloning and expression of a high affinity L-proline transporter expressed in putative glutamatergic pathways of rat brain. *Neuron*, 1992. **8**:915–26.

151. Renick S. E., Kleven D. T., Chan J., *et al.* The mammalian brain high-affinity L-proline transporter is enriched preferentially in synaptic vesicles in a subpopulation of excitatory nerve

terminals in rat forebrain. *J Neurosci*, 1999. **19**:21–33.

152. Goff D. C., Coyle J. T. The emerging role of glutamate in the pathophysiology and treatment of schizophrenia. *Am J Psychiatry*, 2001. **158**:1367–77.

153. Hahn C. G., Wang H. Y., Cho D. S., *et al.* Altered neuregulin 1-erbB4 signaling contributes to NMDA receptor hypofunction in schizophrenia. *Nat Med*, 2006. **12**:824–8.

154. Paterlini M., Zakharenko S. S., Lai W. S., *et al.* Transcriptional and behavioral interaction between 22q11.2 orthologs modulates schizophrenia-related phenotypes in mice. *Nat Neurosci*, 2005. **8**:1586–94.

155. Maxwell S. A., Davis G. E. Differential gene expression in p53-mediated apoptosis-resistant vs. apoptosis-sensitive tumor cell lines. *Proc Natl Acad Sci USA*, 2000. **97**:13009–14.

156. Williams H. J., Williams N., Spurlock G., *et al.* Detailed analysis of PRODH and PsPRODH reveals no association with schizophrenia. *Am J Med Genet B Neuropsychiatr Genet*, 2003b. **120**:42–6.

157. Jacquet H., Rapoport J. L., Hecketsweiler B., *et al.* (2006) Hyperprolinemia is not associated with childhood onset schizophrenia. *Am J Med Genet B Neuropsychiatr Genet*, 2006. **141**:192.

158. Williams H. J., Williams N., Spurlock G., *et al.* Association between PRODH and schizophrenia is not confirmed. *Mol Psychiatry*, 2003a. **8**:644–5.

159. Raux G., Bumsel E., Hecketsweiler B., *et al.* (2006) Involvement of hyperprolinemia in cognitive and psychiatric features of the 22q11 deletion syndrome. *Hum Mol Genet*, 2007. **16**:83–91. [Epub Nov 29, 2006.]

160. El-Husseini A. E., Craven S. E., Chetkovich D. M., *et al.* Dual

palmitoylation of PSD-95 mediates its vesiculotubular sorting, postsynaptic targeting, and ion channel clustering. *J Cell Biol*, 2000. **148**:159–72.

161. Chen W. Y., Shi Y. Y., Zheng Y. L., *et al*. Case-control study and transmission disequilibrium test provide consistent evidence for association between schizophrenia and genetic variation in the 22q11 gene ZDHHC8. *Hum Mol Genet*, 2004a. **13**:2991–5.

162. De L. A., Pasini A., Amati F., *et al*. Association study of a promoter polymorphism of UFD1L gene with schizophrenia. *Am J Med Genet*, 2001. **105**:529–33.

163. Srivastava D., Yamagishi H. Reply: role of the dHAND-UFD1L pathway. *Trends Genet*, 1999. **15**:253–4.

164. Yagi H., Furutani Y., Hamada H., *et al*. Role of TBX1 in human del22q11.2 syndrome. *Lancet*, 2003. **362**:1366–73.

165. Paylor R., Glaser B., Mupo A., *et al*. Tbx1 haploinsufficiency is linked to behavioral disorders in mice and humans: implications for 22q11 deletion syndrome. *Proc Natl Acad Sci USA*, 2006. **103**:7729–34.

166. Maynard T. M., Haskell G. T., Peters A. Z., *et al*. (2003) A comprehensive analysis of 22q11 gene expression in the developing and adult brain. *Proc Natl Acad Sci USA*, 2003. **100**:14433–8.

167. Braff D. L., Geyer M. A., Swerdlow N. R. Human studies of prepulse inhibition of startle: normal subjects, patient groups, and pharmacological studies. *Psychopharmacology (Berl)*, 2001. **156**:234–58.

168. Lindsay E. A., Botta A., Jurecic V., *et al*. Congenital heart disease in mice deficient for the DiGeorge syndrome region. *Nature*, 1999. **401**:379–83.

169. Long J. M., Laporte P., Merscher S., *et al*. Behavior of mice with mutations in the conserved region deleted in velocardiofacial/ DiGeorge syndrome. *Neurogenetics*, 2006. 7:247–57.

170. Paylor R., McIlwain K. L., McAninch R., *et al*. Mice deleted for the DiGeorge/velocardiofacial syndrome region show abnormal sensorimotor gating and learning and memory impairments. *Hum Mol Genet*, 2001. **10**:2645–50.

171. Gogos J. A., Santha M., Takacs Z., *et al*. The gene encoding proline dehydrogenase modulates sensorimotor gating in mice. *Nat Genet*, 1999. **21**:434–9.

172. Hiroi N., Zhu H., Lee M., *et al*. A 200-kb region of human chromosome 22q11.2 confers antipsychotic-responsive behavioral abnormalities in mice. *Proc Natl Acad Sci USA*, 2005. **102**:19132–7.

173. Jurata L. W., Gallagher P., Lemire A. L., *et al*. Altered expression of hippocampal dentate granule neuron genes in a mouse model of human 22q11 deletion syndrome. *Schizophr Res*, 2006. **88**:251–9.

174. Altar C. A., Jurata L. W., Charles V., *et al*. Deficient hippocampal *Neuron*, expression of proteasome, ubiquitin, and mitochondrial genes in multiple schizophrenia cohorts. *Biol Psychiatry*, 2005. **58**:85–96.

Organic syndromes of schizophrenia: *genetic disorders related to SLP*

Psychosis in Prader-Willi Syndrome

Stewart L. Einfeld, Sophie Kavanagh, Arabella Smith, and Bruce J. Tonge

Facts box

- Prader-Willi Syndrome (PWS) is a congenital disorder characterized by infantile hypotonia, hypogonadism, mild intellectual disability, short stature, small hands and feet, and characteristic facies.

- DNA studies have shown that PWS may arise by three different mechanisms acting within the imprinted region of chromosome 15(q11–13). The three mechanisms are paternal deletion, maternal uniparental disomy (UPD), and a rare abnormality within the imprinting control mechanism.

- The true rate of psychotic disorder in this population remains to be determined, but all reported rates are high, between 10% and 30%.

- Psychotic episodes begin in adolescence or early adulthood. Most studies describe the psychosis in PWS as having an intermittent relapsing course, with full recovery between episodes

- Individuals with PWS because of UPD have about five times the risk of developing psychosis compared with those with a deletion. The mechanism of this increased risk is unknown.

- Other types of psychopathology and problem behaviors in this population include severe hyperphagia and associated behaviors including stealing food and pica; depression; temper tantrums, impulsivity, stubbornness; and skin-picking and obsessive or compulsive-like symptoms.

What is Prader-Willi Syndrome?

PWS is a congenital disorder characterized by infantile hypotonia, hypogonadism, mild intellectual disability,

short stature, small hands and feet, and characteristic facies. Early onset of obesity is associated with hyperphagia and the development of other maladaptive behaviors [1, 2, 3]. Hypothalamic dysfunction is evidenced by deficiency of growth hormone [4] and leutinising hormone [5]. A reduced number of oxytocin-producing cells has been found [6]. DNA studies have shown that PWS may arise by three different mechanisms acting within the imprinted region of chromosome 15(q11–13) [7, 8]. A functional paternal PWS gene is essential for normal development. The three mechanisms are paternal deletion of the PWS locus on chromosome 15(q11–13) in about 74% of cases (most clearly seen on FISH), maternal uniparental disomy (UPD) in approximately 24%, and a rare abnormality within the imprinting control mechanism in 1%–2% of cases [8]. High resolution cytogenetic testing alone is unreliable for the diagnosis of PWS compared with DNA studies [9]. A DNA methylation test can differentiate the maternal and paternal chromosomes by their methylation pattern and is the definitive diagnostic test, although it does not provide the mechanism.

Psychosis in PWS

There have been a number of reports of psychotic illness in those with PWS, suggesting that there may be an association between these conditions. Some authors have attempted to determine the prevalence of psychotic symptoms in those with PWS. Clarke [10] surveyed the caregivers of 95 people with PWS. There was a known genetic diagnosis in 40 cases (42%). They found that 6.3% of 95 subjects had experienced a possible psychotic disorder in the preceding month. Boer and colleagues [11] found that 6 of 54 adults (11%) with genetically proven PWS could be given a diagnosis of psychotic illness. Beardsmore and colleagues [12] found that 21.7% of a sample of 23 adults with PWS had current psychotic symptoms. However, this sample may have been over representative of those with psychiatric problems because some cases were recruited from a psychiatric service. Descheemaeker and colleagues [13] followed up on 53 people with confirmed PWS seen at a genetic clinic, for 15 years. They found that 4 (7.5%) of these people developed psychotic symptoms. Vogels and colleagues [14] also followed up on a group with confirmed PWS through a genetic clinic; 59 patients were followed for 10 years; 6 (10.2%) experienced a psychotic episode. Bray and colleagues [15], in describing a series of 40 patients with PWS, reported that 2 had required hospitalization for brief psychotic episodes. Whitman and Accardo [16] assessed a nonclinical sample of 35 adolescents with PWS. They found that psychotic symptoms were commonly reported: 11% reported visual hallucinations as "very true/often," whereas 11% reported strange ideation and 29% reported paranoid/suspicious as "very true/often." Bartolucci and Younger [17] reported 4 of 9 people with PWS referred for psychiatric consultation as having symptoms of psychosis. The present authors found 16% of their PWS subjects forming part of the Australian Child to Adult Development study [18] to have a history of psychosis. Soni and colleagues [19] found 29% of 119 individuals with PWS had a history of psychotic symptoms. The true rate of psychotic disorder in this population remains to be determined, but all reported rates are high, between 10 and 30%.

Other psychopathology in PWS

PWS has been shown to be associated with a range of symptoms of psychopathology apart from symptoms of psychosis. Most prominent is the severe hyperphagia and associated behaviors including stealing food and pica [3]. Affective symptoms are also commonly reported. In the study of Soni and colleagues [19], 23% had a history of depressive disorder, and 10% bipolar disorder. Verhoeven and colleagues [20] described the symptoms in their cohort as "cycloid psychosis." That is, a sudden onset of delusions and/ or hallucinations accompanied by depressive symptoms that resolve without residual dysfunction. Dykens and Cassidy [21] found that severe temper tantrums, impulsivity, and stubbornness were reported as significant problems in a high proportion of individuals with PWS. Ninety-seven percent had persistent skin-picking, and 71% had obsessive or compulsive-like symptoms. These findings were broadly replicated in an independent sample by Einfeld and colleagues [3].

Course and treatment of psychosis in PWS

Psychotic episodes begin in adolescence or early adulthood. Most studies describe the psychosis in PWS as having an intermittent relapsing course, with full recovery between episodes [19, 22, 23]. The best description of the psychosis in PWS may be an intermittent schizo-affective disorder. There have been no controlled studies of antipsychotic medications in individuals with PWS. In the authors' experience, psychotic symptoms have resolved rather quickly with small doses of antipsychotic medication. There are conflicting case reports regarding the efficacy of sodium valproate to manage the affective symptoms in PWS.

Influence of genetic subtype on psychosis in PWS

Does the genetic type of PWS determine the risk of developing psychosis? We summarized the findings in all studies [10, 11, 12, 13, 14, 23, 24] that have reported interpretable data. These studies have tended to show that UPD and imprinting defects are more likely to be associated with psychosis, but this finding has been inconsistent. In all the reported series taken together, there were 78 adults with PWS due to a deletion, of whom 11 had suffered a psychosis, 38 subjects with UPD of whom 26 had suffered psychosis, and 5 with imprinting defects of whom 4 had suffered psychosis. This means that the relative risk for psychosis for deletion: UPD: imprinting defect is approximately 1:5:6.

Why is psychotic illness more common in the uniparental disomy subtype of PWS?

What could account for the increased risk of psychosis when PWS is caused by UPD? The genetic defects causing PWS all feature loss of the paternal region by deletion, imprinting center defect, or UPD. The deletions take out specific defined regions of chromosome 15, the common large deletion (from bands q11–13), or the imprinting center microdeletions (exons within the SNRPN gene). On the other hand, UPD is of the whole chromosome 15 (only rarely has partial UPD been described in PWS [25]). Any hypothesis to explain a preponderance of PWS in patients with UPD must acknowledge that another gene(s) on chromosome 15 is maternally imprinted and when no paternal copy is present leads to deleterious effects on brain function.

For this purpose, putative genes could be within the critical 15(q11–13) region or outside this region. The genes within the region that encode a protein comprise SNRPN (controlling RNA splicing), SNURF (a ring finger protein that can bind DNA), the P gene (which codes for tyrosinase positive albinism), GABRA B3, A5, G3 (GABA receptor subunit genes), E6AP (UBE3A) (the Angelman Syndrome gene), Necdin (encodes a DNA binding protein), and Marko-rin 3 (also known as ZNF127, a zinc finger protein that is able to bind DNA). The role of most of these genes is to control expression. The GABA genes act in brain and are good candidates theoretically for brain dysfunction, but this is mostly evidenced by epilepsy, which is not associated with PWS and furthermore the GABA genes are not imprinted.

Of the many genes outside the critical region, none is currently known to be maternally imprinted, and none has been conclusively linked to psychosis. It has been a suggestion that a gene is associated with growth on chromosome 15 outside the q(11–13) region because patients with Angelman Syndrome due to UPD have enhanced growth compared to those with deletion; but here, the UPD is paternal. Another difficulty is that UPD may uncover the effect of an autosomal recessive gene, as found in a child with Bloom Syndrome (BS), and PWS, where the mother was a carrier of BS (localized to 15(q25–26)) [25].

The genetic component to the psychosis in PWS is unclear and why maternal UPD of 15(q11–13) should predispose to psychosis is unresolved. Recent studies suggest that epigenetic factors on chromosome 18 may play an etiopathological role in schizophrenia and bipolar affective disorders [26]. In PWS, maternal UPD may contribute to psychosis in patients predisposed to these disorders, due either to disomy for a given "deleterious" maternal gene or nullisomy for a "necessary" paternal gene [27]. Our current level of understanding of the link between psychosis and PWS is less advanced than for the velo-cardio-facial syndrome [28]. However, in that condition the effects are a consequence of a deletion. In PWS, genomic defects produce their consequences through abnormalities of imprinting, in which abnormalities of gene function may be less apparent.

Conclusion

PWS is associated with a much-increased rate of psychotic disorder, which presents as an intermittent schizo-affective disorder. When all reports of psychosis in PWS are considered, maternal uniparental disomy appears to increase the risk of psychosis by five to six times compared with the deletion form. The mechanism of such increased risk is as yet unknown. However, studies to investigate this are indicated not just for their relevance to PWS, but because of their potential to elucidate the pathogenesis of psychosis in general.

Acknowledgments

The Australian Child to Adult Development Study was supported by the National Health and Medical Research Council grant number 113844. Part of this work was carried out while Stewart Einfeld and Sophie Kavanagh were at the School of Psychiatry, University of New South Wales.

Thanks to Siân Horstead for editing assistance.

References

1. Prader A., Labhart A., Willi H. Ein Syndrom von Adipositas, Kleinwuchs, Kryptorchismum und Oligophrenie nach myatonieartigem Zustand im Neugeborenenalter. *Schweiz Med Wschr*, 1956. **86**:1260–1.

2. Greenswag L. R. Adults with Prader-Willi syndrome: a survey of 232 cases. *Dev Med Child Neurol*, 1987. **29**:145–52.

3. Einfeld S. L., Smith A., Durvasula S., *et al*. Behavior and emotional disturbance in Prader-Willi Syndrome. *Am J Med Genet A*, 1999. **82**:123–7.

4. Farber R. S., Kerrigan J. R. The multiple indications for growth hormone treatment of pediatric patients. *Pediatric Annals*, 2006. **35**:926–32.

5. Goldstone A. P. Prader-Willi syndrome: advances in genetics, pathophysiology and treatment. *Trends in Endocrinology & Metabolism*, 2004. **15**:12–20.

6. Swaab D. F. Prader-Willi syndrome and the hypothalamus. *Acta Paediatrica Supplement*, 1997. **423**:50–4.

7. Robinson W. P., Bottani A., Xie Y. G., *et al*. Molecular, cytogenetic, and clinical investigations of Prader-Willi syndrome patients. *Am J Hum Genet*, 1991. **49**:1219–34.

8. Nicholls R. D. New insights reveal complex mechanisms involved in genomic imprinting. *Am J Hum Genet*, 1994. **54**:733–40.

9. Smith A., Prasad M., Deng Z. M., *et al*. Comparison of high resolution cytogenetics, fluorescence in situ hybridisation, and DNA studies to validate the diagnosis of Prader-Willi and Angelman's Syndromes. *Arch Dis Child*, 1995. **72**:397–402.

10. Clarke D. Prader-Willi syndrome and psychotic symptoms: 2. A preliminary study of prevalence using the Psychopathology Assessment Schedule for Adults with Developmental Disability checklist. *J Intellect Disabil Res*, 1998. **42**:451–4.

11. Boer H., Holland A., Whittington J., *et al*. Psychotic illness in people with Prader Willi Syndrome due to Chromosome 15 maternal uniparental disomy. *Lancet*, 12 2002. **359**:135–6.

12. Beardsmore A., Dorman T., Cooper S-A., *et al*. Affective psychosis and Prader-Willi syndrome. *J Intellect Disabil Res*, 1998. **42**:463–71.

13. Descheemaeker M. J., Vogels A., Govers V., *et al*. Prader-Willi Syndrome: new insights in the behavioral and psychiatric spectrum. *J Intellect Disabil Res*, 2002. **46**:41–50.

14. Vogels A., Matthijs G., Legius E., *et al*. Chromosome 15 maternal uniparental disomy and psychosis in Prader-Willi Syndrome. *J Med Genet*, 2003. **40**(1):72–3.

15. Bray G. A., Dahms W. T., Swerdloff R. S., *et al*. The Prader-Willi syndrome: a study of 40 patients and a review of the literature. *Medicine*, 1982. **62**:59–80.

16. Whitman B. Y., Accardo P. Emotional symptoms in Prader-Willi Syndrome adolescents. *Am J Med Genet*, 1987. **28**:897–905.

17. Bartolucci G., Younger J. Tentative classification of neuropsychiatric disturbances in Prader-Willi syndrome. *J Intellect DisabiliRes*, 1994. **38**:621–9.

18. Einfeld S. L., Piccinin A. M., Mackinnon A., *et al*. Psychopathology in young people with intellectual disability. *JAMA*, 2006. **296**:1981–9.

19. Soni S., Whittington J., Holland A. J., *et al*. The course and outcome of psychiatric illness in people with Prader-Willi syndrome: implications for management and treatment. *J Intellect Disabili Res*, 2007. **51**:32–42.

20. Verhoeven W. M., Curfs L. M., Tuinier S. Prader-Willi syndrome and cycloid psychoses. *J Intellect Disabili Res*, 1998. **42**:455–62.

21. Dykens E. M., Cassidy S. B. Correlates of maladaptive behavior in children and adults with Prader-Willi syndrome. *Neuropsychiatric Genetics*, 1995. **60**:546–9.

22. Verhoeven W. M., Tuinier S. Prader-Willi syndrome: atypical psychoses and motor dysfunctions. *Int Rev Neurobiol*, 2006. **72**:119–30.

23. Clarke D. J., Boer H., Webb T., *et al*. Prader-Willi syndrome and psychotic symptoms: 1. Case descriptions and genetic studies. *J Intellect Disabili Res*, 1998. **42**:159–65.

24. Verhoeven W. M. A., Tuinier S., Curfs L. M. G. Prader-Willi syndrome: the psycho-pathological phenotype in uniparental disomy. *J Med Genet*, 2003. **40**(10):112e.

25. Woodage T., Prasad M., Dixon J. W., *et al*. Bloom syndrome and maternal uniparental disomy for chromosome 15. *Am J Hum Genet*, 1994. **55**(1):74–80.

26. Petronis A. The genes for major psychosis: aberrant sequence or regulation? *Neuropsycho-pharmacology*, 2000. **23**:1–12.

27. Smith A. Why is there no diploid overdose effect in Prader-Willi syndrome due to uniparental disomy? *Acta Geneticae Medicae et Gemellologiae*, 1996. **45**:179–89.

28. Einfeld S. L. Behaviour phenotypes of genetic disorders. *Curr Opin Psychiatry*, 2004. **17**:343–8.

26 Friedreich's Ataxia and schizophrenia-like psychosis

Perminder S. Sachdev

Facts box

- Friedreich's Ataxia (FRDA) is an autosomal recessive neurodegenerative disorder that is the most common cause of inherited ataxia. It is caused by triplet GAA expansion on chromosome 9q13.

- It is characterized by onset at the age 5–25 years, with neurological features (progressive gait and limb ataxia; dysarthria; areflexia, loss of vibration, and proprioceptive sense; abnormal eye movements; pyramidal weakness of feet and cognitive dysfunction); cardiomyopathy; diabetes; scoliosis; and pes cavus.

- It is associated with cognitive dysfunction and intellectual impairment in a minority, personality disturbance, and depression.

- Cases of schizophrenia-like psychosis with paranoid delusions and hallucinations have been reported that respond to antipsychotic drugs. The reports are too few to determine prevalence or establish a specific relationship between FRDA and schizophrenia.

FRDA is an autosomal recessive neurodegenerative disorder that is the most common cause of inherited ataxia. Nicholaus Friedreich first described it in a series of papers in 1863–1877 [1], but it is only recently, since the discovery of the underlying genetic abnormality, that its full spectrum is becoming clear. Its symptoms relate to the central nervous system, heart, and pancreas. Its prevalence is estimated at about 1 in 50,000 individuals in European populations [2].

Clinical features

Age of onset

The typical onset is in the first two decades of life. The Quebec Cooperative Study criteria [3] suggested that the onset must be before age 20 years. The Harding [2] criteria extended the upper limit to 25 years. In the large Dürr and colleagues [4] series, the mean age of onset was 15.5 ± 8 years, with 19/140 (13.6%) having an age of onset after 25 years, which is generally regarded as late-onset. The number of repeats on the abnormal gene relates to the age of onset (discussed later), and late onset is associated with an atypical presentation. The discovery of the FRDA gene has extended the range of ages of onset from 2 to 51 years [4].

Signs and symptoms

Neurological features

FRDA primarily involves the ascending and descending tracts of the spinal cord, in particular the spinocerebellar tracts, the pyramidal tracts, and posterior columns. This, combined with involvement of the cerebellum, peripheral nerves, dorsal roots of the spinal cord and the tracts and nuclei of the lower brain stem (including the optic nerve), explains the diverse neurological features. The frequency of the clinical features in two series is summarized in Table 26.1.

In almost all cases, the initial symptom is gait ataxia, although in a few cases, scoliosis may be present before ataxia becomes manifest. Ataxia was present in all patients in the Dürr and colleagues [4] series. This may appear as clumsiness in the early stages, but the ataxia gradually worsens, with the development of a broad-based and lurching gait, and spreads to the arms, leading to action tremor. Cervical involvement leads to titubation and, in the

Table 26.1 Signs and symptoms of FRDA: data from two large studies. Patients in the Dürr *et al.* study were all homozygous for GAA expansion.

Clinical Feature	Dürr *et al.*, 1996 (n = 140) %	Harding, 1981 (n = 115) %
Age (mean ±SD) year	31 ± 13	–
Age of onset (mean ±SD)	15.5 ± 8	10.5
Neurological Feature		
Gait ataxia	100	–
Limb ataxia	99	99
Lower limb areflexia	87	99
knee jerk present	12	0.9
Loss of vibration sense	78	73
Extensor plantar response	79	89
Dysarthria	91	97
Horizontal nystagmus	40	20
Muscle weakness in lower limbs	67	88
Muscle wasting		
lower limbs	39	39
upper limbs	25	49
Saccadic pursuit eye movement	30	12
Sphincter disturbance	23	–
Swallowing difficulty	27	–
Reduced visual activity	13	18
Hearing loss	13	8
Axonal neuropathy	98 (n = 63)	96
Abnormal brain-stem ERPs	61 (n = 29)	–
Abnormal visual ERPs	34 (n = 34)	–
Musculoskeletal		
Scoliosis	60	79
Pes Cavus	55	55
Other Features		
Cardiomyopathy	63 (on ECG)	–
Diabetes or abnormal glucose tolerance	32	10
Facial dysmorphia	3.6	
Seizures	1.4	
Dystonia	1.4	
Myoclonus	3.6	
Postural Tremor	1.4	
Mental Retardation	3.6	

* Adapted from Dürr *et al.* (1996).

later stages, truncal involvement may make even sitting difficult.

With time, weakness and wasting develop in the muscles of the feet, lower legs, and hands, resulting in deformities. Loss of reflexes in the lower limbs is common, with knee jerks being present in only 1% [2] and 12% [4] of cases in two series. There is gradual loss of sensation, vibration, and position sense in the extremities. The plantar response is up-going, suggesting pyramidal tract involvement. The Romberg sign is usually positive. Dysarthria is common and horizontal nystagmus may be present, consistent with cerebellar and spinocerebellar involvement. Sphincter disturbance and swallowing difficulties are absent until late in the disease. Decreased visual acuity and hearing loss are also late features.

Kyphoscoliosis and pes cavus may be early signs and are common. Other deformities include flexion of the toes, hammertoes, or foot inversion.

Other features

Cardiac involvement was evident on electrocardiography in 67% in the Dürr and colleagues [4] series. This includes cardiomyopathy of the hypertrophic nonobstructive type, myocardial fibrosis, and cardiac failure. Patients develop symptoms such as chest pain, shortness of breath, and heart palpitations. About 30% develop impaired glucose tolerance and 10% diabetes mellitus. Less common features are facial dysmorphia, seizures, dystonic postures, myoclonus, and postural tremor that may not have a causal link with the genetic abnormality.

Psychiatric features

These have been variably reported. Although Friedreich [1] did not report intellectual impairment in his cases, early reports noted the presence of intellectual impairment in about a quarter of cases in one series [5] and 15% in another [6], which varied in degree from mild to severe. This high prevalence was not supported by Davies [7], who did not find an excess of mental retardation in FDRA, although some patients showed impairments in recent memory, attention, and concentration. Davies concluded that these patients had mild but significant cognitive deficits that set in early but were nonprogressive. Dürr and colleagues [4] reached a somewhat similar conclusion that mental retardation was uncommon (5/140 = 3.6% in their series) and probably not a feature of the disease.

Personality abnormalities have also been reported, but the specificity of these is doubted. Irritability, antisociality, episodes of mute or resentful behavior, denial of illness, and excessive preoccupation with religion or mysticism have all been reported [7, 8]. The relative contribution of neurologic deficits and environmental factors in this is unclear. The presence of psychosis is discussed later.

Late-onset FRDA

This is defined as onset after 25 years, and the disease in these cases is milder overall. Gait and limb ataxia are present in all cases; dysarthria, loss of posterior column sensations, and abnormal eye movements are also common [4, 9]. These patients are more likely to have lower limb spasticity and retained reflexes. Cardiomyopathy is usually absent [9].

Laboratory investigations

Electrocardiography shows features of cardiomyopathy, with T-wave inversion, hypertrophy of the interventricular septum and the left ventricular wall, and heart rhythm abnormalities, such as tachycardia and heart block. Axonal neuropathy of predominantly sensory type is evident on nerve conduction studies in many patients. There is often abnormal central motor conduction velocity. Visual and brain-stem auditory evoked potentials may be abnormal. Glucose tolerance is impaired in a proportion of cases (Table 26.1). MRI shows that atrophy of the cervical cord, atrophy of the cerebellum, in particular the vermis, is not uncommon [9, 10, 11]. Mild generalized cerebral atrophy may be seen in some cases [12]. Genetic testing is diagnostic of the disease (discussed later).

Course of illness

In most cases, the disease is slowly progressive, with the person being confined to a wheelchair in 10–15 years (range 1–25 years) after onset. There are individual variations, however, and cases occur with long stationary periods or very slow progression. Death often occurs within 20 years of onset, often from heart disease, but some sufferers live into their 60s and 70s.

Genetic abnormality

FDRA is an autosomal recessive disorder with a genetic defect mapped to chromosome 9 in the region

now known to code for the protein *frataxin*. The causative mutation is an unstable expansion of a GAA repeat in the first intron [13]. The vast majority of sufferers are homozygous for the GAA repeat, but compound heterozygotes have been described [13]. The number of expansions varies considerably, within patients as well as families. In the Dürr and colleagues [4] study, the number of repeats varied from 120 to 1,700. The size of the expansion correlated with the age of onset and rate of progression of the disease [4], with smaller expansions leading to later onset (>25 years) and slower progression, often with atypical features such as retained tendon reflexes or hyperreflexia.

GAA expansion leads to the formation of a "sticky" triplex DNA structure causing reduced levels of frataxin, a protein that localizes in mitochondrial membranes and crests [14]. Studies in yeast as well as animal models have shown that this low frataxin levels lead to intramitochondrial iron accumulation and impaired mitochondrial oxidative phosphorylation, contributing to increased oxidative stress and cellular damage [15]. However, the precise function of frataxin remains unknown.

Psychosis in FRDA

A number of case reports of psychosis in FRDA have appeared in the literature, but the anecdotes are too few to come to any firm opinion on a specific relationship between the two. One of the earliest case reports was by Davies in 1949 [8], who reported the case of a 15-year-old boy who developed motor symptoms at the age of 13 years and became irritable, aggressive toward his parents, developed persecutory ideas and visual hallucinations, and had episodes of rage. His EEG showed abnormality over the right temporo-occipital region. Davison and Bagley [16] reviewed the evidence for a "Friedreich's psychosis" in 1969 and concluded few cases existed and the etiology was possibly heterogeneous, thereby not supporting a special relationship. Sporadic reports have continued to appear. Salbenblatt and colleagues [17] reported a 36-year-old man who had a gradual onset of persecutory delusions and auditory and visual hallucinations in the later stages of his illness. He died 6 weeks after the initiation of antipsychotic medication. A more recent report in a 37-year-old female emphasized delusions of reference as the major symptoms of psychosis [18]. Such reports are insufficient to extrapolate from FRDA to the

pathogenesis of schizophrenia, although some specu-
lation in this regard has been published [19].

Treatment

The treatment of FRDA has until recently been mainly
symptomatic. Considering the likely role of oxidative stress in the pathogenesis, antioxidants have been
tried. A four-year open study of a combination of coenzyme Q_{10} and vitamin E reported improvement in
cardiac function and stabilization or slowed decline
in neurological symptoms [20]. A synthetic analogue
of coenzyme Q_{10} has been shown to show reduction in cardiac hypertrophy but was not found to
help neurological symptoms of the disease [21, 22].
A novel approach suggested recently is to use a histone deacetylase inhibitor to restore the transcriptional activity of the silenced frataxin gene [23],
but clinical studies for these drugs have not been
performed.

The presence of psychosis usually warrants the
use of an antipsychotic drug. The likelihood of motor
symptoms in FRA would support the use of atypical
in preference to classical antipsychotic drugs. Reports
of the successful use of risperidone 2 mg/day [17] and
aripiprazole 10 mg/day [18] attest to the benefit of
these drugs in controlling psychotic symptoms. Long-
term use of these drugs has not been reported in the
literature.

Other autosomal recessive cerebellar ataxias

FRDA is one of a group of hereditary ataxias recently
reviewed by Fogel and Perlman [24] that are autosomal
recessive and involve spinocebellar degeneration. The
clinical features include cerebellar syndeoms, sensorimotor neuropathy, eye signs, movement abnormalities, seizures, skeletal abnormalities, and skin disorders. Cognitive impairment is an important feature in
some of the early onset disorders such as ataxia telang-
iectasia, ataxia with oculomotor apraxia, infantile-
onset spinocerebellar ataxia, Marinesco-Sjogren's Syndrome, and so on. Psychosis has been reported in some
of these syndromes, in particular, late-onset Tay-Sachs
Disease, cerebrotendinous xanthomatosis, and mitochondrial recessive ataxia, which are discussed elsewhere in this book.

References

1. Friedreich N. Über degenerative Atrophie der spinalen Hinterstränge. *Virchows Arch Path Anat*, 1863. **26**:391–419.

2. Harding A. E. Friedreich's ataxia: a clinical and genetic study of 90 families with an analysis of early diagnostic criteria and intrafamilial clustering of clinical features. *Brain*, 1981. **104**:589–620.

3. Geoffroy G., Barbeau A., Breton G., *et al.* Clinical description and roentgenologic evaluation of patients with Friedreich ataxia. *Can J Neurol Sci*, 1976. **3**:279–86.

4. Dürr A., Cossee M., Agid Y., *et al.* Clinical and genetic abnormalities in patients with Friedreich's ataxia. *N Engl J Med*, 1996. **335**:1169–75.

5. Bell J., Carmichael E. A. On hereditary ataxia and spastic paraplegia. *The Treasury of Human Inheritance*, 1939. **4**:141–281.

6. Sjogren T. Klinische und erbbiologische Untersuchungen über die Heredoataxien. *Acta Psychiatrica et Neurologica*, 1943. **27** (Suppl):1–200.

7. Davies D. L. The intelligence of patients with Friedreich's ataxia. *J Neurol Neurosurg Psychiatr*, 1949. **12**:34–8.

8. Davies D. L. Psychiatric changes associated with Friedreich's ataxia. *J Neurol Neurosurg Psychiatr*, 1949. **12**:246–50.

9. Bhidayasiri R. , Perlman S. L., Pulst S.-M., *et al.* Late-onset Friedreich Ataxia: phenotypic analysis, magnetic resonance imaging findings, and review of the literature. *Arch Neurol*, 2005. **62**:1865–9.

10. Wullner U., Klockgether T., Petersen D., *et al.* Magnetic resonance imaging in hereditary and idiopathic ataxia. *Neurology*, 1993. **43**:318–25.

11. De Michele G., Disalle F., Filla A., *et al.* Magnetic resonance imaging in typical and late-onset Friedreich's disease and early onset cerebellar ataxia with retained tendon reflexes. *Ital J Neurol Sci*, 1995. **16**:303–8.

12. Junck L., Gilman S., Gebarski S. S., *et al.* Structural and functional brain imaging in Friedreich's ataxia. *Arch Neurol*, 1994. **51**:349–55.

13. Campuzano V., Montermini L., Molto M. D., *et al.* Friedreich's ataxia: autosomal recessive disease caused by an intronic GAA triplet repeat expansion. *Science*, 1996. **271**:1423–7.

14. Babcock M., DeSilva D., Oaks R., *et al.* Regulation of mitochondrial iron accumulation by Yfh1p, a putative homolog of frataxin. *Science*, 1997. **276**:1709–12.

15. Koutnikova H., Campuzano V., Foury F., *et al.* Studies of human, mouse and yeast homologoues indicate a mitochondrial function for frataxin. *Nat Genet*, 1997. **16**:345–51.

16. Davison K., Bagley C. R. (1969). Schizophrenia-like psychoses associated with organic disorders of the nervous system: a review of the literature. In *Current problems in neuropsychiatry*, Herrington R. N. (Ed.). *British Journal of Psychiatry Special Publication No 4*. Ashford, Kent: Headley Brothers.

17. Salbenblatt M. J., Buzan R. D., Dubovsky S. L. Risperidone treatment for psychosis in end-stage Friedreich's ataxia. *Am J Psychiatry*, 2000. **157**:303.

18. Chan Y.-C. Aripiprazole treatment for psychosis associated with Freidreich's ataxia. *Gen Hosp Psychiatry*, 2005. **27**:372–8.

19. Fischer K. M. Expanded (CAG)$_n$, (CGG)n and (GAA)n trinucleotide repeat microsatellite, and mutant purine synthesis and pigmentation genes cause schizophrenia and autism. *Med Hypoth*, 1998. **51**:223–33.

20. Hart P. E., Lodi R., Rajagopalan B., *et al.* Antioxidant treatment of patients with Friedreich ataxia. *Arch Neurol*, 2005. **62**:621–6.

21. Buyse G., Mertens L., Di Salvo G., *et al.* Idebenone treatment in Friedreich's ataxia: neurological, cardiac, and biochemical monitoring. *Neurology*, 2003. **60**:1679–81.

22. Mariotti C., Solari A., Torta D., *et al.* Idebenone treatment in Friedreich patients: one-year-long randomized placebo-controlled trial. *Neurology*, 2003. **60**:1676–9.

23. Herman D., Jenssen K., Burnett R., *et al.* Histone deacetylase inhibitors reverse gene silencing in Friedreich's ataxia. *Nat Chem Biol*, 2006 Oct. 2. **10**:551–8.

24. Fogel B. L., Perlman S. Clinical features and molecular genetics of autosomal cerebellar ataxias. *Lancet neurol*, 2007. **6**:245–57.

27

Wilson's Disease

Edward C. Lauterbach and Leslie Lester-Burns

Facts box

- Wilson's Disease (WD) is an autosomal recessive disorder involving multiple mutations of the gene ATP7B on chromosome 13q14.3, a gene critical to hepatic copper excretion.
- It leads to copper deposition primarily in the liver and the basal ganglia lenticular nucleus (putamen and globus pallidus), leading to the alternative name of *hepatolenticular degeneration*.
- Reported prevalence rates of psychosis are quite variable, from 2%–11%.
- Beyond the typical positive symptoms of hallucinations, delusions, and thought disorders, a wide diversity of psychiatric features are observed, including silliness, euphoria, sexual preoccupation, hebephrenia, catatonia, occasional hallucinations, "hysterical" behavior, and "narrowing of mental horizons."
- Cognitive disorders occur in somewhat less than 25% of patients.
- At times, psychotic features emerge within several months after commencing anticopper therapy due to rapid copper mobilization, but persistent treatment usually leads to remission.
- For treatment of psychosis, conventional psychopharmacological approaches should be applied with special consideration of the effects of copper deposition on the brain, liver, kidney, heart, and bone marrow.
- The risk of extrapyramidal side effects, including neuroleptic malignant syndrome, is higher.
- ECT should only be administered with extreme caution in WD, given the capacity for prolonged seizures and the dearth of studies reporting safety and efficacy.
- The pathophysiology of psychosis in WD is poorly understood.

Introduction

Wilson's Disease (WD) is an autosomal recessive disorder involving multiple mutations of the gene ATP7B on chromosome 13q14.3, a gene critical to hepatic copper excretion [1]. WD therefore results in an accumulation and deposition of copper throughout the body, including the liver, brain, musculoskeletal system, heart, kidneys, endocrine system, red blood cells, skin, and other tissues. Wilson [2] was the first to link liver cirrhosis with basal ganglia movement disorders in this illness. Copper deposition occurs primarily in the liver and the basal ganglia lenticular nucleus (putamen and globus pallidus), leading to the alternative name for WD, *hepatolenticular degeneration*. Widespread copper deposition can produce a variety of psychiatric and medical manifestions of WD [3] but, with early detection, WD responds well to currently available decoppering agents.

In this chapter, we first consider WD in general, including its epidemiology, presentation, prognosis, genetics, pathogenetic mechanisms, neuropathology, diagnosis, neuroradiology, clinical features, and treatment. We then consider psychosis arising in the context of WD, other psychiatric features that are associated with primary schizophrenia, and important clinical issues that must be considered in treating the psychosis of WD. Finally, we conclude with pathophysiological considerations and directions for future research in WD psychoses.

General considerations

The prevalence of WD approximates 1 case per 30,000 [4]. About one-third of patients with WD present with each of the three primary disease presentations: hepatic (hepatic WD), neurological (neurological WD), and psychiatric (psychiatric WD). Severe mutations result in childhood and adolescent onset of hepatic WD, whereas less severe mutations usually result in onset in the second through fourth decade of life with neurological or psychiatric presentations. The prognosis depends upon the clinical manifestations present at the time treatment is begun. Without treatment, patients may die within 6 months to 5 years of WD onset. With treatment, however, patients can live fairly normal lives. Thus, early recognition and treatment are critical in WD.

The gene (ATP7B) is located on chromosome 13q14 band 14.1–21.1 [5]. The gene product appears to be a copper-containing P-type ATPase. Copper is incorporated into apoceruloplasmin by this ATP7B P-type ATPase localized in the trans-Golgi network [6]. Normally, apoceruloplasmin binds copper to form holoceruloplasmin, which is then packaged in vesicles and excreted into the biliary system, but apoceruloplasmin in WD fails to bind copper [6]. Holoceruloplasmin is therefore lacking in the biliary system [7], reflecting impaired copper transport from the hepatocyte to the biliary system. ATP7B mutations produce an abnormal interaction between the ATPase and copper chaperone proteins such as Atox1, preventing copper incorporation into apoceruloplasmin to form holocerulosplasmin [8], impairing hepatobiliary copper excretion. Biliary excretion normally accounts for 10% of copper loss each day [9], and impaired biliary excretion soon leads to copper accumulation. More than 200 mutations of the WD gene are known [4], some associated with ethnicity, severity, age of onset, or presentation [5, 10]. Highly dysfunctional mutations lead to early-onset severe hepatic WD, whereas milder mutations lead to late-onset neurological WD [11]. A cytosine-adenine transversion may be responsible for 30% of North American WD cases [12]. Animal models include the Bedlington terrier, Long Evans Cinnamon rat, toxic milk mouse, and the murine ATP7B gene deletion model [4].

Pathophysiology and pathology

The physiological importance of copper is critical. Copper is integral to cytochrome c oxidase in the mitochondrial electron transport chain, catecholamine metabolism (tyrosine metabolism, dopamine beta-hydroxylase, and monoamine oxidase), melanin formation, collagen and elastin cross-linkage, and free radical deactivation (superoxide dismutase). Excessive copper accumulation can lead to cellular demise through a number of potential mechanisms. These include free radical-induced cellular oxidation, inhibited protein synthesis, poisoning of enzymes (in mitochondria, cytosol, and cell membrane), intracellular failure (of mitochondria, peroxisomes, microtubules, plasma membranes, enzymes, and DNA cross-linking), and induction of cellular injury, inflammation, and cell death due to unbound ionic copper [9, 10]. Mitochondrial copper accumulation can also produce premature oxidative aging and mitochondrial DNA mutations, further impairing cell function [13]. A thorough review of normal copper metabolism can be found elsewhere [9]. Copper overload in WD induces CD95 (APO-1/Fas)-mediated apoptosis [14], and both increased degradation and functional inactivity of the X-linked inhibitor of apoptosis, XIAP, reducing its ability to inhibit caspase-3 [15].

Brain pathology can include widespread copper deposition, gliosis, and astrocytic proliferation, especially in grey matter. Spongy necrosis, demyelination, and denervation may be evident in frontal, parietal, and occipital cortical areas. Macroscopically, ventricular dilatation, lenticular atrophy, yellowish or reddish brown discoloration, softening, and spongy degeneration are seen. Cavitation is especially apparent in rapidly progressive juvenile dystonic forms of WD, whereas atrophy is more common in more slowly progressive adult forms. The pathology of hepatic encephalopathy is similar to WD pathology and is occasionally superimposed [16]. Liver failure can increase pallidal manganese concentrations.

Diagnosis and clinical features

Clinical suspicion is imperative in diagnosing WD. Initial presentation with hepatic, neurological, or psychiatric symptoms, particularly when accompanied by a family history of WD or the presence of Kayser-Fleischer rings (KFRs) on slit lamp exam, warrants a diagnostic workup to exclude WD. KFRs result from corneal-copper deposition, but they may often be absent in WD associated with psychiatric manifestations [17]. WD is diagnosed by determining low blood ceruloplasmin (< 20 mg/dl) and high 24-hour urinary copper levels (> 50 µg/dl) and is confirmed by elevated copper levels on liver biopsy (> 150 µg/g) [3]. In cases involving ambiguous results, the presence of KFRs and low serum copper can add diagnostic confidence.

Putaminal increased signal on MRI T2 images is supportive of the diagnosis, although increased signal is also often seen in the pons [18, 19] and sometimes in the thalamus, globus pallidus, caudate, cerebellum, subcortical white matter, and midbrain. T1 signal is often reduced in affected structures, but can be increased in the globus pallidus in liver disease with portocaval shunting [20]. Common CT findings are ventricular dilatation, basal ganglia hyperdensities, and atrophy of the cerebral cortex, brainstem, or cerebellum. Basal ganglia MRI hypointensity and CT hypodensity are consistent with cavitation in more aggressive WD. On positron emission tomography (PET), glucose metabolism may be reduced in the cerebellum and striatum, as well as cortical and thalamic regions [21]. Neurological severity correlates with reduced striatal glucose metabolism [22] and dopamine D2 receptor binding on SPECT imaging [22, 23].

Initial neurological signs are subtle and include mild tremor, speech difficulties, or micrographia. In a study of 19 patients with a duration of WD of at least a decade, 17 (89%) had basal ganglia signs, whereas 2 (11%) had oculomotor or cerebellar signs [24]. In a Chinese study of 71 patients with WD hospitalized over an 11-year period, 52 patients (73.2%) had neurologic symptoms at the time of diagnosis, including tremors (66.2%), dysarthria (56.3%), gait disturbances (46.5%), generalized or multifocal dystonia (42.3%), decreased facial expression (40.8%), and rigidity (33.8%) [25]. Akinetic-rigid syndrome was seen in nine patients. Personality changes (38%) were not uncommon. Other less-frequent presentations were increased deep-tendon reflexes (23.9%), epileptic seizures (5.6%), and hypokalemic periodic paralysis (1.4%); tremor was mainly kinetic and postural and 32 (45%) of the 71 patients had the classic wing beating tremor [25]. As neurological features progress, however, common findings in order of decreasing frequency include dysdiadochokinesia, dysarthria, bradykinesia, postural tremor, parkinsonism, hyperkinesia, and ataxia [26]. Although relatively rare in adults [26], dystonia and chorea are particularly common in children [24]. Seizures occur in a minority of patients, often remitting with WD treatment. Patients with neurological WD can die within 6 months if treatment is not initiated. Without treatment, patients with WD progress to become dysarthric, bedridden, and unable to function.

Psychiatric symptoms occur in isolation in approximately 20%, are the predominant presenting manifestation in 33%, and are present at initial presentation in 67% [2, 27, 28, 29]. The predominant psychiatric features evident across the WD literature include personality changes, cognitive disturbances, and mood disorders [3, 30, 31]. Half of patients undergo psychiatric hospitalization before WD is first diagnosed [32, 33]. Tragically, the diagnosis of WD is often missed [34, 35]. Psychiatrists are not alone in missing the diagnosis. A retrospective Chinese study of 1,011 cases of WD found that 516 cases had been originally misdiagnosed as more than 100 different systemic diseases as well as primary psychosis [36].

Treatment

A full explication of treatment is beyond the scope of this chapter and is elaborated elsewhere [3]. Gene therapies are currently under development [37, 38]. Treatment considerations include selection of anticopper therapies and the treatment of specific manifestations [3, 8, 39]. Early recognition and treatment of WD are imperative because improvement with treatment is limited to the first 5 years of symptomatic illness and the first 2 years of treatment [27, 40]. Copper-chelating agents (penicillamine and trientine) increase urinary copper excretion. Trientine is also known as triethylene tetramine dihydrochloride. Copper-depleting agents (zinc and tetrathiomolybdate) reduce copper absorption and induce copper sequestration into a hepatic nontoxic pool. Consideration must be given to the various indications, dosing, side effects, and other factors in administering these agents, discussed elsewhere [3, 8, 39]. Copper chelators have been recommended for hepatic WD, whereas copper depletors have been recommended for neurological WD [3, 8, 39]. Improvement with anticopper agents often occurs only after 6 months of treatment. Exacerbations of neurological and psychiatric symptoms sometimes occur during the first several months of therapy due to rapid copper mobilization. A variety of treatment techniques have been advocated in the context of such exacerbations [3, 35, 41, 42], but the basic concept is to switch to a less aggressive agent. Liver transplantation is curative and has its own special indications [3, 10, 16, 43]. Patient survival after transplant exceeds 80% [3, 44]. Plasma exchange and peritoneal dialysis have been used in fulminant WD and WD hemolytic anemia, but are rarely necessary.

Good results have been reported with tetra-thiomolybdate in patients with psychiatric WD [45]. Incongruous behavior and cognitive impairment have been found to improve more than irritability and depression after WD treatment [40]. Other conditions reported to improve with WD treatment include amnestic disorder, dementia, hypersexuality, aggression, hyperactivity, and disinhibition. Psychiatric symptoms may resolve more often in patients lacking dysarthria, incongruous behavior, and hepatic symptoms.

Against this backdrop of understanding WD in general, we first consider psychosis within the context of WD, then review other WD psychiatric features that have been documented in schizophrenia, and finally discuss critical issues in treating WD psychosis.

Psychosis in Wilson's Disease

Psychotic features

Wilson reported two cases of psychosis (cases 2 and 3) in his original paper, including auditory hallucinations, control delusions of made action, and delusions of reference [2]. Psychotic features can be the presenting sign of WD, hence, the clinical admonition to exclude WD in first-onset psychosis. Psychotic features appear to be more prevalent in neurological WD than in hepatic WD [28, 31, 32, 35]. Although an increased prevalence of psychosis in WD is the subject of debate, clinical evidence suggests WD as an etiology of psychotic manifestations.

Although early studies suggested an association of psychosis and WD related to basal ganglia pathology [46], Beard maintained that coincidental primary schizophrenia and improper diagnosis of schizophrenia in cases that later manifested dementia fully accounted for psychosis in WD [47]. Davison and Bagley pointed out, however, that subsequent development of dementia by no means invalidated the initial diagnosis of schizophrenia but rather strengthened the supposition that the original psychosis was attributable to underlying WD pathology [48].

Prevalence studies have produced mixed findings. Davison and Bagley found 8 (1.5%) "acceptable" cases and 11 (2.1%) questionable cases of schizophrenia among 520 reported WD cases, exceeding the accepted

normative prevalence of 0.2%–0.5% based on contemporary nosology [48], but reporting biases are possible. Dening and Berrios retrospectively studied a series of 195 WD patients undergoing an initial neurological hospital admission. Two raters reviewed charts. Definite delusions occurred in two (1%), possible delusions in one (0.5%), definite hallucinations in one (0.5%), and possible hallucinations in one (0.5%), and the prevalence of schizophreniform psychosis was not increased above normative rates [28].

Other studies, however, suggest higher prevalences. In a series of 34 consecutive patients with confirmed diagnoses of WD, one patient (2.9%) had been previously diagnosed with schizophrenia [33]. In a Chinese study of 71 patients with WD (45 male and 26 female) hospitalized over an 11-year period, 8 (11.3%) were found to have hallucinations [25]. In patients with neurological WD, psychosis and catatonia each occurred in 8% of the patients [35].

Longitudinal studies also observe higher prevalences. In a retrospective longitudinal case history review of 24 WD patients presenting with psychiatric symptoms at the time of WD diagnosis, psychosis was present in 2 patients (8.3%), including 1 with catatonia [32]. Oder and colleagues prospectively studied 45 patients with WD (27 had neurological features), finding prominent delusions in 3 patients (6.7%) [26], whereas the expected combined age-adjusted life prevalence of schizophrenia and schizophreniform disorder together would be ≤ 2.0% [49].

Prevalence studies to date suffer from inconsistent selection factors, referral biases, reporting biases, are often of limited sample size, and are usually retrospective in nature. Case reports, however, reveal antipsychotic-refractory [50, 52, 54, 56], anticopper therapy-responsive [26, 41, 50, 51, 52, 53, 54] psychoses that develop in parallel with the evolution of WD neurological features [50, 51, 54, 56], suggesting that WD can induce schizophreniform psychoses.

A number of case reports indicate that the psychosis of WD is frequently misdiagnosed as schizophrenia or some other primary psychosis despite the presence of WD neurological features [50, 51, 54]. Sometimes these neurological features have been misinterpreted as antipsychotic side effects [51].

Presenting psychotic features have included auditory [54, 55] and visual [56] hallucinations, delusions [52, 54, 55], paranoia [53], incoherence [52], inappropriate and derailing speech [55], neologisms [55], catatonia [54, 56], disinhibited [55] and disorganized [56] behavior, suicide attempts [55], mannerisms [52], social withdrawal [53], and dysphoria [53]. Delusions have involved nihilistic [54], persecutory [54, 55], and somatic [55] themes. Depressive [53, 54, 56] and anxiety [53] symptoms have sometimes attended these psychoses. At times, psychotic features emerge within several months after commencing anticopper therapy due to rapid copper mobilization, but persistent treatment usually leads to remission (see the section on treating psychosis in WD, discussed later).

Associated neurological features in WD psychosis have included parkinsonism [50, 54, 56], dysarthric speech [51], gait disorders [50], and upper motor neuron signs (Babinski, hypertonia, hyperreflexia) [56]. Radiological correlates of WD psychosis have included bilateral putaminal cavitation with delusions [51] and T1 and T2 hyperintensities in the putamen, caudate, and pallidum with delusions and auditory and visual hallucinations [56].

Other features of schizophrenia observed in Wilson's Disease

Beyond the typical positive symptoms of hallucinations, delusions, and thought disorders, a wide diversity of psychiatric features are observed in schizophrenia, and many of these are evident in WD. Wilson observed prominent psychiatric symptoms in his patients, including silliness, euphoria, sexual preoccupation, hebephrenia, catatonia, occasional hallucinations, "hysterical" behavior, and "narrowing of mental horizons." He concluded that "facility, docility, childishness, and emotional overaction form the chief features of the more chronic cases" [2]. Other studies indicate that personality disturbances, irritability, depression, and academic or employment failure are common psychiatric manifestations [27, 40].

Personality changes are the most common psychiatric disorders in WD, occur in about half of patients [30, 34], and include mainly irritability and aggression, but also apathy, disinhibition, and impulsivity, [2, 30], sometimes leading to marital disruption and criminality [32], and tend to be associated with neurological or hepatic features [33]. In a series of 34 consecutive patients with confirmed diagnoses of WD, irritability correlated with the presence of neurological or hepatic features of WD and was less apparent among asymptomatic WD patients [33]. Irritability, incongruous behavior, and personality disturbances have been associated with brainstem signs and dystonia but not tremor [28]. Personality syndromes also correlate with dyskinesia, dysarthria, and putaminal and pallidal lesions [58]. Psychopathic features are associated with dysarthria [59]. Incongruous, disinhibited, aggressive, hyperactive, and hypersexual behaviors, but not irritability, have improved with treatment of the underlying WD [27, 40].

Cognitive disorders occur in somewhat less than 25% of WD patients and cognitive impairments, memory, and IQ can improve after WD is treated [27, 30]. WAIS-R IQ score impairments have been associated with neurological and hepatic features [33]. Attentional deficits are associated with dropping out of school and loss of employment [27]. Diminished functional capacity correlates with ataxia, tremor, and focal thalamic lesions [58].

Mania, manic features including hypersexuality, hyperactivity, and aggression, emotional lability, pathological laughing and crying, depression, anxiety, and substance abuse [27, 40] can develop in WD. Mania has been observed, as have isolated manic behaviors, including hypersexuality, hyperactivity, and aggression [27, 40]. Major depression occurs in at least 30% of patients with WD, and may affect nearly all patients at some point in the illness [3, 26, 28, 32, 59]. Depression has correlated with cognitive impairment, parkinsonian rigidity, bradykinesia, gait disorders, and dilatation of the third ventricle [3, 58, 59]. Suicidal behavior has been documented in as many as 16% of patients across studies [26, 27, 30], with the risk potentially compounded by disinhibited and impulsive personality changes. Isolated manic symptoms and some cases of depression improve with anticopper treatment.

Treating psychosis in Wilson's Disease

In using psychotropics to treat psychoses arising in WD, it is important to determine the origin of the psychotic features. For example, psychotic features may arise from primary psychiatric disorders coexisting with WD, from WD itself, from WD treatment, or from secondary complications of WD such as delirium, dementia, bipolar disorder, depression, seizures (ictal or interictal psychoses), and so on. There is some evidence that the benzodiazepine antagonist flumazenil may have utility in the delirium of hepatic encephalopathy [60].

As in other neuropsychiatric illnesses, medicines should be started at low doses and gradually titrated upward to avoid evoking serious side effects. Controlled studies of psychotropic treatment in psychiatric WD have not been reported.

The clinician must also stay alert for atypical presentations and atypical responses in WD. Neuroleptic-refractory psychosis responding to lithium [61] and nortriptyline-refractory depression responding to levodopa [62] have been reported in lenticular disease. Otherwise, conventional psychopharmacological approaches should be applied with special consideration of the effects of copper deposition on the brain, liver, kidney, heart, and bone marrow.

Basal ganglia cuprification may lead to a heightened susceptibility to psychotropic-induced dystonia and other movement disorders [63]. Neuroleptic malignant syndrome, parkinsonism, and severe extrapyramidal reactions [16] are more likely in WD, and atypical antipsychotics may be safer in this regard [53]. Cortical actions of atypical antipsychotics may still be viable even when subcortical dopaminergic systems are unresponsive to antipsychotics. Capacities to worsen cognitive impairment and gait disorders must be considered. Clozapine can attenuate parkinsonian and dystonic features in non-WD patients, although bone marrow suppression and seizure risks, already intrinsic to WD, should be considered. A single case report indicated improvement in delirium and a persecutory delusion in WD during treatment with clozapine 100mg/d, which had failed to respond to penicillamine and zinc [64]. Vigilance for cognitive impairment, cardiac dysrhythmia, and hypotension is of course necessary with antipsychotics possessing anticholinergic and alpha-blocking properties because WD patients are already at risk for these conditions due to the disease itself. Psychotropics that lower seizure threshold, such as clozapine, may increase the likelihood of seizures in WD, especially during WD treatment [59]. Patients on anticonvulsants are at risk for the many drug interactions that can occur between these agents and psychotropics [65]. Liver disease in WD hepatic and renal involvement may affect the metabolism of psychotropics, leading to dose accumulation and toxic blood levels. Use of shorter half-lived drugs, lower doses, and drugs that are minimally metabolized before elimination may circumvent this problem. Renal dysfunction in WD may lead to elevated lithium concentrations. Cardiac copper deposition can affect conduction pathways and produce dysrhythmias, including tachycardia or bradycardia with reduced cardiac efficiency [66]. EKG abnormalities occur in about 30% of patients with WD, and orthostatic hypotension and sudden death sometimes occur. Therefore, psychotropics with low dysrhythmogenic and hypotensive potentials will be critical in some cases [65]. Bone marrow suppression can occur with certain psychotropics as well as in WD. Attention must also be given to drug-drug interactions. Given the potentially lethal treatment effects, a thorough discussion of benefits, risks, and side effects should be undertaken as part of the informed consent process.

The case report literature reveals that psychotic features are sometimes unresponsive [50, 52, 54, 56] to or actually aggravated [54] by antipsychotic therapy, yet responsive to anticopper therapies [26, 41, 50, 51, 52, 53, 54]. Treatment failures have occurred with haloperidol [54, 56], chlorpromazine [54], thioridazine [56], and a variety of other neuroleptics, presumably due to cuprification of circuits mediating antipsychotic response. In the prospective study of Oder and colleagues [26], the authors noted that delusions in their three patients responded well to anticopper therapy. Catatonia has also responded to anticopper therapy [54].

Case reports reveal occasional worsening of psychosis after commencing anticopper therapies, analogous to WD treatment-related neurological exacerbations [41, 51]. In one case, the patient developed *de novo* bizarre behavior, visual hallucinations, paranoid delusions, referential thinking, and heightened sensory awareness within several months of starting penicillamine treatment [41]. With persistent anticopper treatment, however, subsequent remission of psychotic symptoms occurred a number of months later [51].

WD patients with psychosis may be particularly prone toward extrapyramidal side effects [53, 63]. At times, extrapyramidal side effects have been refractory to treatment with antimuscarinics [53] and dopamine agonists [53], presumably related to putaminal cuprification [53] or cuprous alteration of striatal muscarinic and dopamine receptor functions. Neuroleptic malignant syndrome in WD has responded to dantrolene and bromocriptine in at least some cases [67].

ECT should only be administered with extreme caution in WD, given the capacity for prolonged seizures [57] and the dearth of studies reporting safety and efficacy [55, 56]. In one case, ECT (six bifrontal treatments, sine wave pulse, 110 V, 0.8 s) along with haloperidol 15 mg/d, were safe and effective in resolving auditory hallucinations, delusions, thought disorder, and suicidal ideation in a paranoid psychosis possibly ascribable to WD [55]. In a second case, the first bilateral treatment (30 s seizure) markedly improved muscular rigidity, and the second treatment (49 s seizure) led to normal ambulation and remission of delusions and auditory command and visual hallucinations [56]. However, in another case, a single bilateral brief pulse ECT (12.4 J of charge) resulted in a 3-minute seizure and mania in a WD patient with persecutory and control delusions, loose associations, disorganized behavior, negativism, cognitive impairment, and major depression, suggesting the need for extreme caution in patients with high copper levels [57]. WD itself carries an increased risk of seizures.

Research considerations

Possible pathophysiological mechanisms for psychosis

Much research is still needed before a tentative pathophysiology of psychosis in WD can be formulated. Copper deposition in specific brain regions may play a role. Candidate structures include the ventral tegmental area, ventral striatum/nucleus accumbens, ventral pallidum/internal pallidum, thalamic nuclei, temporal cortex, amygdala, other limbic structures, and other regions, and copper deposition in regions such as these should be evaluated in prospective studies. Copper may affect energy metabolism, leading to reduced activity in salient brain regions. Copper might have effects on primary firing of monoamine nuclei, such as ventral tegmental mesolimbic projections, or on cortical and other feedback acting on monoamine systems. Copper might also affect neurotransmitter receptor efficacy or may turn on or off genes amplifying postsynaptic receptor effects through G protein coupling or postreceptor effector signaling. Copper could also affect enzymes involved in neurotransmitter degradation. Copper may have effects on ligand and voltage gated ion channels, thus influencing neuronal membrane potentials and modulating neuronal firing. Single cell studies and functional imaging may elucidate these or other mechanisms. Similarly, the phenomenon of antipsychotic-refractory psychotic features may represent copper deposition in target ventral striatum, or cuprous transection of corticostriatopallidothalamocortical circuits, preventing antipsychotics

from restoring a more normal physiology to systems involved in psychosis.

Future directions

Against this backdrop of unknowns described above, an agenda for research is offered. Pursuit of this agenda can produce information relevant to understanding and effectively treating psychosis in WD. It can also inform our understanding of pathogenetic mechanisms involved in schizophrenia and other primary psychoses. A research agenda includes:

1. Large multicenter studies to obtain adequate sample size and to average out selection factors
2. Prospective determinations of psychosis prevalence in WD, taking into account sample selection and referral biases, with particular attention to:
   a) Visual, auditory, and other modalities of hallucinations
   b) Specific types of delusions
   c) Formal thought disorders
   d) Inappropriate affect
   e) Bizarre or inappropriate behavior
   f) Catatonia
   g) Negative symptoms
   h) Cognitive impairment
   i) Functional impairment in WD psychosis
   j) Psychotic syndromes using DSM-IV-TR criteria and structured clinical interviews
3. Prospective evaluation of WD patients to determine risk factors and disease correlates, including neurological signs and hepatic status, in those developing psychosis
4. Determination of the correlates of specific psychotic symptoms and functional decline
5. Systematic evaluation and reporting of MRI structural imaging correlates in WD patients presenting with WD psychotic features, specifying precisely the psychotic feature under investigation, with close attention to:
   a) The specific pattern of regional involvement in striatal and pontine copper deposition
   b) Involvement of specific corticostriatopallido-thalamocortical circuits
   c) The pattern of midbrain copper deposition
   d) The pattern of cerebral cortical, subcortical, temporo-limbic, brainstem, and cerebellar

copper deposition, with special attention to structures that have been implicated in functional and structural imaging studies [68, 69], including:

(1) Middle prefrontal gyrus (especially Brodmann areas 6 and 8), inferior prefrontal gyrus (especially area 44), and dorso-medial thalamus, implicated in schizophrenia

(2) Broca's area, implicated in hallucinating patients with schizophrenia

(3) Anterior thalamic nuclei, implicated in psychosis

(4) Hippocampus, and medio-temporal and frontal cortices, implicated in negative symptoms

6. Similar investigations with functional magnetic resonance (fMR), single photon emission computed tomography (SPECT), and PET, with close attention to particular structures and systems implicated in schizophrenia and psychosis [68, 69, 70], including:

a) Glucose metabolism and cerebral blood flow correlates of WD psychosis

b) Presynaptic release and receptor binding studies of dopamine, glutamate, GABA, norepinephrine, and serotonin in WD psychosis

7. Studies of variables of treatment outcome would be informative, including:

a) Controlled studies of antipsychotic treatment in WD psychosis

b) The role of clozapine (and other antipsychotics) in treating psychosis in WD in terms of safety in regard to seizures, bone marrow suppression, and cognition vs. safety in the context of extrapyramidal disorders

c) Risk factors for NMS and other EPS developing with antipsychotic use in WD

d) Copper deposition correlates of:

(1) Anticopper therapy-induced psychosis

(2) Anticopper therapy-responsive psychosis

(3) Antipsychotic-refractory psychosis

(4) Novel psychotropic-responsive psychosis

(5) Antimuscarinic-refractory and dopamine agonist-refractory EPS in WD

(6) ECT safety and efficacy

WD represents a prototypic neuropsychiatric disorder. The prevalence and correlates of psychosis still remain to be defined despite more than a century of experience with this disease. Understanding psychosis in WD not only promises to improve our treatment of patients with this disease, but also carries the potential to expand our understanding of psychosis in general, and schizophrenia in particular.

References

1. Roelofsen H., Wolters H., Van Luyn M. J., *et al.* Copper-induced apical trafficking of ATP7B in polarized hepatoma cells provides a mechanism for biliary copper excretion. *Gastroenterology*, 2000. **119**:782–93.

2. Wilson S. A. K. Progressive lenticular degeneration, a familial nervous disease associated with cirrhosis of the liver. *Brain*, 1912. **34**:295–507.

3. Lauterbach E. C. (2000). Wilson's disease (hepatolenticular degeneration). In *Psychiatric Management in Neurological Disease*, Lauterbach E. C. (Ed.). Washington, DC: American Psychiatric Press Inc., pp. 93–136.

4. Gitlin J. D. Wilson Disease. *Gastroenterology*, 2003. **125**:1868–77.

5. Nanji M. S., Nguyen V. T., Kawasoe J. H., *et al.* Haplotype and mutation analysis in Japanese patients with Wilson's disease. *Am J Hum Genet*, 1997. **60**:1423–9.

6. Kojimahara N., Nakabayashi H., Shikata T., *et al.* Defective copper binding to apo–ceruloplasmin in a rat model and patients with Wilson's disease. *Liver*, 1995. **15**:135–42.

7. Chowrimootoo G. F., Andoh J., Seymour C. A. Western blot analysis in patients with hypocaeruloplasminaemia. *QJM*, 1997. **90**:197–202.

8. El-Youssef M. Wilson's disease. *Mayo Clin Proc*. 2003. **78**:1126–36.

9. Hoogenraad T. U., Van Den Hamer C. J. A. (1996). Copper metabolism, copper toxicity and pathogenesis of Wilson's Disease. In *Wilson's Disease*, Hoogenraad T. U. (Ed.). London: WB Saunders, pp. 25–44.

10. Walshe J. M. Copper: not too little, not too much, but just right. Based on the triennial Pewterers Lecture delivered at the National Hospital for Neurology, London, on 23 March 1995. *J R Coll Physicians Lond*, 1995. **19**:280–8.

11. Houwen R. H., Juyn J., Hoogenraad T. U., *et al.* H714Q mutation in Wilson's disease is associated with late, neurological presentation. *J Med Genet*, 1995. **32**:480–2.

12. Hoogenraad T. U., Houwen R. H. J. (1996). Prevalence and genetics. In *Wilson's Disease*, Hoogenraad T. U. (Ed.). London: WB Saunders, pp. 14–24.

13. Mansouri A., Gaou I., Fromenty B., *et al.* Premature oxidative aging of hepatic mitochondrial DNA in Wilson's disease. *Gastroenterology*, 1997. **113**: 599–605.

14. Strand S., Hofmann W. J., Grambihler A., *et al.* Hepatic failure and liver cell damage in acute Wilson's disease involve CD95 (APO-1/Fas) mediated apoptosis. *Nat Med*, 1998. **4**:588–93.

15. Mufti A. R., Burstein E., Csomos R. A., *et al.* XIAP is a copper binding protein deregulated in Wilson's disease and other copper toxicosis disorders. *Mol Cell*, 2006. **21**:775–85.

16. Hoogenraad T. U. (Ed). *Wilson's Disease* (1996). London: WB Saunders.

17. Makharia G. K., Nandi B., Garg P. K., *et al.* Wilson's disease with neuropsychiatric manifestations and liver disease but no Kayser-Fleischer ring. *J Clin Gastroenterol*, 2002. **35**:101–2.

18. King A. D., Walshe J. M., Kendall B. E., *et al.* Cranial MR imaging in Wilson's disease. *AJR Am J Roentgenol*, 1996. **167**:1579–84.

19. Saatci I., Topcu M., Baltaoglu F. F., *et al.* Cranial MR findings in Wilson's disease. *Acta Radiol*, 1997. **38**:250–8.

20. van Wassenaer-van Hall H. N., van Den Heuvel A. G., Algra A., *et al.* Wilson disease: findings at MR imaging and CT of the brain with clinical correlation. *Radiology*, 1996. **198**:531–6.

21. Kuwert T., Hefter H., Scholz D., *et al.* Regional cerebral glucose consumption measured by positron emission tomography in patients with Wilson's disease. *Eur J Nucl Med*, 1992. **19**:96–101.

22. Schlaug G., Hefter H., Engelbrecht V., *et al.* Neurological impairment and recovery in Wilson's disease: evidence from PET and MRI. *J Neurol Sci*, 1996. **136**:129–39.

23. Oder W., Brucke T., Kollegger H., *et al.* Dopamine D2 receptor binding is reduced in Wilson's disease: correlation of neurological deficits with striatal 123I – iodobenzamide binding. *J Neural Transm*, 1996. **103**:1093–103.

24. Arendt G., Hefter H., Stremmel W., *et al.* The diagnostic value of multi-modality evoked potentials in Wilson's disease. *Electromyogr Clin Neurophysiol*, 1994. **34**:137–48.

25. Huang C. C., Chu N. S. Wilson's Disease: clinical analysis of 71 cases and comparison with previous Chinese series. *J Formos Med Assoc*, 1992. **91**:502–7.

26. Oder W., Grimm G., Kollegger H., *et al.* Neurological and neuropsychiatric spectrum of Wilson's disease: a prospective study of 45 cases. *J Neurol*, 1991. **238**:281–7.

27. Akil M., Brewer G. J. Psychiatric and behavioral abnormalities in Wilson's disease. *Adv Neurol*, 1995. **65**:171–8.

28. Dening T. R., Berrios G. E. Wilson's disease: psychiatric symptoms in 195 cases. *Arch Gen Psychiatry*, 1989. **46**:1126–34.

29. Schwartz M., Fuchs S., Polak H., *et al.* Psychiatric manifestation in Wilson's disease. *Harefuah*, 1993. **124**:75–7.

30. Lauterbach E. C., Cummings J. L., Duffy J., *et al.* Neuropsychiatric

correlates and treatment of lenticulostriatal diseases: a review of the literature and overview of research opportunities in Huntington's, Wilson's and Fahr's diseases. *J Neuropsychiatry Clin Neurosci*, 1998. **10**:249–66.

31. Lauterbach E. C. Wilson's disease. *Psychiatr Ann*, 2002. **32**:114–20.

32. Akil M., Schwartz J. A., Dutchak D., *et al*. The psychiatric presentations of Wilson's disease. *J Neuropsychiatry Clin Neurosci*, 1991. **3**:377–82.

33. Rathbun J. K. Neuropsychological aspects of Wilson's Disease. *Int J Neurosci*, 1996. **85**:221–9.

34. Walshe J. M., Yealland M. Wilson's disease: the problem of delayed diagnosis. *J Neurol Neurosurg Psychiatry*, 1992. **55**:692–6.

35. Brewer G. J., Yuzbasiyan-Gurkan V. Wilson disease. *Medicine* (Baltimore), 1992. **71**:139–64.

36. Hu J., Lu D., Wang G. Study on the clinical misdiagnosis of hepatolenticular degeneration. *Zhonghua Yi Xue Za Zhi*, 2001. **81**:642–4.

37. Meng Y., Miyoshi I., Hirabayashi M., *et al*. Resotration of copper metabolism and rescue of hepatic abnormalities in LEC rats, an animal model of Wilson's disease, by expression of human ATP7B gene. *Biochim Biophys Acta*, 2004. **1690**:208–19.

38. Ha-Hao D., Merle U., Hofmann C., *et al*. Chances and shortcomings of adenovirus-mediated ATP7B gene transfer in Wilson's disease: proof of principle demonstrated in a pilot study with LEC rats. *J Gastroenterol*, 2002. **40**:209–16.

39. Brewer G. J. Neurologically presenting Wilson's disease: epidemiology, pathophysiology and treatment. *CNS Drugs*, 2005. **19**:185–92.

40. Dening T. R., Berrios G. E. Wilson's disease: a longitudinal study of psychiatric symptoms. *Biol Psychiatry*, 1990. **28**:255–65.

41. McDonald L. V., Lake C. R. Psychosis in an adolescent patient with Wilson's disease: effects of chelation therapy. *Psychosom Med*, 1995. **57**:202–4.

42. Huang C. C., Chu N. S. Wilson's disease: resolution of MRI lesions following long-term oral zinc therapy. *Acta Neurol Scand*, 1996. **93**:215–18.

43. Cuthbert J. A. Wilson's disease: a new gene and an animal model for an old disease. *J Investig Med*, 1995. **43**:323–36.

44. Bellary S., Hassanein T., Van Thiel D. H. Liver transplantation for Wilson's disease. *J Hepatol*, 1995. **23**:373–81.

45. Brewer G. J. Interactions of zinc and molybdenum with copper in therapy of Wilson's disease. *Nutrition*, 1995. **11**(1 Suppl): 114–16.

46. Slater E., Cowie V. (Eds.). (1971). *The Genetics of Mental Disorders*. London: Oxford University Press.

47. Beard A. W. The association of hepatolenticular degeneration with schizophrenia. *Acta Psychiatr Neurol Scand*, 1959. **34**:411–28.

48. Davison K., Bagley C. R. (1969). Schizophrenia-like psychoses associated with organic disorders of the central nervous system: a review of the literature. In *Current Problems in Neuropsychiatry. Schizophrenia, Epilepsy, the Temporal Lobe*, Herrington R. N. (Ed.). *Br J Psychiatry* Special Publication No. 4. Ashford, Kent: Headley Brothers Ltd., pp. 113–84.

49. Keith S. J., Regier D. A., Rae D. S. (1991). Schizophrenic disorders. In *Psychiatric Disorders in America*, Robins L. N. and Regier D. A. (Eds.). New York: The Free Press, pp. 33–52.

50. Saint-Laurent M. Schizophrenia and Wilson's Disease. *Can J Psychiatry*, 1992. **37**:358–60.

51. Garnier H., Diederich N., Pilloy W., *et al*. Late form with psychiatric presentation of Wilson's disease, with pseudo-compulsive stereotyped movements. Neuro-radiological correlations. *Rev Neurol* (Paris), 1997. **153**:124–8.

52. Modai I., Karp L., Liberman U. A., *et al*. Penicillamine therapy for schizophreniform psychosis in Wilson's disease. *J Nerv Ment Dis*, 1985. **173**:698–701.

53. Chroni E., Lekka N. P., Tsibri E., *et al*. Acute, progressive akinetic-rigid syndrome induced by neuroleptics in a case of Wilson's disease. *J Neuropsychiatry Clin Neurosci*, 2001. **13**:531–2.

54. Chung Y. S., Ravi S. D., Borge G. F. Psychosis in Wilson's disease. *Psychosomatics*, 1986. **27**:65–6.

55. Shah N., Kumar D. Wilson's disease, psychosis, and ECT. *Convuls Ther*, 1997. **13**:278–9.

56. Rodrigues A. C., Dalgalarrondo P., Banzato C. E. Successful ECT in a patient with a psychiatric presentation of Wilson's disease. *J ECT*, 2004. **20**:55.

57. Negro Junior P. J., Louza Neto M. R. Results of ECT for a case of depression in Wilson's disease [letter]. *J Neuropsychiatr Clin Neurosci*, 1995. **7**:384.

58. Oder W., Prayer L., Grimm G., *et al*. Wilson's disease: evidence of subgroups derived from clinical findings and brain lesions. *Neurology*, 1993. **43**:120–4.

59. Dening T. R., Berrios G. E. Wilson's disease: a prospective study of psychopathology in 31 cases. *Br J Psychiatry*, 1989. **155**:206–13.

60. Bostwick J. M., Masterson B. J. Psychopharmacological treatment of delirium to restore mental capacity. *Psychosomatics*, 1998. **39**:112–7.

61. Munir K. M. The treatment of psychotic symptoms in Fahr's

disease with lithium carbonate. *J Clin Psychopharmacol*, 1986. **6**:36–8.

62. Jaeckle R. S., Nasrallah H. A. Major depression and carbon monoxide-induced parkinsonism: diagnosis, computerized axial tomography, and responsive to L-dopa. *J Nerv Ment Dis*, 1985. **173**:503–8.

63. Tu J. The inadvisability of neuroleptic medication in Wilson's disease. *Biol Psychiatry*, 1981. **16**:963–8.

64. Krim E., Barroso B. Psychiatric disorders treated with clozapine in a patient with Wilson's disease. *Presse Med*, 2001. **30**: 738.

65. Stoudemire A., Moran M. G., Fogel B. S. (1995). Psychopharmacology in the medically ill patient. In *APA Textbook of Psychopharmacology*, Schatzberg A. F. and Nemeroff C. B. (Eds.). Washington, DC: American Psychiatric Press, pp. 783–801.

66. Hilz M. J., Druschky K. F., Bauer J., *et al.* Wilson's disease – critical deterioration under high-dose parenteral penicillamine therapy. *Dtsch Med Wochenschr*, 1990. **115**:93–7.

67. Kontaxakis V., Stefanis C., Markidis M., *et al.* Neuroleptic malignant syndrome in a patient with Wilson's disease [letter].

J Neurol Neurosurg Psychiatry, 1988. **51**:1001–2.

68. Kandel E. R., Schwartz J. H., Jessell T. M. (Eds.). (2000). *Principles of Neural Science*. 4th ed. New York: McGraw-Hill.

69. McIntosh A. M., Job D. E., Moorhead T. W., *et al.* Voxel-based morphometry of patients with schizophrenia or bipolar disorder and their unaffected relatives. *Biol Psychiatry*, 2004. **56**:544–52.

70. Carlsson A., Waters N., Holm-Waters S., *et al.* Interactions between monoamines, glutamate, and GABA in schizophrenia: new evidence. *Ann Rev Pharmacol Toxicol*, 2001. **41**:237–60.

28

Huntington's Disease and related disorders and their association with schizophrenia-like psychosis

Perminder S. Sachdev

Facts box

- The development of suspiciousness and ideas of reference is seen in many patients with Huntington's Disease (HD).
- Rates of schizophrenia-like psychosis (SLP) in HD ranging from 5% to 16% have been reported.
- It is not uncommon for some patients with HD to have received a diagnosis of schizophrenia, possibly for years, before their accurate diagnosis.
- The HD patients who develop psychosis do not have repeat numbers different from those without psychosis.
- It is possible that, despite their differences, HD patients may develop neuropsychological deficits that resemble those in schizophrenia and this might provide the substrate for the development of psychotic symptoms in HD.
- Psychosis is uncommon in spinocerebellar ataxia, but other psychiatric disorders are common.
- Triplet repeats do not appear to have a major role in the genetics of schizophrenia, but a minor role in a minority of cases cannot be ruled out.

Huntington's Disease (HD) is a progressive neurodegenerative disease with a classical autosomal dominant pattern of inheritance. It has conferred eponymous fame on George Huntington who described the typical clinical triad of movement disorder, cognitive impairment, and psychiatric features, and emphasized its familial nature [1]. The disorder is uncommon, with a reported prevalence of about 4 to 7 per 100,000 in most Western countries [2, 3, 4] but much lower rates in Asian and African countries

[4]. Pockets of very high prevalence of HD have been described in places like Tasmania in Australia and the Moray Firth area of Scotland [5]. It was one such pocket in the Venezuelan villages of Barranquitas and Lagunetas that the early work toward the discovery of the HD gene was carried out by the U.S.-Venezuela Huntington's Disease Collaborative Research Project [6]. The linkage of the HD gene to chromosome 4p in 1983 [7] and its eventual discovery as a trinucleotide repeat 10 years later [8] are landmark events in the history of neurogenetics.

Clinical features

Age of onset

The usual age of onset is in the fourth or fifth decade, with the median age in the mid-40s. However, onset has been described in early childhood as well as in the 80s. The disease tends to be more severe if the onset is early, and premonitory psychiatric features are more common in such cases. The age of onset is also somewhat related to the motor features, with striate rigidity prominent in the early 20s, chorea in midlife, and intention tremor more common for a later onset. In siblings, onset seems to be closer together, but still with considerable variability. Onset before the age of 20 occurs in about 10% of cases and is regarded as "juvenile onset." Age of onset is said to show "anticipation," in other words, the disorder becomes manifest at an earlier age as it is passed on to the next generation, especially for paternal transmission.

Signs and symptoms

The initial symptoms are equally likely to be neurological or psychiatric, and no general rule can be described for their chronology. Typically, choreiform movements are the first manifestation and cognitive and psychiatric symptoms follow. However, the psychiatric symptoms may sometimes precede the movement disorder or cognitive dysfunction by many years.

Neurological symptoms

The choreiform movements initially appear in the hands and face and make the patient appear clumsy and nervous. These are usually in the form of twitching and grimacing. Gradually, these spread to the rest of the musculature, making movements jerky and rapid, and, in the late stages, the patient is continuously displaying these movements. The movements have a stereotyped quality, and in the later stages may become more athetoid. The patient cannot hold the protruded tongue (*impersistence*), and this phenomenon is observed in other muscle groups as well. The gait may be affected by a curious dance-like ataxia (*choreic dance*). The speech becomes dysarthric and explosive. Eye movements are affected in most patients, with impaired initiation and slowness of saccades and distractibility of ocular fixation. The muscle tone is variable. There may be hypotonia, or varying degree of rigidity, associated with tremor and bradykinesia. Striate rigidity rather than chorea is an important feature of some cases of early-onset HD (*Westphal variant*). In later stages, the diaphragm and bulbar muscles may be involved, resulting in jerky breathing, staccato speech, and dysphagia. After 10 to 15 years, the patient is no longer able to stand or walk and deteriorates into a vegetative state.

Cognitive symptoms

The early features are a general inefficiency at work and in managing daily routines, with the patient becoming disorganized and slipshod, suggesting executive deficits. Thinking becomes slow and rigid, with delayed reaction time and poor working memory [9]. The patient makes more perseverative errors on the Wisconsin Card Sorting Test [10]. Concentration is poor and abstraction and judgment are affected. Memory is not prominently disturbed, unlike Alzheimer's Disease, although problems have been noted in both declarative and procedural memory [9, 11, 12]. Language, gnosis, and praxis are usually spared [12, 13], at least in the early stages, although word finding difficulties, paraphasias, and decreased speech production are seen in later stages. Visuospatial functioning has been less well studied, but deficits were reported in one study in tasks that required the manipulation of personal space [14]. The presence of cognitive deficits in the absence of typical cortical disturbances such as dysphasia, agnosia, and apraxia has suggested the term "subcortical dementia" to describe it. In late stages, the patient is severely impaired and may show akinetic mutism. The degree of cognitive impairment is related to the duration of the disease and degree of caudate nucleus and generalized atrophy. Mild cognitive deficits have been reported in asymptomatic carriers [15], and an inverse relationship between cognitive function and the length of triplet repeats has been noted [16].

Psychiatric symptoms

The initial changes are often subtle alterations in personality. Patients are usually described as irritable, suspicious, annoying, impulsive, or eccentric. They may become excessively religious or grandiose. Poor self-control with alcohol abuse and sexual promiscuity are also described, and rates of criminal behavior are reportedly increased. Other patients become morose and apathetic and neglectful of themselves. Personality change has been reported in about one-half of HD patients. In one recent study using a structured assessment [17], a DSM-IV diagnosis of personality disorder was present in 10 of 21 (47%) of HD patients (mean age 52.1 years), with the following subtypes: labile, disinhibited, paranoid and apathetic, as well as a disorder characterized by child-like regressive behavior. Twenty percent of the patients with personality disorder did not meet DSM-IV criteria for cognitive disorder or dementia. Personality disorder may sometimes be present for many years before the development of the movement disorder.

Affective disorder is also common in HD. In a survey by Folstein and colleagues [18], 41% showed major mood disturbance, 32% being depressed and 9% bipolar, with the mood disorder predating the motor symptoms by 2 to 20 years. The mood disorder appeared to be confined to certain families, with higher rates of mood disorder in the relatives of affected individuals. In a recent survey [17], major depression was reported in 28%, minor depression in 14%, and mania in 5%. Suicide was found to account for 7% of deaths in nonhospitalized patients [19]. Psychosis in HD is discussed later.

Longitudinal course

The disease is slowly but relentlessly progressive, with the mean duration being 21.4 (range 1.2 to 40.8) in one study [16]. The progression of symptoms is variable, and some patients remain cognitively intact in spite of severe motor deficits. The duration is shorter in those with an onset of < 20 years and > 50 years. Over a 3-year period, the cumulative incidence in non-symptomatic carriers was 3% if neurological examination was normal, 23% if mildly abnormal, and 60% if highly abnormal [20].

Diagnosis

The diagnosis is strongly suggested by the characteristic clinical features and family history and established by genetic testing (discussed in a later section). Neuroimaging may play a role in diagnosis and determining the severity of cerebral involvement. CT and MRI characteristically show dilated ventricles, with frontal atrophy, and particularly atrophy of the heads of the caudate nuclei. Significant reduction in the thalamus and the medial temporal structures is also seen [21]. The characteristic finding on PET scanning is bilateral hypometabolism in the caudate and putamen, which may be seen in at-risk individuals [22]. Single photon emission computed tomography (SPECT) scanning replicates this finding, with reduced blood flow in the caudate [23]. Some disorders that may resemble HD are summarized in Table 28.1.

Given that the genetic abnormality predicts the disease with great accuracy, *presymptomatic diagnosis* has received much attention and guidelines have been established [24]. Great care must be taken in ensuring accuracy and laboratories have different practices to ensure this. Preimplantation diagnosis has been successfully applied [25].

Genetics

Huntington's Disease is the prototypical autosomal disease caused by an expanded CAG repeat at the 5' end of the hungtingtin (Htt) gene that is located on chromosome 4p16.3 [8]. It is one of a number of trinucleotide repeat neurological disorders listed in Table 28.2. In healthy individuals, the gene carries 6–35 CAG repeats, and no individuals with repeat lengths < 36 have been diagnosed to have HD. Repeat lengths > 39 definitely result in the disease, with > 98% sensitivity and > 99% specificity [26]. Repeats in the range 36–39 are variably penetrant, and the probability of disease for 36 or 37 triplets is about 50% [27]. Repeats < 27 triplets are stable during meiosis, whereas 27–35 triplets may rarely expand. Triplets in the abnormal range are unstable, with bias toward longer repeats in paternal transmission. This results in anticipation from father to child, with children developing the disease about 8 years earlier [28]. Repeat lengths are related to age of onset, explaining about 50%–60% of the variance [29]. Juvenile onset is generally related to > 60 repeats [29]. Genetic modifiers of age of onset have been reported, for example, polymorphism on the kainite receptor (GluR6) gene for a younger onset [30] and the APOE*4 gene for a later onset [31]. Lack of family history may occur in as high as 8% of affected individuals. This may be on the basis of new mutations, considered to be 1–3%, anticipation, early death or misdiagnosis of parent, adoption, or false paternity.

The abnormal CAG repeat sequence leads to a polyglutamine (polyQ) stretch near the N-terminus resulting in a mutant Htt. The functions of normal Htt, a 3140 amino acid protein, are incompletely understood, but it is highly conserved in evolution and Htt knockout mice die at 8–10 days of gestation [32]. It may have a role in intracellular transport. Mutant Htt results in toxic gain of function with interference with cytoskeletal and vesicular functions and effects on gene expression leading to apoptosis [33]. This may be due to aggregation of the protein or its interaction with other proteins. The mutant Htt is expressed throughout the body. Its levels in the brain are higher in the cortex and the cerebellum than the striatum, but the latter is more vulnerable to the damage. The mechanism of degeneration is an important area of investigation if treatments are to be developed to delay or prevent the onset of the disease.

Huntington's Disease and schizophrenia-like psychosis

The association of schizophrenia-like psychosis (SLP) with HD has been reported by many authors and has been examined from a number of perspectives:

Epidemiological association

The development of suspiciousness and ideas of reference is seen in many patients with HD, and these characteristics have been described as the features of personality change in patients that sometimes predate the typical features of the disorder by many years. Rates of SLP in HD from 5% to 16% have been reported [34, 35]. If all psychotic symptoms are included, the rates may be as high as 25% [36]. The symptoms are usually

Table 28.1 Disorders in the differential diagnosis of Huntington's Disease (adapted from [26])

Disorder	Comment
Acquired Disorders	
Infections/postinfections	
– Sydenham's chorea	Poststreptococcal in 20% of cases of rheumatic fever
– Neurosyphilitis	
Drug-related	
– Tardive dyskinesia	Secondary to chronic antipsychotic drug use
– Drug-induced chorea	L-dopa, dopamine agonists, stimulants, anti-epileptic drugs, lithium
Basal ganglia lesions	Stroke, tumors, infections, hypoxia
Others	
– Senile chorea	Late onset; may resemble late onset HD
– Pregnancy	Rare cause of chorea
– Polycythemia vera	0.5%–5.0% of cases
– Systemic lupus erythematosus	1%–7% of cases
Genetic Disorders	
Autosomal dominant	
– Spinocerebellar ataxia (SCA)	Chorea may be present in SCA17, SCA2, SCA3 and some othe types; (CAG) in expansion
– Dentatorubral-pallidoluysian atrophy (DRPLA)	(CAG) in expansion in atrophin 1; more common in Japan
– Benign hereditary chorea	Childhood onset; linkage to chromosome 14q
– Fahr's Disease	Idiopathic basal ganglia calcification; linkage to chromosome 14q
– Hereditary Creutzfeldt-Jakob Disease	15% of C-J Disease; RP gene mutation in chromosome 20p
– Huntington's Disease-like 2	Resembles HD clinically and pathologically; CTG expansion Junctophilin-3; African ethnicity
Autosomal recessive	
– Wilson's Disease	Abnormal Cu metabolism; mutation in ATP 7B
– Neuronal ceroid lipofuscinosis (NCL)	Liposomal storage disorder; mutations in 8 different genes (CLN1-CLN8); adult form may be dominant or recessive
– Pantolthenate kinase-associated neurodegeneration	Abnormal Fe accumulaton; 50% of cases form PANK2 mutations
Other genetic disorders	
– Mitochondrial disorders	Multiple types; maternal inheritance
– Neuro-acanthocytosis	Several conditions:
	Choreo-acanthocytosis – recessive mutation in chorein;
	McCleod Syndrome – X-linked mutation in Xk gene
	Dominant forms

hallucinations and delusions, the latter generally persecutory, referential, or grandiose in nature. McHugh and Folstein [37] described the typical evolution of SLP in an HD patient as being preceded by a delusional mood from which hallucinations and delusions well up rather acutely and tend to last many months. Apathy is a common feature and may be conceptualized as a negative symptom of SLP. In many patients, perplexity, negativism, and stereotypic movements may be seen. It is not uncommon for some patients with HD to have received a diagnosis of schizophrenia, possibly for years, before their accurate diagnosis, a situation more common in the pre-1993 era before the gene had been identified. The author has encountered a

Table 28.2 Trinucleotide repeat disorders

I. Translated (poly Q or polyglutamine) triplet repeat disorders	Triplet sequence
a. Huntington's Disease (HD)	CAG
b. Dentatorubral-Pallidoluysian atrophy (DRPLA)	CAG
c. Spinocerebellar ataxia, types 1, 2, 3, 6, 7, 17	CAG
d. Kennedy's Disease (x-linked spinal and bulbar muscular atrophy)	CAG
II. Untranslated triplet repeat disorders	
a. Spinocerebellar ataxia	CIG
type 8	CAG
type 12	
b. Friedreich's ataxia (FRDA)	GAA
c. Mytomic dystrophy*	CIG
d. Fragile X syndrome*	CGG

* Not associated with neurodegeneration.

number of such cases. Many factors have been described as determining psychosis in HD. Early age of onset is related to a higher incidence [34]. Family history of schizophrenia is increased, and there are a number of reports of familial aggregation of SLP in HD [35, 38, 39, 40]. Correa and colleagues [41] reported the association of HD and psychosis in three generations in one family.

Genetics

Because of the high prevalence of psychotic symptoms, the frequency of trinucleotide repeats has been examined in schizophrenia. The phenomenon of anticipation has been reported in pedigrees of schizophrenia [42]. Repeat Expansion Detection techniques have suggested an increased number of triplet repeats in schizophrenia [43, 44]. Studies of (CAG)n in schizophrenia have however not reported an increase of repeats [45, 46]. Moreover, the HD patients who develop psychosis do not have repeat numbers different from those without psychosis [47, 48]. The only reported association of (CAG)n with schizophrenia is that with the gene for dominant spinocerebellar ataxia 1 at chromosome 6pter-p22 [49], but this awaits replication. Other proteins with (CAG)n that are candidate genes for schizophrenia are Pim-1 proto-oncogene, alkaline phosphatase, TATA-binding protein, and brain natriuretic protein [50].

Another aspect of the genetics of schizophrenia in relation to HD is the familial aggregation of the two disorders mentioned above. This may suggest an associated genetic abnormality that predisposes the individuals to psychosis, or perhaps some other vulnerability factor that may be epigenetic or environmental. It could also mean that the nature of the disorder in these individuals is such that they develop a vulnerability to psychosis owing to it. The investigation of these factors could result in important insights into the pathogenesis of schizophrenia.

Pathology

If the neuropathology of HD creates a vulnerability for SLP, it would be useful to examine this to understand the nature of pathology that might underlie psychosis. In particular, the early changes in HD are of interest, as psychosis or a personality change toward suspiciousness is often an early manifestation. Striatal degeneration has been described as an early manifestation, which begins in the medial aspect and spreads but tends to spare the nucleus accumbens. The small spiny neurons appear to be affected before the larger ones, with loss of dendrites being an early finding. In more advanced cases, changes have been described in the globus pallidus, subthalamic nucleus, red nucleus, substantia nigra, and the cerebellum. The medium spiny neurons are GABA-ergic and provide inhibitory input from the striatum to the globus pallidus. How their degeneration could lead to psychosis can only be speculated upon. It is possible that striatal sensitivity to dopamine changes as a consequence, and such a change in the medial aspects may be related to the development of psychosis. The development of chorea has been related to increased dopaminergic activity, as is suggested by similar involuntary movements produced by dopaminergic drugs. However, loss of GABA inhibition may produce the same result. The loss of GABA in the striatum also alters this activity in fronto-subcortical circuits that underlie behavioral syndromes [51]. In children and young adults with chorea and behavioral disorders, the subthalamic nucleus had been reported to be markedly affected.

In the cortex, layers 3, 5, and 6 suffer neuronal loss, with reduced numbers as well as neuronal size, and an increase in glial numbers [52]. In schizophrenia, there is a downward shift in neuronal size in layer 3, with an increased density of small neurons [52]. This change is evident in the frontal cortex but not in the occipital cortex. There is no evidence that degenerative cell loss occurs in the schizophrenic cortex. There are therefore significant differences in the pathology of the two disorders, although some similarities exist, possibly in the early stages of the disorders. Further work on the pathology of schizophrenia is necessary to understand the significance of any similarities. Furthermore, the neuropathological correlates of psychosis in HD may shed some light into the pathomechanisms of schizophrenia.

Neuropsychology

The cognitive deficits of schizophrenia resemble the subcortical cognitive syndrome of HD. Schizophrenics have deficits in executive function, they have memory problems that are not the most salient of their deficits, they show slowing in their thinking, and their motor skills are impaired [53, 54]. Rates of depression are higher in schizophrenia, just as they are in subcortical syndromes [51]. Not all authors agree, however, that schizophrenia is characterized by subcortical dysfunction, and many investigations suggest that the cognitive dysfunction of schizophrenia is better accounted for by fronto-temporal dysfunction [55]. It is possible that, despite their differences, HD patients may develop neuropsychological deficits that resemble those in schizophrenia and this might provide the substrate for the development of psychotic symptoms in HD.

Treatment

The psychosis associated with HD usually responds to neuroleptic medication, which is also known to suppress the involuntary movements of HD [56]. Haloperidol, a potent dopamine D2 antagonist, has been one of the more commonly used drugs in the past. Because of its propensity for extrapyramidal side effects, a number of atypical drugs such as risperidone [56, 57], olanzapine [58] and sulpiride [59] have been tried, with good results generally reported in the literature. Doses of risperidone used are typically 2–4 mg/day, and equivalent doses are recommended for the other drugs. Clozapine may be used to treat the psychosis, but it has little beneficial effect on chorea except in high doses. Because adverse reactions are often encountered, clozapine should be used

with restraint in this patient group [60]. Patients generally need long-term treatment. Because the longitudinal course of psychosis in patients has not been well charted, firm recommendations are difficult to make. Irritability may also respond to atypical neuroleptics. HD patients may need treatment with other drugs such as antidepressants or antiepileptic drugs. GABA-ergic drugs such as benzodiazepines, baclofen, and valproic acid have not been noted to be beneficial for psychosis, motor disorder, or cognition. Newer drugs being developed for the disorder target the pathophysiological process. One such drug is cystamine, which is an inhibitor of transglutaminase and has been shown to reduce tremors and prolong life in mice with the mutant HD gene [61]. There are many other substances in clinical trials for HD, which include the antibiotic minocycline and the dietary supplement creatine [61].

Other trinucleotide repeat disorders

The trinucleotide disorders are broadly divided into two categories [33]: (i) the polyglutamine (polyQ) repeat disorders, in which the expanded polyQ component of the protein results in a toxic gain of function leading to neurodegeneration, the classic example being HD discussed above; and (ii) disorders in which the triplet repeats occur in an untranslated region of the gene, leading to various mechanisms, including gene suppression. These are summarized in Table 28.2.

The spinocerebellar ataxias (SCA) are a group of 25 disorders, eight of which are due to a triplet repeat disorder [33]. The SCA gene codes for ataxin. There has been much interest in the psychiatric features of SCA, which stems from the appreciation that the cerebellum makes a significant contribution to cognition [62, 63]. In a report of 133 patients with cerebellar degeneration, 30% had cognitive deficits and 41% had noncognitive psychiatric symptoms [64]. In a further report from the same group, 31 patients with spinocerebellar degeneration were compared with 29 healthy subjects [17]. The rate of all psychiatric disorders in the former was 77%, being predominantly mood disorder. One case of schizophrenia and two cases of psychotic disorder not otherwise specified were noted. The authors suggested that the psychosis might be a consequence of the cerebellar dysfunction leading to a "dysmetria" of thinking and pointed out to the studies of cerebellar dysfunction in schizophrenia [65]. Psychosis in cerebellar degenerative disorders has been reported by other authors as well [66], although the literature on this topic is limited.

The association of SCA with SLP further raises the issue of triplet repeats and their role in the genetics of schizophrenia. As mentioned above, this associa-tion has been of interest to geneticists and the field was reviewed in 2000 [67]. This review ruled out a major role for triplet repeats in the etiology of schizophre-nia, but did not rule out a modest role in a minority of cases. The field needs further work, as was discussed in Chapter 23 of this book.

References

1. Huntington G. On chorea. *Med Surg Rep*, 1872. **26**:317–21.

2. Folstein S. E., Chase G., Wahl W. E., *et al.* Huntington's disease in Maryland: clinical aspects of racial variation. *Am J Hum Genet*, 1987. **41**:168–79.

3. Bolt J. M. W. Huntington's chorea in the West of Scotland. *Br J Psychiatry*, 1970. **116**:259–70.

4. Evers-Kiebooms G., Nys K., Harper P., *et al.* Predictive DNA-testing for Huntington's disease and reproductive decision making: a European collaborative study. *Eur J Hum Genet*, 2002. **10**:167–76.

5. Lyon R. L. Huntington's chorea in the Moray Firth area. *Br Med J*, 1962. **1**:1301–6.

6. Wexler N. S., Bonilla E., Young A. B., *et al.* Huntington's disease in Venezuela and gene linkage. *Cytogenet Cell Genet*, 1984. **37**:605. (Abstract).

7. Gusella J. F., Wexler N. S., Conneally P. M., *et al.* A polymorphic DNA marker genetically linked to Huntington's disease. *Nature*, 1983. **306**:234–8.

8. Huntington's Disease Collaborative Research Group. A novel gene containing a trinucleotide repeat that is expanded and unstable on Huntington's disease chromosomes. *Cell*, 1993. **72**:971–83.

9. Morris M. Dementia and cognitive changes in Huntington's disease. *Adv Neurol*, 1995. **65**:187–200.

10. Saint-Cyr J. A., Taylor A. E., Lang A. E. Procedural learning and neostriatal dysfunction in man. *Brain*, 1988. **111**:941–59.

11. Shoulson I. Huntington's disease: cognitive and psychiatric features. *Neuropsychiatry Neuropsychol Behav Neurol*, 1990. **3**:15–22.

12. Butters N., Wolfe J., Granholm E., *et al.* An assessment of verbal recall, recognition and fluency abilities in patients with Huntington's disease. *Cortex*, 1986. **22**:11–32.

13. Brandt J., Folstein S. E., Folstein M. F. Differential cognitive impairment in Alzheimer's disease and Huntington's disease. *Ann Neurol*, 1988. **23**:555–61.

14. Brouwers P., Cox C., Martin A., *et al.* Differential perceptual-spatial impairment in Huntington's and Alzheimer's dementias. *Arch Neurol*, 1984. **41**:1073–6.

15. Diamond R., White R. F., Myers R. H., *et al.* Evidence of presymptomatic cognitive decline in Huntington's disease. *J Clin Exp Neuropsychol*, 1992. **14**:961–75.

16. Foroud T., Siemers E., Kleindorfer D., *et al.* Cognitive scores of carriers of Huntingont's disease gene compared to non-carriers. *Ann Neurol*, 1995. 37:657–64.

17. Leroi I., O'Hearn E., Marsh L., *et al.* Psychopathology in patients with degenerative cerebellar diseases: a comparison to Huntington's disease. *Am J Psychiatry*, 2002. **159**:1306–14.

18. Folstein S. E., Abbott M. H., Chase G. A., *et al.* The association of affective disorder with Huntington's disease in a case series and in families. *Psychol Med*, 1983. **13**:537–42.

19. Reed T. E., Chandler J. H. Huntington's chorea in Michigan: I. Demography and genetics. *Am J Hum Genet*, 1958. **10**:210–25.

20. Young A. B., Shoulson I., Penney J. B., *et al.* Huntington's disease in Venezuela: neurologic features and functional decline. *Neurology*, 1986. **36**:244–9.

21. Jernigan T. L., Salmon D. P., Butters N., *et al.* Cerebral structure on MRI. Part II: specific changes in Alzheimer's and Huntington's diseases. *Biol Psychiatry*, 1991. **29**:68–81.

22. Mazziotta J. C., Phelps M. E., Pahl J. J., *et al.* Reduced cerebral glucose metabolism in asymptomatic subjects at risk for Huntington's disease. *New Engl J Med*, 1987. **316**:357–62.

23. Smith F. W., Besson J. A. O., Gemmell H. G., *et al.* The use of technetium-99m-HMPAO in the assessment of patients with dementia and other neuropsychiatric conditions. *J Cereb Blood Flow Metab*, 1988. **8**:S116–22.

24. International Huntington Association (IHA) and the World Federation of Neurology (WFN) Research Group on Huntington's Chorea. Guidelines for the molecular genetics predictive test in Huntington's disease. *Neurology*, 1994. **44**:1533–6.

25. Schulman J. D., Black S. H., Handyside A., *et al.* Preimplantation genetic testing for Huntington disease and certain other dominantly inherited disorders. *Clin Genet*, 1996. **49**:57–8.

26. Kremer B., Goldberg P., Andrew S. E., *et al.* A worldwide study of the Huntington's disease mutation. The sensitivity and sensitivity of measuring CAG repeats. *N Engl J Med*, 1994. **330**:1401–6.

27. Margolis R. L., Ross C. A. Diagnosis of Huntington disease. *Clin Chem*, 2003. **49**:1726–32.

28. McInnis M. G. Anticipation: an old idea in new genes. *Am J Hum Genet*, 1996. **59**:973–9.

29. Duyao M., Ambrose C., Myers R., *et al.* Trinucleotide repeat length instability and age of onset in Huntington's disease. *Nat Genet*, 1993. **4**:387–92.

30. MacDonald M. E., Vonsattel J. P., Shrinidhi J., *et al.* Evidence for the GluR6 gene associated with younger onset age of Huntington's disease. *Neurology*, 1999. **47**:155–60.

31. Panas M., Avramopoulos D., Karadima0 G., *et al.* Apolipoprotein E and presenilin-1 genotypes in Huntington's disease. *J Neurol*, 1999. **246**:574–7.

32. Duyao M. P., Auerbach A. B., Ryan A., *et al.* Inactivation of the mouse Huntington's disease gene homolog Hdh. *Science*, 1995. **269**: 407–10.

33. Everett C. M., Wood N. W. Trinucleotide repeats and neurodegenerative disease. *Brain*, 2004. **127**:2385–405.

34. Folstein S. E., Chase G. A., Wahl W. E., *et al.* Huntington disease in Maryland: clinical aspects of racial variation. *Am J Hum Genet*, 1987. **41**:168–79.

35. Shiwach R. Psychopathology in Huntington's disease patients. *Acta Psychiatr Scand*, 1994. **90**:241–6.

36. Beckson M., Cummings J. L. Psychosis in basal ganglia disorders. *Neuropsychiatry Neuropsychol Behav Neurol*, 1992. **5**:126–31.

37. McHugh P. R., Folstein M. F. (1975). Psychiatric syndromes of Huntington's chorea. In *Psychiatric Aspects of Neurological Disease*, Benson D. F., Bulmer D. (Eds.). New York: Grune & Stratton, pp. 267–86.

38. Lovestone S., Hodgson S., Sham P., *et al.* Familial psychiatric presentation of Huntington's disease. *J Med Genet*, 1996. **33**:128–31.

39. Tsuang D., DiGiacomo L., Lipe H., *et al.* Familial aggregation of schizophrenia-like symptoms in Huntington's disease. *Am J Med Genet*, 1999. **81**:323–7.

40. Tsuang D., Almqvist E., Lipe H., *et al.* Familial aggregation of psychotic symptoms in Huntington's disease. *Am J Psychiatry*, 2000. **157**:1955–9.

41. Correa B. B., Xavier M., Guimaraes J. Association of

Huntington's Disease and schizophrenia-like psychosis in a Huntington's disease pedigree. *Clin Pract Epidemiol Ment Health*, 2006. **2**:1.

42. Basset A. S., Honer W. G. Evidence for anticipation in schizophrenia. *Am J Hum Genet*, 1994. **54**:864–70.

43. ODonovan M. C., Guy C., Craddock N., *et al.* Expanded CAG repeats in schizophrenia and bipolar disorder. *Nat Genet*, 1995. **10**:380–1.

44. Morris A. G., Gaitonde E., McKenna P. J., *et al.* CAG repeat expansions and schizophrenia: association with disease in females and with early age-at-onset. *Hum Mol Genet*, 1995. **4**:1957–61.

45. Rubinsztein D. C., Leggo J., Goodburn S., *et al.* Huntington's Disease (HD) gene CAG repeats in schizophrenic patients shows overlap of the normal and HD affected ranges but absence of correlation with schizophrenia. *J Med Genet*, 1994. **31**:690–3.

46. Jain S., Leggo J., De Lisi L. E., *et al.* Analysis of thirteen trinucleotide repeat loci as candidate genes for schizophrenia and bipolar disorder. *Am J Med Genet (Neuropsychiatr Genet)*, 1996. **67**:139–46.

47. MacMillan J. C., Snell R. G., Tyler A., *et al.* Molecular analysis and clinical correlations of the Huntington's disease mutation. *Lancet*, 1993. **342**:954–8.

48. Weigell-Weber M., Schmid W., Spiegel R. Psychiatric symptoms and CAG expansion in Huntington's disease. *Am J Med Genet*, 1996. **67**:53–7.

49. Wang S., Sun C. E., Walczak C. A., *et al.* Evidence for a susceptibility locus for schizophrenia on chromosome 6pter-p22. *Nat Genet*, 1995. **10**:41–6.

50. Riggins G. J., Lokey L. K., Chastain J. L., *et al.* Human genes containing polymorphic

trinucleotide repeats. *Nat Genet*, 1992. **2**:186–91.

51. Cummings J. L. Frontal-subcortical circuits and human behaviour. *Arch Neurol*, 1993. **50**:873–80.

52. Rajkowska G., Selemon L. D., Goldman-Rakic P. S. Neuronal and glial somal size in the prefrontal cortex: a postmortem morphometric study of schizophrenia and Huntington's disease. *Arch Gen Psychiatry*, 1998. **55**:215–24.

53. Gold J. M., Goldberg T. E., Weinberger D. R. Prefrontal function and schizophrenic symptoms. *Neuropsychiatry Neuropsychol Behav Neurol*, 1992. **5**:253–61.

54. Tamlyn D., McKenna P. J., Mortimer A. M., *et al.* Memory impairment in schizophrenia: its extent, affiliations and neuropsychological character. *Psychol Med*, 1992. **22**:101–15.

55. Hanes K. R., Andrewes D. G., Pantelis C., *et al.* Subcortical dysfunction in schizophrenia: comparison with Parkinson's disease and Huntington's disease. *Schizophr Res*, 1996. **19**: 121–8.

56. Dallocchio C., Buffa C., Tinelli C., *et al.* Effectiveness of risperidone in Huntington chorea patients. *J Clin Psychopharmacol*, 1999. **19**:101–3.

57. Parsa M. A., Szigethy E., Voci J. M., *et al.* Risperidone in treatment of choreoathetosis of Huntington's disease. *J Clin Psychopharmacol*, 1997. **17**:134–5.

58. Bogelman G., Hirschmann S., Modai I. Olanzapine and Huntington's disease. *J Clin Psychopharmacol*, 2001. **21**:245–6.

59. Reveley M. A., Dursum S. M., Andrews H. A. Comparative trial use of sulpiride and risperidone in Huntington's disease: a pilot study. *J Clin Psychopharmacol*, 1996. **10**:162–5.

60. van Vugt J., Siesling S., Vergeer M., *et al.* Clozapine versus placebo in Huntington's disease: a double blind randomised comparative study. *J Neurol Neurosurg Psychiatry*, 1997. **63**:35–9.

61. Karpuj M. V., Becher M. W., Springer J. E., *et al.* Prolonged survival and decreased abnormal movements in transgenic model of Huntington's Disease, with administration of the transglutaminase inhibitor cystamine. *Nat Med*, 2002. **8**:143–9.

62. Schmahmann J. D., Pandya D. N. The cerebrocerebellar system. *Int Rev Neurobiol*, 1997. **41**:31–60.

63. Schmahmann J. D., Sherman J. C. Cerebellar cognitive affective syndrome. *Int Rev Neurobiol*, 1997. **41**:433–40.

64. Leroi I., O'Hearn E., Margolis R. L. Psychiatric syndromes in cerebellar degeneration. *Int Rev Psychiatry*, 2001. **13**:323–9.

65. Andreasen N. C., Nopoulos P., O'Leary D. S., *et al.* Defining the phenotype of schizophrenia: cognitive dysmetria and its neural mechanisms. *Biol Psychiatry*, 1999. **46**:908–20.

66. Kutty I. N., Prendes J. L. Psychosis and cerebellar degeneration. *J Nerv Ment Dis*, 1981. **169**:390–1.

67. Vincent J. B., Paterson A. D., Strong E., *et al.* The unstable trinucleotide repeat story of major psychosis. *Am J Med Genet*, 2000. **97**:77–97.

29

Fahr's Disease and psychosis

Kim Burns and Henry Brodaty

Facts box

- Fahr's Syndrome and Fahr's Disease are characterized by radiological, neurological, cognitive, and psychiatric abnormalities, although variable presentations are described.

- Symmetrical, bilateral basal ganglia calcification (BGC) occurs without physical abnormalities.

- The underlying etiology and pathogeneses remain unclear.

- BGC occurs in many other conditions, suggesting a common pathogenic pathway.

- Psychotic symptoms include auditory and visual hallucinations, paranoid delusions or paranoid trends, ideas of reference, ideas of influence, catatonia, fugue states, and atypical features, such as complex perceptual distortions.

- Although a link between psychotic symptoms and basal ganglia pathology is supported, symptoms appear to be variable after the onset of neuronal damage and remission has been reported.

- Treatment is largely symptomatic.

- Patients may be particularly susceptible to neuroleptic malignant syndrome and extrapyramidal side effects with antipsychotic medication.

Fahr's Disease (FD) or idiopathic basal ganglia calcification (IBGC) is also known as bilateral striatopallidodentate calcinosis [1], morbus Fahr, striatopallidodentate calcification, and calcinosis nucleorum cerebri [2]. Manyam [3] quotes 35 different names for this syndrome. It is described as symmetrical, bilateral BGC without parathyroid dysfunction or physical abnormalities, generally hereditary with an autosomal dominant transmission [4]. IBGC is characterized by radiological, neurological, cognitive, and psychiatric abnormalities. However, a form of the disorder in which calcification is inherited independently of neurological, cognitive, and psychiatric symptoms has also been identified [5].

Fahr's Disease is variably differentiated from Fahr's Syndrome (FS), in which BGC occurs secondary to another disorder. The distinction may be immaterial, however, as psychiatric symptoms in both FD and syndrome are possibly mediated by basal ganglia (BG) dysfunction rather than the effects of the primary disorder. Intracranial calcification on CT scanning is indistinguishable between the two conditions [6, 7, 8] and FS and FD are also differentiated from "radiological" BGC without clinical features [9].

Prevalence and incidence

Fahr's Disease is a rare disorder [3], and an incidental finding of BGC does not equal FS [10]. BGC is a common finding on routine CT brain scans, estimated to occur in 0.93% of cases presenting for neuroimaging. Before the availability of CT scans, diagnosis was made based on skull roentgenogram or autopsy. The number of cases of intracranial calcifications diagnosed has increased with the advent of head CT scans [1].

Lauterbach [11] reviewed seven studies and found BGC in 274 of 29,484 cases [10, 12, 13, 14, 15, 16]. Kobari [17] reviewed three studies and found brain calcification in approximately 0.3 to 1.2% [12, 18, 19]. Reported rates of neurological abnormalities in patients with CT evidence of BGC vary between 0% [10] and 20% [13]. Logically, the prevalence of FS in the general population should be less than the 0.5% prevalence reported in patients receiving CT scans [2]. Although the true prevalence of FD is unknown, it is highly probable that it must be rarer still.

Basal ganglia

The basal ganglia are large subcortical nuclear masses grouped on the basis of their interconnections. Although there is some debate as to which structures should be included within the basal ganglia, it is generally agreed that the core components include the caudate nucleus, nucleus accumbens, putamen, and globus pallidus. The caudate nucleus and putamen together are called the striatum; the putamen and globus pallidus are together described as the lentiform nucleus [9, 20].

The basal ganglia play an important role in the regulation of mood, emotion, motivation, and cognition as well as motor control [20, 21]. They have a high metabolic rate, a peculiar vascular supply, and autoregulation facilitating increased vascular permeability [22, 23]. Functions include motor learning, sequencing and movements, attentional allocation and filtering, working memory, implicit learning, memory [9] and possibly reward processes [24].

Psychiatric symptoms, frequently seen in diseases of the basal ganglia such as Fahr's, Parkinson's, Wilson's, and Huntington's Diseases, are thought to be due to disruption of cortical-subcortical circuits mediated by the basal ganglia [25]. BGC may reflect or cause dysfunction of the basal ganglia-thalamo-cortical circuit that leads to these symptoms [26].

Etiology

Although FD has generally been considered to be idiopathic, genetics appears to play a part. An autosomal dominant pattern of inheritance has been described in 10 out of 11 families with familial IBGC [17, 27, 28, 29] and possibly an autosomal recessive pattern in one family [3, 30]. A linkage to chromosome 14q in a family with multiple affected members has been described, in which genetic anticipation was also found [31]. The associations between these abnormal phenotypes and abnormal genes remain unclear despite the mapping to chromosome 14q of a susceptibility locus for FD [5].

Pathogenesis and pathology

The key feature of FD is mineralization, especially calcification. Although other minerals are present, the calcium is radiopaque and present in the greatest quantities [3]. The cause of this is not known, although genetics play a part.

Lowenthal [32] set down criteria for the definition of FS (including FD), but these have not gained currency. The calcification must (i) have a characteristic distribution, involving at least the globus pallidus, with or without cerebellar calcification; (ii) be evident on CT, and (iii) be of sufficient size to be detected on a macroscopic pathological exam.

Although calcifications tend to occur in the dentate nuclei and basal ganglia, as well as the cerebellar and cerebral white matter [27], the most common distribution of calcification in FD is limited to the globus pallidus [25].

Chabot [4] subdivided FD according to the severity of the pathology: massive, affecting the pallidum, striatum, dentate nuclei; medium, affecting the pallidum and striatum; and mild, affecting the pallidum only.

Microscopically, calcifications generally develop within vessel walls and the perivascular space, ultimately extending toward neurons, which can remain undamaged for some time [4]. Progressive basal ganglia mineralization can compress the vessel lumen, thus initiating a cycle of impaired blood flow, neural tissue injury, and mineral deposition [22, 23]. The calcifications of the finer cerebral vessels are concentrated in the walls of arterioles and capillaries as well as in the perivascular parenchyma of the grey and white matter [Bamberger 1855 in 27, 33, 34, 35].

Calcifications are composed of not only calcium but also iron, zinc, and aluminum [36]. Additionally, basal ganglia concretions contain copper, magnesium, and potassium within an organic matrix [Hurst 1926 in 33, 37, 38, 39]. The mineral composition varies by anatomic site and proximity to vasculature [40]. Defective iron transport and free radical production may damage tissue, initiating calcification [41]. Calcium deposits appear to be deposited secondarily around a nidus composed of mucopolysaccharides and related substances [33, 34, 35]. When mineral deposits are extensive, "brain stones" develop [37].

At the microscopic level, basal ganglia (BG) concretions are recognized as basophilic globules tracking the vessel walls of arteries, arterioles, capillaries, and veins. Scanning electron microscopy has shown a connection between some of the spherical and hemispherical bodies that were formed in the adventitial cells of blood vessels and surrounding glial cells [42]. The intima of involved vessels is usually preserved but occasionally proliferates to narrow the lumen [37]. The pathophysiological mechanisms leading to calcification formation are unclear [32, 36]. Fahr-type calcification has been reported in several neurodegenerative disorders, such as diffuse neurofibrillary tangles with calcification and Alzheimer's Disease [43].

Clinical features

There is great variability in the presentation of FD. Although the condition presents most commonly with motor deficits, approximately 40% of those with the disease present with primarily cognitive and other psychiatric symptoms [11]. Clinical features are reported as individual or family case studies because the condition is rare. Inconsistency and latency of clinical features are thought to occur because calcification is often present for an extended period before neuronal impairment is evident [4]. In a study of 38 cases with FD, Manyam [1] found a significantly greater degree of calcification in symptomatic patients when compared to those who were asymptomatic. Konig [14] suggests that the time of occurrence of calcification may be important so that early-life depositions are associated with oligophrenia, later dates with various mood changes, and still later dates with dementia syndromes. Clinical features are described in the subsections that follow.

Psychiatric features

Psychosis and/or mood disorders may occur in combination with neurological symptoms [9]. Alternatively, subcortical lesions may appear with psychiatric symptoms without the concurrent involvement of motor circuits that produce clinically significant motor symptoms [44]. Psychotic symptoms include auditory and visual hallucinations, paranoid delusions or paranoid trends, ideas of reference, ideas of influence, catatonia, fugue states, and atypical features such as complex perceptual distortions [45, 46, 47, 48]. Although a link between psychotic symptoms and basal ganglia pathology is supported, symptoms appear to be variable after the onset of neuronal damage and remission has also been reported [4]. IBGC is also associated with a schizophrenia-like-psychosis [4, 7, 45, 49]. Chabot and colleagues [4] found that the risk of psychosis was proportional to the extent of calcification although Brodaty and colleagues [50] reported no significant association between the extent of BGC and psychiatric status.

Although the psychiatric manifestations of FD are varied, the most prominent are mood disorders occurring in 20%–30% of patients. These can include depression, mania, or bipolar disorder. Anxiety disorders are common, with up to 30% of patients presenting with obsessive-compulsive disorders [14, 51].

Neurological features

A variety of neurological manifestations have been described. Movement disorders such as parkinsonism, paresis, dystonia, and speech impairment are often present [9]. Extrapyramidal symptoms commonly include chorea and ataxia, although individuals may present with mixed extrapyramidal symptoms [37]. Pyramidal signs can also occur [27]. Other neurological features can include stroke-like events, tremor, myoclonus, spasticity, epileptic seizures, and coma [9]. The location of the calcification does not necessarily correlate with the neurological signs [7, 19, 28, 52, 53].

Cognitive features

Cognitive disorders such as apathy, amnesia, and dementia may be present [36]. FD may present as neurologically asymptomatic with pronounced cognitive and behavioral abnormalities [44, 54]. The dementia found in individuals with FD differs clinically, neuropsychologically, and pathologically from Alzheimer's Disease [21, 50], and, although typically progressive, it is of the fronto-subcortical type [4, 7, 9, 45]. The neuropathology of dementia associated with FD involves fronto-temporal atrophy, neocortical neurofibrillary tangles, and neuronal loss in the nucleus basalis of Meynert but senile plaques are absent [55]. Other features include calcareous deposition, white-matter demyelination, and fibrous gliosis [14]. Dementia has also been associated with centrum semiovale calcification [56].

Cognitive abnormalities include slow mentation, poor concentration and attention, as well as mild to moderate impairment of verbal and nonverbal memory with normal language, abstraction, construction, and praxis [57, 58]. Palilalia and dysarthria may be prominent [59]. Anterograde amnesia, attentional impairment, and severe disexecutive syndrome, including impairment in planning, problem solving, set shifting, flexibility, and divergent thinking, have also been reported [44]. Brodaty and colleagues [50] found no significant relationship between IBGC status and cognitive impairment or dementia. Konig [14] reported no direct associations in etiology, localization, volume, or symptoms except that extensive

BG sclerosis is associated with more severe mental deterioration.

Differential diagnosis

FD should be distinguished from incidentally found BGC with or without associated clinical neuropsychiatric features [11]. Principal causes of bilateral BGC include hypoparathyroidism, pseudohypoparathyroidism, and Albright's hereditary osteodystrophy [4]. Developmental defects should also be ruled out [27]. Brain CT scan is considered standard clinical practice and is sensitive in demonstrating minimal BGC calcification [60]. CT appears to be superior to MRI for evaluating the presence of mineral deposits in brain tissue. Radiological findings vary from barely detectable dust-like opacification to significant radiodensities [32]. Recognition of calcifications on CT scan is straightforward due to the high resolving capability of CT and because calcifications consist of hydroxyapatite similar to that of bones [27, 61]. Although MRI correlates better with functional impairment [27, 56], calcification signals may remain undetected on MRI scans when they are at an intermediary stage [62]. Hyperintense T2-weighted images may reflect a slowly progressive metabolic or inflammatory process that subsequently calcifies and is probably responsible for neurological deficits [56].

Causes of basal ganglia calcification

Basal ganglia calcification can occur in numerous different disorders (see Table 5, p. 75 in [37] for a comprehensive list). A summary of these falls into the following categories:

1. Neurological conditions, including CNS lupus [63, 64], tuberous sclerosis [65], early-onset Alzheimer's Disease [66], atypical senile dementia [67], motor neuron disease [68], myotonic muscular distrophy [69] and mitochondrial encephalopathies [70, 71].
2. Chemically induced or iatrogenic conditions, including therapeutic radiation [15, 65, 72], carbon monoxide poisoning [73, 74], lead intoxication [73], methotrexate treatment [15], and long-term anticonvulsant therapy [13, 75].
3. Metabolic conditions, including hypercalcemia [12, 29], hypoparathyroidism [76], pseudohypoparathyroidism [32, 59, 77], pseudo-pseudohypoparathyroidism [32, 59, 78],

Addison's Disease [74], and an inborn error of vitamin D metabolism (i.e., reduced 25-OH vitamin D_3 with normal levels of 1–25(OH)2 vitaminD_3) [79].
4. Genetic/congenital conditions, including birth anoxia [51, 80], oculocraniosomatic disease [81], and Down's Syndrome [66, 82]. Microencephaly, pigmentary macular degeneration, progeria, and abnormal calcium metabolism can also be associated with infantile and juvenile BGC [11].
5. Infectious and inflammatory conditions associated with BGC, including neurobrucellosis [83], congenital rubella [73], toxoplasmosis [73, 80], chorea [74], cerebral malaria [74], and encephalitis [74, 80]. BGC can also occur in patients with abnormal calcium metabolism in AIDS [84, 85].

Natural history and prognosis

Three forms of the disease have been described: a childhood form with onset in infancy and death within the first few years of life [86, 87]; an early-adult-onset type with presentation between 20 and 40 years of age and manifesting initially as a psychosis; and a late-onset variety typically presenting between the ages of 40 and 60 [7, 88].

The course of FD is characteristically slow and progressive. Neurological or psychiatric symptoms such as psychosis tend to precede cognitive decline. BGC may be detected before clinical symptoms develop. Individuals presenting with psychosis, for example, may develop dementia and motor disturbances later in life [58].

Treatment

Selective removal of deposited calcium from brain tissue is not possible; although calcium is the major mineral deposited, other minerals are also implicated [3]. Treatments with CNS-specific calcium channel blocking agents have been unsuccessful [Manyam unpublished in 3]. Likewise, no specific treatments to limit calcification progression are available apart from a theoretically appealing, yet unconfirmed report of improvement using chelators (xydifon, penicillamine, deferoxamine), antioxidants, and calcium antagonists [89]. Loeb [90] reports sustained symptomatic improvement in a case of familial idiopathic cerebral calcification with disodium etidronate, a bisphosphonate, without reduction in calcification. Although specific treatment for FD is unavailable, in the case of FS the primary causes should be treated [9].

Limited literature and few data on the appropriate treatment of psychiatric symptoms in FD are available to guide clinicians [11]. Patients may be particularly susceptible to neuroleptic malignant syndrome [88, 91] and extrapyramidal side effects with antipsychotic medication [92]. As yet, there are no systematically conducted controlled psychotropic treatment studies in FD [11].

Management

Aspects of management can be categorized according to symptoms. Testing and counseling for genetic susceptibility may be warranted; prenatal testing is unavailable and linkage testing is available on a research basis only [93].

For psychiatric symptoms, antipsychotics, antidepressants, general support, and psychotherapy, as indicated, may be helpful. Psychosis responds unpredictably to treatment and is, on occasion, unresponsive [7, 88, 94]. Neuroleptic medication should be used with caution as it may potentiate extrapyramidal symptoms [7]. Some success has been achieved with lithium in individuals whose symptoms have proven refractory to haloperidol [95]. Patients with IBGC and depression have been shown to respond to antidepressant treatments, including imipramine and ECT [11]. However, given the variable presence of increased intracranial pressure and the risk of seizures in this group, ECT may be ill advised [11]. Appropriate pharmacological treatment may improve symptoms of anxiety and obsessive-compulsive disorder [93].

Management of cognitive symptoms follows the general lines of dementia care, including support for families and referral to Alzheimer's associations. No reports are available on the use of cholinesterase inhibitors or memantine in FS or FD.

For neurological symptoms, physiotherapy and rehabilitation may be helpful. The response of parkinsonian features to levodopa therapy is generally poor, possibly because the parkinsonism arises from postsynaptic receptor site dysfunction and not decreased dopamine turnover [8]. A positive response to levodopa in limited cases has been attributed to the coexistence of IBGC and idiopathic Parkinson's Disease

[1]. Pharmacologic therapies typically used for movement disorders may alleviate dystonia and other involuntary movements. Appropriate antiepileptic medications should be prescribed for seizure control [93].

Implications for clinical practice

Fahr's Disease is an uncommon condition. Clinicians should consider the diagnosis in patients who present with (i) the characteristic triad of neurological, cognitive, and psychiatric symptoms; (ii) some of these symptoms and BGC on CT scan; or (iii) some of these symptoms, extrapyramidal signs, and poor response to antiparkinsonian treatment. A detailed family history can assist with diagnosis and may have implications for genetic counseling.

Suggestions for future research

Although FD is uncommon, it may provide a heuristic window. Further investigation of FD may contribute to the understanding of psychosis through the study of correlations between localized lesions, clinical symptoms, and cerebral imaging abnormalities in a homogeneous group. Such study is likely to further knowledge of the pathophysiology of the psychotic symptoms [4].

Research may focus on correlations between neuropsychiatric symptoms and genes, neuropathology and neuroimaging. Little is known about the longitudinal course of the disease, and long-term follow-up could elucidate the relationship between radiological changes and neuropsychiatric manifestations. Correlation of neuropsychiatric findings with disease stage, clinical signs, and radiologic, metabolic, physiologic, and pathologic markers of disease may add to the understanding of this condition [11].

Additionally, the efficacy and risks of neuropharmacologic and psychopharmacologic interventions in FD and the correlates of good and poor outcomes with these interventions remain to be defined [11]. Given the substantial number of conditions associated with BGC, it is likely that more conditions will be identified in the future. The importance of distinguishing chance associations from causal relationships should not be underestimated. Future research may determine which of these conditions cause FD [2].

References

1. Manyam B. V., Walters A. S., Narla K. R. Bilateral striopallidodentate calcinosis: clinical characteristics of patients seen in a registry. *Movement Disord*, 2001. **16**(2):258–64.

2. Lauterbach E. C. (2000). Fahr's syndrome. In *Psychiatric Management in Neurological Disease*, Lauterbach E. C. (Ed.). Washington, DC: American Psychiatric Publishing, Inc., pp. 137–78.

3. Manyam B. V. What is and what is not 'Fahr's disease.' *Parkinsonism Relat Disord*, 2005. **11**(2):73–80.

4. Chabot B., Roulland C., Dollfus S. Schizophrenia and familial idiopathic basal ganglia calcification: a case report. *Psychol Med*, 2001. **31**(4):741–7.

5. Brodaty H. M. P., Luscombe G., Kwok J. B., *et al.* Familial idiopathic basal ganglia calcification (Fahr's disease) without neurological, cognitive and psychiatric symptoms is not linked to the BGC1 locus on chromosome 14q. *Hum Genet*, 2002. **110**:8–14.

6. Cohen C. R., Duchesneau P. M., Weinstein M. A. Calcification of the basal ganglia as visualized by computed tomography. *Radiology*, 1980. **134**(1):97–9.

7. Cummings J. L., Gosenfeld L. F., Houlihan J. P., *et al.* Neuropsychiatric disturbances associated with idiopathic calcification of the basal ganglia. *Biol Psychiatry*, 1983. **18**(5): 591–601.

8. Klawans H. L., Lupton M., Simon L. Calcification of the basal ganglia as a cause of levodopa-resistant parkinsonism. *Neurology*, 1976. **26**(3):221–5.

9. Ring H. A., Serra-Mestres J. Neuropsychiatry of the basal ganglia. *J Neurol Neurosurg Psychiatry*, 2002. **72**(1):12–21.

10. Vles J. S. H., Lodder J., Van Der Lugt P. J. M. Clinical significance of basal ganglia calcifications detected by CT: A retrospective study of 33 cases. *Clin Neurol Neurosurg*, 1981. **83**(4):253–6.

11. Lauterbach E. C., Cummings J. L., Duffy J., *et al.* Neuropsychiatric correlates and treatment of lenticulostriatal diseases: a review of the literature and overview of research opportunities in Huntington's, Wilson's, and Fahr's diseases. A report of the ANPA Committee on Research. American Neuropsychiatric Association. [See comment.] *J Neuropsych Clin Neurosci*, 1998. **10**(3):249–66.

12. Harrington M. G., Macpherson P., McIntosh W. B., *et al.* The significance of the incidental finding of basal ganglia calcification on computed tomography. *J Neurol Neurosurg Psychiatry*, 1981. **44**(12):1168–70.

13. Kazis A. D. Contribution of CT scan to the diagnosis of Fahr's syndrome. *Acta Neurol Scand*, 1985. **71**(3):206–11.

14. Konig P. Psychopathological alterations in cases of symmetrical basal ganglia sclerosis. *Biol Psychiatry*, 1989. **25**(4):459–68.

15. Murphy M. J. Clinical correlations of CT scan-detected calcifications of the basal ganglia. *Ann Neurol*, 1979. **6**(6):507–11.

16. Stellamor K., Stellamor V. Roentgen diagnosis of Fahr's disease. *Rontgen-Blatter*, 1983. **36**(6):194–6.

17. Kobari M., Nogawa S., Sugimoto Y., *et al.* Familial idiopathic brain calcification with autosomal dominant inheritance. *Neurology*, 1997. **48**(3):645–9.

18. Forstl H., Krumm B., Eden S., *et al.* Neurological disorders in 166 patients with basal ganglia calcification: a statistical evaluation. *J Neurol*, 1992. **239**(1):36–8.

19. Koller W. C., Cochran J. W., Klawans H. L. Calcification of the basal ganglia: computerized tomography and clinical correlation. *Neurology*, 1979. **29**(3):328–33.

20. Pierri J. N., Lewis D. A. (2005). Functional neuroanatomy. In *Kaplan and Sadock's Comprehensive Textbook of Psychiatry*, Sadock B. J. and Sadock V. A. (Eds.). Philadelphia: Lippincott Williams & Wilkins.

21. Cummings J. L., Benson D. F. Subcortical dementia. Review of an emerging concept. *Arch Neurol*, 1984. **41**(8):874–9.

22. Bhimani S., Sarwar M., Virapongse C., *et al.* Computed tomography of cerebrovascular calcifications in postsurgical hypoparathyroidism. *J Comput Assist Tomogr*, 1985. **9**(1): 121–4.

23. Sarwar M., Ford K. Rapid development of basal ganglia calcification. *AJNR: Am J Neuroradiol*, 1981. **2**(1): 103–4.

24. Schultz W., Tremblay L., Hollerman J. R. Reward prediction in primate basal ganglia and frontal cortex. *Neuropharmacology*, 1998. **37**(4–5):421–9.

25. Shakibai S., Johnson J., Bourgeois J. Paranoid delusions and cognitive impairment suggesting Fahr's disease. *Psychosomatics*, 2005. **46**(6):569–72.

26. Aarsland D., Litvan I., Larsen J. P. Neuropsychiatric symptoms of patients with progressive supranuclear palsy and Parkinson's disease. *J Neuropsych Clin Neurosci*, 2001. **13**(1): 42–9.

27. Manyam B. V., Bhatt M. H., Moore W. D., *et al.* Bilateral stiopallidodentate calcinosis: cerebrospinal fluid, imaging, and electrophysiological studies. *Ann Neurol*, 1992. **31**:379–84.

28. Ellie E., Julien J., Ferrer X. Familial idiopathic striopallidodentate calcifications. *Neurology*, 1989. **39**(3):381–5.

29. Flint J., Goldstein L. H. Familial calcification of the basal ganglia: a case report and review of the literature. *Psychol Med*, 1992. **22**(3):581–95.

30. Smits M. G., Gabreels F. J., Thijssen H. O., *et al.* Progressive idiopathic strio-pallido-dentate calcinosis (Fahr's disease) with autosomal recessive inheritance. Report of three siblings. *Eur Neurol*, 1983. **22**(1):58–64.

31. Geschwind D. H., Loginov M., Stern J. M. Identification of a locus on chromosome 14q for idiopathic basal ganglia calcification (Fahr disease). *Am J Hum Genet*, 1999. **65**(3):764–72.

32. Lowenthal A. (1986). Striopallidodentate calcifications. In *Handbook of Clinical Neurology*, Vol 5(49), Vinken P. J. and Bruyn G. W. (Eds.). Amsterdam: John Wiley & Sons, Inc., pp. 417–36.

33. Adachi M., Wellmann K. F., Volk B. W. Histochemical studies on the pathogenesis of "idiopathic non-arteriosclerotic cerebral calcification." *J Neuropathol Exper Neurol*, 1968. **27**(1):153–4.

34. Friede R. L., Magee K. R., Mack E. W. Idiopathic nonarteriosclerotic calcification of cerebral vessels. Fahr's disease – a clinical and histochemical study. *Arch Neurol*, 1961. **5**:279–86.

35. Neumann M. A. Iron and calcium dysmetabolism in the brain with special predilection for globus pallidus and cerebellum. *J Neuropath Exp Neurol*, 1963. **22**:184–68.

36. Lowenthal A., Bruyn G. W. (1968). Calcification of the striopallidodendate system. In *Handbook of Clinical Neurology, Disease of the Basal Ganglia*, Vol 6, Vinken P. J. and Bruyn G. W. (Eds.). Amsterdam: North-Holland Publishing Company, pp. 703–25.

37. Casanova M. F., Araque J. M. Mineralization of the basal ganglia: implications for neuropsychiatry, pathology and neuroimaging. *Psychiatry Res*, 2003. **121**(1):59–87.

38. Duckett S., Galle P., Escourolle R., *et al.* Presence of zinc, aluminum, magnesium in striopalledodentate (SPD) calcifications (Fahr's disease): electron probe study. *Acta Neuropathol*, 1977. **38**(1):7–10.

39. Smeyers-Verbeke J., Michotte Y., Pelsmaeckers J., *et al.* The chemical composition of idiopathic nonarteriosclerotic cerebral calcifications. *Neurology*, 1975. **25**(1):48–57.

40. Bouras C., Giannakopoulos P., Good P. F., *et al.* A laser microprobe mass analysis of trace elements in brain mineralizations and capillaries in Fahr's disease. *Acta Neuropathol*, 1996. **92**(4):351–7.

41. Beall S. S., Patten B. M., Mallette L., *et al.* Abnormal systemic metabolism of iron, porphyrin, and calcium in Fahr's syndrome. *Ann Neurol*, 1989. **26**(4):569–75.

42. Kobayashi S., Yamadori I., Miki H., *et al.* Idiopathic nonarteriosclerotic cerebral calcification (Fahr's disease): an electron microscopic study. *Acta Neuropathol*, 1987. **73**(1):62–6.

43. Fujita D., Terada S., Ishizu H., *et al.* Immunohistochemical examination on intracranial calcification in neurodegenerative diseases. *Acta Neuropathol*, 2003. **105**(3):259–64.

44. Benke T., Karner E., Seppi K., *et al.* Subacute dementia and imaging correlates in a case of Fahr's disease. *J Neurol Neurosurg Psychiatry*, 2004. **75**(8):1163–5.

45. Lauterbach E. C., Spears T. E., Prewett M. J., *et al.* Neuropsychiatric disorders, myoclonus, and dystonia in calcification of basal ganglia pathways. *Bio Psychiatry*, 1994. **35**(5):345–51.

46. Rosenberg D. R., Neylan T. C., el-Alwar M., *et al.* Neuropsychiatric symptoms associated with idiopathic calcification of the basal ganglia. *J Nerv Ment Dis*, 1991. **179**(1):48–9.

47. Wodarz N., Becker T., Deckert J. Musical hallucinations associated with post-thyroidectomy hypoparathyroidism and symmetric basal ganglia calcifications. [See comment.] *J Neurol Neurosurg Psychiatry*, 1995. **58**(6):763–4.

48. Hall P. Calcification of the basal ganglia apparently presenting as a schizophreniform psychosis. *Postgrad Med J*, 1972. **48**:636–9.

49. Fernandez-Bouzas A., Angrist B., Hemdal P., *et al.* Basal ganglia calcification in schizophrenia. *Biol Psychiatry*, 1990. **27**(6):682–5.

50. Brodaty H., Mitchell P., Luscombe G., *et al.* Familial idiopathic basal ganglia calcification (Fahr's disease) without neurological, cognitive and psychiatric symptoms is not linked to the IBGC1 locus on chromosome 14q. *Hum Genet*, 2002. **110**:8–14.

51. Lopez-Villegas D., Kulisevsky J., Deus J., *et al.* Neuropsychological alterations in patients with computed tomography-detected basal ganglia calcification. *Arch Neurol*, 1996. **53**(3):251–6.

52. Henkelman R. M., Watts J. F., Kucharczyk W. High signal intensity in MR images of calcified brain tissue. *Radiology*, 1991. **179**(1):199–206.

53. Taxer F., Haller R., Konig P. Clinical early symptoms and CT findings in Fahr syndrome. *Nervenarzt*, 1986. **57**(10):583–8.

54. Modrego P. J., Mojonero J., Serrano M., *et al.* Fahr's syndrome presenting with pure and progressive presenile dementia. *Neurol Sci*, 2005. **26**(5):367–9.

55. Shibayama H., Kobayashi H., Nakagawa M., *et al.* Non-Alzheimer non-Pick dementia with Fahr's syndrome. *Clin Neuropathol*, 1992. **11**(5): 237–50.

56. Avrahami E., Cohn D. F., Feibel M., *et al.* MRI demonstration and CT correlation of the brain in patients with idiopathic intracerebral calcification. *J Neurol*, 1994. **241**(6):381–4.

57. Chiu H. F., Lam L. C., Shum P. P., *et al.* Idiopathic calcification of the basal ganglia. *Postgrad Med J*, 1993. **69**(807):68–70.

58. Cummings J. L., Benson D. F. (1992). *Dementia: a Clinical Approach*. Boston: Butterworth-Heinemann.

59. Boller F., Boller M., Denes G., *et al.* Familial palilalia. *Neurology*, 1973. **23**(10):1117–25.

60. Puvanendran K., Low C. H., Boey H. K., *et al.* Basal ganglia calcification on computer tomographic scan. A clinical and radiological correlation. *Acta Neurol Scand*, 1982. **66**(3):309–15.

61. Faria A. V., Pereira I. C., Nanni L. Computerized tomography findings in Fahr's syndrome. *Arq neuropsiquiatr*, 2004. **62**(3B): 789–92.

62. Scotti G., Scialfa G., Tampieri D., *et al.* MR imaging in Fahr Disease. *J Comput Assist Tomogr*, 1985. **9**(4):790–2.

63. Matsumoto R., Shintaku M., Suzuki S., *et al.* Cerebral perivenous calcification in neuropsychiatric lupus erythematosus: a case report. *Neuroradiology*, 1998. **40**(9): 583–6.

64. Nordstrom D. M., West S. G., Andersen P. A. Basal ganglia calcifications in central nervous system lupus erythematosus. *Arthritis Rheum*, 1985. **28**(12):1412–6.

65. Legido A., Zimmerman R. A., Packer R. J., *et al.* Significance of basal ganglia calcification on computed tomography in children. *Pediatr Neurosci*, 1988. **14**(2):64–70.

66. Mann D. M. Calcification of the basal ganglia in Down's syndrome and Alzheimer's disease. *Acta Neuropathol*, 1988. **76**(6):595–8.

67. Tsuchiya K., Nakayama H., Iritani S., *et al.* Distribution of basal ganglia lesions in diffuse neurofibrillary tangles with calcification: a clinicopathological study of five autopsy cases. *Acta Neuropathol*, 2002. **103**(6):555–64.

68. Eleopra R., Accurti I., Neri W., *et al.* Unusual case of Fahr syndrome with motoneuron disease. *Ital J Neurol Sci*, 1991. **12**(6):597–600.

69. Kusunose Y., Taniguchi T., Yamada M., *et al.* Two siblings of myotonic muscular dystrophy associated with basal ganglia calcification. *Rinsho Shinkeigaku – Clinical Neurology*, 1987. **27**(10):1276–9.

70. Markesbery W. R. Lactic acidemia, mitochondrial myopathy, and basal ganglia calcification. *Neurology*, 1979. **29**(7):1057–60.

71. Yoda S., Terauchi A., Kitahara F., *et al.* Neurologic deterioration with progressive CT changes in a child with Kearns-Shy syndrome. *Brain Dev*, 1984. **6**(3):323–7.

72. Lee K. F., Suh J. H. CT evidence of grey matter calcification secondary to radiation therapy. *Comput Tomogr*, 1977. **1**(1): 103–10.

73. Philpot M. P., Lewis S. W. The psychopathology of basal ganglia calcification. *Behav Neurol*, 1989. **2**:227–34.

74. Kalamboukis Z., Molling P. Symmetrical calcification of the brain in the predominance in the basal ganglia and cerebellum. *J Neuropathol Exp Neurol*, 1962. **21**:364–71.

75. Ogata A., Ishida S., Wada T. A survey of 37 cases with basal ganglia calcification (BGC): CT-scan findings of BGC and its relationship to underlying diseases and epilepsy. *Acta Neurol Scand*, 1987. **75**(2):117–24.

76. Palubinskas A. J., Davies H. Calcification of the basal ganglia of the brain. *Am J Roentgenol, Radium Ther Nucl Med*, 1959. **82**:806–22.

77. Macgregor M. E., Whitehead T. P. Pseudo-hypoparathyroidism; a description of three cases and a critical appraisal of earlier accounts of the disease. *Arch Dis Child*, 1954. **29**(147):398–418.

78. Foley J. Calcification of the corpus stiatum and dentate nuclei occurring in a family. *J Neurol Neurosurg Psychiatry*, 1951. **14**(4):253–61.

79. Martinelli P., Giuliani S., Ippoliti M., *et al.* Familial idiopathic strio-pallido-dentate calcifications with late onset extrapyramidal syndrome. *Mov Disord*, 1993. **8**(2):220–2.

80. Moskowitz M. A., Winickoff R. N., Heinz E. R. Familial calcification of the basal ganglions: a metabolic and genetic study. *New Engl J Med*, 1971. **285**(2):72–7.

81. Seigel R. S., Seeger J. F., Gabrielsen T. O., *et al.* Computed tomography in oculocranio-somatic disease (Kearns-Sayre syndrome). *Radiology*, 1979. **130**(1):159–64.

82. Takashima S., Becker L. E. Basal ganglia calcification in Down's Syndrome. *J Neurol Neurosurg Psychiatry*, 1985. **48**(1):61–4.

83. Mousa A. M., Muhtaseb S. A., Reddy R. R., *et al.* The high rate of prevalence of CT-detected basal ganglia calcification in neuropsychiatric (CNS) brucellosis. *Acta Neurol Scand*, 1987. **76**(6):448–56.

84. Fenelon G., Gray F., Paillard F., *et al.* A prospective study of patients with CT detected pallidal

calcifications. *J Neurol Neurosurg Psychiatry*, 1993. **56**(6):622–5.

85. Belman A. L., Lantos G., Horoupian D., *et al.* AIDS: calcification of the basal ganglia in infants and children. *Neurology*, 1986. **36**:1192–9.

86. Babbitt D. P., Tang T., Dobbs J., *et al.* Idiopathic familial cerebrovascular ferrocalcinosis (Fahr's disease) and review of differential diagnosis of intracranial calcification in children. *Am J Roentgenol Radium Ther Nucl Med*, 1969. **105**(2):352–8.

87. Melchoir J. C., Bende C. E., Yakovlev P. I. Familial idiopathic cerebral calcifications in childhood. *Am Med Assoc J Dis Child*, 1960. **99**:787–803.

88. Francis A. F. Familial basal ganglia calcification and schizophreniform psychosis. *Br J Psychiatry*, 1979. **135**:360–2.

89. Skvortsov I. A., Rudenskaia G. E., Karaseva A. N., *et al.* Effectiveness of the therapeutic use of complexones in various diseases of the extrapyramidal system in children. *Zh Nevropatol Psikhiat Im S S Korsakova*, 1987. **87**(10):1457–62.

90. Loeb J. A. Functional improvement in a patient with cerebral calcinosis using a bisphosphonate. *Mov Disord*, 1998. **13**(2):345–9.

91. Francis A., Freeman H. Psychiatric abnormality and brain calcification over four generations. *J Nerv Ment Dis*, 1984. **172**(3):166–70.

92. Trautner R. J., Cummings J. L., Read S. L., *et al.* Idiopathic basal ganglia calcification and organic mood disorder. *Am J Psychiatry*, 1988. **145**(3):350–3.

93. Sobrido M. J., Hopfer S., Geschwind D. H. Familial idiopathic basal ganglia calcification, 2004

94. Callender J. S. Non-progressive familial idiopathic intracranial calcification: a family report. *J Neurol Neurosurg Psychiatry*, 1995. **59**(4):432–4.

95. Munir K. M. The treatment of psychotic symptoms in Fahr's Disease with lithium carbonate. *J Clin Psychopharmacol*, 1986. **6**(1):36–8.

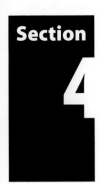

Related concepts

The Charles Bonnet Syndrome

30

William Burke

- The syndrome is named after Charles Bonnet who first described complex visual hallucinations in a normal person, his grandfather.
- The essential feature is the occurrence of simple and complex visual hallucinations (VHs) in the absence of a psychiatric disorder.
- Most cases are due to damage to some part of the visual system.
- A deafferentation hypersensitivity model best explains the syndrome.
- There are reasons to believe that complex hallucinations are generated in a part of the cerebral cortex extending from superior temporal cortex ventrally to the parahippocampal gyrus.
- The hallucinations are usually pleasant or neutral and eventually disappear, although complex hallucinations may last several years.
- In some cases, the hallucinations seem to be the first signs of dementia.

Introduction

The syndrome takes its name from Charles Bonnet, a biologist and philosopher of science, who in 1760 described the hallucinations experienced by his grandfather Charles Lullin [1]. Lullin had cataracts removed from both eyes and, although the operations were at first successful, eventually at the age of 89 years he became completely blind in one eye and had very little sight in the other. He then developed visual hallucinations (VHs). As described by Bonnet, Lullin saw before him "figures of men and women, birds, carriages, battlements…He saw these figures make different movements, approach, move

away, vanish…he saw battlements rise up before his eyes…The tapestries in his apartment seemed to him to change suddenly into tapestries of a different style…All the images seemed…made of a perfect clarity…as if the objects were actually there…But no sound reached his ears…This…respectable…old man…full of health…of intact memory…does not at all take these visions for reality" [1]. Bonnet stressed the mental normality of his grandfather.

Although there were many reports of visual hallucinations in the nineteenth century, most of these were due to lesions of the brain and were often associated with other signs such as epilepsy and stroke [2]. In the twentieth century, interest in this phenomenon slowly increased. The eponym "Charles Bonnet Syndrome" was introduced in 1936 by de Morsier in recognition of the contribution of his fellow Genovese [3]. In 1967, de Morsier [4] summarized the main papers up to that time (18 cases), but even as late as 1989, only about 46 cases had been reported [5]. Since then, there has been an escalation of interest, research, and publications on the topic. In recent years, there have been several reviews of the literature [6, 7, 8, 9].

Definition

The simplest definition of Charles Bonnet Syndrome (CBS) is that it consists of VHs in a patient who is psychologically normal and has full cognition and insight, that is, realizes that the hallucinations are not real, even if initially he is fearful that he might be "going mad." These cases can be subdivided into three groups. The largest group (group A) consists of cases in which there is visual impairment and apparently no other contributory factor. In the second group (group B), there is visual impairment but the occurrence of VHs is dependent on another factor or "trigger." In the third group (group C), there is no visual impairment but VHs are triggered in a variety of ways. There are many other classifications [4, 8, 10].

Visual impairment includes any injury from retina to extrastriate cortex but also includes light restriction as in corneal scarring or cataract. The commonest conditions are age-related macular degeneration (AMD), glaucoma, and cataract [8, 11]. Other conditions are optic neuritis [12], enucleation of the eye [13], retinitis pigmentosa [14], diabetic retinopathy [11], corneal disease [11], destruction of optic nerves by tumor [15], macular photocoagulation [16], macular translocation [17], and occipital lobe damage [18, 19].

Three other types of visual "hallucinations" may be included in group A. Photopsias are flashes of light or the appearance of small simple discs of light, usually white but sometimes colored, generally ascribed to some irritation in the retina. Palinopsia refers to the abnormal persistence of a visual image. This is not an after-image, however, because there is no reversal of luminance or color. Although palinopsia occurs in patients with visual impairment, it has also been reported in people with normal vision [20]. Visual "auras" occur in association with migraine but can also occur independently [21, 22, 23]. The commonest type is referred to as "fortifications" because of a fancied resemblance to castles. The multicolored zigzags spread from the point of gaze out to the periphery of the visual field in 20 to 30 minutes. It is believed to be due to a form of "spreading depression," partly because there is total blindness in the wake of the zigzags [22]. Photopsias, palinopsia, and auras are not usually included in the CBS category.

Trigger factors capable of generating VHs in patients with visual impairment include: tramadol (an opioid) in a patient with diabetic retinopathy [24], opioids (morphine) in a patient with retinitis pigmentosa [25], laser iridotomy in a patient with glaucoma [26], brimonidine in eye drops used for glaucoma [27], social isolation [28], and strong emotional states, for example, bereavement [29].

Finally, group C consists of cases without visual impairment but in which VHs occur. Of course, there are many drugs (hallucinogens) whose main effect is to cause hallucinations [30]. In addition, several other drugs, not regarded as hallucinogens, may cause VHs in certain circumstances. Very often, they are medicaments being given for another condition, for example, drugs acting on the GABAergic system of the brain such as digoxin [31, 32], estrogen [33], or drugs used to treat Parkinson's, such as amantadine [34] or amitriptyline [28]. Certain nonvisual diseases are capable of inducing VHs, for example, migraine

[35], HIV [36], predementia Alzheimer's [6], Parkinsons's [37, 38, 39], and pineal tumor [40]. Whole brain radiation therapy following removal of a metastatic adenocarcinoma near the right cuneus caused the emergence of hallucinations consisting of memories of distinct people and events [41]. These were unlike the typical CBS hallucinations and more like the experiential recollections described by Penfield and Perot [42]. Perceptual isolation can lead to VHs [43, 44, 45]. Isolation and life-threatening stress (e.g., among hostages) can also cause hallucinations [46]. De Morsier [4] thought that CBS was a disease of old age. However, there are now several well-attested cases of CBS in children [47, 48, 49]. Nevertheless, because visual disease is commoner in old people, likewise, CBS is more evident.

Some investigators would restrict CBS to groups A and B [8]. This is a matter of choice. The existence of group C is not in doubt. The clearest example of this is the occurrence of VHs in normal people who have been blindfolded for a day or more [50, 51, 52].

Attempts have been made to exclude visual defects as a critical factor [4, 6]. For example, some CBS patients have normal visual acuity, such as in some cases of cerebral infarct [53] and cases of glaucoma. This argument is faulty because acuity is not an adequate measure of visual impairment [54]. The lists of conditions given here for groups A, B, and C are not exhaustive.

Simple and complex hallucinations

Most writers [6, 8, 55] specify that the VHs be "complex" to be regarded as CBS. By this is meant that the patient sees elaborate visions of people, animals, various identifiable objects, scenery, buildings, text, and so on. It is now clear that simpler visions also occur, such as rotating discs of light and simple auras, leaves, branching structures, geometrical arrangements, such as chess boards, netting, egg crates, and tessellations – often depicted as lines crisscrossing at right angles (Figure 30.1). Sometimes the elements separate into lozenges or tiles. These simpler hallucinations are less obvious to the patient and may not be very different to after-images. Because they are less dramatic than the complex hallucinations, do not move, may be small or faint, and may be short lasting, they are not always reported by the patient. Nevertheless, many patients experience both simple and complex VHs and it is possible that they have a common origin. The patient

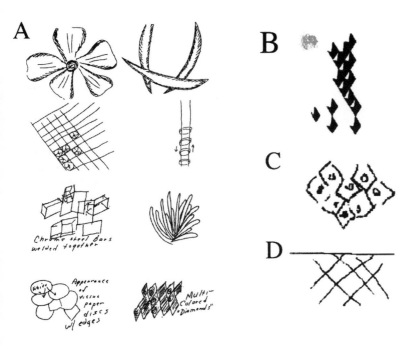

Figure 30.1 Examples of simple hallucinations. A. Sketches by patient with occipital lobe damage (from [19]). B. Sketch by patient with right occipital infarct; rhomboids are about 0.5° in size and appear in the left visual field (from [56]). C. Hallucinations from two patients with eye disease (from [57]).

should be carefully questioned and shown some examples of these "simple" hallucinations.

An important feature of central visual pathways is that the lower-order cortical areas, especially V1 to V5, are strictly visuotopic (retinotopic). This is true but to a much coarser degree for the higher-order areas [58, 59], where cells become specialized for the detection of complex features, such as faces, buildings, tools, text, and scenery. The cells in these areas may not be insensitive to simpler stimuli, but they are much more sensitive to particular objects. It is likely, therefore, that the simpler geometric hallucinations have closer ties with the lower-order visual areas. This idea finds support in my own observations [60]. These were made following the occurrence of a macular hole (foveal retinal detachment) in each of my eyes at the same time. These hallucinations (Figure 30.2) were small and faint but quite clear and occurred in overlapping sequence A → B → C over a period of 10 to 12 days.

When the primate visual area V1 is stained for cytochrome oxidase, it is characterized by orderly rows of "blobs" with an arrangement both qualitatively and quantitatively similar to that of the "spots" shown in Figure 30.2B. Similarly, when visual area V2 is stained, it reveals an arrangement of stripes closely resembling in dimensions the brickwork shown in Figure 30.2A. Cytochrome oxidase is an indicator of high metabolic rate and might be expected to signal the

areas where spontaneous activity was high. The conclusion may therefore be reached that these geometric hallucinations are due to increased activity in V1 and V2, even if the perceptive process occurs at a higher level.

An extension of this line of thought is that the observed hallucination will be determined by the highest level in the visual pathway at which there is "marked" spontaneous activity. In some way, the brain must distinguish this "marked" activity from ordinary ongoing spontaneous activity. It may be that the "marking" is achieved by a "bursting" pattern, which is capable of reaching a threshold in the perceptual process that cannot be reached by the ordinary spontaneous activity [9]. Bursty firing is well known to exert powerful transmission effects [61]. The electroencephalogram during hallucinations in patients with damage to the occipital lobe may [62] or may not [19, 63] show epileptiform discharges. Nevertheless, it has been repeatedly shown that isolated cortex becomes epileptogenic [64, 65].

A further elaboration of these ideas is to suggest that the more extensive the damage to the visual system, the higher in the visual hierarchy does the increased spontaneous activity extend and the more likely it is that the hallucinations will be complex. Leaves and branching structures might be located higher than brick walls; people and buildings would be

A

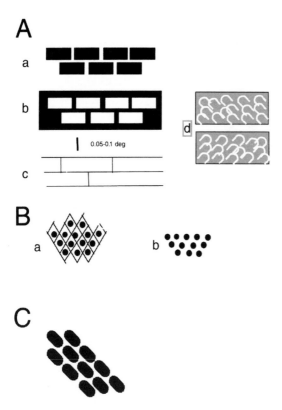

B

C

Figure 30.2 Sketches of portions of hallucinations seen by the author over a period of 10–12 days following a macular hole in each eye. The hallucinations appeared in the sequence A, B, C with some overlap. Those shown in Ad have persisted for several years and may be generated in the lateral geniculate nucleus where reinnervation may occur less readily. (From [60], with permission.)

in the highest regions. However, the evidence to date does not support this idea [66, 67]. It may be that the progression through the visual cortex from simple to complex is dependent on the ability of the cortical neurons to emit marked spontaneous discharges, and this ability would vary in different individuals.

Theories of hallucination generation

There are two broad theories of hallucination generation [68]. The first theory, the "Perception and Attention Deficit Model" [69], proposes that there is both impaired attention and poor sensory activation and the interaction between the two leads to hallucinations. This model may be appropriate for the hallucinations of schizophrenia and some other hallucinations, although a case has been made out for a deafferentation model here also [70]. The second model emphasizes the "deafferentation syndrome" aspect [18, 68, 71]. It

is this second model, which is appropriate for CBS, and which I will explore in detail. Simply stated, the deafferentation theory proposes that deafferentation leads to hypersensitivity at the deafferented synapses and this leads to increased spontaneous activity that is the neural basis of the hallucinations. The fact that low contrast sensitivity is a strong risk factor for CBS also supports this theory [72].

The deafferentation syndrome model has been most successful when applied to the somatosensory system, the best example being the "phantom limb" phenomenon. When a patient loses a limb, the neurons in the cerebral cortex that normally receive input from the limb are still there and undamaged. Therefore, if by any means they are excited, they will signal that the limb is being touched or stimulated in some way. It is irrelevant how the cortical neurons are excited; as a result of deafferentation, they are likely to become spontaneously active and this activity will create the phantom. The theory was probably even more successful in explaining the anomalies in pain sensation, for example, how pain can be increased when the number of pain receptors is decreased [73]. Deafferentation in the auditory system can lead to tinnitus and hallucinations [74, 75, 76]. Occasionally, a combination of visual and hearing loss leads to both visual and auditory hallucinations [77]. The fact that hallucinations can occur in other sensory modalities in the absence of psychiatric involvement suggests that the term "CBS" might reasonably be applied to these occurrences also but this is not the case at present.

Hallucinations could depend on a purely excitatory effect or there could be removal of a maintained inhibition, a "disinhibition." Cogan [35] classified visual hallucinations into "irritative" and "release." The former were compared to an "epileptic" or "ictal" attack, whereas the latter was presumably a disinhibition. In fact, we do not usually have enough information to decide between these two alternatives or even to determine if they are alternatives. For convenience, I will concentrate on the purely excitatory model, always remembering that other possibilities exist.

Several synapses, some from the mammalian central nervous system, some from elsewhere, have been studied in great detail under conditions in which the inputs have been varied widely. There has been a large measure of agreement between the different reports. Total silencing of the input to a synapse leads to the following presynaptic changes: increases in the size of the terminal bouton, in the total number of vesicles, in

Table 30.1 Cortical areas with increased sensitivity to specific visual stimuli

Name of area	Acronym	Anatomy	Stimulus/function	Reference
Fusiform face area	FFA	Fusiform gyrus	Faces	Kanwisher et al., 1997 [84]
Parahippocampal place area	PPA	Parahippocampal gyrus	Scenery	Epstein and Kanwisher, 1998 [85]
Superior temporal sulcus face area	STS-FA	Superior temporal sulcus	Movements of the eyes and mouth	Perrett et al., 1982, 1985 [86, 87] Puce et al., 1998 [88]
Extrastriate body area	EBA	Lateral occipitotemporal cortex	Whole body	Downing et al., 2001 [89]
Lateral occipital complex	LOC	Lateral and ventral occipital cortex	Analysis of object structure	Kourtzi and Kanwisher, 2000 [90]
Visual word form area	VWFA	Left ventral occipitotemporal sulcus	Text	Cohen and Dehaene, 2004 [91]

the number of docked vesicles, in the size of the release zone, in the size of the readily releasable pool, and in the release probability [72]. Postsynaptically silencing of the synapse causes "externalization" of synaptic receptors that become "internalized" when synaptic traffic increases [79, 80, 81, 82]. The postsynaptic membrane also shows greater electric excitability during disuse of the synapse [65]. All of these changes point in the same direction: increased excitability of the synapse during deafferentation. In certain conditions, this may lead to increased spontaneous activity.

Most neurons in the visual system are binocular. Therefore, these are deafferented only when the inputs from the corresponding parts of both eyes are lost. However, most neurons in the lateral geniculate nucleus are monocular, and in cortical area V1, there are monocular neurons activated only from contralateral nasal retina. Before the extent of deafferentation can be judged, it is necessary to have a detailed knowledge of the position and size of the lesion. This is seldom possible. When the damage is in the cerebral cortex, the more anterior the lesion, the less likely will there be any hallucinations [63]; this may be because the chance of deafferentation is less.

Site of complex hallucinations

There is now evidence from separate types of study strongly suggesting that complex VHs are generated in visual areas in the temporal lobe of the cerebral cortex and some adjacent regions. The evidence is threefold. First, electrical stimulation of the ventral superior, middle, and inferior temporal gyri; of the inferior parietal lobule; and of the fusiform and parahippocampal gyri in the conscious patient causes an awakening of memories of people, animals, and scenes [42].

Second, functional magnetic resonance imaging (fMRI) from hallucinating patients has revealed increased activity in ventral temporal lobe, with one patients hallucinating faces showing heightened activity in the fusiform gyrus of the ventral occipital lobe [83].

Lastly, in this general region, several areas have been delineated as containing neurons with increased sensitivity to specific visual stimuli (Table 30.1). These areas have been mapped using fMRI or positron emission tomography (PET) technology or direct recording from individual neurons.

The FFA seems to be the same as the area mentioned in the last-but-one paragraph and is probably concerned with facial recognition, whereas the STS-FA is more related to facial expression [92]. The areas described by Wicker and colleagues [93] as concerned with gaze would have included STS-FA. Lesion of the VWFA causes alexia but may also lead to VHs consisting of grammatically correct, meaningful written sentences or phrases [94]. The patient cannot read but can hear and write correctly what she hears. There is evidently an area in this region deafferented by the lesion in the VWFA, possibly the anterior fusiform area described by Nobre and colleagues [95] or part of the cortical area associated with auditory hallucinations because of the resemblance of the hallucinations to those experienced by schizophrenics [94].

The conclusion from these three separate approaches is that complex VHs are closely associated with increased activity in a region of cortex extending from superior temporal cortex ventrally to the parahippocampal gyrus and probably originate in one or other part of this region. There is no reason why this conclusion should not apply to all VHs, whatever their etiology. However, each patient has a unique pattern of hallucinations and it is not surprising that these differ from the images created by the highly abnormal electrical stimulation of the brain or from mental imagery [52]. The view presented here is radically different from that of Weinberger and Grant [66], who denied any localization of hallucinations to anatomy or any association with the blind field. An important aspect of the anatomy underlying the occurrence of VH is the set of connections between the different areas. This hodological feature is discussed at length by ffytche [96].

What determines the total duration of hallucinations and why do they usually eventually cease?

Associated with the degree of complexity of the hallucinations is the total period over which they are manifest. In general, it is the case that complex hallucinations persist for a long time, sometimes years, whereas simple hallucinations last days or weeks. To take again the extreme cases of Bonnet's grandfather and myself, his hallucinations lasted for several months, whereas mine lasted for 10 to 12 days. Another example of a mild deafferentation associated with a short-lasting manifestation of VHs is the linkage of these two features during macular translocation [17].

According to the deafferentation theory, a deafferented neuron becomes hyperexcitable and may develop an increased spontaneous activity. It follows that re-afferentation (re-innervation) should reverse this sequence. The nervous system has this universal property that denervation or disuse causes sprouting of nearby neurons [98]. In the visual system, there are several examples of this, for example, a retinal lesion causes sprouting of cortical neurons in the vicinity of the deafferented synapses [98, 99]. It would be expected that sprouting would occur at all deafferented synapses. However, sprouting is a fairly localized process and, if the lesion is extensive, there may be few or no nearby intact afferent neurons. On the other hand, a small injury would create few deafferented synapses and a speedy recovery could be expected.

Prevalence and incidence

The published estimates are unreliable for several reasons:

1. There is no agreed definition of CBS.
2. The available data are derived from highly selected populations of patients, for example, ophthalmology clinics.
3. Patients experiencing complex hallucinations may not report them for fear of being treated as insane.
4. Patients with simple hallucinations may not report them because they are short lasting, regarded as insignificant, or are not even noticed.

Within selected groups (mostly of people with visual disease), the estimates vary from 10% to 51% [67, 100, 101, 102, 103, 104]. Visual impairment (even total blindness) does not necessarily lead to VHs [100]. Also, with a progressive disease such as AMD, hallucinations may commence long after the initial diagnosis of the disease [105].

Course and outcome

CBS hallucinations are usually not unpleasant and in virtually all cases eventually disappear. They do not normally require treatment although, of course, the underlying cause of the hallucinations must be determined and treated. Patients are generally relieved when they are told that they have no mental illness. CBS has been treated successfully with antiepileptic medication, for example, carbamazepine [106], and with serotonin reuptake inhibitors [107]. The successful treatment of VH using a steroid in a patient with temporal arteritis without effect on the loss of vision emphasizes the importance of cerebral ischemia in the development of VH [108]. The same conclusion is reached when VH occurs after strokes [109]. In one case CBS resulting from a stroke was completely suppressed by transcranial magnetic stimulation of the occipital cortex, an effect not understood but obviously of therapeutic importance [110].

Implications for clinical practice

Correct diagnosis is most important. The first step is to establish that there is no psychiatric condition. The second step is to get some evidence about the likely cause of the hallucinations (visual impairment, drugs, other diseases). The patient should then be referred to the appropriate specialist. Walterfang and colleagues provide a very useful discussion of psychiatric consultation [111].

Suggestions for future research

Whenever the opportunity presents itself, an imaging technique should be used at the time of a hallucination in order to localize the relevant anatomy. There is some evidence that Single Photon Emission Computed Tomography (SPECT) may be the most sensitive technology [112].

There is evidence that VHs may be an early sign of dementia [2, 113, 114, 115]. The occurrence of VHs without peripheral visual pathology may indicate a central defect not restricted to the visual system. It is advisable to keep track of all such cases. In particular, if dementia does develop, it should be asked whether the antecedent hallucinations give any predictive clue, for example, were they simple or complex?

Patients should be encouraged to make careful notes and sketches of their hallucinations, especially if they are of the simple (geometric) type. For example, an attempt should be made to determine the size of the hallucination and of its component parts. This can be done by superimposing the hallucination against a feature in the room, for example, a picture on the wall. Three measurements are needed: the dimensions of the feature (picture), the fraction occupied by the hallucination, and the distance of the patient from the feature. From these data, the size of the VH and its component parts (in degrees) can be determined from trigonometric tables. Size should always be reported in degrees because the size in centimeters will vary with the distance at which the eyes are focused. The position of the VH in relation to the point of gaze (above, below, left, right) should be noted. These data may help to relate the hallucination to an anatomical feature.

References

1. Bonnet C. (1760). *Essai Analytique sur les facultés de l'âme.* Copenhagen: Philibert.

2. Johnson T. H. Visual hallucinations accompanying organic lesions of the brain, with special reference to their value as localizing phenomena. *Trans Am Ophthalmol Soc,* 1933. 31:344–94.

3. de Morsier G. Les automatismes visuels (Hallucinations visuelles rétro-chiasmatiques). *Schweizerische Medizinische Wochenscrift,* 1936. 29:700–3.

4. de Morsier G. Le syndrome de Charles Bonnet: hallucinations visuaelles des vieillards sans deficience mentale. *Ann Med Psychol (Paris),* 1967. 2(5):677–702.

5. Podoll K. Osterheider M, Noth J. Das Charles Bonnet-Syndrom. *Fortschr Neurol Psychiatr,* 1989. 57:43–60.

6. Gold K., Rabins P. V. Isolated visual hallucinations and the Charles Bonnet Syndrome: a review of the literature and presentation of six cases. *Compr Psychiatry,* 1989. 30:90–8.

7. Fernandez A., Lichtshein G., Vieweg V. R. W. The Charles Bonnet Syndrome: a review. *J Nerv Ment Dis,* 1997. 185(3): 195–200.

8. Menon G. J., Rahman I. , Menon S. J., *et al.* Complex visual hallucinations in the visually impaired: the Charles Bonnet syndrome. *Surv Ophthalmol,* 2003. 48(1):58–72.

9. ffytche D. H. Visual hallucinations in eye disease. *Curr Opin Neurol,* 2009. 22:28–35.

10. Needham W. E., Taylor R. E. Atypical Charles Bonnet hallucinations. An elf in the woodshed, a spirit of evil, and the cowboy malefactors. *J Nerv Ment Dis,* 2000. 188:108–15.

11. Teunisse R. J., Cruysberg J. R., Hoefnagels W. H., *et al.* Visual hallucinations in psychologically normal people: Charles Bonnet's syndrome. *Lancet,* 1996. 347: 794–7.

12. Chen C. S., Lin S. F. Charles Bonnet syndrome and multiple sclerosis. *Am J Psychiatry,* 2001. 158:1158–9.

13. Gross N. D., Wilson D. J., Dailey R. A. Visual hallucinations after enucleation. *Ophthal Plast Reconstr Surg,* 1997. 13:221–5.

14. Gonzalez-Delgado M., Tunin A., Salas P. Sindrome de Charles Bonnet. *Neurologia,* 2004. 19(2):80–2.

15. Plesnicar B. K., Zolar B., Bocic M. B. The Charles Bonnet syndrome: A case report. *Wien Klin Wochenschr,* 2004. 116(Suppl. 2): 75–7.

16. Cohen S. Y., Safran A. B., Tadayoni T., *et al.* Visual hallucinations immediately after macular photocoagulation. *Am J Ophthalmol,* 2000. 129:815–6.

17. Au Eong K-G., Fujii G. Y., Ng E. W. M., *et al.* Transient formed visual hallucinations following macular translocation for subfoveal choroidal neovascularization secondary to age-related macular degeneration. *Am J Ophthalmol,* 2001. 131: 664–6.

18. Lance J. W. Simple formed hallucinations confined to the area of a specific visual field defect. *Brain,* 1976. 99:719–34.

19. Anderson S. W., Rizzo M. Hallucinations following occipital lobe damage: the pathological activation of visual representations. *J Clin Exp Neuropsychol,* 1994. 16:651–63.

20. Pomeranz H. D., Lessell S. Palinopsia and polyopia in the absence of drugs or cerebral disease. *Neurology,* 2000. 54(4):855–9.

21. Richards W. The fortification illusions of migraines. *Sci Am,* 1971. 224(5):88–96.

22. Grüsser O. J. Migraine phosphenes and the retino-cortical magnification factor. *Vision Res,* 1995. 35(8):1125–34.

23. Wilkinson F. Auras and other hallucinations: windows on the visual brain. *Prog Brain Res,* 2004. 144:305–20.

24. Mascaro J., Formiga F., Pujol R. Charles-Bonnet syndrome exacerbated by tramadol. *Aging* (Milano), 2003. 15:518–9.

25. Benítez del Rosario M. A., Montón F., Salinas A., *et al.* Charles Bonnet Syndrome and opioids. *J Am Geriatr Soc,* 2001. 49(2):235–6.

26. Tan C. S. H., Yong V. K. Y., Au Eong K. G. Onset of Charles Bonnet syndrome (formed visual hallucinations) following bilateral laser peripheral iridotomies. *Eye,* 2004. 18:647–9.

27. Tomsak R., Zaret C. R., Weidenthal D. Charles Bonnet syndrome precipitated by brimonidine tartrate eye drops. *Br J Ophthalmol,* 2003. 87:917.

28. Teunisse R. J., Zitman F. G., Raes D. C. M. Clinical evaluation of 14 patients with the Charles Bonnet Syndrome (Isolated Visual Hallucinations). *Compr Psychiatry,* 1994. 35:70–5.

29. Alroe C. J., McIntyre J. N. M. Visual hallucinations. The Charles Bonnet syndrome and bereavement. *Med J Aust,* 1983. 2:674–5.

30. Nicholls D. E. Hallucinogens. *Pharmacol Ther,* 2004. 101:131–81.

31. Gödecke-Koch T., Schlimme T., Fada D., *et al.* Charles-Bonnet-Syndrom bei einer älteren Patientin mit beidseitigem Visusverlust, Hyperthyreose und relativer Digitalis-Überdosierung. *Nervenarzt,* 2002. Ü73: 471–4.

32. Stofler P. M., Franzoni A. S., Di´Fazio I., *et al.* Charles Bonnet Syndrome and GABAergic

drugs – a case report. *J Am Geriatr Soc*, 2004. **52**:646–7.

33. Fernandes L. H. S., Scassellati-Sforzolin B., Spaide R. F. Estrogen and visual hallucinations in a patient with Charles Bonnet syndrome. *Am J Ophthalmol*, 2000. **129**:407.

34. Ebersbach G. An artist's view of drug-induced hallucinosis. *Mov Disord*, 2003. **18**:833–4.

35. Cogan D. G. Visual hallucinations as release phenomena. *Albrecht v Graefes Arch klin exp Ophthal.* 1973. **188**:139–50.

36. Maricle R. A., Turner L. D., Lehman K. D. The Charles Bonnet Syndrome: a brief review and case report. *Psychiatr Serv*, 1995. **46**:289–91.

37. Barnes J., David A. S. Visual hallucinations in Parkinson's disease: a review and phenomenological survey. *J Neurol Neurosurg Psychiatry*, 2001. **70**:727–33.

38. Holroyd S., Currie L., Wooten G. F. Prospective study of hallucinations and delusions in Parkinson's disease. *J Neurol Neurosurg Psychiatry*, 2001. **70**:734–8.

39. Onofrj M., Bonanni L., Albani G., *et al.* Visual hallucinations in Parkinson's disease: Clues to separate origins. *J Neurol Sci*, 2006. **248**:143–50.

40. Miyazawa T., Fukui S., Otani N., *et al.* Peduncular hallucinosis due to a pineal meningioma – Case report. *J Neurosurg*, 2001. **95**:500–2.

41. Faber K. M., Johnson L. N. Hallucinating the past: a case of spontaneous and involuntary recall of long-term memories. Perspectives on the hemispheric organization of visual memory. *J Neurol*, 2003. **250**:55–62.

42. Penfield W., Perot P. The brain's record of auditory and visual experience. A final summary and discussion. *Brain*, 1963. **86**(4): 595–694.

43. Bexton W. H., Heron W., Scott T. H. Effects of decreased variation in the sensory environment. *Can J Psychol*, 1954. **8**(2):70–6.

44. Heron W., Dooane B. K., Scott T. H. Visual disturbances after prolonged perceptual isolation. *Can J Psychol*, 1956. **10**:13–8.

45. Zuckerman M., Cohen N. Sources of reports of visual and auditory sensations in perceptual-isolation experiments. *Psychol Bull*, 1964. **62**:1–20.

46. Siegel R. K. Hostage hallucinations. Visual imagery induced by isolation and life-threatening stress. *J Nerv Ment Dis*, 1984. **172**(5):264–72.

47. White C. P., Jan J. E. Visual hallucinations after acute visual loss in a young child. *Dev Med Child Neurol*, 1992. **34**: 259–61.

48. Schwartz T. L., Vahgei L. Charles Bonnet Syndrome in children. *J AAPOS*, 1998. **2**:310–3.

49. Mewasingh L. D., Kornreich C., Christiaens F., *et al.* Pediatric phantom vision (Charles Bonnet syndrome). *Pediatr Neurol*, 2002. **26**:143–5.

50. Pascual-Leone A., Hamilton R. (2001). The metamodal organization of the brain. In *Vision: from Neurons to Cognition*, Casanova C., Pitto M. (Ed.). Amsterdam: Elsevier Science BV, pp. 427–45.

51. Merabet L. B., Maguire D., Warde A., *et al.* Visual hallucinations during prolonged blindfolding in sighted subjects. *J Neuroophthalmol*, 2004. **24**:109–13.

52. Sireteanu R., Oertel V., Mohr H., *et al.* Graphical illustration and functional neuroimaging of visual hallucinations during prolonged blindfolding: A comparison to visual imagery. *Perception*, 2008. **37**:1805–21.

53. Ashwin P. T., Tsaloumas M. D. Complex visual hallucinations (Charles Bonnet syndrome) in the hemianopic visual field following occipital infarction. *J Neurol Sci*, 2007. **263**:184–6.

54. Madill S. A., ffytche D. H. Charles Bonnet syndrome in patients with glaucoma and good acuity. *Br J Ophthalmol*, 2005. **89**:785–6.

55. Damas-Mora J., Skelton-Robinson M., Jenner F. A. The Charles Bonnet Syndrome in perspective. *Psychol Med*, 1982. **12**:251–61.

56. Kölmel H. W. Coloured patterns in hemianopic fields. *Brain*, 1984. **107**:155–67.

57. ffytche D. H., Howard R. J. The perceptual consequences of visual loss: 'positive' pathologies of vision. *Brain*, 1999. **122**: 1247–60.

58. Levy I., Hasson U., Avidan G., *et al.* Center-periphery organization of human object areas. *Nat Neurosci*, 2001. **4**:533–9.

59. Levy I., Hasson U., Harel M., *et al.* Functional analysis of the periphery effect in human building-related areas. *Hum Brain Mapp*, 2004. **22**:15–26.

60. Burke W. The neural basis of Charles Bonnet hallucinations: a hypothesis. *J Neurol Neurosurg Psychiatry*, 2002. **73**:535–41.

61. Swadlow H. A., Gusev A. G. The impact of 'bursting' thalamic impulses at a neocortical synapse. *Nat Neurosci*, 2001. **4**:402–8.

62. Tonon C., Stracciari A., Garutti C., *et al.* A case of occipital epilepsy in an elderly woman. *Arch Gerontol Geriatr*, 2001. (Suppl) 7: 395–400.

63. Vaphiades M. S., Celesia G. G., Brigell M. G. Positive spontaneous visual phenomena limited to the hemianopic field in lesions of central visual pathways. *Neurology*, 1996. **47**:408–17.

64. Echlin F. A., Arnett V., Zoll J. Paroxysmal high voltage discharges from isolated and

377

partially isolated human and animal cerebral cortex. *EEG Clin Neurophysiol*, 1952. **4**:147–64.

65. Prince D. A., Tseng G-F. Epileptogenesis in chronically injured cortex: in vitro studies. *J Neurophysiol*, 1993. **69**:1276–90.

66. Weinberger L. M., Grant F. C. Visual hallucinations and their neuro-optical correlates. *Arch Ophthalmol* (Chicago), 1940. **23**:166–99.

67. Abbott E. J., Connor G. B., Artes P. H., *et al.* Visual loss and visual hallucinations in patients with age-related macular degeneration (Charles Bonnet Syndrome). *Invest Ophthalmol Vis Sci*, 2007. **48**(3):1416–23.

68. ffytche D. H. Two visual hallucinatory syndromes. *Behav Brain Sci*, 2005. **28**(6):763–4.

69. Collerton D., Perry E., McKeith L. Why people see things that are not there: a novel Perception and Attention Deficit model for recurrent complex visual hallucinations. *Behav Brain Sci*, 2005. **28**:737–57.

70. Bennett M. R. Consciousness and hallucinations in schizophrenia: the role of synapse regression. *Aust N Z J Psychiatry*, 2008. **42**:915–31.

71. Schultz G., Melzack R. The Charles Bonnet syndrome: 'phantom visual images.' *Perception*, 1991. **20**: 809–25.

72. Jackson M. L., Bassett K., Nimalan P. V., Sayre E. C. Contrast sensitivity and visual hallucinations in patients referred to a low vision rehabilitation clinic. *Br J Ophthalmol*, 2007. **91**:296–8.

73. Oaklander A. L. The density of remaining nerve endings in human skin with and without postherpetic neuralgia after shingles. *Pain*, 2001. **92**:139–45.

74. Berrios G. E. Musical hallucinations. A historical and clinical study. *Br J Psychiatry*, 1990. **156**:188–94.

75. Griffiths T. D. Musical hallucinosis in acquired deafness. Phenomenology and brain substrate. *Brain*, 2000. **123**: 2065–76.

76. Cerrato P., Imperiale D., Giraudo M., *et al.* Complex musical hallucinosis in a professional musician with a left subcortical haemorrhage. *J Neurol Neurosurg Psychiatry*, 2001. **71**:280–1.

77. Patel H. C., Keshavan M. S., Martin S. A case of Charles Bonnet Syndrome with musical hallucinations. *Can J Psychiatry*, 1987. **32**:303–4.

78. Murthy V. N., Schikorski T., Stevens C. F., *et al.* Inactivity produces increases in neurotransmitter release and synapse size. *Neuron*, 2001. **32**:673–82.

79. Rao A., Craig A. M. Activity regulates the synaptic localization of the NMDA receptor in hippocampal neurons. *Neuron*, 1997. **19**:801–12.

80. O'Brien R. J., Kamboj S., Ehlers M. D., *et al.* Activity-dependent modulation of synaptic AMPA receptor accumulation. *Neuron*, 1998. **21**:1067–78.

81. Li G-H., Lee E. M., Blair D., *et al.* The distribution of P2X receptor clusters on individual neurons in sympathetic ganglia and their redistribution on agonist activation. *J Biol Chem*, 2000. **275**: 29107–12.

82. Dutton J. L., Poronnik P., Li G. H., *et al.* P2X$_1$ receptor membrane redistribution and down-regulation visualized by using receptor-coupled green fluorescent protein chimeras. *Neuropharmacology*, 2000. **39**:2054–66.

83. ffytche D. H., Howard R. J., Brammer M. J., *et al.* The anatomy of conscious vision: an fMRI study of visual hallucinations. *Nat Neurosci*, 1998. **1**:738–42.

84. Kanwisher N., McDermott J., Chun M. M. The fusiform face area – a module in human extrastriate cortex specialized for face perception. *J Neurosci*, 1997. **17**:4302–11.

85. Epstein R., Kanwisher N. A cortical representation of the local visual environment. *Nature* (London), 1998. **392**:598–601.

86. Perrett D. I., Rolls E. T., Caan W. Visual neurones responsive to faces in the monkey temporal cortex. *Exp Brain Res*, 1982. **47**:329–42.

87. Perrett D. I., Smith P. A. J., Potter D. D., *et al.* Visual cells in the temporal cortex sensitive to face view and gaze direction. *Proc Biol Sci*, 1985. **223**:293–317.

88. Puce A., Allison T., Bentin S., *et al.* Temporal cortex activation in humans viewing eye and mouth movements. *J Neurosci*, 1998. **18**:2188–99.

89. Downing P. E., Jiang Y. H., Shuman M., *et al.* A cortical area selective for visual processing of the human body. *Science* (Washington, DC), 2001. **293**:2470–3.

90. Kourtzi Z., Kanwisher N. Cortical regions involved in perceiving object shape. *J Neurosci*, 2000. **20**:3310–8.

91. Cohen L., Dehaene S. Specialization within the ventral stream: the case for the visual word form area. *Neuroimage*, 2004. **22**:466–76.

92. Hoffman E. A., Haxby J. V. Distinct representations of eye gaze and identity in the distributed human neural system for face perception. *Nat Neurosci*, 2000. **3**:80–4.

93. Wicker B., Michel F., Henaff M. A., *et al.* Brain regions involved in the perception of gaze: a PET study. *Neuroimage*, 1998. **8**: 221–7.

94. ffytche D. H., Lappin J. M., Philpot M. Visual command

hallucinations in a patient with pure alexia. *J Neurol Neurosurg Psychiatry*, 2004. **75**:80–6.

95. Nobre A. C., Allison T., McCarthy G. Word recognition in the human inferior temporal lobe. *Nature*, 1994. **372**:260–3.

96. ffytche D. H. The hodology of hallucinations. *Cortex*, 2008. **44**(8):1067–83.

97. Scott I. U., Schein O. D., Feuer W. J., Folstein M. F. Visual hallucinations in patients with retinal disease. *Am J Ophthalmol*, 2001. **131**:590–8.

98. Florence S. L., Taub H. B., Kaas J. H. Large-scale sprouting of cortical connections after peripheral injury in adult macaque monkeys. *Science* (Washington, DC), 1998. **282**:1117–21.

99. Darian-Smith C., Gilbert C. D. Axonal sprouting accompanies functional reorganization in adult cat striate cortex. *Nature* (London), 1994. **368**:737–40.

100. Fitzgerald R. G. Visual phenomenology in recently blind adults. *Am J Psychiatry*, 1971. **127**:1533–9.

101. Lepore F. E. Spontaneous visual phenomena with visual loss: 184 patients with lesions of retinal and afferent pathways. *Neurology*, 1990. **40**:444–7.

102. Brown G. C., Murphy R. P. Visual synptoms associated with choroidal neovascularization. Photopsias and the Charles Bonnet syndrome. *Arch Ophthalmol*, 1992. **110**:1251–6.

103. Holroyd S., Rabins P. V., Finkelstein D., *et al.* Visual hallucinations in patients with macular degeneration. *Am J Psychiatry*, 1992. **149**:1701–6.

104. Crumbliss K. E., Taussig M. J., Jay W. M. Vision rehabilitation and Charles Bonnet Syndrome. *Semin Ophthalmol*, 2008. **23**:121–6.

105. Jacob A., Prasad S., Boggild M., *et al.* Charles Bonnet Syndrome – elderly people and visual hallucinations. *Br Med J*, 2004. **328**:1552–4.

106. Hosty G. Charles Bonnet Syndrome: a description of two cases. *Acta Psychiatr Scand*, 1990. **82**:316–7.

107. Lang U. E., Stogowski D., Domula M., Schmidt E., Gallinat J., Tugtekin S. M., *et al.* Charles Binnet Syndrome: successful treatment of visual hallucinations due to vision loss with selective serotonin reuptake inhibitors. *J Psychopharmacol*, 2007. **21**(5):553–5.

108. Razavi M., Jones R. D., Manzel K. *et al.* Steroid-responsive Charles Bonnet syndrome in temporal arteritis. *J Neuropsychiatry Clin Neurosci*, 2004. **16**:505–8.

109. De Haan E., Nys G. M., van Zandvoort M. J., Ramsey N. F. The physiological basis of visual hallucinations after damage to the primary visual cortex. *Neuro Report*, 2007. **18**:1177–80.

110. Merabet L. B., Kobayash M., Barton J., Pascual-Leone A. Suppression of complex visual hallucinatory experiences by occipital transcranial magnetic stimulation: a case report. *Neurocase*, 2003. **9**(5):436–40.

111. Walterfang M., Mocellin R., Velakoulis D. Visual hallucinations in consultation-liaison neuropsychiatry. *Acta Neuropsychiatrica*, 2007. **19**:330–7.

112. Kishi T., Uegaki J., Kitani M., *et al.* The usefulness of single photon emission computed tomography in Charles Bonnet Syndrome: a case with occipital lobe involvement. *Gen Hosp Psychiatry*, 2000. **22**:132–5.

113. Crystal H. A., Wolfsom L. I., Ewing S. Visual hallucinations as the first symptom of Alzheimer's Disease. *Am J Psychiatry*, 1988. **145**:1318.

114. Haddad P. M., Benbow S. M. Visual hallucinations as the presenting symptom of senile dementia. *Br J Psychiatry*, 1982. **161**:263–5.

115. Pliskin N. H., Kiolbasa T. A., Towle V. L., *et al.* Charles Bonnet Syndrome: an early marker for dementia? *J Am Geriatr Soc*, 1996. **4**(9):1055–61.

31

Acute brief psychosis – an organic syndrome?

Anand K. Pandurangi

Facts box

- Acute Psychotic Disorders (APDS) have been described for more than a hundred years.
- APDs may represent 8%–20% of nonaffective, nonorganic psychotic presentations.
- APDs are more prevalent in developing countries.
- Most or all APDs resolve in 12 weeks or less.
- In 50% of patients, there is recurrence of one or more psychotic episode.
- Long-term prognosis is good, both from symptom and functional points of view.
- APDs often occur after fever, during puerperium, concomitant with systemic infections, and in association with many medical and neurological disorders.
- There is modest evidence linking APDs to demonstrable pathology, including changes in EEG, brain scan, viral antibody titers, and so on.
- APDs may be a result of a genetic or developmental vulnerability interacting with physiological or psychological stress.
- APDs are best treated with low- to medium-dose antipsychotics in combination with supportive therapy and psychoeducation of patient and family.

Current description of acute psychotic disorders in ICD and DSM

Acute Psychotic Disorders (APDs) are a group of "functional" disorders with unknown etiology categorized separately from schizophrenia and bipolar disorders. Their relation to the latter disorders remains unclear. APDs are characterized by sudden (acute) onset and florid psychotic symptoms that resolve in days to weeks [1]. They are reportedly more prevalent in developing countries than developed countries [2], thereby receiving greater recognition in the International Classification of Diseases (ICD) than the Diagnostic and Statistical Manual of Mental Disorders (DSM) of the American Psychiatric Association.

The ICD provides many terms to capture the various presentations, whereas the DSM has only two categories for this group. For example, in the ICD-9 [3] these conditions were conceptualized as reactions to emotional and environmental stress and subcategorized into syndromes, such as depressive, excitative, paranoid, confusional and mixed [3]. In ICD-10, however, the conditions were renamed as Acute Transient Psychotic Disorders (ATPDs), and any association with a psychological stressor was less emphasized. The current subtypes are ATPD with and ATPD without schizophrenia symptoms, and ATPD with prominent delusions [1]. Classic schizophrenia symptoms such as prominent auditory hallucinations, well-formed delusions, and formal thought disorder may be present or absent depending on the subtype. Often the symptoms and signs are unstable, changing considerably even during the short course. To highlight this aspect of the disorders, the term "polymorphic" has been used within the voluminous diagnostic terms, i.e., "acute transient polymorphic psychosis with (or without) schizophrenia-like symptoms." Nonspecific psychotic symptoms may include regressed behaviors such as withdrawal, posturing, mutism, and poor self-care, or dramatic behaviors such as hyperactivity, stereotypy, emotional volatility, anxiety, paranoia, dysphoria, fleeting delusions, fleeting hallucinations. There are many more possible presentations and some are culture specific. All these subtypes are conceived to be brief or transient – typically lasting from a few days to about 2 weeks, although they may last as long as 12 weeks. When a condition diagnosed as APD outlasts this duration, the diagnosis is revised to a chronic condition such as schizophrenia, delusion disorder, or a mood disorder with psychosis.

In DSM-IV, the equivalent terms are Brief Psychotic Disorder (BPD) and Schizophreniform Disorder [4]. These terms are self-explanatory and the underlying concepts are very similar to those in the ICD. Disorders presenting with classic schizophrenia symptoms but of short duration are to be diagnosed as Schizophreniform Disorder, whereas all other psychotic presentations are referred to as Brief Psychotic Disorder or Psychosis NOS.

Brief history of acute psychotic disorders

Acute psychotic disorders [5] have a rather interesting history. Although Kraepelin formulated Dementia Praecox and Manic-Depressive Illness as the two major psychoses [6], it is well known that other terms continued to be used for various acute psychotic disorders, such as Bouffeé Delirante [7], Cycloid Psychosis [8], Manic Delirium [9], Atypical Psychosis [10], Schizophreniform Psychosis [11], and so on. Earlier, the Scandinavians led by Wimmer had recognized a "Third Psychosis" based largely on Jaspers' description of criteria for psychogenic psychoses [12, 13]. The term Reactive Psychosis was used for these conditions for many years [14, 15]. The term Hysterical Psychosis was also used to describe similar psychoses in England and the United States [16]. As noted earlier, the ICD-9 included Reactive Psychosis with depressive, excitement, paranoid, confusional, and mixed subtypes [3]. The DSM-III described these as Brief *Reactive* Psychosis [17] and in the DSM-IV, the term *reactive* was dropped to Brief Psychotic Disorder [4]. As noted earlier, in the DSM-III and -IV, some cases of APD may be diagnosed as Schizophreniform Disorder and others as Psychosis NOS [18].

Incidence, prevalence, risk factors, course, and outcome

There are no true community-based epidemiological studies of APD and hence no estimate of true incidence. Their incidence may vary significantly based on the setting, such as hospitals, clinics, and practices, and between developed and developing countries. Within treatment-seeking samples, as many as 8%–20% of patients with a nonaffective, nonorganic psychosis may appropriately be diagnosed as APD [2, 19, 20, 21]. There is typically a female preponderance in contrast to schizophrenia and bipolar disorder where the gender distribution (over time) is more or less equal. Onset is typically in the third or fourth decade but may be at any age. A psychological or environmental stress factor is frequently but not always present. Acute psychotic disorders are more common in immigrants. Both ICD and DSM consider APD to have good prognosis for the episode with virtually complete recovery, but neither comment definitively on the course such as recurrence rates nor on the long-term outcome and prognosis. It is known from various studies that a full resolution of the psychosis occurs in almost all cases within 12 weeks, with most cases resolving in 2–6 weeks, and in some cases the psychosis may even resolve in days. About 50% of the cases relapse within 2–3 years [2, 22, 23, 24].

Differential diagnoses of APDs include schizophrenia, psychotic depression, mania, substance-induced psychosis, delirium, psychosis due to general medical condition, and dissociative disorders. Rapid changes in delusions and mood have been found to distinguish APD from schizophrenia and bipolar disorder [25]. Malhotra and colleagues [26, 27] found APD, in comparison to schizophrenia, to be more common in females, more frequently associated with stress, such as childbirth and fever, and to have a more frequent family history of APD but not schizophrenia. In contrast to mood disorders, sustained mood changes are infrequent in APD [28]. The long-term prognosis is considered very good, in relation to schizophrenia, schizoaffective disorder, and bipolar disorders [2, 22]. However, the disorders are not a homogeneous group. For example, in about 30% of patients, there may be persistent behavioral, affective, or perceptual changes of a mild kind, although these do not interfere much with overall function [22]. Likewise, much variability in the long-term course and prognosis was noted by Singh and colleagues [29] in patients who initially presented with an APD. In a 20-year follow-up study of "atypical psychoses," Otsuka and colleagues [30] observed that there were three patterns of course and outcomes. Whereas descriptions of Group II and Group III are similar to manic depression and schizophrenia, respectively, Group I had an interesting course. Patients recurrently presented with confusion, dream-like states, and paranoid hallucinatory symptoms, which lasted a few days to 4 weeks, and were completely improved between episodes. Thus, the phenomenology of this group of psychoses is very different from schizophrenia and manic depression and often consists of an acute crescendo onset, confusion, dream-like state, visual hallucinations, transient paranoid states, and rapidly changing mood states, all of which resolve in a relatively short period of time. It is reasonable to conclude from this literature that the term "APD" encompasses a heterogeneous group of disorders.

Biological abnormalities in acute psychotic disorders

The ICD and DSM require that organicity including delirium be ruled out before making the diagnosis of APD; however, this is often an arbitrary judgment on the part of the clinician. For example, fever is commonly associated with APD [27, 31, 32], and, puerperium, with its well-recognized physiologic changes, is an especially vulnerable period for APD [27, 33]. Within ATPD as defined by the ICD-10, Marneros and Pillman [22] found about 35% of patients to have a comorbid somatic disorder, including endocrine, neurological, and cardiovascular disorders, although there was no particular pattern of somatic comorbidity nor could they assign any etiological role to the medical disorder. Further, the somatic comorbidity was no different in comparison cohorts with schizophrenia or schizoaffective disorder [22]. Some patients (in all three groups) had abnormal thyroid and B12 levels. In the same study, about 28% of ATPD patients had nonspecific radiological findings with head CT or MRI but again not significantly different from schizophrenia or schizoaffective disorder. Other studies looking for possible neurobiological abnormalities in APD have reported variably positive findings. Hoffler and colleagues found increased cerebral atrophy in patients with cycloid psychoses [34]. Srikanth and colleagues reported a good correlation of BPRS scores with increased viral antibody titers, suggesting a possible etiological role for the infection [35]. In a later prospective study of APD from the same center, Janakiramaiah and colleagues [36] reported elevated antibody titers to CMV, HSV-1, Mumps, Measles, Varicella, or Japanese encephalitis in 50% of 22 cases of brief psychotic disorder.

Common symptoms of APD such as perplexity, confusion, dream-like states, and so on, are reminiscent of epileptic phenomena. Epileptic discharges have been noted from the amygdala during intracranial recording coincident with acute psychosis [37]. Sharp and Hendren [38] raise the possibility that acute psychosis is a limbic ictal phenomena occurring in brains vulnerable to hyperexcitable states and may not be reflected in increased electrical activity but nevertheless is accompanied by increased metabolic activity and blood flow. These authors implicate a dysfunctional glutamate system resulting from lower inhibitory activity of the reticular nucleus in the thalamus, leading to increased firing from the anterior thalamic nucleus – this in turn induces increased firing by neurons in the cingulated cortex and, eventually, injury to the limbic cortical neurons. Sharp and Hendren [38] cite phencyclidine and ketamine studies as well as the effects of GABAergic anticonvulsants in preventing such injury in support of this proposal. Earlier, Monroe [39], Tucker and colleagues [40], and Innui and colleagues [41] also reported EEG evidence supportive of a relation between seizure pathology and ATPD. Mitsuda [42] and Hatotani [43], in the context of the Japanese concept of atypical psychoses, believe such psychoses to be positioned between schizophrenia and epilepsy. Rottig and colleagues [44] (part of the studies summarized by Marneros and Pillman [22]) did not find EEG evidence to support this notion. About 30% of their patients did show nonspecific EEG abnormalities but these abnormalities were not different from the comparison groups of schizophrenia and schizoaffective disorder. These authors concluded there was no support for an epileptic or cerebral irritable pathology unique to ATPD. However, there was no healthy or nonpsychotic control group, and it is plausible that the pathology they found is shared by many psychotic disorders. Further, standard scalp EEG may not be the best way of assessing limbic irritability.

Acute psychosis in general medical and neurological conditions

Acute psychosis sometimes occurs as part of a general medical or neurological disorder and if judged to be directly due to the medical condition, a diagnosis of "Organic Psychosis" is made in the ICD and "Psychosis Secondary to a General Medical Condition" in the DSM. It is beyond the scope of this chapter to catalog all medical disorders known to present with psychosis. The relation between the primary medical condition and the psychosis is not always clear and, unlike the Jasperian criteria for psychogenic psychoses, no clear criteria have been laid down in either system to assist

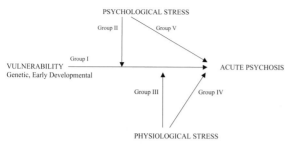

Figure 31.1 Vulnerability–stress model of APD.

the clinician in making this judgment. In any case, as more has been learned about the neurobiology of psychoses, the organic-versus-functional dichotomy has become increasingly outdated. We discuss in the next section a classification of acute psychoses based in part on overlapping etiopathology including biological and organic causes (Figures 31.1 and 31.2).

Acute psychotic disorders are seen during or after infectious diseases such as typhoid, malaria, and influenza, and many case series and reports have been published of acute psychosis in various infectious disorders [45, 46, 47, 48, 49, 50, 51]. Likewise, disorders with systemic effects, including the nervous system such as endocrine disorders [52, 53, 54], metabolic syndromes [55, 56, 57], and connective tissue disorders [58], are known to manifest with acute psychosis. A more direct association of APD with brain pathology is evident in certain neurological disorders. These include but are not restricted to congenital and developmental conditions [59, 60, 61],

seizure disorder [62, 63], demyelinating disorders [64, 65, 66], infectious disorders, including meningitis-encephalitis [35, 67, 68], vascular conditions including migraine [69, 70, 71, 72, 73], and degenerative disorders, including Parkinson's Disease [74]. A group of less-recognized disorders manifest acute psychosis, albeit not in any consistent manner. Primary phospholipid syndrome (PAPS), in which antiphospholipids and other antibodies may induce coagulopathies, causing arterial thrombosis and ischemic brain disorders may include acute psychosis as a prominent manifestation [75]. Likewise, disorders with anticardiolipin production may also manifest psychosis. Conversely, Schwartz and colleagues [76] have shown that in their cohort, 32% (11/34) of the unmedicated acute psychotic patients had antiphospholipid antibodies, including IgG-anti cardiolipin compared to 0% controls. The recently identified syndrome of MELAS, which includes stroke-like phenomena, is also known to present with psychosis [77, 78]. The pathologic mechanism in these disorders may be intermittent and transient vascular insufficiency to critical brain areas.

Pathophysiology of acute psychotic disorder and proposed etiopathological subgroups

The exact pathophysiology of either the so-called "functional APDs" or those occurring in the context of general medical and neurological disorder is

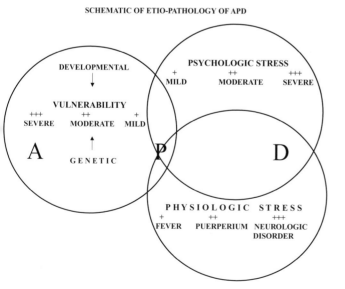

Figure 31.2 Schematic of etiopathology of APD.

unknown. However, there may either be coarse brain disease and/or a dysfunction in critical pathways serving higher order cognitive processing and integration, leading to psychosis. It may be argued reasonably that the same pathways implicated in the pathogenesis of the positive symptoms of schizophrenia may be involved in both functional and organic APDs.

It appears that as heterogeneous as APDs are, they might be conceived of as falling into the following five etiopathological groups:

1. Vulnerability Group with genetic or developmentally induced vulnerability to psychosis
2. Vulnerability – Psychologic Stress Group
3. Vulnerability – Physiologic Stress Group
4. Neurotoxic Group
5. Catastrophic – Psychosocial Stress Group

The first group is best denoted by those cases that may spontaneously manifest psychosis – this may be recurrent, and the vulnerability likely arises from genetic or early developmental factors and is enduring. For the second group, vulnerability exists but is not a sufficient factor and psychological stress is necessary to induce the acute psychosis – this group includes the most common "reactive psychoses" cases. The third group is the physiologic counterpart of the second group with additional burden from marginal physiologic resources, anemia, for example, to combat common physical stress. The physical stress interacts with the inherent vulnerability to induce the acute psychosis. This group would include people who develop an acute psychosis after fever, puerperium, or infections common in developing countries such as typhoid and malaria. Some (probable) cases of "psychosis secondary to a general medical condition" in the DSM could fall under this group. Group 4 consists of cases likely to be diagnosed as clearly organic in ICD or psychosis secondary to a general medical condition in DSM. These medical-neurological conditions appear to have direct neurotoxic effects that produce psychosis depending on the severity of the neurotoxicity. Group 5 consists of patients who experience acute psychosis in the face of catastrophic stress such as in prisoners of war or in victims of earthquakes, floods, tsunamis, and so on, and may truly be a "psychogenic" condition. It should be noted that to some extent, these five groups are overlapping but they can also be unique. Das and colleagues [79] found empirical

support for such a vulnerability-stress model in that patients with APD and without a family history of schizophrenia had a greater number of stressful events before the acute psychosis. It also becomes evident that for four of the five groups, the acute psychosis may be described as partially or wholly biological in origin.

Further, it is likely that as far as the pathophysiology of the core psychosis is concerned, it is common to all five groups, which substantially overlaps with the pathophysiology of the two functional psychoses of schizophrenia and psychotic mood disorders. In attempting to dissect the crucial anatomy of psychosis in these disorders, it may be posited that there is a "psychosis circuit" involving the thalamus-prefrontal cortex-anterior cingulated cortex – hippocampus – entorhinal cortex – paleostriatum – thalamus [71, 80]. This is not to imply that other structures in the brain are not involved in psychosis but to emphasize that at the current time this circuit has been most robustly related to psychosis. Other subcircuits and links may and probably do exist – for example, the cerebellum – reticular-activating system – thalamus, or subcircuits within the paleostriatum, and so on, and these may contribute to unique aspects of an individual's psychosis. Further, we now know that higher cortical functions are best understood as served by "distributed" circuits in the brain and the same dysfunction may result from damage to any one of a number of different (and interlinked) circuits [81]. The best analogy is that of an interstate roadway system, wherein a destination may be reached by numerous permutations and combinations of roads, but a primary expressway serves as the most direct path. Thus, in the case of psychosis, the greater the involvement of the psychosis circuit, the greater the chances that psychosis will result. This anatomical understanding begins to inform us that the so-called "functional APDs" may be manifestations of neurobiological dysfunction, which may be anatomical, physiological, or chemical in nature, or some combination thereof. The vascular lesions seen in certain strokes are particularly informative. Ischemia from any cause in the areas supplied by the anterior cerebral artery is particularly associated with perceptual and cognitive disturbances [72, 82].

In the case of acute brief psychoses, organicity may be invoked, because molecular or metabolic dysfunction is likely. One possible way out of the organic-functional terminology conundrum is to use the term "neurobiological" for all disorders wherein there is reasonable suspicion of neurological and/or biological dysfunction as demonstrated by currently available technologies. This term better captures current conceptions of pathologies in psychosis and should be substituted for the older term "organic." The term "neurobiological," then, is a more accurate term for APDs than "organicity." Many of them occur under conditions of altered physiology, and in others, the neural circuits implicated in psychosis are very likely involved [83, 84]. However, there is indeed not a significant literature on this topic. One suspects this is a result of the focus of most biological investigations on schizophrenia with the belief, rightly or wrongly, that much of what we find in schizophrenia may be extrapolated to the other psychoses.

Clinical management of acute psychotic disorder

The treatment of APD typically involves the use of antipsychotic medications. Clinical experience suggests that APDs respond well to such medications. Both typical and atypical antipsychotic medications may be used and there is no literature to suggest that any particular class of medications is to be preferred over others. It has become the standard, though, to use atypical medications as first-line therapy to avoid acute neuromuscular side effects. The literature does suggest that despite the florid nature of the psychosis, it is not necessary to use large doses of antipsychotics for the relief of symptoms in APDs [85, 86]. This is similar to the experience with the traditional organic psychosis. Patients with the latter are more prone to extrapyramidal adverse effects as well as other toxicities of these drugs. Sometimes, it may be sufficient to conservatively treat the associated symptoms such as fever, dehydration, infections, and so on, and to provide supportive psychotherapy for integration and healing of the break in the ego to avoid the need to aggressively prescribe antipsychotics. This is not as much a recommendation as simply an observation. Further, it may be reassuring to patients that they do not need "stronger" antipsychotic medications typically associated with the more severe illnesses such as schizophrenia or bipolar disorder. This treatment plan would be consistent with the quick recompensation that is the

rule in APD, and fits the notion that in many APDs, there are nonspecific medical factors at work on a vulnerable "neurobiological" system, and supporting the system is as important as the use of antipsychotics. The patient and the family need to be reassured about the brief duration of psychotic symptoms despite their florid and dramatic nature. Supportive psychotherapy to support the fragile ego functions during and immediately after the psychosis is critical. Psychoeducation on the illness nature of the condition, stress reduction, coping skills, and early detection in case of recurrence, is an important part of management [85, 87].

Suggestions for future research

Whereas the literature on the phenomenology and course of APD is rich, the research on the epidemiology, biology, and treatment of these disorders is limited. Much is extrapolated from the literature on schizophrenia, and treatment practices remain untested. With the availability of technology for functional imaging, chemical spectroscopy, and genomics, APDs offer a fertile ground for research into the pathophysiology of psychosis. With their well-known cross-cultural differences, APDs offer a unique opportunity for studying the core pathology of psychosis and possibly untangling genetic–environmental risk factors. The role of specific psychological, social, and cultural factors in the risk-protection equation needs to be studied.

Conclusions

Acute psychotic disorders are a commonly seen group of psychoses, with acute onset, short course, and full resolution of symptoms. They seem to be more prevalent in developing countries and in other vulnerable populations, both psychosocially (e.g., immigrants) and physiologically (e.g., puerperium and fevers). They may be best understood as a transient dysfunction in the psychosis circuit of the nervous system in the face of (i) inherent vulnerability, (ii) psychosocial stress, (iii) neurotoxic pathology, or some combination thereof, particularly in populations with marginal physiological resources. There is modest evidence of demonstrable neurobiological abnormalities in these disorders. They may share a common dysfunction in the "psychosis circuit" with schizophrenia and psychotic mood disorders and may justifiably be considered as "neurobiological" disorders. Like other psychotic disorders, they are best treated with antipsychotic medications, supplemented with symptomatic and supportive medical and psychological therapies. Although recurrence of the psychosis is to be expected in a proportion of cases, the long-term prognosis is good with preserved function at or close to baseline. They offer a very useful and unique window into the study of the major psychoses and should become the focus of more studies.

References

1. World Health Organization. (1992). *The ICD-10 Classification of Mental and Behavioral Disorders: Clinical Descriptions and Diagnostic Guidelines.* Geneva: WHO.

2. Susser E., Fennig S., Jandorf L., *et al.* Epidemiology, diagnosis, and course of brief psychoses. *Am J Psychiatry*, 1995. **152**:1743–8.

3. World Health Organization (1972). *ICD-9 CM.* Geneva: WHO.

4. APA Task Force on Nomenclature and Classification. (1994). *DSM-IV.* Washington, DC: APA Press.

5. Pillmann F., Marneros A. Brief and acute psychoses: the development of concepts. *Hist Psychiatry*, 2003. **14**:161–77.

6. Kraepelin E., Robertson G M. (1989). *Dementia Praecox and Paraphrenia, Together with Manic-Depressive Insanity and Paranoia.* Special ed. Birmingham, Alabama: Classics of Medicine Library.

7. Ey H. (1954). 'Bouffees delirantes' et psychoses hallucinatories aigus. etudes psychiatriques. Vol 3. Paris: Desclee de Brouwer, pp. 203–324.

8. Leonhard K. Cycloid psychoses – endogenous psychoses which are neither schizophrenic nor manic-depressive. *J Ment Sci*, 1961. **107**:633–48.

9. Kraeplin E. (1990). Psychiatry: *a Textbook for Students and Physicians* (Original in German. English Translation of the 6th Edition 1899), Quen J. M. (Ed.). Canton, Mass.: Science History Publications.

10. Kususowa R. Untersuchung der atypischen endogen psychosen (periodische psychosen). *Psychiatr, Neurol Med Psychol*, 1961. **13**:364–70.

11. Langfeldt G. (1939). *The Schizophrenifom States.* Kopenhagen: Munksgaard.

12. Wimmer A. (2003). *Psychogenic Psychoses (1916) Ed.* Australia: Adelaide Academic Press.

13. Jaspers K. (1913, 1997). *General Psychopathology.* Berlin: Springer. Translated by Hoenig J. and Hamiltom M. W. Johns Hopkins. Baltimore: University Press.

14. Strömgren E. (1986). Reactive (psychogenic) psychoses and their relation to schizoaffective psychoses. In *Schizoaffective Psychoses*, Marneros A., Tsuang M. T. (Eds.). Heidelberg: Springer, pp. 260–71.

15. Ungvari G. S., Mullen P. E. Reactive psychoses revisited. *Aust NZ J Psychiatr*, 2000. **54**:621–4.

16. Hollender M. H., Hirsch S. J. Hysterical psychosis. *Am J Psychiatry*, 1964. **120**:1066–74.

17. APA Task Force on Nomenclature and Classification. (1987). DSM-III-R. Washington, DC: APA Press.

18. Fennig S., Bromet E. J., Craig T., *et al.* Psychotic patients with unclear diagnoses. A descriptive analysis. *J Nerv Ment Dis*, 1995. **183**:207–13.

19. Castagnini A., Bertelsen A., Munk-Jorgensen P., *et al.* The relationship of reactive psychosis and ICD-10 acute and transient psychotic disorders: evidence from a case register-based comparison. *Psychopathology*, 2007. **40**:47–53.

20. Jager M., Bottlender R., Strauss A., *et al.* The classification of functional psychoses: The impact of ICD-10 diagnoses (research diagnostic criteria) for the prediction of the long-term course. *Fortschr Neurol Psychiatr*, 2004. **72**:70–8.

21. Allodi F. Acute paranoid reaction (bouffee delirante) in Canada. *Can J Psychiatry*, 1982. **27**:366–73.

22. Marneros M., Pillman F. (2004). *Acute and Transient Psychoses.* Cambridge: Cambridge University Press.

23. Tohen M., Strakowski S. M., Zarate C., Jr., *et al.* The McLean-Harvard first-episode project: 6-month symptomatic and functional outcome in affective and non-affective psychosis. *Biol Psychiatry*, 2000. **48**:467–76.

24. Varma V. K., Malhotra S., Yoo E. S., *et al.* Course and outcome of acute non-organic psychotic states in India. *Psychiatr Q*, 1996. **67**: 195–207.

25. Marneros A., Pillmann F., Haring A., *et al.* Is the psychopathology of acute and transient psychotic disorder different from schizophrenic and schizoaffective disorders? *Eur Psychiatry*, 2005. **20**:315–20.

26. Malhotra S., Malhotra S. Acute and transient psychotic disorders: Comparison with schizophrenia. *Curr Psychiatry Rep*, 2003. **5**:178–86.

27. Malhotra S., Varma V. K., Misra A. K., *et al.* Onset of acute psychotic states in India: a study of sociodemographic, seasonal and biological factors. *Acta Psychiatr Scand*, 1998. **97**: 125–31.

28. Susser E., Varma V. K., Malhotra S., *et al.* Delineation of acute and transient psychotic disorders in a developing country setting. *Br J Psychiatry*, 1995. **167**:216–19.

29. Singh S. P., Burns T., Amin S., *et al.* Acute and transient psychotic disorders: Precursors, epidemiology, course and outcome. *Br J Psychiatry*, 2004. **185**:452–9.

30. Otsuka K., Kato S., Abe T., *et al.* Classification of long-term clinical course of 'atypical psychosis': a 20-year follow-up study at a medical school hospital. *Seishin Shinkeigaku Zasshi*, 2002. **104**:1069–90.

31. Farooq S., Khawaja M. Y. Fever and acute brief psychosis in developing countries. *Br J Psychiatry*, 1999. **175**:586.

32. Collins P. Y., Varma V. K., Wig N. N., *et al.* Fever and acute brief psychosis in urban and rural settings in North India. *Br J Psychiatry*, 1999. **174**:520–4.

33. Rehman A. U., St Clair D., Platz C. Puerperal insanity in the 19th and 20th centuries. *Br J Psychiatry*, 1990. **156**:861–5.

34. Hoffler J., Braunig P., Kruger S., *et al.* Morphology according to computed tomography of first episode cycloid psychosis and its long term course – differences compared to schizophrenia. *Acta Psychiatr Scand*, 1997. **96**:184–7.

35. Srikanth S., Ravi V., Poornima K. S., *et al.* Viral antibodies in recent onset, non-organic psychoses: Correspondence with symptomatic severity. *Biol Psychiatry*, 1994. **36**:517–21.

36. Jankiramaiah N., Gangadhar B. N., Pandit L. V., *et al.* Viral infection in drug naive DSM-IV brief psychotic disorder patients. *Biol Psychiatr*, 1998. **43**:43S–43S.

37. Takeda Y., Inoue Y., Tottori T., *et al.* Acute psychosis during intracranial EEG monitoring: Close relationship between psychotic symptoms and discharges in amygdala. *Epilepsia*, 2001. **42**:719–24.

38. Sharp F. R., Hendren R. L. Psychosis: atypical limbic epilepsy versus limbic hyperexcitability with onset at puberty? *Epilepsy Behav*, 2007. **10**:515–20.

39. Monroe R. Episodic behavior disorders – schizophrenia or epilepsy. *Arch Gen Psychiatry*, 1959. **1**:205–14.

40. Tucker G. J., Price T. R., Johnson V. B., *et al.* Phenomenology of temporal lobe dysfunction: a link to atypical psychosis – a series of cases. *J Nerv Ment Dis*, 1986. **174**:348–56.

41. Innui K., Motomura E., Okushima R., *et al.* EEG findings in patients with DSM-IV mood disorder, schizophrenia and other psychotic disorders. *Biol Psychiatry*, 1998. **43**:69–75.

42. Mitsuda H. The concept of atypical psychoses from the aspect of clinical genetics. *Acta Psychiatr Scand*, 1965. **41**:372–7.

43. Hatotani N. The concept of 'atypical psychoses': Special reference to its development in Japan. *Psychiatr Clin Neurosci*, 1996. **50**:1–10.

44. Rottig S., Pillmann F., Bloink R., *et al.* Is there evidence in the EEG for increased epileptiform activity in ICD-10 acute and transient psychotic disorder? *Psychopathology*, 2005. **38**:281–4.

45. de Ronchi D., Faranca I., Forti P., *et al.* Development of acute psychotic disorders and HIV-1 infection. *Int J Psychiatry Med*, 2000. **30**:173–83.

46. Koch J., Strik W. K., Becker T., *et al.* Acute organic psychosis after malaria tropica *Nervenarzt*, 1996. **67**:72–6.

47. Sowunmi A. Psychosis after cerebral malaria in children. *J Natl Med Assoc*, 1993. **85**:695–6.

48. Jarvis M. R., Wasserman A. L., Todd R. D. Acute psychosis in a patient with Epstein-Barr virus infection. *J Am Acad Child Adolesc Psychiatry*, 1990. **29**;468–9.

49. Rottgers H. R., Weltermann B. M., Evers S., *et al.* Acute psychiatric symptoms as the initial manifestation of HIV-infection: Differential diagnosis, therapy and medico-legal issues. *Nervenarzt*, 2000. **71**:404–10.

50. Nguyen T. H., Day N. P., Ly V. C., *et al.* Post-malaria neurological syndrome. *Lancet*, 1996. **348**:917–21.

51. Doyle M. E., Labbate L. A. Incidence of HIV infection among patients with new-onset psychosis. *Psychiatr Serv*, 1997. **48**:237–8.

52. Brownlie B. E., Rae A. M., Walshe J. W., *et al.* Psychoses associated with thyrotoxicosis – 'thyrotoxic psychosis.' A report of 18 cases, with statistical analysis of incidence. *Eur J Endocrinol*, 2000. **142**:438–44.

53. Krishna K., Singh P., Pradhan A. B. Atypical presentations of Sheehan's syndrome. *J Assoc Physicians India*, 2006. **54**:747–8.

54. Gruber E., Algermissen C., Ebel H. Organic schizophreniform disorder with pre-existing autoimmune thyroiditis. *Nervenarzt*, 2003. **74**:1012–5.

55. Burgovne K., Swartz R., Ananth J. Porphyria: Reexamination of psychiatric implications. *Psychother Psychosom*, 1995. **64**:121–30.

56. Hift R. J., Meissner P. N. An analysis of 112 acute porphyric attacks in Cape Town, South Africa: Evidence that acute intermittent porphyria and variegate porphyria differ in susceptibility and severity. *Medicine (Baltimore)*, 2005. **84**:48–60.

57. Jiang W., Gagliardi J. P., Raj Y. P., *et al.* Acute psychotic disorder after gastric bypass surgery: Differential diagnosis and treatment. *Am J Psychiatry*, 2006. **163**:15–19.

58. Rogers M. P., Reich P., Kelly M. J., *et al.* Psychiatric consultation among hospitalized arthritis patients. *Gen Hosp Psychiatry*, 1980. **2**:89–94.

59. Iwawaki A., Fujiya K., Kobayashi K. Acute polymorphic psychosis in adults with mild intellectual deficits. *Psychiatry Clin Neurosci*, 1996. **50**:109–13.

60. Oner O., Oner P., Deda G., *et al.* Psychotic disorder in a case with Hallervorden-Spatz disease. *Acta Psychiatr Scand*, 2003. **108**:394–7; discussion 397–8.

61. Vogels A., De Hert M., Descheemaeker M. J., *et al.* Psychotic disorders in Prader-Willi syndrome. *Am J Med Genet*, 2004. **127**:238–43.

62. Cockerell O. C., Moriarty J., Trimble M., *et al.* Acute psychological disorders in patients with epilepsy: a nation-wide study. *Epilepsy Res*, 1996. 25:119–31.

63. Roy A. K., Rajesh S. V., Iby N., *et al.* A study of epilepsy-related psychosis. *Neurol India*, 2003. 51:359–60.

64. Jongen P. J. Psychiatric onset of multiple sclerosis. *J Neurol Sci*, 2006. 245:59–62.

65. Habek M., Brinar M., Brinar V. V., *et al.* Psychiatric manifestations of multiple sclerosis and acute disseminated encephalomyelitis. *Clin Neurol Neurosurg*, 2006. 108:290–4.

66. Rodriguez-Gomez D., Gonzalez-Vazquez E., Perez-Carral O. Acute psychosis as the presenting symptom of multiple sclerosis. *Rev Neurol*, 2005. 41:255–6.

67. Kalra H., Allet L., Tiwari S. C., *et al.* Psychiatric manifestations of neurocysticercosis. *Psychiatr Danub*, 2006. 18:200–4.

68. Schlitt M., Lakeman F. D., Whitley R. J. Psychosis and herpes simplex encephalitis. *South Med J*, 1985. 78:1347–50.

69. Berthier M., Starkstein S. Acute atypical psychosis following a right hemisphere stroke. *Acta Neurol Belg*, 1987. 87:125–31.

70. Fuller G. N., Marshall A., Flint J., *et al.* Migraine madness: Recurrent psychosis after migraine. *J Neurol Neurosurg Psychiatry*, 1993. 56:416–18.

71. McGilchrist I., Goldstein L. H., Jadresic D., *et al.* Thalamo-frontal psychosis. *Br J Psychiatry*, 1993. 163:113–15.

72. Hall D. P., Young S. A. Frontal lobe cerebral aneurysm rupture presenting as psychosis. *J Neurol Neurosurg Psychiatry*, 1992. 55:1207–8.

73. Spranger M., Spranger S., Schwab S., *et al.* Familial hemiplegic migraine with cerebellar ataxia and paroxysmal psychosis. *Eur Neurol*, 1999. 41:150–2.

74. Factor S. A., Molho E. S. Emergency department presentations of patients with Parkinson's disease. *Am J Emerg Med*, 2000. 18:209–15.

75. Kalashnikova L. A. Non-ischemic neurological manifestations in patients with primary antiphospholipid syndrome. *Zh Nevrol Psikhiatr Im S S Korsakova*, 2005. 105:18–23.

76. Schwartz M., Rochas M., Weller B., *et al.* High association of anticardiolipin antibodies with psychosis. *J Clin Psychiatry*, 1998. 59:20–3.

77. Iizuka T., Sakai F., Kan S., *et al.* Slowly progressive spread of the stroke-like lesions in MELAS. *Neurology*, 2003. 61:1238–44.

78. Sharfstein S. R., Gordon M. F., Libman R. B., *et al.* Adult-onset MELAS presenting as herpes encephalitis. *Arch Neurol*, 1999. 56:241–3.

79. Das S. K., Malhotra S., Basu D., *et al.* Testing the stress-vulnerability hypothesis in ICD-10-diagnosed acute and transient psychotic disorders. *Acta Psychiatr Scand*, 2001. 104:56–8.

80. Tekin S., Cummings J. L. Frontal-subcortical neuronal circuits and clinical neuropsychiatry: an update. *J Psychosom Res*, 2002. 53:647–54.

81. Hoffman R. E. Neural network simulations, cortical connectivity, and schizophrenic psychosis. *MD Comput*, 1997. 14:200–8.

82. Rabins P. V., Starkstein S. E., Robinson R. G. Risk factors for developing atypical (schizophreniform) psychosis following stroke. *J Neuropsychiatry Clin Neurosci*, 1991. 3:6–9.

83. Poirier M. F. Biological approaches to acute psychoses. *Encephale*, 1999. 25 Spec No 3:33–9.

84. Mitsuda H., Fukuda T. (1974). *Biological Mechanisms of Schizophrenia and Schizophrenia-like Psychoses*. Tokyo: Igaku Shoin.

85. Douki S., Taktak M. J., Ben Zineb S., *et al.* Therapeutic strategies in the first psychotic episode. *Encephale*, 1999. 25 Spec No 3:44–51.

86. Lambert M., Conus P., Lambert T., *et al.* Pharmacotherapy of first-episode psychosis. *Expert Opin Pharmcother*, 2003. 4:717–50.

87. Gaebel W., Marder S. Conclusions and treatment recommendations for the acute episode in schizophrenia. *Int Clin Psychopharmacol*, 1996. 11:93–100.

Treatment

Drug treatment of secondary schizophrenia

Michael D. Jibson and Rajiv Tandon

Facts box

- Treatment of a primary disorder with secondary psychosis may improve, have no effect on, or complicate treatment of the psychotic symptoms.
- Antipsychotic medications are nonspecific agents that improve hallucinations, delusions, and thought disorganization irrespective of cause and without addressing underlying pathology.
- Clozapine has significantly greater efficacy for primary psychotic disorders than other antipsychotics, but also carries greater risk.
- Antipsychotics other than clozapine may have minor differences in efficacy, but these are overshadowed by major differences in side effects.
- Treatment selection among the antipsychotics will usually be determined by side-effect risk for individual patients, rather than by efficacy differences for specific disorders.

Introduction

Schizophrenia is characterized by psychosis and long-term functional impairment, generally accompanied by affective disturbance, loss of volition, interpersonal deficits, and cognitive dysfunction. Secondary schizophrenia is the occurrence of these symptoms as a direct result of a diagnosable medical condition, such as seizure disorder or drug intoxication. Primary schizophrenia refers to a condition in which these disease manifestations cannot be directly explained by identifiable medical pathology or intoxicants.

The symptoms of schizophrenia may be conceptualized as falling into four basic categories. Posi-

tive symptoms refer to active psychosis, as manifested by hallucinations, delusions, suspiciousness, and disorganized thought or behavior. Negative symptoms include blunted affect, reduced-speech production, loss of interest in personal relationships, lack of motivation or volition, anhedonia, and social inattention. Cognitive impairments involve the full range of attention, memory, language, and executive function. Mood symptoms include aberrations in affective expression as well as a predilection for depression associated particularly with acute episodes of illness.

Each of these domains is likely to be involved to some degree in all schizophrenia patients, but none is pathognomonic for the illness. Thus, the diagnosis of primary schizophrenia is made by the exclusion of other diagnosable conditions that give rise to a similar cluster of symptoms. The length of the differential diagnosis, and the rarity of many of the conditions to be considered, make it impractical to systematically eliminate every possible medical diagnosis. Evaluation instead focuses on general screening procedures and the observation of symptoms atypical for the primary disorder.

Among the findings that would suggest the presence of a medical condition giving rise to psychotic symptoms are a positive drug screen, focal neurological signs, seizure activity, a history of brain injury, endocrine abnormalities, evidence of infection or inflammatory process, or a family history of a genetic disorder such as Huntington's or Wilson's Disease. More ambiguous is the presence of a movement disorder, which might suggest a neurologic condition, but could also be the result of antipsychotic treatment or may simply be associated with primary schizophrenia. Clinical features and diagnostic tests for the more common causes of secondary schizophrenia are beyond the scope of this chapter and are described elsewhere in this book; the appropriate treatment of secondary schizophrenia begins with a comprehensive diagnostic assessment.

General principles of drug treatment

Drug treatment of primary schizophrenia is symptomatic, without the expectation of improvement in underlying core pathology. Medications are judged on their efficacy in each symptom domain, with their greatest effect on positive symptoms. They affect the overall course of illness primarily by managing these symptoms and reducing their impact on the patient's functional ability and quality of life.

Treatment of secondary schizophrenia, in contrast, may include drug therapy directed at the primary pathology: this may be curative of both medical and psychiatric symptoms, may alleviate psychosis by controlling medical symptoms, may be required for control of medical symptoms and have little impact on the secondary psychiatric disorder, or may be in direct conflict with treatment of the psychotic symptoms. The following examples illustrate these possible interactions between treatment of the primary disorder and the secondary psychosis.

In 1900, approximately 5% of institutionalized mental patients were diagnosed with general paresis of the insane [1]. Symptoms included active psychosis accompanied by progressive dementia and characteristic motor signs. With the identification of *Treponema pallidium* as the causative agent, the diagnosis was changed to tertiary syphilis and the focus of treatment shifted from psychosis to the underlying central nervous system infection. Definitive antibiotic treatment in the form of penicillin cured the primary illness and alleviated psychosis and dementia in 80% of patients with mild disease. Although patients with advanced disease continued to experience symptoms associated with neuronal damage, 30% of patients who had suffered psychiatric symptoms for several years recovered from those symptoms sufficiently to return to the community and even resume employment [2]. In this context, penicillin might be considered the first, and among the most successful, psychiatric medications.

Temporal lobe epilepsy is among the most common causes of partial complex seizures and has a high correlation with intermittent or chronic psychosis. It is not known if the seizure activity of the disorder or the underlying brain lesion is associated with development of psychosis [3]. Surgical resection of the temporal lobe brings about remission of seizures in a majority of cases, but rarely leads to improvement of the psychosis, and may even result in an increase in these symptoms [4]. In this case, treatment of the underlying disorder must be carried on in parallel with treatment of the psychosis.

Parkinson's Disease is an idiopathic degeneration of motor pathways within the brain. In its advanced stages, it may be associated with psychosis and cognitive decline, as well as its characteristic tremor and bradykinesia [5]. Treatment of the primary disorder is symptomatic, focusing on relief of rigidity and other motor symptoms by augmentation of endogenous dopamine with dopaminergic medication. As is generally true of dopamine agonists, these agents may initiate or worsen psychotic symptoms [6], placing the treatment of the primary diagnosis in direct conflict with that of the secondary psychosis. Conversely, use of antipsychotic medications with even a low risk of motor side effects may worsen the parkinsonian symptoms [7].

Generally, in cases in which underlying pathology is identified and is treatable, treatment should focus on the primary diagnosis. Antipsychotic medications should be brought to bear whenever these treatments are not adequate to address the secondary psychiatric symptoms or when they may worsen such symptoms.

Antipsychotic medications

A large body of evidence demonstrates the efficacy of antipsychotic medications in the treatment of primary schizophrenia, schizoaffective disorder, and bipolar mania. The primary effect of the medications is reduction of delusions, hallucinations, disorganization, and acute agitation associated with any of these disorders. In bipolar disorder, the medications have demonstrated broad efficacy against the elevated mood symptoms of manic episodes, and to a lesser extent against bipolar depression. They are often helpful for the depressive symptoms associated with schizophrenia. There is little evidence that they are effective for depression in contexts other than schizophrenia or bipolar disorder. They have modest benefits for the negative symptoms of schizophrenia and minimal benefit for its cognitive symptoms. They do not appear to address underlying pathology in any of these disorders but are limited entirely to symptom reduction.

Antipsychotics are widely used for primary and secondary psychotic symptoms in other contexts, such as brief psychotic disorder, dementia, drug-induced states, and major depression. Most data support the use of the medications as nonspecific agents effective for psychosis irrespective of the clinical situation. In a few cases, specific studies support such use.

Antipsychotic medications will be reviewed briefly, followed by specific evidence of their efficacy in selected types of secondary schizophrenia.

Conventional antipsychotic medications

Older drugs with higher risk of extrapyramidal side effects (bradykinesia, rigidity, tremor, and akathisia; EPS) and tardive dyskinesia (TD) are classified as conventional antipsychotics, neuroleptics, or first-generation antipsychotics (FGAs). These drugs show good efficacy against psychotic symptoms such as delusions and hallucinations, but less benefit for the negative symptoms and functional deterioration that often accompany these symptoms. They remain important because of their widespread availability, low cost, and useful routes of administration, including oral, intramuscular, intravenous, and depot formulations.

The risk of movement disorders with these drugs is relatively high. Tardive dyskinesia occurs at a rate of 5% of patients per year of exposure to the conventional drugs. TD risk also rises with age, such that patients over 70 years old have a 25%–30% risk of TD after 1 year of drug exposure [8].

Low-potency conventional antipsychotics

Neuroleptics with lower potency tend to be highly sedating and strongly anticholinergic, but to have somewhat less risk of EPS. These drugs include chlorpromazine, thioridazine, and mesoridazine. The latter two drugs have recently been implicated in sudden cardiac deaths apparently related to prolongation of the qT interval of heart conductivity. Consequently, they are no longer recommended for first-line antipsychotic treatment. The drugs within this class show few differences from one another in efficacy; they do differ in terms of their propensity to cause a variety of side effects such as cardiac risk.

Medium- and high-potency conventional antipsychotics

Conventional antipsychotics with higher potency are less sedating than their low-potency counterparts and are only mildly anticholinergic, but carry a higher risk of EPS. Haloperidol, fluphenazine, thiothixene, and perphenazine are among the common members of this class. The recent CATIE study, which included perphenazine, highlighted the strengths and weaknesses

of this class [9]. In the schizophrenic CATIE study population, perphenazine was as effective as newer antipsychotics, but resulted in more treatment discontinuation because of EPS. Although TD was not a problem with perphenazine in the study, it should be noted that patients with pre-existing movement disorders were not randomized to the drug, thus limiting the predictive value of the study for these side effects. Perphenazine carries a slightly lower risk of EPS than the other drugs of this class, but there are few other substantive differences among them. Many members of this class (including fluphenazine, perphenazine, and haloperidol) are available in a long-acting injectable (depot) formulation.

Atypical antipsychotic medications

Newer drugs with lower risk of EPS and TD are classified as atypical or second-generation antipsychotics. With the exception of clozapine, which will be discussed separately, they are not more effective than the older drugs, but have a more benign side-effect profile with regard to abnormal movements. Tardive dyskinesia risk with the newer drugs is estimated at 0.5% per year of exposure, and patients over 70 years old have a 5%–10% risk during 1 year of treatment [10].

These drugs differ significantly from one another in side effects, including risk of EPS, weight gain and metabolic dysregulation, sedation, anticholinergic effects, and cardiac effects. They have not been shown to differ from one another in efficacy as established in randomized, placebo-controlled trials [11]. They may, however, differ in effectiveness in community settings, as represented in the CATIE study. They also have significant differences in mechanism of action, pharmacokinetics, and route of administration. Consequently, each drug will be reviewed briefly, in alphabetical order.

Aripiprazole is unique among the antipsychotics as a dopamine D_2 partial agonist, binding the receptor, but eliciting a reduced response compared with intrinsic dopamine. The drug has clearly demonstrated efficacy for primary schizophrenia and acute bipolar mania and mixed episodes [12], with less evidence available for other uses. Aripiprazole is available as standard tablets, orally disintegrating tablets, and sterile solution for intramuscular injection. In clinical trials among schizophrenia patients, the average dose found to be effective was 15 mg/day, with a range of 10–30 mg/day. Among manic patients, the modal dose was

395

30 mg/day, the highest recommended by the manufacturer. The drug is absorbed slowly following either oral or injectable administration and has a 75-hour clearance half-time. Drug–drug interactions are uncommon with aripiprazole, but because of its metabolism via the cytochrome P450 system, it may require dose adjustment if given concurrently with carbamazepine, fluoxetine, or ketoconazole. The most common side effects with aripiprazole are headache, nausea, vomiting, akathisia, tremor, and constipation. Weight gain and other metabolic dysregulation are generally minimal, as are cardiac effects.

Olanzapine has been shown to be effective for schizophrenia, acute and maintenance treatment of bipolar mania, and acute agitation [13]. A smaller body of evidence supports its efficacy for behavioral disturbance in dementia [14, 15, 16], delirium [17, 18], Tourette's syndrome [19], and borderline personality disorder [20]. Olanzapine is available as standard tablets, orally disintegrating tablets, and sterile solution for intramuscular injection. Clinical trials of the oral drug have generally limited doses to 20 mg/day, the highest recommended by the manufacturer, but doses up to 30 mg/day of the injectable drug have been well tolerated in controlled studies [21]. The drug is absorbed slowly, reaching peak serum concentration at 5 hours with either standard or disintegrating tablets. It is cleared with a half-time of 30 hours by the cytochrome P450 system. Of special note is a 30% drop in serum levels among smokers. Its most common side effects are weight gain, sedation, akathisia, hypotension, dry mouth, and constipation [22, 23]. Its risk of metabolic dysregulation appears higher than that of other conventional or atypical agents [24, 25]. Its major advantages are extensive clinical experience and possibly superior effectiveness in community settings related to its greater ease of dosing.

Quetiapine has demonstrated efficacy for schizophrenia [26, 27], acute bipolar mania [28], bipolar depression [29], and acute agitation [30]. The drug has also been used for delirium [31], dementia [32, 33], and has been broadly used for mood and anxiety disorders [34], obsessive-compulsive disorder, aggression, hostility, posttraumatic stress disorder, borderline personality disorder, and comorbid substance abuse [35]. Its low risk of movement disorder make it especially useful in Parkinson's Disease and Lewy-body dementia. Quetiapine is available in standard tablets only. Clinical trials have focused on somewhat different dose ranges for different

disorders, 300 mg/day for bipolar depression, 400–800 mg/day for schizophrenia, and 600 mg/day for mania. The manufacturer recommends doses no higher than 800 mg/day for any condition. The drug has an intermediate time to peak concentration and is cleared with a relatively rapid 6–7 hour half-time. Although twice daily dosing is recommended by the manufacturer, at least one study found no difference in efficacy when the drug was given once per day [36]. Drug–drug interactions are uncommon with quetiapine, but its levels are affected by inhibitors or inducers of the cytochrome P450 system. The most prominent side effects with the drug are sedation, orthostatic hypotension, akathisia, dry mouth, and weight gain. Sedation and hypotension may limit the rate of titration of the medication, although increases as rapid as 100 mg/day may be well tolerated. Its side effects are noteworthy for the absence of EPS in most studies, making it the preferred drug in patients at risk for movement disorders.

Risperidone is the oldest of this group of drugs, and has accumulated a substantial body of evidence for its efficacy in schizophrenia [37], bipolar mania [38], agitation [39], and behavioral disturbances in autism [40]. It has also been used for behavioral problems in dementia [41], bipolar maintenance therapy [42], and delirium [43]. Risperidone is available in standard tablets, orally disintegrating tablets, liquid concentrate, and long-acting injectable formulation. Although approved for use at oral doses up to 16 mg/day, it is typically administered in the 2–6 mg/day range, and is rarely used at doses higher than 8 mg/day because of dose-dependent EPS. The long-acting injectable formulation is recommended at doses up to 50 mg every 2 weeks. The drug has rapid oral uptake and is cleared with a 20-hour half-time. Drug–drug interactions are uncommon and only slight changes in serum levels occur with inducers or inhibitors of the cytochrome P450 system. The most common side effects of risperidone are mild sedation, hypotension, akathisia, prolactin elevation, and weight gain. Compared with other atypical agents, its risk of EPS is somewhat higher, although well below that of conventional drugs. Although prolactin elevation occurs in more than half of patients, clinical effects, such as galactorrhea or sexual dysfunction are less common [44, 45]. Important advantages of risperidone include its extensive clinical experience and availability of a long-acting formulation.

Ziprasidone has demonstrated efficacy for schizophrenia [46], acute bipolar and mixed mania [47], and psychotic agitation [48]. Case reports are also available describing its use in dementia, delirium, and borderline personality disorder. The medication is available in capsules and intramuscular injectable formulations. The highest dose recommended by the manufacturer is 160 mg/day, but doses up to 240 mg/day are common in the community. The medication is absorbed slowly, and then metabolized with a 7-hour clearance half-time, hence twice daily dosing is recommended. Its bioavailability is 60% when taken with a meal, compared with only 30% when taken alone. Side effects include mild sedation early in treatment, nausea, weakness, nasal congestion, and mild qT prolongation (~10 msec) [49]. It shows only mild interactions with inducers and inhibitors of the cytochrome P450 system, but should be used with caution in conjunction with cardiac medications that prolong qT interval. Post-marketing surveillance has found no evidence of increased mortality or morbidity in the absence of a concurrent cardiac problem or administration of another drug that extends the qT interval [50]. Its primary advantage is its low risk of weight gain.

Clozapine

Although clozapine is the prototype atypical drug, it is sufficiently unique to merit separate classification and consideration. It has well-established efficacy for schizophrenia [51] and bipolar disorder [52, 53], including those patients who do not respond to other medications. Among these treatment-refractory individuals, 30%–50% respond to clozapine. It has also been used for aggression and behavioral problems associated with dementia, brain injury, mental retardation, and personality disorders, intermittent explosive disorder, and posttraumatic stress disorder [54, 55]. Because of the potential for life-threatening agranulocytosis, the medication is recommended only for treatment-refractory cases, generally after at least three other medications have been tried, including at least one conventional and one atypical drug. Agranulocytosis occurs in 1%–2% of patients, usually in the first 6 months of treatment. More common side effects include orthostatic hypotension, tachycardia, weight gain and metabolic dysregulation, sialorrhea, sedation, and constipation. Seizure risk is dose dependent, increasing from 2% per year at 300 mg/day to 6% per year at 900 mg/day. In contrast to other antipsychotic

medications, clozapine's side effects tend to be prominent and enduring. Clozapine is most commonly used at doses between 300 and 600 mg/day. In addition to its unique effectiveness, clozapine carries no risk of EPS or TD, and is the only proven treatment for TD caused by other drugs [56].

Antipsychotics for secondary schizophrenia

A limited body of evidence is available for secondary psychosis, including a few small, randomized trials, but consisting mostly of case series and open-label trials. In general, these data support the use of antipsychotic agents for symptomatic relief of psychotic symptoms in the context of other medical conditions. An important consideration, however, is the potential of the drugs to worsen certain underlying conditions, such as seizure disorders, movement disorders, or anticholinergic delirium. They may also pose a threat to certain populations, including patients with Alzheimer's Disease, cardiac arrhythmias, or metabolic derangements such as diabetes or hyperlipidemia.

Antipsychotics for schizophrenia secondary to neurological disorders
Dementia

Antipsychotics have been studied more extensively in dementia than in other neurological disorders, and have been widely used for psychotic symptoms in the context of Alzheimer's Disease and other types of dementia. Despite their general acceptance for treatment of this population, several recent studies have suggested that they offer little benefit and may cause significant problems. This was the conclusion of the CATIE-AD study, which found no advantage of olanzapine, quetiapine, or risperidone over placebo, but noted that 16%–24% of the 421 patients enrolled in the study discontinued antipsychotics due to side effects [57]. A large study comparing risperidone to placebo had similar results [58]. Two recent meta-analyses, in contrast, found a small but significant positive effect size for risperidone [59], and for both risperidone and olanzapine [60]. The latter study, however, also found significantly increased risk of cerebrovascular events and extrapyramidal side effects with both drugs, for which the entire class of drugs now carries an FDA-mandated warning. Polled experts nevertheless recommend atypical antipsychotics for control of psychosis and behavioral disturbances in dementia [61].

Parkinson's Disease

Studies of Parkinson's Disease have examined both antipsychotic efficacy and the effect of the drugs on movement symptoms. Clozapine has proven effective in reducing psychotic symptoms and has not shown a risk of worsening parkinsonian symptoms [62, 63]. Quetiapine has received attention because of its low risk of movement disorders in schizophrenia patients, and has generally proven effective in Parkinson patients [64, 65, 66]. Some studies, however, show it to be less effective than clozapine, [67, 68] and one study found no efficacy for quetiapine [69]. Risperidone [70] and olanzapine [71] have been the subject of fewer and smaller studies, and have generally been found to carry higher risk of parkinsonian symptoms. Ziprasidone and aripiprazole are represented only by case studies.

Current recommendations for antipsychotic use in Parkinson's Disease favor quetiapine or clozapine as a first-line agent, and clozapine for treatment-refractory cases.

Seizure disorder

Antipsychotics have shown benefit in small, open-label, and retrospective studies of psychosis in the context of various seizure disorders. The largest of these studies involved 21 children and adolescents treated with risperidone and showed a response rate comparable to that seen for primary psychotic disorders [72]. Although the antipsychotic clozapine is known to lower seizure threshold, there was no increase in seizure activity in a series of six patients treated for severe psychosis unresponsive to other interventions [73]. Perhaps most intriguing have been studies showing normalization of brain function in epilepsy-related psychosis with antipsychotic medications [74, 75]. More common, however, is the finding that the psychosis can only be adequately treated after the seizures have been controlled [76].

Antipsychotics for schizophrenia secondary to systemic disorders

Systemic lupus erythematosus

Psychosis is among the more common and severe symptoms of systemic lupus erythematosus (SLE), sometimes presenting as the initial manifestation of the disease and always requiring intervention [77]. Although the preferred approach to treatment is to address the underlying disorder, antipsychotics may be useful as adjunctive agents or in treatment-refractory cases [78]. No single antipsychotic drug has emerged as uniquely effective, and survey data indicate that all agents are widely used with equally fair results [79].

Complicating the diagnostic and therapeutic approach to psychosis in SLE is the risk of psychosis with steroid treatment, one of the standard therapies of the disorder. Recommended approaches to differentiate SLE-related psychosis from steroid-induced symptoms are manipulation of the dose of corticosteroid to determine if the psychosis improves or worsens with increased doses of the drug [79]. Because psychotic symptoms respond promptly to effective treatment of the underlying disorder, they should improve with more aggressive steroid treatment [80].

Human immunodeficiency virus

Psychosis and negative symptoms similar to those seen in primary schizophrenia have long been noted in human immunodeficiency virus (HIV) patients. The differential diagnosis of these symptoms is complicated by the increased risk of individuals with pre-existing psychotic disorders to contract HIV. As with other forms of schizophrenia, psychotic symptoms respond more favorably to antipsychotic treatment than do negative symptoms.

HIV patients are particularly at risk for extrapyramidal side effects from antipsychotic medications [81]. Atypical antipsychotics in general are recommended on that basis for this population [82]. Thus far, no single agent has demonstrated unique efficacy or tolerability in this population.

As in the case of SLE, certain treatments of HIV infection may place patients at increased risk of psychosis. Specifically, antiretroviral agents have been associated with onset or worsening of psychosis [83]. In these cases, alteration of the antiretroviral regimen is the preferred approach.

Antipsychotics for schizophrenia secondary to genetic disorders

Huntington's Disease

Huntington's Disease is a genetically acquired degenerative disorder of the basal ganglia [84]. As in the case of Parkinson's Disease, patients may manifest psychosis, choreoform movements, and cognitive decline. Because there is no effective treatment for the underlying disorder, antipsychotic medications are the first-line therapy for psychotic symptoms and may be useful for other symptoms of the disease. A recent critical review of treatments found modest support for the use of antipsychotics to treat psychotic symptoms, behavioral disturbance, and choreoform movements [85]. Specifically, studies are available on the use of risperidone for psychosis, olanzapine for behavioral disturbance and movement disorder, and haloperidol for psychosis and chorea. Current thinking regarding the increased risk of extrapyramidal symptoms with conventional drugs suggests the preferential use of atypical agents. For this reason, clozapine has been widely used to control both psychosis and motor symptoms [86], but with the availability of other, more benign, antipsychotics with low risk of EPS, clozapine should be considered only one of several viable options.

Wilson's Disease

A rare flaw in copper metabolism gives rise to the deposition of metallic copper in brain, liver, and other tissues, leading to the psychiatric and medical manifestations of Wilson's Disease. Because psychosis is so often an early manifestation of the disease, many of these patients are diagnosed with schizophrenia and treated with antipsychotic medications, with limited benefit [87]. Definitive treatment involves chelation of excess copper. Psychotic symptoms may improve as copper levels normalize, especially in cases treated early in the course of illness. A specific role for antipsychotic medications has not been established with formal studies, and there are few data to guide clinicians in this area.

Antipsychotics for substance-induced schizophrenia

Drugs of abuse

Most studies of antipsychotic treatment of substance-induced psychosis focus on the pharmacology of both the precipitating and the treating agents. Hallucinogens and psychostimulants have been used extensively in human and animal models to provoke or stimulate psychotic symptoms for study. Despite this interest from a research perspective, few studies of clinical efficacy are available. Expert guidelines recommend the use of antipsychotics and benzodiazepines to control symptoms until detoxification from the offending agent is complete [88].

Dopaminergic drugs

Dopaminergic agents used to treat movement disorders, such as in Parkinson's Disease, carry a well-

known risk of psychosis. Several antipsychotic agents have been reported to be effective in these cases, though only a few have been the subject of carefully conducted studies. The emphasis in these cases is on reduction of psychosis without exacerbation of the movement disorder. Consequently, agents with low risk of parkinsonian side effects, particularly clozapine and quetiapine, have been the focus of most studies.

Clozapine has been shown to improve psychotic symptoms induced by levodopa treatment of Parkinson's patients, with complete amelioration of psychosis in about half of patients [89, 90, 91]. Clozapine doses in these studies were well below those used in primary schizophrenia, typically around 50 mg/day. More recently, low to moderate doses of quetiapine have shown similar efficacy [92, 93, 94, 95]. Neither of these agents caused a worsening of the movement disorder or dementia. In contrast, both olanzapine [96] and ziprasidone [97] have been reported in small studies to reduce the effectiveness of levodopa treatment in Parkinson's patients, thus limiting their utility in these cases.

Corticosteroids

Glucocorticoids are a rare, but well-established cause of psychosis, often in conjunction with mood elevation [98]. No controlled studies of individual antipsychotics are available in this population, but numerous case reports support the use of risperidone [99, 100, 101] or conventional antipsychotics [102, 103]. The mood-stabilizing agent valproic acid has also been used prophylactically against both psychosis and mood disturbance [104].

Implications for clinical practice

The pattern that emerges in these cases is sufficient to recommend the use of antipsychotic medications for control of hallucinations, delusions, and thought disorganization irrespective of the origin of the symptoms. Although in a few cases other symptomatic treatments may be useful, antipsychotics remain the agents of choice in most cases. In those conditions for which medical treatment of the primary disorder is possible, antipsychotics may be used in addition to, but never in place of, treatment of the underlying pathology.

Antipsychotic treatment selection

Although limited efficacy studies are available for some of these conditions, in most instances they are not

Table 32.1 Comparison of antipsychotic side effects

	Anticholinergic symptoms	EPS	Hypotension	Prolactin elevation	qTc prolongation	Sedation	Wt gain
Aripiprazole	+/−	+/−	+/−	+/−	+/−	+/−	+/−
Olanzapine	+	+/−	+/−	+/−	+/−	+	+++
Quetiapine	++	+/−	++	+/−	+/−	+++	+
Risperidone	+/−	+	+	++	+/−	+	+
Ziprasidone	+/−	+/−	+/−	+/−	+	+/−	+/−
Clozapine	+++	0	+++	+/−	+/−	+++	+++
Low Potency Neuroleptics	+++	+	+++	++	+	+++	++
High Potency Neuroleptics	+/−	+++	+	++	+/−	+	+

\+/−: Rarely significant or encountered only at high doses
+: Mild severity or low frequency at average doses
++: Moderate severity or frequency at average doses
+++: Often clinically significant across the entire dose range

sufficient to dictate drug choice. To an even greater degree than with primary schizophrenia, selection of an antipsychotic requires attention not only to efficacy data, but more particularly to side-effect profiles. In contrast to the paucity of information on effectiveness, side-effect profiles are well known and often directly pertinent to the patient's conditions. Among the prominent side-effect differences shown by these medications are risk of movement disorder, sedation, anticholinergic effects, hypotension, weight gain, metabolic dysregulation, and seizure. As these may adversely affect the patient's underlying disorder, they should generally be considered first in treatment selection. A comparison of risk for these side effects is given in Table 32.1 as a guide to the clinician in treatment selection.

Abnormal movements are common in neurological disorders and must be a principal consideration in drug selection among these patients. The antipsychotics with the most benign EPS profiles are quetiapine and clozapine. Because clozapine carries additional side effects and mortality risks, quetiapine will be the drug of choice in most of these cases. In contrast, conventional agents will generally be avoided.

A similar review of side effects will drive treatment choices in other cases as well. Aripiprazole and ziprasidone are most favorable when somnolence is a problem, but quetiapine or a low-potency conventional agent may be preferred when sedation is desirable. Weight gain and metabolic dysregulation are least problematic with aripiprazole and ziprasidone, but olanzapine or clozapine may be indicated to assist a

patient in maintaining sufficient weight. Despite its superior efficacy, clozapine may need to be avoided because of seizure risk. In each case, awareness of side-effect risks is a primary consideration of treatment choice.

Summary and conclusions

Sustained psychosis may arise in a variety of contexts, all of which are manifest as delusions, hallucinations, disorganization, and functional deterioration. Antipsychotic medications are the mainstay of treatment for these symptoms in primary schizophrenia, the pathophysiology of which is poorly understood and not remediable with current therapies. These drugs also have a place in the treatment of secondary schizophrenia, although in conjunction with therapies addressing the primary condition, if it is known and treatable. Antipsychotics have generally been shown to be effective in both primary and secondary conditions for control of active psychosis and behavioral difficulties. The current state of knowledge supports the use of antipsychotics for symptom control, but not to the exclusion of more definitive treatment of underlying conditions, and always with caution regarding their complicating side effects. There are more substantive differences among the side effects of the antipsychotic medications than their efficacy; hence, side-effect profiles will generally guide treatment choices. More carefully conducted efficacy studies involving this treatment population would be a welcome addition to the medical literature.

References

1. Hare E. H. The origin and spread of dementia paralytica. *J Ment Sci*, 1959. **105**:594–626.

2. Hahn R. D., Webster B., Weickhardt G., *et al.* Penicillin treatment of general paresis (dementia paralytica). *Arch Neurol Psychiatry*, 1959. **81**:557–90.

3. Sachdev P. Schizophrenia-like psychosis and epilepsy: the status of the association. *Am J Psychiatry*, 1998. **155**:325–36.

4. Blumer D., Wakhlu S., Davies K., *et al.* Psychiatric outcome of temporal lobectomy for epilepsy: incidence and treatment of psychiatric complications. *Epilepsia*, 1998. **39**:478–86.

5. Weintraub D., Stern M. B. Psychiatric complications in Parkinson disease. *Am J Geriatr Psychiatry*, 2005. **13**:844–51.

6. Aarsland D., Larsen J. P., Cummings J. L., *et al.* Prevalence and clinical correlates of psychotic symptoms in Parkinson disease. *Arch Neurol*, 1999. **56**:595–601.

7. Friedman J. H., Factor S. A. Atypical antipsychotics in the treatment of drug-induced psychosis in Parkinson's disease. *Mov Disord*, 2000. **15**:201–11.

8. Kane J. M., Woerner M., Lieberman J. Tardive dyskinesia: prevalence, incidence, and risk factors. *J Clin Psychopharmacol*, 1988. **8**(4 Suppl):52S–56S.

9. Lieberman J. A., Stroup T. S., McEvoy J. P., *et al.* Clinical Antipsychotic Trials of Intervention Effectiveness (CATIE) Investigators. Effectiveness of antipsychotic drugs in patients with schizophrenia. *New Eng J Med*, 2005. **353**:1209–23.

10. Correll C. U., Leucht S., Kane J. M. Lower risk for tardive dyskinesia associated with second-generation antipsychotics: a systematic review of 1-year studies. *Am J Psychiatry*, 2004. **161**:414–25.

11. Tandon R., Jibson M. D. Efficacy of newer generation antipsychotics in the treatment of schizophrenia. *Psychoneuroendocrinology*, 2003. **28**:9–26.

12. Kane J. M., Carson W. H., Saha A. R., *et al.* Efficacy and safety of aripiprazole and haloperidol versus placebo in patients with schizophrenia and schizoaffective disorder. *J Clin Psychiatry*, 2002. **63**:763–71.

13. Battaglia J., Lindborg S. R., Alaka K., *et al.* Calming versus sedative effects of intramuscular olanzapine in agitated patients. *Am J Emerg Med*, 2003. **21**:192–8.

14. Gareri P., Cotroneo A., Lacava R., *et al.* Comparison of the efficacy of new and conventional antipsychotic drugs in the treatment of behavioral and psychological symptoms of dementia (BPSD). *Arch Gerontol Geriatr*, 2004. **9**(Suppl):207–15.

15. De Deyn P. P., Carrasco M. M., Deberdt W., *et al.* Olanzapine versus placebo in the treatment of psychosis with or without associated behavioral disturbances in patients with Alzheimer's disease. *Int J Geriatr Psychiatry*, 2004. **19**:115–26.

16. Fontaine C. S., Hynan L. S., Koch K., *et al.* A double-blind comparison of olanzapine versus risperidone in the acute treatment of dementia-related behavioral disturbances in extended care facilities. *J Clin Psychiatry*, 2003. **64**:726–30.

17. Breitbart W., Tremblay A., Gibson C. An open trial of olanzapine for the treatment of delirium in hospitalized cancer patients. *Psychosomatics*, 2002. **43**:175–82.

18. Skrobik Y. K., Bergeron N., Dumont M., *et al.* Olanzapine vs haloperidol: treating delirium in a critical care setting. *Intens Care Med*, 2004. **30**:444–9.

19. Stephens R. J., Bassel C., Sandor P. Olanzapine in the treatment of aggression and tics in children with Tourette's syndrome – a pilot study. *J Child Adol Psychopharmacol*, 2004. **14**:255–66.

20. Zanarini M. C., Frankenburg F. R., Parachini E. A. A preliminary, randomized trial of fluoxetine, olanzapine, and the olanzapine-fluoxetine combination in women with borderline personality disorder. *J Clin Psychiatry*, 2004. **65**:903–7.

21. Wright P., Birkett M., David S. R., *et al.* Double-blind, placebo-controlled comparison of intramuscular olanzapine and intramuscular haloperidol in the treatment of acute agitation in schizophrenia, *Am J Psychiatry*, 2001. **158**:1149–51.

22. Beasley C. M. Jr., Hamilton S. H., Crawford A. M., *et al.* Olanzapine versus haloperidol: acute phase results of the international double-blind olanzapine trial. *Eur Neuropsychopharmacol*, 1997. 7:125–37.

23. Tran P. V., Dellva M. A., Tollefson G. D., *et al.* Extrapyramidal symptoms and tolerability of olanzapine versus haloperidol in the acute treatment of schizophrenia. *J Clin Psychiatry*, 1997. **58**:205–11.

24. Bobes J., Rejas J., Garcia-Garcia M., *et al.* Weight gain in patients with schizophrenia treated with risperidone, olanzapine, quetiapine or haloperidol: results of the EIRE study. *Schizophr Res*, 2003. **62**:77–88.

25. Leslie D. L., Rosenheck R. A. Incidence of newly diagnosed diabetes attributable to atypical antipsychotic medications. *Am J Psychiatry*, 2004. **161**:1709–11.

26. Borison R. L., Arvanitis L. A., Miller B. G. ICI 204,636, an

atypical antipsychotic: efficacy and safety in a multicenter, placebo-controlled trial in patients with schizophrenia. U.S. SEROQUEL Study Group. *J Clin Psychopharmacol*, 1996. **16**:158–69.

27. Small J. G., Hirsch S. R., Arvanitis L. A., *et al.* Quetiapine in patients with schizophrenia: a high- and low-dose double-blind comparison with placebo. Seroquel Study Group. *Arch Gen Psychiatry*, 1997. **54**:549–57.

28. Sachs G., Chengappa K. N., Suppes T., *et al.* Quetiapine with lithium or divalproex for the treatment of bipolar mania: a randomized, double-blind, placebo-controlled study. *Bipolar Disord*, 2004. **6**:213–23.

29. Calabrese J. R., Keck P. E. Jr., Macfadden W., *et al.* A randomized, double-blind, placebo-controlled trial of quetiapine in the treatment of bipolar I or II depression. *Am J Psychiatry*, 2005. **162**:1351–60.

30. Chengappa K. N., Goldstein J. M., Greenwood M., *et al.* A post hoc analysis of the impact on hostility and agitation of quetiapine and haloperidol among patients with schizophrenia. *Clin Ther*, 2003. **25**:530–41.

31. Kim K. Y., Bader G. M., Kotlyar V., *et al.* Treatment of delirium in older adults with quetiapine. *J Geriatr Psychiatry Neurol*, 2003. **16**:29–31.

32. Reddy S., Factor S. A., Molho E. S., *et al.* The effect of quetiapine on psychosis and motor function in parkinsonian patients with and without dementia. *Mov Disord*, 2002. **17**:676–81.

33. Fernandez H. H., Trieschmann M. E., Burke M. A., *et al.* Quetiapine for psychosis in Parkinson's disease versus dementia with Lewy bodies. *J Clin Psychiatry*, 2002. **63**:513–15.

34. Hirschfeld R. M., Weisler R. H., Raines S. R., *et al.* Quetiapine in the treatment of anxiety in patients with bipolar I or II depression: a secondary analysis from a randomized, double-blind, placebo-controlled study. *J Clin Psychiatry*, 2006. **67**:355–62.

35. Adityanjee Schulz S. C. Clinical use of quetiapine in disease states other than schizophrenia. *J Clin Psychiatry*, 2002. **63**(Suppl 13):32–8.

36. Thase M. E., Macfadden W., Weisler R. H., *et al.* Efficacy of quetiapine monotherapy in bipolar I and II depression: a double-blind, placebo-controlled study (the BOLDER II study). *J Clin Psychopharmacol*, 2006. **26**:600–9.

37. Marder S. R., Meibach R. C. Risperidone in the treatment of schizophrenia. *Am J Psychiatry*, 1994. **151**:825–35.

38. Hirschfeld R. M., Keck P. E. Jr., Kramer M., *et al.* Rapid antimanic effect of risperidone monotherapy: a 3-week multicenter, double-blind, placebo-controlled trial. *Am J Psychiatry*, 2004. **161**:1057–65.

39. Currier G. W., Chou J. C., Feifel D., *et al.* Acute treatment of psychotic agitation: a randomized comparison of oral treatment with risperidone and lorazepam versus intramuscular treatment with haloperidol and lorazepam. *J Clin Psychiatry*, 2004. **65**:386–94.

40. McCracken J. T., McGough J., Shah B., *et al.* Research units on pediatric psychopharmacology autism network. Risperidone in children with autism and serious behavioral problems. *New Eng J Med*, 2002. **347**:314–21.

41. Fontaine C. S., Hynan L. S., Koch K., *et al.* A double-blind comparison of olanzapine versus risperidone in the acute treatment of dementia-related behavioral disturbances in extended care facilities. *J Clin Psychiatry*, 2003. **64**:726–30.

42. Vieta E., Brugue E., Goikolea J. M., *et al.* Acute and continuation risperidone monotherapy in mania. *Human Psychopharmacol*, 2004. **19**:41–5.

43. Mittal D., Jimerson N. A., Neely E. P., *et al.* Risperidone in the treatment of delirium: results from a prospective open-label trial. *J Clin Psychiatry*, 2004. **65**:662–7.

44. Bobes J., Garc A-Portilla M. P., Rejas J., *et al.* Frequency of sexual dysfunction and other reproductive side-effects in patients with schizophrenia treated with risperidone, olanzapine, quetiapine, or haloperidol: the results of the EIRE study. *J Sex Marital Ther*, 2003. **29**:125–47.

45. Kelly D. L., Conley R. R. A randomized double-blind 12-week study of quetiapine, risperidone or fluphenazine on sexual functioning in people with schizophrenia. *Psychoneuroendocrinology*, 2006. **31**:340–6.

46. Daniel D. G., Zimbroff D. L., Potkin S. G., *et al.* Ziprasidone 80 mg/day and 160 mg/day in the acute exacerbation of schizophrenia and schizoaffective disorder: a 6-week placebo-controlled trial. Ziprasidone Study Group. *Neuropsychopharmacology*, 1999. **20**:491–505.

47. Keck P. E. Jr., Versiani M., Potkin S., *et al.* Ziprasidone in Mania Study Group. Ziprasidone in the treatment of acute bipolar mania: a three-week, placebo-controlled, double-blind, randomized trial. *Am J Psychiatry*, 2003. **160**:741–8.

48. Daniel D. G., Potkin S. G., Reeves K. R., *et al.* Intramuscular (IM) ziprasidone 20 mg is effective in

reducing acute agitation associated with psychosis: a double-blind, randomized trial. *Psychopharmacology*, 2001. **155**:128–34.

49. Tandon R., Harrigan E, Zorn S. Ziprasidone: a novel antipsychotic with unique pharmacology and therapeutic potential. *J Serotonin Res*, 1997. **4**:159–77.

50. Weiden P. J., Iqbal N., Mendelowitz A. J., *et al.* Best clinical practice with ziprasidone: update after one year of experience. *J Psychiatr Pract*, 2002. **8**:81–98.

51. Kane J., Honigfeld G., Singer J., *et al.* Clozapine for the treatment-resistant schizophrenic: a double-blind comparison with chlorpromazine. *Arch Gen Psychiatry*, 1988. **45**:789–96.

52. Suppes T., Webb A., Paul B., *et al.* Clinical outcome in a randomized 1-year trial of clozapine versus treatment as usual for patients with treatment-resistant illness and a history of mania. *Am J Psychiatry*, 1999. **156**:1164–9.

53. Green A. I., Tohen M., Patel J. K., *et al.* Clozapine in the treatment of refractory psychotic mania. *Am J Psychiatry*, 2000. **157**:982–6.

54. Kant R., Chalansani R., Chengappa K. N., *et al.* The off-label use of clozapine in adolescents with bipolar disorder, intermittent explosive disorder, or posttraumatic stress disorder. *J Child Adol Psychopharmacol*, 2004. **14**:57–63.

55. Fava M. Psychopharmacologic treatment of pathologic aggression. *Psychiatric Clin N Am*, 1997. **20**:427–51.

56. Spivak B., Mester R., Abesgaus J., *et al.* Clozapine treatment for neuroleptic-induced tardive dyskinesia, parkinsonism, and chronic akathisia in schizophrenic patients. *J Clin Psychiatry*, 1997. **58**:318–22.

57. Schneider L. S., Tariot P. N., Dagerman K. S., *et al.* Effectiveness of atypical antipsychotic drugs in patients with Alzheimer's disease. *N Engl J Med*, 2006. **355**:1525–38.

58. Mintzer J., Greenspan A., Caers I., *et al.* Risperidone in the treatment of psychosis of Alzheimer disease: results from a prospective clinical trial. *Am J Geriatr Psychiatry*, 2006. **14**:280–91.

59. Schneider L. S., Dagerman K., Insel P. S. Efficacy and adverse effects of atypical antipsychotics for dementia: meta-analysis of randomized, placebo-controlled trials. *Am J Geriatr Psychiatry*, 2006. **14**:191–210.

60. Ballard C., Waite J. The effectiveness of atypical antipsychotics for the treatment of aggression and psychosis in Alzheimer's disease. *Cochrane Database Syst Reviews*, 2006. CD003476.

61. Alexopoulos G. S., Jeste D. V., Chung H., *et al.* The expert consensus guideline series. Treatment of dementia and its behavioral disturbances. Introduction: methods, commentary, and summary. *Postgrad Med*, 2005. Spec No:6–22.

62. Pollak P., Tison F., Rascol O., *et al.* Clozapine in drug induced psychosis in Parkinson's disease: a randomised, placebo controlled study with open follow up. *J Neurol Neurosurg Psychiatry*, 2004. **75**:689–95.

63. The Parkinson Study Group. Low-dose clozapine for the treatment of drug-induced psychosis in Parkinson's disease. *N Engl J Med*, 1999. **340**:757–63.

64. Morgante L., Epifanio A., Spina E., *et al.* Quetiapine and clozapine in parkinsonian patients with dopaminergic psychosis. *Clin Neuropharmacol*, 2004. **27**:153–6.

65. Morgante L., Epifanio A., Spina E., *et al.* Quetiapine versus clozapine: a preliminary report of comparative effects on dopaminergic psychosis in patients with Parkinson's disease. *Neurol Sci*, 2002. **23**(Suppl 2): S89–90.

66. Prohorov T., Klein C., Miniovitz A., *et al.* The effect of quetiapine in psychotic Parkinsonian patients with and without dementia. An open-labeled study utilizing a structured interview. *J Neurol*, 2006. **253**:171–5.

67. Merims D., Balas M., Peretz C., *et al.* Rater-blinded, prospective comparison: quetiapine versus clozapine for Parkinson's disease psychosis. *Clin Neuropharmacology*, 2006. **29**:331–7.

68. Klein C., Prokhorov T., Miniovich A., *et al.* Long-term follow-up (24 months) of quetiapine treatment in drug-induced Parkinson disease psychosis. *Clin Neuropharmacology*, 2006. **29**: 215–19.

69. Ondo W. G., Tintner R., Voung K. D., *et al.* Double-blind, placebo-controlled, unforced titration parallel trial of quetiapine for dopaminergic-induced hallucinations in Parkinson's disease. *Mov Disord*, 2005. **20**:958–63.

70. Ellis T., Cudkowicz M. E., Sexton P. M., *et al.* Clozapine and risperidone treatment of psychosis in Parkinson's disease. *J Neuropsychiatry Clin Neurosci*, 2000. **12**:364–9.

71. Breier A., Sutton V. K., Feldman P. D., *et al.* Olanzapine in the treatment of dopamimetic-induced psychosis in patients with Parkinson's disease. *Biol Psychiatry*. 2002. **52**:438–45.

72. Gonzalez-Heydrich J., Pandina G. J., Fleisher C. A., *et al.* No seizure exacerbation from risperidone in youth with comorbid epilepsy and psychiatric disorders: a case series.

J Child Adol Psychopharmacol, 2004. **14**:295–310.

73. Langosch J. M., Trimble M. R. Epilepsy, psychosis and clozapine. *Hum Psychopharmacol*, 2002. **17**:115–19.

74. Ishii R., Canuet L., Iwase M., *et al.* Right parietal activation during delusional state in episodic interictal psychosis of epilepsy: a report of two cases. *Epilepsy Beha*, 2006. **9**:367–72.

75. Oner O., Unal O., Deda G. A case of psychosis with temporal lobe epilepsy: SPECT changes with treatment. *Pediatr Neurol*, 2005. **32**:197–200.

76. Brewerton T. D. The phenomenology of psychosis associated with complex partial seizure disorder. *Ann Clin Psychiatry*, 1997. **9**:31–51.

77. Sibbitt W. L. Jr., Brandt J. R., Johnson C. R., *et al.* The incidence and prevalence of neuropsychiatric syndromes in pediatric onset systemic lupus erythematosus. *J Rheumatol*, 2002. **29**:1536–42.

78. Bodani M., Kopelman M. D. A psychiatric perspective on the therapy of psychosis in systemic lupus erythematosus. *Lupus*, 2003. **12**:947–9.

79. Tincani A., Brey R., Balestrieri G., *et al.* International survey on the management of patients with SLE. II. The results of a questionnaire regarding neuropsychiatric manifestations. *Clin Exp Rheumatol*, 1996. **14**(Suppl 16):S23–9.

80. Sanna G., Bertolaccini M. L., Khamashta M. A. Neuropsychiatric involvement in systemic lupus erythematosus: current therapeutic approach. *Curr Pharm Des*, 2008. **14**: 1261–9.

81. Sewell D. D., Jeste D. V., McAdams L. A., *et al.* Neuroleptic treatment of HIV-associated

psychosis. HNRC group. *Neuropsychopharmacology*, 1994. **10**:223–9.

82. Dolder C. R., Patterson T. L., Jeste D. V. HIV, psychosis and aging: past, present and future. *AIDS*, 2004. **18**(Suppl 1):S35–4.

83. Foster R., Olajide D., Everall I. P. Antiretroviral therapy-induced psychosis: case report and brief review of the literature. *HIV Med*, 2003. **4**:139–44.

84. Rosenblatt A., Leroi I. Neuropsychiatry of Huntington's disease and other basal ganglia disorders. *Psychosomatics*, 2000. **41**:24–30.

85. Bonelli R. M., Wenning G. K. Pharmacological management of Huntington's disease: an evidence-based review. *Curr Pharm Des*, 2006. **12**:2701–20.

86. Factor S. A., Friedman J. H. The emerging role of clozapine in the treatment of movement disorders. *Mov Disord*, 1997. **12**:483–96.

87. Akil M., Brewer G. J. Psychiatric and behavioral abnormalities in Wilson's disease. *Adv Neurol*, 1995. **65**:171–8.

88. Leweke F. M., Gerth C. W., Klosterkotter J. Cannabis-associated psychosis: current status of research. *CNS Drugs*, 2004. **18**:895–910.

89. Pollak P., Tison F., Rascol O., *et al.* Clozapine in drug induced psychosis in Parkinson's disease: a randomised, placebo controlled study with open follow up. *J Neurol Neurosurg Psychiatry*, 2004. **75**:689–95.

90. Trosch R. M., Friedman J. H., Lannon M. C., *et al.* Clozapine use in Parkinson's disease: a retrospective analysis of a large multicentered clinical experience. *Mov Disord*, 1998. **13**:377–82.

91. Widman L. P., Burke W. J., Pfeiffer R. F., *et al.* Use of clozapine to treat levodopa-induced psychosis in Parkinson's disease:

retrospective review. *J Geriatr Psychiatry Neurol*, 1997. **10**:63–6.

92. Juncos J. L., Roberts V. J., Evatt M. L., *et al.* Quetiapine improves psychotic symptoms and cognition in Parkinson's disease. *Mov Disord*, 2004. **19**:29–35.

93. Fernandez H. H., Trieschmann M. E., Burke M. A., *et al.* Long-term outcome of quetiapine use for psychosis among Parkinsonian patients. *Mov Disord*, 2003. **18**:510–14.

94. Reddy S., Factor S. A., Molho E. S., *et al.* The effect of quetiapine on psychosis and motor function in parkinsonian patients with and without dementia. *Mov Disord*, 2002. **17**:676–81.

95. Fernandez H. H., Friedman J. H., Jacques C., *et al.* Quetiapine for the treatment of drug-induced psychosis in Parkinson's disease. *Mov Disord*, 1999. **14**:484–7.

96. Molho E. S., Factor S. A. Worsening of motor features of parkinsonism with olanzapine. *Mov Disord*, 1999. **14**:1014–16.

97. Schindehutte J., Trenkwalder C. Treatment of drug-induced psychosis in Parkinson's disease with ziprasidone can induce severe dose-dependent off-periods and pathological laughing. *Clin Neurol Neurosurg*, 2007. **109**:188–91.

98. Wolkowitz O. M., Reus V. I., Canick J., *et al.* Glucocorticoid medication, memory and steroid psychosis in medical illness. *Ann N Y Acad Sci*, 1997. **823**:81–96.

99. Herguner S., Bilge I., Yavuz Y. A., *et al.* Steroid-induced psychosis in an adolescent: treatment and prophylaxis with risperidone. *Turk J Pediatr*, 2006. **48**:244–7.

100. DeSilva C. C., Nurse M. C., Vokey K. Steroid-induced psychosis treated with risperidone. *Can J Psychiatry*, 2002. **47**:388–9.

101. Kramer T. M., Cottingham E. M. Risperidone in the treatment of steroid-induced psychosis. *J Child Adolesc Psychopharmacol*, 1999. **9**:315–16.

102. Ingram D. G., Hagemann T. M. Promethazine treatment of steroid-induced psychosis in a child. *Ann Pharmacother*, 2003. 37:1036–9.

103. Ahmad M., Rasul F. M. Steroid-induced psychosis treated with haloperidol in a patient with active chronic obstructive pulmonary disease. *Am J Emerg Med*, 1999. 17:735.

104. Abbas A., Styra R. Valproate prophylaxis against steroid induced psychosis. *Can J Psychiatry*, 1994. **39**:188–9.

33 Nonpharmacological interventions in secondary schizophrenia

David J. Kavanagh, Jennifer M. Connolly, and Kim T. Mueser

Facts box

- Irrespective of etiology, there is significant room for psychological treatments to target cognitive or behavioral triggers for psychotic symptoms and for strategies to improve outcomes.

- There is a substantial body of literature targeting the treatment of substance use in schizophrenia because of its important association with this disorder.

- Insomnia may complicate the management of psychosis or be its trigger, and nonpharmacological strategies for its management may have an important clinical role.

- Strategies to manage residual psychotic symptoms include cognitive behavior therapy, social skills training, cognitive remediation, and family intervention – and these could possibly be applied to both primary and secondary schizophrenia.

- There have not as yet been controlled trials on averting potential psychosis using either a substance use or insomnia intervention, although substance use is addressed in multicomponent studies on early episodes of psychosis.

Introduction

Because the primary focus of this book is on psychoses arising from specific organic syndromes, it may at first seem odd that a chapter on psychological interventions for these problems should be included, as there is no psychological treatment that directly targets their organic basis.

However, there is significant room for psychological treatments to target cognitive or behavioral triggers for psychotic symptoms and for strategies to improve

outcomes. Up to now, little research has focused solely on psychological treatment for unequivocally secondary psychosis. As a consequence, we must rely on extrapolations from work on psychoses in general, on schizophrenia or affective psychosis, or even on the management of the behavioral risk in nonpsychotic populations. Although the treatments and methods discussed here have an evidence base in primary psychosis, the evidence supporting their application to secondary psychosis is yet to be established. Much of this chapter must therefore be speculative.

Because of the importance of substance use as a risk for psychotic symptoms, this chapter emphasizes research on that topic. However, that is not the only potential target of psychological intervention. Among potential determinants, insomnia has been addressed in its own right within the general population. Features and sequelae of psychosis – positive symptoms, cognitive deficits, and functional skills-have also had research attention, as have factors that may improve outcomes, such as adherence, family interventions, and early detection of relapse. Although this work has not been specific to secondary psychosis, aspects may be applicable to it.

Substance use

As previously discussed in this volume (Chapters 14–22), use of some psychoactive substances can not only trigger a temporary psychotic reaction [1, 2] but can initiate a potentially lifelong disorder in vulnerable individuals [3, 4]. Because substance use is very common in patients with psychosis [5, 6], and because it is often hard to know whether it has a primary role in the psychosis at early stages of the disorder, substance use needs to be routinely assessed and addressed in patients with psychosis.

Treatment of substance misuse in people with psychotic disorders has often relied on a parallel or sequential approach. In *parallel* treatments, the mental illness and substance misuse are treated by different clinicians, usually from different agencies. In *sequential* treatments, efforts initially focus on treating or stabilizing one disorder and then addressing the second. Problems arise with each of these strategies [7, 8]. Parallel or sequential treatments by different agencies are subject to differing policies and procedures in each agency and to problems with communication and coordination [9]. At worst, this can result in the patient missing treatment for one or more of their problems (e.g., because they do not fulfill priority criteria for service or do not receive assertive follow-up) or receiving inconsistent advice.

There is another, potentially critical problem with the separation of treatments: unless both treating clinicians have the knowledge and skills to treat both types of problem, the treatment may not be sufficiently modified to suit this population. Furthermore, except where psychotic symptoms remain secondary to the substance misuse, each problem is likely to exacerbate the other [10]. Accordingly, current treatments for substance misuse and psychotic symptoms typically have a single clinician or clinical team assuming responsibility for management of both problem areas [11]. Based on the theme of integration, a number of treatment programs have been developed for comorbidity [12, 13, 14, 15, 16]. These programs have considerable differences, but they typically share emphases on engagement and motivation enhancement, harm reduction, assertive outreach, and comprehensiveness.

Some of the engagement and motivational challenges with substance users who have psychotic symptoms are similar to those faced by opportunistic interventions for others with negative sequelae to substance use. It is now well established that confrontational methods in those contexts are ineffective [17]. The sensitivity of people with psychosis to interpersonal stress [18] presents a further reason to avoid such approaches in this population. Instead, motivational interviewing [19] is typically used. This approach empathically elicits the patient's own ambivalence and concern about their substance use and potential behavior change. It also addresses low self-efficacy about their ability to carry out change and helps them develop their own goals and plans. Whereas cognitive deficits in people with psychosis present significant challenges for this technique, a version with several short sessions, simplified questions, visual aids, more-frequent summaries and greater rehearsal can be used [20, 21]. This work can even occur during an acute psychotic episode, provided the person can maintain attention on a single subject for a few minutes. In fact, engagement during an inpatient stay has some advantages – high availability for brief discussions and salience of negative consequences (e.g., unpleasant symptoms, being on a psychiatric ward, receiving a psychiatric diagnosis, receipt of medication, medication side effects, involuntary treatment). Motivation to maintain session attendance and remain symptom free may be augmented by contingent reinforcement [22, 23, 24, 25], although care needs to be taken to ensure that this reinforcement is not so great as to undermine intrinsic motivation [26].

Most current approaches also incorporate harm reduction as well as abstinence goals. Any ongoing use of psychoactive substances heightens the risk of a return to problematic substance use [27], and in some cases, the risk of psychotic relapse [10]. However, many patients are initially unwilling or unable to adopt an abstinence goal. Commitment to addressing potential risks, to partial reductions, or to stopping use of one drug is often easier to elicit, and has the advantages of consolidating collaborative engagement, building confidence, and addressing urgent threats to the patient's life and welfare. Those who choose to adopt intermediate goals are encouraged to evaluate whether achieving these goals effectively addresses their substance-related problems. As a result, many do then adopt an abstinence goal. In this way, therapists provide support for patient-identified goals, without compromising their commitment to best outcomes.

Even with effective engagement processes, assertive outreach is often needed. Frequently, patients are only tenuously engaged in treatment or have difficulty keeping appointments, especially during symptom exacerbations [28]. Like other mental health services, integrated programs for people with substance use and psychotic symptoms typically trace and contact people in community settings when they miss appointments [29]. Rapid follow-up helps to retain these people in treatment and avert relapse.

In common with other community mental health services, most integrated treatments for substance use and psychosis address a wide range of needs, including housing, work, education, social skills, recreation, and clinical problems. Dealing with these needs can consolidate motivations for abstinence, address some triggers for consumption (e.g., dysphoria, social pressure), and develop activities and social networks that are inconsistent with substance use [30].

Randomized controlled trials on substance misuse and psychosis

Research into the management of substance use and psychosis has typically focused on co-occurring disorders rather than on psychosis that is clearly secondary to substance use, although (partly because of diagnostic uncertainties at initial episodes) some studies do include people who have received a diagnosis of substance-induced psychosis [20]. However, data on people with separable disorders that are often linked by ties of mutual influence [10, 31] should have direct bearing on strategies that would be effective in secondary psychosis.

A systematic search for randomized controlled trials on psychosis and substance misuse using research databases, reference lists of published papers, and personal communications with researchers resulted in identification of 17 randomized controlled trials (Table 33.1). Studies that focused solely on program engagement or forensic outcomes were excluded, as were quasi-experimental and within-subject designs, and those having only a small proportion with psychosis. Nine studies (53%) were conducted in the United States, six in Australia, and one [32] was from the United Kingdom. Most studies (11, 65%) recruited outpatient participants (including two on homeless people [33, 34]), and another two studies included both outpatients and inpatients [35, 36]. Fifteen studies (88%) had mixed samples with serious mental illness or with schizophrenia spectrum disorders: of the remaining two, one was on bipolar disorder [37] and the other was on schizophrenia [35]. Participants varied from ones experiencing their first episode [38], to people with chronic and disabling disorders. Most studies had a majority of men (48%–97%, median = 74%). Sample sizes ranged from 25 to 485, and the median sample size of 120 gives confidence that most studies have power exceeding 0.80 of detecting a post-treatment difference between means of moderate size $(d = .50)$.

As Table 33.1 shows, a wide range of interventions is represented. Contact time ranged from one session of 30–45 minutes [39, 40] to intensive case management over 3 years [29, 41]. Overall durations of the studies varied from 3 months to 5 years post-baseline, with a satisfactory median duration of 12 months. No standardized intervention has yet been examined in more than one published study. Furthermore, an as-yet unpublished test of the intervention by the first author,

controlling for therapist contact, failed to find a significant effect from the intervention [42].

Based on published data, we awarded a point for each of 10 methodological criteria ($> 50\%$ of the eligible sample entering the study, confirmation of diagnosis by standard interview, appropriate randomization procedure, baseline equivalence or statistical control, equivalence of contact time, $\leq 33\%$ loss from attrition, independent checks on protocol adherence, corroboration of substance use reports, blind ratings, and intention to treat analyses). Scores rose from 2.0 in 1993, to an average of 7.1 in 2006. Four studies had a score ≥ 8 [37, 38, 41, 43], three of which were published in 2006 or 2007.

Eleven of the studies (65%) [20, 22, 29, 32, 33, 35, 36, 37, 39, 40, 44] had at least some substance-use outcomes in an experimental group that were better than controls, although in almost all cases, these results were inconsistent across substance-use targets, were not obtained at all assessment points, or were not obtained on intention-to-treat analyses.

One problem with detection of treatment appears to be that improvements may only be seen on some substances, symptoms, or functional domains, and are often unstable over time. Setbacks may occur, even when the overall trajectory is positive. Existing research may often underestimate the true impact of treatment when it focuses on being completely substance free, on days to first substance use, or similar indices of ultimate success. More sensitive indices of transition toward better control of substance use (e.g., percentage of assessments that were substance free, or showed reductions in substance use [22]) may be required, especially at early stages. Similarly, continuous measures of symptoms or of functioning may be required to detect the full impact of interventions on these outcomes.

A further challenge for existing studies was that over half (N = 9, 53%) [20, 29, 34, 37, 38, 39, 41, 45, 46] reported at least some substance-related improvements across the whole sample. For example, this was true for five of the six studies that did not find significantly superior substance-related results for experimental groups over those found in controls [34, 38, 41, 45, 46]. These apparent improvements may reflect regression to the mean, since people are more likely to enter treatment when their problems are worse than usual, and later assessments on average will tend to be better. However, it is important to recognize that the control interventions in most cases were active

Table 33.1 Studies included in a review of randomized controlled trials for treatment of substance misuse and psychosis

Study	Design	Quality Score/10
Lehman et al. (1993) [99]	TAU vs. ICM + Gp	2
Burnam et al. (1995) [33]	S-I Control vs. NRes vs. Res (NResRes: P-Ed + S-H + Gp + CM + Rec)	4
Hellerstein et al. (1995, 2001) [45, 100]; Miner et al. (1997) [28] [45, 100, 28]	TAU (Par) vs. Int (Gp + P-Ed + S-H)[1]	6
Herman et al. (1997, 2000) [44, 101]	TAU vs. Int (P-Ed + R-Ed + S-H + Gp)	4
Drake et al. (1998) [29]	CM vs. ACT	7.5
Barrowclough et al. (2001); Haddock et al. (2003) [32, 58]	TAU vs. Int (MI + CBT-S + FI)	6
Baker et al. (2002) [39, 102]	Ad vs. MI	4.5
Hulse and Tait (2002, 2003) [40, 103]	Inf vs. MI	5
Graeber et al. (2003) [35]	P-Ed vs. MI	4
James et al. (2004) [36]	P-Ed (SUD) vs. Gp (P-Ed, MI, CBT)	4.5
Kavanagh et al. (2004) [20]	TAU vs. MI	6
Calsin et al. (2005); Morse et al. (2006) [34, 57]	TAU vs. ACT vs. Int ACT	6
Baker et al. (2006) [46]	TAU vs. MI + Int CBT	7
Bellack et al. (2006) [22]	Support + P-Ed vs. MI + CBT for SUD	5.5
Edwards et al. (2006) [38]	TAU[2] + P-Ed vs. MI + P-Ed + Int. CBT	8
Essock et al. (2006) [41]	Int CM vs. Int ACT	8
Weiss et al. (2007) [37]	Int Gp vs. SUD Gp	9

Notes:
TAU: Treatment as usual or routine care
Ad: Advice (may include referral to parallel service)
S-I Control: Service information only
Par: Parallel treatment for psychosis, alcohol/drug problems
Int: Integrated treatment for comorbidity
Ed: Education (P-Ed: Patient; R-Ed: Relatives/carers)
Inf: Written information
Res: Residential treatment (NRes: Nonresidential)
Wk: Work program
Gp: Group intervention
S-H: AA or other self-help groups
CM: Standard case management (ICM: Intensive)
ACT: Assertive community treatment
MI: Motivational interviewing
Inc: Incentives
CBT: Cognitive-behavior therapy (CBT-S: for psychotic symptoms)
Rec: Development of recreational activities
RI: Relatives/carers intervention
FI: Family intervention (patient and relative(s))
SUD: Substance use disorder
1. Gp was a manualized support group, with issues and skill foci modified according to individual needs. Housing, medical, prevocational, family interventions were also offered as needed.
2. Case management, mobile assessment and treatment, family intervention, group programs, and a recovery clinic for early psychosis was received by all participants.

treatments (e.g., parallel or sequential interventions, or standard case management). Furthermore, where the control treatment was a brief intervention, results may also be due to some participants only requiring an intervention of minimal intensity. This is consistent with observations of brief interventions for substance misuse having substantial impact in the general population [17], and with many people with psychosis and substance misuse making temporary modifications to their consumption after having a single negative experience with the substance [47]. The challenge for researchers is to discover treatments that are clearly better than these control group responses, which in some studies were substantial [20].

Effects on symptoms, relapses, or rehospitalizations are more difficult to demonstrate, given that each may have other contributing factors, especially in a mixed psychotic sample. Accordingly, only six studies (35%) [22, 32, 36, 37, 39, 41] showed at least some symptomatic effects that were superior to controls. These did not always include positive symptoms of psychosis and were not necessarily seen over all assessment periods. However, there are examples of controlled trials on similar samples (not included in Table 33.1 because they did not report on substance use), which found significant impacts on hospitalization or forensic outcomes [48, 49]. Both trials used a substantial integrated intervention, comparing it with either parallel treatment [49] or referral for case management and housing assistance [48]. Also absent from Table 33.1 is a randomized controlled trial on first-episode psychosis, where the sample included 27% with substance-related harm or dependence [50, 51]. In that study, an integrated assertive community treatment with an offer of multiple family group intervention showed superior symptomatic and substance use outcomes to standard case management at both 1 and 2 years post-baseline.

Although reviews that also included quasi-experimental designs and program evaluations have suggested a much more positive view of the current state of treatments in this area [52, 53], the randomized controlled trials do not give cause for a high degree of confidence in our ability to make substantial differences to the two primary treatment targets in people with psychotic symptoms and substance use. Furthermore, results may well be better for people with psychotic symptoms that are clearly secondary to substance use, although to our knowledge this hypothesis has not been examined.

Despite many limitations to the available data, they do now permit some tentative conclusions.

Brief interventions have limited impact on substance use as stand-alone treatments [54]. This observation is true of three of four published studies [20, 39, 40]. It is also consistent with an as yet unpublished study by the first author, which compared a brief motivational intervention with a therapist-contact control incorporating rapport building, articulation of life goals, and substance assessment [42]. The one positive trial of brief intervention [35] had a relatively small sample size (N = 30).

The current data are even equivocal over the impact of motivational interviewing on sustained engagement in treatment, with at least one study finding that brief advice gave similar effects [39]. However, motivational components may have contributed to the impact of combination treatments in Table 33.1, and other studies not in Table 33.1 have found effects on initial engagement in treatment [55]. Within the reviewed studies, incentives for participation and assertive follow-up may be masking the true impact of motivational procedures on engagement. Furthermore, brief intervention trials do not reflect the impact of ongoing motivational components that may be integrated into longer-term treatments [56], because most brief intervention studies only had one to three sessions, with no subsequent follow-up reminders. A potential effect from brief advice is consistent with the empirical support for this approach in alcohol treatments for the general population [17]. People who can make sustained changes in response to brief motivational interventions may also be the ones who respond to even less intensive intervention, such as a passing comment from their doctor.

The foregoing observations are based on studies that include people who have a diagnosis of an independent DSM-IV psychotic disorder – that is, one that may be exacerbated by substance use but is also present when substances are not used. Brief interventions for people with psychosis that is clearly secondary to substance use may well show greater impact, especially when other indices of substance disorder severity are mild.

Greater intensity of case management per se has little added effect. Integrated treatment using more intensive and assertive community treatment offers little or no additional benefit over a similar intervention within less intensive case management [34, 41, 43, 57]. At present, it seems that a standard intensity of case management may be sufficient.

Better outcomes may potentially come from extended cognitive behavioral therapy (CBT). At present, there are no randomized controlled trials of extended CBT versus other forms of extended, integrated treatment. Studies with CBT for substance use and psychosis that extend over several months appear to have somewhat stronger outcomes than in other studies [22, 32], although the only long-term follow-up published to date [58] suggests that significant substance use effects may not be maintained. Further refinement of CBT approaches to comorbidity may have significant potential.

Integrated treatment appears superior. In both the randomized controlled trials and in research with less rigorous methodology, integrated programs tend to have superior outcomes to nonintegrated controls, although findings are mixed [52, 59]. However, it is not yet clear what features of integrated treatments produce these effects. For example, is it an overall coherence and compatibility of treatment, a more flexible application or modified content of treatment components, selection of strategies with multiple benefits (e.g., pleasurable, nondrug activities), more effective titration of concurrent demands on the patient, or simply an assurance that assertive treatment for both psychotic symptoms and substance use is accessed? Future research needs to go beyond the concept of integration per se, to identify these key features, and how their impact might be maximized.

Once again, it is not yet clear whether these comments are applicable to people whose psychotic symptoms are clearly secondary to substance use. It may be that this population will respond well to an intervention that has a primary focus on the substance use, without ignoring management of the psychotic symptoms or their effect on cognitive processing.

Although the combination of substance use and psychosis presents significant challenges for any psychological intervention, the foregoing review suggests that there may be room for increasing the effect of existing treatments. Potential features, which existing treatments include to varying extent, include:

1. Whether other potential comorbidities that may influence substance use are effectively addressed (e.g., antisocial personality disorder [60], depression, physical disorders)
2. Whether all substances are addressed at some point in the treatment (since multiple substance use is the norm [5])
3. Whether relapse risks are addressed [61, 62, 63, 64], and participants are effectively re-engaged after any temporary reversions to previous substance use
4. Whether the intervention helps participants to develop new, rewarding roles, social networks, and activities [65] that are inconsistent with

substance use and consolidate natural reinforcers for positive change
5. Whether negative attitudes of others toward the person are altered (because these attitudes are likely to impact on ability to maintain change, and on risk of symptom recurrence [66]
6. Whether cognitive and other performance demands at each point in treatment are within the ability of the patients [67] and do not cause distress
7. Whether treatment strategies maximize impact by affecting multiple problem areas for the individual
8. Whether there is a focus on building functional strengths and self-efficacy [68] and on recovery [69] rather than a sole or primary emphasis on functional deficits

Suggestions for future research

1. Given that several trials saw positive changes in control groups, future outcome trials need to have substantial samples (i.e., totaling 200 or more), in order to be able to detect small- to medium-effect sizes with confidence.
2. Future research needs to examine more closely
   - Whether people with psychosis that is clearly secondary to substance use have different responses to interventions than those with two or more comorbid disorders;
   - Whether a program that focuses on substance use can prevent episodes of psychosis from emerging;
   - Relative impact of extended CBT and alternate interventions, in participants who did not fully respond to brief intervention;
   - Effective components of integrated treatment;
   - Optimal timing of interventions (e.g., at or between psychotic episodes, or in relation to stage of change);
   - Maintenance of a positive change trajectory and prevention of relapse, and more sensitive assessments of change.

Implications for clinical practice

At this stage, any recommendations for practice must necessarily be tentative. However:

1. Because many people with psychotic symptoms that are secondary to substance use are only in contact with health services for the short periods

when symptoms are present, and motivation for extended treatment is often low, practicalities will usually demand an initial focus on brevity, motivation, and immediate planning.

2. People with repeated episodes of psychotic symptoms after substance use may require a more extended intervention, which may need concrete incentives for attendance and initial attempts at change [22, 23, 24], with attention to problem solving and skills training that focus on high-risk situations for relapse or recurrence [62], and which builds roles and activities for sustained recovery.

Psychological management of insomnia

Although sleep disturbance can be caused by psychosis, sleep deprivation may also trigger psychotic symptoms [70, 71]. Insomnia therefore offers a second potential trigger of psychotic symptoms that may be addressed by psychological intervention.

There appear to be no controlled trials on the psychological management of insomnia in schizophrenia or other psychoses, whether primary or secondary. Only two case series were identified in serious mental disorder [72, 73], and there are several trials with mixed psychiatric diagnoses [74]. These studies found that cognitive-behavioral methods that are used to treat primary insomnia were also effective in achieving positive sleep outcomes in patients with mental illness [72, 73, 74]. Evidence also suggests that psychological treatments for primary insomnia provide better short- and long-term outcomes than pharmacological treatments [75].

Not everyone with sleep deprivation would describe themselves as having difficulty in getting to sleep. People with a decreased perceived need for sleep in manic states, for example, are unlikely to think of it as insomnia and may not see it as a problem. As with substance abuse, motivational interviewing [19] may be needed in some cases where treatment is voluntary, in order to gain engagement in a sleep-related intervention. In bipolar patients, case study evidence suggests that interventions to reset circadian rhythms and provide greater sleep duration (extended bed rest and darkness) [76] may prove helpful. Some strategies in standard insomnia treatment (e.g., relaxation or meditation to reduce arousal, and progressive changes to sleep schedules) should in principle have some

impact in mania, although reductions in total sleep time during sleep scheduling should probably be avoided.

Suggestions for future research

1. Randomized trials are required for the psychological management of insomnia in people with serious mental disorder, including trials on psychosis that may be secondary to insomnia.
2. Research is needed into the most effective components of psychological interventions for insomnia in people with serious mental disorders, and into changes required to maximize the impact of treatment in this population.

Implications for clinical practice

Given that the current, limited data suggest that the same psychological strategies for insomnia may be applied as in the general population, the following may be recommended [76]:

1. *Stimulus Control.* The bed and bedroom are associated with sleep, rather than other activities such as watching TV or reading. The patient is instructed to only go to bed when it is time to sleep and to get out of bed and leave the room if sleep has not been achieved within 20 minutes. Other distracting stimuli, such as TVs and computers are also removed from the bedroom.
2. *Relaxation Training and Biofeedback.* In the former, patients are taught progressive muscular relaxation, abdominal breathing, or similar strategies, and encouraged to use them when trying to sleep. In the latter, somatic arousal is addressed by providing the patient with feedback on parameters such as muscle tension.
3. *Sleep Scheduling.* Sleep time is restricted to gradually bring hours of sleep more in line with normal parameters. Patients are initially instructed to go to bed when they usually are getting to sleep, and to rise at a certain time, regardless of how much sleep they had. Naps during the day are eliminated to ensure fatigue is experienced during the evening. The time to bed is gradually brought forward, until an acceptable sleep routine is established.
4. *Cognitive Therapy.* Dysfunctional beliefs and attitudes about the patient's insomnia are

challenged, using Socratic questioning and behavioral experiments.

5. *Paradoxical Intention.* Patients with sleep initiation insomnia may be instructed to remain passively awake and avoid any effort to fall asleep. This therapy addresses the activating effects of excessive efforts to go to sleep.

6. *Sleep Hygiene Therapy.* Another popular strategy in multicomponent treatments that requires further support before recommendation as a stand-alone intervention is *Sleep Hygiene Therapy.* Patients are educated about lifestyle factors that may exacerbate insomnia, such as diet and exercise. Recommendations are also made to avoid sleep-incompatible behaviors such as caffeine use or exercise in the hours before bedtime.

Management of psychotic symptoms and their sequelae

Although pharmacological treatments will likely always hold the front line in the management of psychosis, there are limitations to the benefits and improvements that can be achieved from pharmacological intervention alone. Many patients are noncompliant with medication, and despite advances in pharmacotherapies, some continue to have symptoms despite high levels of adherence. Nor does medication directly address the social and functional impact of the psychosis. Given these limitations, there has been substantial recent interest in the development of psychological interventions to address the symptoms and consequences of psychosis. Extensive research has been conducted and has been subject to multiple reviews and meta-analysis [e.g. 77, 78, 79, 80, 81]. Overall, current evidence supports the use of a range of psychological interventions, in comparison with a control intervention.

Cognitive Behavioral Therapies (CBTs) are the leading nonpharmacological approaches to positive symptoms, and currently yield moderate effect sizes on symptom severity [81]. Although there is no universally accepted CBT, treatments typically share some common elements [79, 82, 83, 84], including:

1. *Psychoeducation* about symptoms and diagnosis allows development of insight into the disorder. The relationship between thoughts and behaviors is explained and leads into identification of the

events and situations that precipitate and perpetuate the symptoms.

2. *Problem solving* is employed to develop strategies to address the contributing factors.

3. *Cognitive restructuring or cognitive therapy* involves identifying the misattributions or distortions related to the symptom and helping the patient to challenge and reappraise these through verbal challenge and evidence testing. Behavioral experiments are also used to test the validity of the beliefs.

4. *Relapse prevention.* Idiosyncratic triggers and early warning signs of relapse are identified, and plans are developed to address them.

CBT can also be applied to *medication adherence* [85]. Although psychoeducation alone is relatively ineffective at producing significant changes in medication adherence in most studies [86], there is evidence that motivational interviewing [87] and cueing techniques [88, 89] can significantly raise adherence.

Social Skills Training (SST), a variety of CBT, addresses the fact that psychosis is commonly associated with diminished social competence, which in turn contributes to family conflict, social isolation, and work disability [90]. SST aims to enhance communication and social coping skills, using education and problem solving, modeling, repetitive practice, corrective feedback, positive reinforcement, and *in vivo* homework assignments [81, 91]. Targeted skills are individually tailored, but may include training in accurate perception of emotions and intentions expressed by others; expressing emotions, intentions, or desires; and basic conversational skills [91]. There is evidence of generalization to the natural environment and an impact on functioning, provided that generalization is specifically addressed in the program [90, 91, 92, 93 cf. 94].

CBTs require cognitive capabilities (including processing speed, attention span, working memory, and verbal learning) that are negatively affected by psychosis [95], and methods to address these deficits may be necessary to maximize the impact of psychological interventions [91]. Whereas the severity and enduring nature of cognitive deficits may not be as pronounced in secondary psychosis, cognitive dysfunction is likely to be experienced when the person is highly symptomatic, and may be ongoing if the secondary psychosis does not remit. In either case, treatments may need to be adapted in cases of cognitive deficit, with

413

short sessions, simpler sentence construction, greater repetition and more frequent summaries, and explicit training for generalization.

Cognitive Remediation attempts to address ongoing cognitive deficits. Several programs for cognitive remediation have been developed [96], but generally involve increasingly demanding paper-and-pencil or computerized tasks with corrective feedback, scaffolding, and errorless learning techniques to teach specific skills, and development of strategies to compensate for deficits (making lists, posting reminders). Recent meta-analyses tend to find small- to moderate-effect sizes from these strategies on a range of cognitive outcomes [81], together with a moderate translation to social functioning [cf. 94].

Family Intervention addresses the risks for symptomatic relapse that are associated with negative or overly intrusive interactions with family members [97] and engages families in provision of appropriate support. Interventions with households that would otherwise present a high risk of relapse result in significantly reduced rates of patient relapse and rehospitalization and greater compliance with medication [81]. Family interventions typically involve psychoeducation, communication training, goal setting, and problem solving [81, 98].

Only one study was identified that examined the impact of family intervention and CBT for psychotic symptoms in people with substance use and psychosis [32]. Because the study combined these strategies with other interventions including motivational interviewing, it is not clear what contribution to the study's impact was provided by these components.

Suggestions for future research

It is not currently clear whether these psychological interventions improve the outcomes of people with psychoses that are triggered or maintained by substance use, insomnia, or other problems. Research into this question is required.

Implications for clinical practice

Where patients with secondary psychoses are suffering from ongoing positive symptoms, social skill, or cognitive deficits, or one or more members of the patient's household display critical attitudes or intrusive behavior toward the patient, the respective psychological strategies should be considered.

Summary and conclusions

Most causes of secondary psychosis constitute cerebral insults that are not directly accessible to psychological intervention. Two exceptions, discussed in the current chapter, are psychoactive substance use and insomnia. Psychological interventions for concurrent substance misuse and psychosis are having a significantly greater impact on substance use (and in some studies, on symptoms and functioning) than are control interventions, although effects on average are weaker in longer-term follow-up. Insomnia has had little attention in people with established psychosis, but the current data suggests that the same strategies that have been effective in the general population will also work in this context. There have not as yet been controlled trials on averting potential psychosis using either a substance use or insomnia intervention, although substance use is addressed in multicomponent studies on early episodes of psychosis [38, 50, 51]. There is evidence to support a range of psychological interventions for the symptoms and sequelae of psychosis, and many of these are likely to be applicable to people with secondary psychoses, particularly where ongoing symptoms or psychological deficits are present. There is, however, substantial opportunity to increase the generalization of trained skills and their impact on overall functioning.

References

1. Georgotas A., Zeidenberg P. Observations on the effects of four weeks of heavy marihuana smoking on group interaction and individual behavior. *Compr Psychiatry*, 1979. **20**:427–32.

2. D'Souza D. C., Perry E., MacDougall L., *et al.* The psychotomimetic effects of intravenous delta-9-tetrahydrocannabinol in healthy individuals: implications for psychosis. *Neuropsychopharmacology*, 2004. **29**:1–15.

3. Arseneault L., Cannon M., Poulton R., *et al.* Cannabis use in adolescence and risk for adult psychosis: longitudinal prospective study. *Br Med J*, 2002. **325**:1212–13.

4. Strakowski S. M., McElroy S. L., Keck P. E. J., *et al.* The effects of antecedent substance abuse on the development of first-episode mania. *J Psychiatr Res*, 1996. **30**:59–68.

5. Kavanagh D. J., Waghorn G., Jenner L., *et al.* Demographic and clinical correlates of comorbid substance use disorders in psychosis: multivariate analyses from an epidemiological sample. *Schizophr Res*, 2004. **66**:115–24.

6. Regier D. A., Farmer M. E., Rae D. S., *et al.* Comorbidity of mental disorders with alcohol and other drug abuse. Results from the epidemiologic catchment area (ECA) study. *JAMA*, 1990. **264**:2511–18.

7. Polcin D. L. Issues in the treatment of dual diagnosis clients who have chronic mental illness. *Prof Psychol Res Pr*, 1992. **23**:30–7.

8. Wallen M. C., Weiner H. D. Impediments to effective treatment of the dually diagnosed patient. *J Psychoactive Drugs*, 1989. **21**:161–8.

9. Kavanagh D. J., Greenaway L., Jenner L., *et al.* Contrasting views and experiences of health professionals on the management of comorbid substance abuse and mental disorders. *Aust NZ J Psychiatry*, 2000. **34**:279–89.

10. Hides L., Dawe S., Kavanagh D. J., *et al.* A prospective study of psychotic symptom and cannabis relapse in recent onset psychosis. *Br J Psychiatry*, 2006. **189**: 137–43.

11. Minkoff K., Drake R. E. (Eds.). (1991). *Dual Diagnosis of Major Mental Illness and Substance Disorder*. San Francisco: Jossey-Bass.

12. Carey K. B. Substance use reduction in the context of outpatient psychiatric treatment: a collaborative, motivational, harm reduction approach. *Community Ment Health J*, 1996. **32**:291–306.

13. Drake R. E., Bartels S. B., Teague G. B., *et al.* Treatment of substance abuse in severely mentally ill patients. *J Nerv Ment Dis*, 1993. **181**:606–11.

14. Kavanagh D. J. An intervention for substance abuse in schizophrenia. *Behav Change*, 1995. **12**:20–30.

15. Minkoff K. An integrated treatment model for dual diagnosis of psychosis and addiction. *Hosp Community Psychiatry*, 1989. **40**:1031–6.

16. Mueser K. T., Noordsy D. L., Drake R. E., *et al.* (2003). *Integrated Treatment for Dual Disorders: a Guide to Effective Practice*. New York: Guilford Press.

17. Miller W. R., Wilbourne P. L. Mesa Grande: A methodological analysis of clinical trials of treatments for alcohol use disorders. *Addiction*, 2002. **97**:265–77.

18. Myin-Germeys I., van Os J., Schwartz J. E., *et al.* Emotional reactivity to daily life stress in psychosis. *Arch Gen Psychiatry*, 2001. **58**:1137–44.

19. Miller W. R., Rollnick S., Eds. (2002). *Motivational Interviewing: Preparing People for Change*. New York: Guilford.

20. Kavanagh D. J., Young R., White A., *et al.* A brief motivational intervention for substance abuse in recent-onset psychosis. *Drug Alcohol Rev*, 2004. **23**:151–5.

21. Martino S., Carroll K. M., Kostas D., *et al.* Dual diagnosis interviewing: a modification of motivational interviewing for substance-abusing patients with psychotic disorders. *J Subst Abuse Treat*, 2002. **23**:297–308.

22. Bellack A., Bennett M. E., Gearon J. S., *et al.* A randomized clinical trial of a new behavioral treatment for drug abuse in people with severe and persistent mental illness. *Arch Gen Psychiatry*, 2006. **63**:426–32.

23. Drebing C. E., Van Ormer E. A., Krebs C. The impact of enhanced incentives on vocational rehabilitation outcomes for dually diagnosed veterans. *J Appl Behav Anal*, 2005. **38**:359–72.

24. Ries R. K., Dyck D. G., Short R., *et al.* Outcomes of managing disability benefits among patients with substance dependence and severe mental illness. *Psychiatr Serv*, 2004. **55**:445–7.

25. Sigmon S. C., Steingard S., Badger G. J., *et al.* Contingent reinforcement of marijuana abstinence among individuals with serious mental illness: A feasibility study. *Exp Clin Psychopharmacol*, 2000. **8**:509–17.

26. Greene D., Lepper M. R. Effects of extrinsic rewards on children's subsequent intrinsic interest. *Child Dev*, 1974. **45**:1141–5.

27. Drake R. E., Wallach M. Moderate drinking among people with severe mental illness. *Hosp Community Psychiatry*, 1993. **44**:780–2.

28. Miner C. R., Rosenthal R. N., Hellerstein D. J., *et al.* Prediction

of compliance with outpatient referral in patients with schizophrenia and psychoactive substance use disorders. *Arch Gen Psychiatry*, 1997. **54**:706–12.

29. Drake R. E., McHugo G. J., Clark R. E., *et al.* Assertive community treatment for patients with co-occurring severe mental illness and substance use disorder: A clinical trial. *Am J Orthopsychiatry*, 1998. **68**:201–15.

30. Drake R. E., Wallach W. A., Alverson H. S., *et al.* Psychosocial aspects of substance abuse by clients with severe mental illness. *J Nerv Ment Dis*, 2002. **190**:100–6.

31. Mueser K. T., Drake R. E., Wallach M. A. Dual diagnosis: a review of etiological theories. *Addict Behav*, 2000. **23**:717–34.

32. Barrowclough C., Haddock G., Tarrier N., *et al.* Randomized controlled trial of motivational interviewing, cognitive behavior therapy, and family intervention for patients with comorbid schizophrenia and substance use disorders. *Am J Psychiatry*, 2001. **158**:1706–13.

33. Burnam M. A., Morton S. C., McGlynn E. A., *et al.* An experimental evaluation of residential and nonresidential treatment for dually diagnosed homeless adults. *J Addict Dis*, 1995. **14**:111–34.

34. Calsin R. J., Yonker R. D., Lemming M. R., *et al.* Impact of assertive community treatment and client characteristics on criminal justice outcomes in dual disorder homeless individuals. *Crim Behav Ment Health*, 2005. **15**:236–48.

35. Graeber D. A., Moyers T. B., Griffith G., *et al.* A pilot study comparing motivational interviewing and an educational intervention in patients with schizophrenia and alcohol use disorders. *Community Ment Health J*, 2003. **39**:189–201.

36. James W., Preston N. J., Koh G., *et al.* A group intervention which assists patients with dual diagnosis reduce their drug use: a randomized controlled trial. *Psychol Med*, 2004. **34**:983–90.

37. Weiss R. D., Griffin M. L., Kolodziej M. E., *et al.* A randomized trial of integrated group therapy versus group drug counseling for patients with bipolar disorder and substance dependence. *Am J Psychiatry*, 2007. **164**:100–7.

38. Edwards J., Elkins K., Hinton M., *et al.* Randomized controlled trial of a cannabis-focused intervention for young people with first-episode psychosis. *Acta Psychiatr Scand*, 2006. **114**:109–17.

39. Baker A., Lewin T., Reichler H., *et al.* Evaluation of a motivational interview for substance use within psychiatric in-patient services. *Addiction*, 2002. **97**:1329–37.

40. Hulse G. K., Tait R. J. Six-month outcomes associated with a brief alcohol intervention for adult inpatients with psychiatric disorders. *Drug Alcohol Rev*, 2002. **21**:105–12.

41. Essock S. M., Mueser K. T., Drake R. E., *et al.* Comparison of ACT and standard case management for delivering integrated treatment for co-occurring disorders. *Psychiatr Serv*, 2006. **57**:185–96.

42. Kavanagh D. J., Young R. M., Shockley N., *et al.* Randomized controlled trial of brief motivational intervention vs a therapist contact control for substance misuse in psychosis. (In submission.)

43. Drake R. E., Mercer-McFadden C., Mueser K. T., *et al.* Review of integrated mental health and substance abuse treatment for patients with dual disorders. *Schizophr Bull*, 1998. **24**:589–608.

44. Herman S. E., BootsMiller B., Jordan L., *et al.* Immediate

outcomes of substance use treatment within a state psychiatric hospital. *J Ment Health Adm*, 1997. **24**:126–38.

45. Hellerstein D. J., Rosenthal R. N., Miner C. R. A prospective study of integrated outpatient treatment for substance-abusing schizophrenic patients. *Am J Addict*, 1995. **4**:33–42.

46. Baker A., Bucci S., Lewin T. J., *et al.* Cognitive-behavioural therapy for substance use disorders in people with psychotic disorders: Randomised controlled trial. *Br J Psychiatry*, 2006. **188**:439–48.

47. Green B., Kavanagh D. J., Young R. M. Predictors of cannabis use in men with and without psychosis. *Addict Behav*, 2007. **32**:2879–87. [Epub May 3, 2007.]

48. Chandler D. W., Spicer G. Integrated treatment for jail recidivists with co-occurring psychiatric and substance use disorders. *Community Ment Health J*, 2006. **42**:405–25.

49. Mangrum L. F., Spence R. T., Lopez M. Integrated versus parallel treatment of co-occurring psychiatric and substance use disorders. *J Subst Abuse Treat*, 2006. **30**:79–84.

50. Petersen L., Jeppeson P., Thorup A., *et al.* A randomised multicentre trial of integrated versus standard treatment for patients with a first episode of psychotic illness. *Br Med J*, 2005. **331**:602–9.

51. Petersen L., Nordentoft M., Jeppeson P., *et al.* Improving 1-year outcome in first-episode psychosis. *Br J Psychiatry*, 2005. **187**(Suppl. 48):S98–S103.

52. Drake R. E., Mueser K. T., Brunette M. F., *et al.* A review of treatments for people with severe mental illnesses and co-occurring substance use disorders. *Psychiatr Rehabil J*, 2004. **27**:360–74.

53. Drake R. E., O'Neal E. A systematic review of research on interventions for people with

co-occurring severe mental and substance use disorders. *J Subst Abuse Treat*, in press.

54. Bechdolf A., Pohlman B., Geyer C., *et al.* Motivational interviewing for patients with comorbid schizophrenia and substance abuse disorders: A review. *Fortsch Neurol Psychiatr*, 2005. **73**:728–35.

55. Steinberg M. L., Ziedonis D. M., Krejci J. A., *et al.* Motivational interviewing with personalized feedback: A brief intervention for motivating smokers with schizophrenia to seek treatment for tobacco dependence. *J Consult Clin Psychol*, 2004. **72**:723–8.

56. Osher F. C., Kofoed L. L. Treatment of patients with psychiatric and psychoactive substance use disorders. *Hosp Community Psychiatry*, 1989. **40**:1025–30.

57. Morse G. A., Calsyn R. J., Klinkenberg D. W., *et al.* Treating homeless clients with severe mental illness and substance use disorders: costs and outcomes. *Community Ment Health J*, 2006. **42**:377–404.

58. Haddock G., Barrowclough C., Tarrier N., *et al.* Cognitive-behavioural therapy and motivational intervention for schizophrenia and substance misuse: 18-month outcomes of a randomised controlled trial. *Br J Psychiatry*, 2003. **183**:418–26.

59. Donald M., Dower J., Kavanagh D. J. Integrated versus non-integrated management and care for clients with co-occurring mental health and substance use disorders: A qualitative systematic review of randomised controlled trials. *Soc Sci Med*, 2005. **60**:1371–83.

60. Mueser K. T., Crocker A. G., Frisman L. B., *et al.* Conduct disorder and antisocial personality disorder in persons with severe psychiatric and substance use disorders. *Schizophr Bull*, 2006. **32**:626–36.

61. Drake R. E., Wallach M. A., McGovern M. P. Future directions in preventing relapse to substance abuse among clients with severe mental illnesses. *Psychiatr Serv*, 2005. **56**:1297–302.

62. Marlatt G. A., Gordon J. R. (Eds.) (1985). *Relapse Prevention: Maintenance Strategies in the Treatment of Addictive Behaviors*. New York: Guilford Press.

63. McGovern M. P., Wrisley B. R., Drake R. E. Relapse of substance use disorder and its prevention among persons with co-occurring disorders. *Psychiatr Serv*, 2005. **56**:1270–3.

64. Xie H., Drake R. E., McHugo G. J. Are there distinctive trajectory groups in substance abuse remission over 10 years? An application of the group-based modeling approach. *Adm Policy Ment Health*, 2006. **33**:423–32.

65. Hunt G. M., Azrin N. H. A community-reinforcement approach to alcoholism. *Behav Res Ther*, 1973. **11**:91–104.

66. Pourmand D., Kavanagh D. J., Vaughan K. Expressed emotion as predictor of relapse in patients with comorbid psychoses and substance use disorder. *Aust NZ J Psychiatry*, 2005. **39**:473–8.

67. Kavanagh D. J., Sitharthan G., Young R. M., *et al.* Addition of cue exposure to cognitive-behaviour therapy for alcohol misuse: a randomized controlled trial with dysphoric drinkers. *Addiction*, 2006. **101**:1106–16.

68. Rapp C. A. (1998). *The Strengths Model: Case Management with People Suffering from Severe and Persistent Mental Illness*. New York: Oxford University Press.

69. Oades L. G., Deane F. P., Crowe T. P., et al. Collaborative Recovery: an integrative model for working with individuals that experience chronic or recurring mental illness. *Australas Psychiatry*, 2005. **13**:279–84.

70. West J. L., Jenzen H. H., Lester B. K. The psychosis of sleep deprivation. *Ann NY Acad Sci*, 1962. **96**:66–70.

71. Chemerinski E., Ho B. C., Flaum M., *et al.* Insomnia as a predictor for symptom worsening following antipsychotic withdrawal in schizophrenia. *Compr Psychiatry*, 2002. **43**:393–6.

72. Dopke C. A., Lehner R. K., Wells A. M. Cognitive-behavioral group therapy for insomnia in individuals with serious mental illnesses: a preliminary evaluation. *Psychiatr Rehabil J*, 2004. **27**:235–42.

73. Biancosino B., Rocchi D., Donà S., *et al.* Efficacy of a short-term psychoeducational intervention for persistent non-organic insomnia in severely mentaly ill patients. *Eur Psychiatr*, 2006. **21**:460–2.

74. Smith M. T., Huang M. I., Manber R. Cognitive behavior therapy for chronic insomnia occurring within the context of medical and psychiatric disorders. *Clin Psychol Rev*, 2005. **25**:559–92.

75. Jacobs G. D., Pace-Schott E. F., Stickgold R., *et al.* Cognitive behavior therapy and pharmacotherapy for insomnia. *Arch Intern Med*, 2004. **164**:1888–96.

76. Wehr T. A., Turner E. H., Shimada J. M., *et al.* Treatment of a rapidly cycling bipolar patient by using extended bed rest and darkness to stabilise the timing and duration of sleep. *Biol Psychiatry*, 1998. **43**:822–8.

77. Morgenthaler T., Kramer M., Alessi C., *et al.* Practice parameters for the psychological and behavioral treatment of insomnia: an update. An American Academy of Sleep Medicine Report. *Sleep* 2006. **29**:1415–19.

78. Pilling S., Bebbington P., Kuipers E., *et al.* Psychological treatment in schizophrenia: I. Meta-analysis

of family interventions and cognitive behavior therapy. *Psychol Med*, 2002. **32**:763–82.

79. Gaudiano B. A. Cognitive behavior therapies for psychotic disorders: current empirical status and future directions. *Clin Psychol Sci Prac*, 2005. **12**:33–50.

80. Zimmerman G., Favrod J., Trieu V. H., *et al*. The effect of cognitive behavioral treatment on the positive symptoms of schizophrenia spectrum disorders: a meta-analysis. *Schizophr Res*, 2005. 77:1–9.

81. Pfammatter M., Junghan U. M., Brenner H. D. Efficacy of psychological therapy in schizophrenia: conclusions from meta-analyses. *Schizophr Bull*, 2006. **32**(Suppl 1):S64–S80.

82. Kingdon A., Turkington D. (1994). *Cognitive-Behavioral Therapy of Schizophrenia*. Hove, UK: Lawrence Erlbaum.

83. Trower P., Birchwood M., Meaden A., *et al*. Cognitive therapy for command hallucinations: randomized controlled trial. *Br J Psychiatry*, 2004. **184**:312–20.

84. Kuipers E., Garety P., Fowler D., *et al*. Cognitive, emotional, and social processes in psychosis: refining cognitive behavioral therapy for persistent positive symptoms. *Schizophr Bull*, 2006. 32(Suppl 1):S24–S31.

85. Donohue G. Adherence to antipsychotic treatment in schizophrenia: what role does cognitive behavioral therapy play in improving outcomes? *Dis Manage Health Outcomes*, 2006. **14**:207–14.

86. Zygmunt A., Olfson M., Boyer C. A., *et al*. Interventions to improve medication adherence in schizophrenia. *Am J Psychiatry*, 2002. 159:1653–64.

87. Kemp R., Hayward P., Applewhaite G., *et al*. Compliance therapy in psychotic patients: randomised controlled trial. *Br Med J*, 1996. **312**:345–9.

88. Boczkowski J. A., Zeichner A., DeSanto N. Neuroleptic compliance among chronic schizophrenic outpatients: an intervention outcome report. *J Consult Clin Psychol*, 1985. **53**:666–71.

89. Cramer J. A., Rosenheck R. Enhancing medication compliance for people with serious mental illness. *J Nerv Ment Dis*, 1999. **187**:53–5.

90. Bellack A. S. Skills training for people with severe mental illness. *Psychiatr Rehabil J*, 2004. 27:375–91.

91. Kopelowicz A., Liberman R. P., Zarate R. Recent advances in social skills training for schizophrenia. *Schizophr Bull*, 2006. 32(Suppl 1):S12–S23.

92. Kurtz M. M., Mueser K. T. A meta-analysis of controlled research on social skills training for schizophrenia. *J Consult Clin Psychol*, 2008. **76**:491–504.

93. Mueser K. T., Penn D. L. Correspondence. *Psychol Med*, 2004. 1365–7.

94. Pilling S., Bebbington P., Kuipers E., *et al*. Psychological treatments in schizophrenia: II. Meta-analyses of randomized controlled trials of social skills training and cognitive remediation. *Psychol Med*, 2004. 32:783–91.

95. Green M. F. (1992). Information processing in schizophrenia. In *Schizophrenia: An Overview and Practical Handbook*, Kavanagh D. J. (Ed). London: Chapman & Hall, pp. 45–58.

96. Delahunty A., Morice R. Rehabilitation of frontal/executive impairments in schizophrenia. *Aust NZ J Psychiatry*, 1996. **30**:760–7.

97. Kavanagh D. J. Recent developments in expressed emotion and schizophrenia. *Br J Psychiatry*, 1992. **160**:601–20.

98. Kavanagh D. (1992). Family interventions in schizophrenia. In *Schizophrenia: an Overview and Practical Handbook*, Kavanagh D. J. (Ed). London: Chapman & Hall, pp. 407–23.

99. Lehman A. F., Herron J. D., Schwartz R. P., *et al*. Rehabilitation for adults with severe mental illness and substance use disorders: a clinical trial. *J Nerv Ment Dis*, 1993. **181**:86–90.

100. Hellerstein D. J., Rosenthal R. N., Miner C. R. Integrating services for schizophrenia and substance abuse. *Psychiatr Q*, 2001. **72**:291–306.

101. Herman S. E., Frank K. A., Mowbray C. T., *et al*. Longitudinal effects of integrated treatment on alcohol use for persons with serious mental illness and substance use disorders. *J Behav Health Serv Res*, 2000. **27**:286–302.

102. Baker A., Lewin T., Reichler H., *et al*. Motivational interviewing among psychiatric in-patients with substance use disorders. *Acta Psychiatr Scand*, 2002. **106**:233–40.

103. Hulse G. K., Tait R. J. Five-year outcomes of a brief psychiatric intervention for adult in-patients with psychiatric disorders. *Addiction*, 2003. **98**:1061–8.

Index